Comprehensive Guide to
URTICARIA

Comprehensive Guide to
URTICARIA

Editors

Sanjeev Gupta MD DNB MNAMS
Professor and Head
Department of Dermatology
MM Institute of Medical Sciences and Research, MMDU
Mullana, Ambala, Haryana, India

Rohit Batra MD
Consultant Dermatologist
Sir Ganga Ram Hospital
Director, Dermaworld
Skin and Hair Clinics
New Delhi, India

Shikha Gupta MD DDVL
Consultant Dermatologist
Skin Konnect Clinics
Delhi & Ghaziabad, Uttar Pradesh, India

Forewords

Seemal R Desai
Kiran V Godse

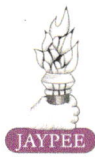

JAYPEE
JAYPEE BROTHERS MEDICAL PUBLISHERS
The Health Sciences Publisher
New Delhi | London

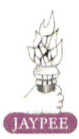 **Jaypee Brothers Medical Publishers (P) Ltd**

Headquarters
EMCA House
23/23-B, Ansari Road, Daryaganj
New Delhi 110 002, India
Landline: +91-11-23272143, +91-11-23272703
+91-11-23282021, +91-11-23245672
E-mail: jaypee@jaypeebrothers.com

Corporate Office
Jaypee Brothers Medical Publishers (P) Ltd.
4838/24, Ansari Road, Daryaganj
New Delhi 110 002, India
Phone: +91-11-43574357
Fax: +91-11-43574314
E-mail: jaypee@jaypeebrothers.com

Overseas Office
JP Medical Ltd.
83, Victoria Street, London
SW1H 0HW (UK)
Phone: +44-20 3170 8910
Fax: +44(0)20 3008 6180
E-mail: info@jpmedpub.com

Website: www.jaypeebrothers.com
Website: www.jaypeedigital.com

© 2025, Jaypee Brothers Medical Publishers

The views and opinions expressed in this book are solely those of the original contributor(s)/author(s) and do not necessarily represent those of editor(s) or publisher of the book.

All rights reserved. No part of this publication may be reproduced, stored or transmitted in any form or by any means, electronic, mechanical, photocopying, recording or otherwise, without the prior permission in writing of the publishers.

All brand names and product names used in this book are trade names, service marks, trademarks or registered trademarks of their respective owners. The publisher is not associated with any product or vendor mentioned in this book.

Medical knowledge and practice change constantly. This book is designed to provide accurate, authoritative information about the subject matter in question. However, readers are advised to check the most current information available on procedures included and check information from the manufacturer of each product to be administered, to verify the recommended dose, formula, method and duration of administration, adverse effects and contraindications. It is the responsibility of the practitioner to take all appropriate safety precautions. Neither the publisher nor the author(s)/editor(s) assume any liability for any injury and/or damage to persons or property arising from or related to use of material in this book.

This book is sold on the understanding that the publisher is not engaged in providing professional medical services. If such advice or services are required, the services of a competent medical professional should be sought.

Every effort has been made where necessary to contact holders of copyright to obtain permission to reproduce copyright material. If any have been inadvertently overlooked, the publisher will be pleased to make the necessary arrangements at the first opportunity.

Inquiries for bulk sales may be solicited at: jaypee@jaypeebrothers.com

Comprehensive Guide to Urticaria / *Sanjeev Gupta, Rohit Batra, Shikha Gupta*
First Edition: **2025**
ISBN: 978-93-6616-543-1
Printed in India

Dedicated to

Our Teachers
For nurturing our academic aspirations

Our Parents
For their belongings, affection and unconditional love

Our Family
Dr Sunita Gupta, Namya and Gauri (Sanjeev Gupta)
Dr Neha Batra and Aarna (Rohit Batra)
Dr Himanshu Gupta, Advit and Viraj (Shikha Gupta)
For their understanding, forbearance, unconditional support and love

Our Patients
For providing us an opportunity to serve them and learn from them

Contributors

Aanchal Bansal MD DNB
Senior Resident
Department of Dermatology,
Venereology and Leprosy
Lady Hardinge Medical College and
Associated Hospitals
New Delhi, India

Aditi Dabhra MD
Resident
Department of Dermatology
Maharishi Markandeshwar Institute of
Medical Sciences and Research, MMDU
Mullana, Ambala, Haryana, India

Aneet Mahendra MD
Professor
Department of Dermatology
Maharishi Markandeshwar Institute of
Medical Sciences and Research, MMDU
Mullana, Ambala, Haryana, India

Anjali Bagrodia MD
Senior Resident
Department of Dermatology,
Venereology and Leprosy
All India Institute of Medical Sciences
Rishikesh, Uttarakhand, India

Anushruti Aggarwal MD
Fellowship in Lasers, Aesthetics and
Dermatosurgery
Consultant Dermatologist
Ludhiana, Punjab, India

Deepti Saxena DNB
Associate Professor
Department of Dermatology and
Venereology
Saraswati Medical College
Hapur, Uttar Pradesh, India

Gagandeep Kaur MD
Senior Resident
Department of Dermatology
Dayanand Medical College and Hospital
Ludhiana, Punjab, India

Geeti Khullar MD DNB
Assistant Professor
Department of Dermatology
Lady Hardinge Medical College and
Associated Hospitals
New Delhi, India

Gouri RP Anand MD
Senior Resident
Dermatology and Venereology
All India Institute of Medical Sciences
New Delhi, India

Himanshu Gupta MD
Consultant Dermatologist
Skin Konnect Clinics
Delhi & Ghaziabad, Uttar Pradesh, India

Kalpana Pathak MD
Consultant Dermatologist
The Skin and Hair Clinic
Ghaziabad, Uttar Pradesh, India

Contributors

Kritika Pandey MD
Consultant Dermatologist
Sculpt Clinic
Gurugram, Haryana, India

Manju Keshari MD
Senior Consultant Dermatologist
Max Super Specialty Hospital
Patparganj, New Delhi
Director, Kemps Skin Clinic
Ghaziabad, Uttar Pradesh, India

Mansak Shishak MD DNB
Consultant
Dr Mansak Skin Clinic
Safdarjung Enclave
New Delhi, India

Namya Gupta MBBS(Student)
Kalpana Chawla Government
Medical College
Karnal, Haryana, India

Naveen K Kansal MD
Additional Professor and Head
Department of Dermatology,
Venereology and Leprosy
All India Institute of Medical Sciences
Rishikesh, Uttarakhand, India

Neeraj Gupta DCH DNB(Pediatrics)
Senior Consultant
Department of Pediatrics
Sir Ganga Ram Hospital
New Delhi, India

Neha Rani MD
Senior Resident
Department of Dermatology
Maharishi Markandeshwar Institute of
Medical Sciences and Research, MMDU
Mullana, Ambala, Haryana, India

Neha Taneja MD
Assistant Professor
Department of Dermatology and
Venereology
All India Institute of Medical Sciences
New Delhi, India

Nidhi Sharma MD
Senior Dermatologist
Skin Health Clinic
Gurugram, Haryana, India

Nitika Nijhara MD
Consultant Dermatologist
Department of Dermatology
BLK-Max Hospital
New Delhi, India

Payal Chauhan MD DNB MNAMS
Associate Professor
Department of Dermatology,
Venereology and Leprosy
All India Institute of Medical Science
Jammu, Jammu and Kashmir, India

Priyadarshini Sahu MD DNB MNAMS
Consultant Dermatologist
Department of Telemedicine
Postgraduate Institute of Medical
Education and Research
Chandigarh, India

Ria Sharma MD
Senior Resident
Department of Dermatology,
Venereology and Leprosy
All India Institute of Medical Science
Jammu, Jammu and Kashmir, India

Riti Bhatia MD
Associate Professor
Department of Dermatology,
Venereology and Leprosy
All India Institute of Medical Sciences
Rishikesh, Uttarakhand, India

Rohit Batra MD
Consultant Dermatologist
Sir Ganga Ram Hospital
Director, Dermaworld
Skin and Hair Clinics
New Delhi, India

Sanjeev Gupta MD DNB MNAMS
Professor and Head
Department of Dermatology
Maharishi Markandeshwar Institute of
Medical Sciences and Research, MMDU
Mullana, Ambala, Haryana, India

Saurabh Swaroop Gupta MD DNB
Assistant Professor
Department of Dermatology
Maharishi Markandeshwar Institute of
Medical Sciences and Research, MMDU
Mullana, Ambala, Haryana, India

Shikha Gupta MD DDVL
Consultant Dermatologist
Skin Konnect Clinics
Delhi & Ghaziabad, Uttar Pradesh, India

Sunita Gupta MD
Professor and Head
Department of Medicine
Maharishi Markandeshwar Institute of
Medical Sciences and Research, MMDU
Mullana, Ambala, Haryana, India

Sunil Kumar Gupta MD
Professor and Head
Department of Dermatology and
Venereology
All India Institute of Medical Sciences
Gorakhpur, Uttar Pradesh, India

Foreword

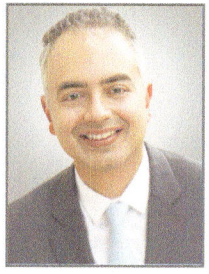

In the era of innovations in dermatology, inflammatory and immunologic skin diseases seem to be on the cusp of so many advances. Urticaria represents the quintessential example of a skin disease with so much complexity and often multiple associated factors. In this textbook, renowned dermatologists Drs Sanjeev Gupta, Rohit Batra and Shikha Gupta have beautifully addressed this intriguing skin condition while simultaneously providing a comprehensive up-to-date diagnostic and therapeutic overview. One of the most exciting things about texts like this book is that you not only find data of traditional long believed studies, but even more importantly to today's practice of medicine, up-to-date recent clinical data. This is of course exceedingly important as we are in a great time of innovation in our beloved dermatology specialty. For example, just 5–10 years ago, who would have ever thought we would have multiple Food and Drug Administration (FDA) approved and internationally recommended treatments for diseases such as vitiligo, alopecia areata, hidradenitis suppurativa and more. In fact, I have told my very own patients that if you had to be suffering from diseases like these, now it is the time to perhaps have these often-devastating conditions since we are in a renaissance period of therapy outcomes and advances in dermatology that can truly transform patients' lives. This is especially true in urticaria, where so many discoveries and translatable therapies are on the cusp of being delivered to you, the practitioner in hopes of further improving the lives of our patients. As you delve into this exciting scientific treasure chest textbook, keep in mind that *"Comprehensive Guide to Urticaria"* is designed to be clinically relevant, practical and usable. This remains a subject area that has gained considerable traction in medical and basic science research, so I sincerely believe this edition will be the first of many!

Happy reading, happy learning, and most importantly let us all use educational assets like this to improve the lives of our patients!

With my personal regards!

Seemal R Desai MD FAAD
President, American Academy of Dermatology, USA

Foreword

सर्वं ज्ञानप्लवेनैव व्याधिं संतरिष्यसि।

"Sarvam jñānaplavenai'va vyādhim santarisyasi."

"With the boat of knowledge, you will overcome all ailments."

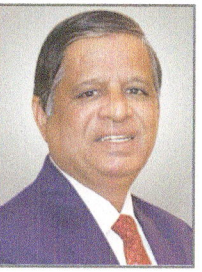

Urticaria commonly known as hives, presents itself in various forms—acute, chronic, spontaneous, and inducible—each with its own set of triggers, symptoms, and treatment responses. Among the different types, autoimmune and autoallergic urticaria add additional layers of complexity. Both types demand a thorough understanding of immunological mechanisms and often necessitate specialized therapeutic strategies. This underscores the importance of a nuanced and individualized approach in effectively managing and treating urticaria in its various forms. These conditions often lead to chronic symptoms that disrupt daily life, causing physical discomfort, sleep disturbances, and significant emotional distress.

One of the primary complexities lies in identifying the triggers. In chronic cases, identifying a specific trigger can be particularly elusive, with many patients showing no identifiable cause at all. This makes diagnosis and treatment a challenging process of elimination, requiring patience and persistence from both the patient and the healthcare provider.

Globally, urticaria presents a significant healthcare challenge. In many countries, it is frequently misdiagnosed or poorly managed, leaving patients in a frustrating cycle of symptoms without relief. In India, the situation is equally concerning. The tropical climate, widespread allergies and varying levels of healthcare access contribute to the complexity of managing urticaria. Many patients experience prolonged discomfort due to a lack of timely and effective treatment options.

The editors deserve immense praise for their dedication and expertise in bringing this book to life. Through meticulous research, clear explanations and practical advice, the author has created a valuable tool that will undoubtedly improve the lives of many.

Kiran V Godse MD PhD FRCP(Glasgow)
Professor, Department of Dermatology
DY Patil Hospital and School of Medicine
Navi Mumbai, Maharashtra, India
President IADVL 2020, President Skin Allergy Society
Best Teacher Award (IADVL), Academic Award IMA (HQs)

About the Editors

Sanjeev Gupta MD DNB MNAMS is working as Professor and Head, Department of Dermatology, MM Institute of Medical Sciences and Research, MMDU, Mullana, Ambala, Haryana, India. He is a member of most national and international academic societies. He has around 170 publications, 8 books and 17 book chapters to his credit. He has invented many dermatological techniques and instruments to simplify the procedures and reduce the cost. Twenty-six of such inventions have been published in one of the most prestigious journals of dermatology—Journal of the American Academy of 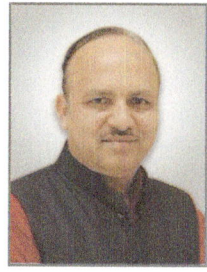 Dermatology USA. He was awarded with "Making a Difference" award by the American Academy of Dermatology, USA. He is the first Indian to be honoured with this prestigious award. He has served his professional association [Indian Association of Dermatologists, Venereologists, and Leprologists (IADVL)] as Executive Committee Member at the state level as Treasurer, Secretary, Vice President, and President and also at the National level as Joint Secretary and Vice President IADVL. He was honoured with the LN Sinha Award by IADVL in 2013 and the ACSI Innovation Award 2021 by the Association of Cutaneous Surgeons of India (ACSI). He is the recipient of Dr BM Ambady Oration awarded at DERMACON 2025 Jaipur.

Rohit Batra MD is a renowned Dermatologist associated with Sir Ganga Ram Hospital, Delhi, and is Head and Founder of Dermaworld Skin and Hair Clinics, New Delhi, India. His areas of interest are clinical dermatology, pediatric dermatology, esthetic dermatology, trichology and multidisciplinary care of dermatological disorders. He has numerous presentations at various national and international conferences. He has been the architect of two of the most famous Dermatology Conclaves— 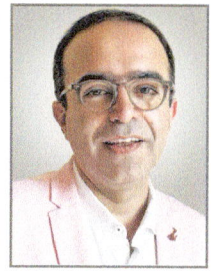 Dermatology and Allied Specialities Summit (DAAS) and Acne India Summit. A prominent organizational guru and a mentor for many, he has held various roles and posts in the IADVL including the President of the IADVL- Delhi State Branch.

Shikha Gupta MD DDVL is a well-known Dermatologist practising in East Delhi and Ghaziabad, India. Her main areas of interest are pediatric dermatology, clinical dermatology and esthetic dermatology including chemical peeling. She was previously associated with Chacha Nehru Bal Chikitsalaya, Delhi, where her interest in pediatric dermatology took shape and she has actively been working in the field ever since. She has given presentations at various national conferences and authored chapters in dermatology textbooks. She has been awarded the "President Appreciation Award" from the IADVL 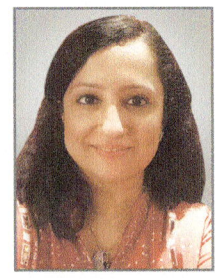 Delhi State Branch during 2023–2024 for her contribution toward the branch and "IWDA-Loreal Leadership Grant" in 2023. She has also won the "XI ISD – Global Education Award" in 2013. She has been actively involved in conducting zonal- and state-level conferences with IADVL-Delhi State Branch and has been coordinating the publishing of the official newsletter of the branch since 2023.

Preface

विद्या ददाति विनयं विनयाद् याति पात्रताम्।
पात्रत्वाद् धनमाप्नोति धनाद्धर्मं ततः सुखम्॥

"Knowledge makes one humble, humility begets worthiness, worthiness creates wealth and enrichment, enrichment leads to right conduct, and right conduct brings contentment"

Urticaria, often referred to as hives, is a widespread condition affecting many individuals. Despite its prevalence, determining the underlying causes and specific triggers can be remarkably challenging. This complexity has given rise to a multitude of treatment options, ranging from well-established scientific approaches to less conventional, unscientific methods available in the market.

Recognizing the need for clarity and effective patient management, this handbook has been meticulously crafted to provide a thorough exploration of urticaria. It encompasses a wide range of topics, including diagnostic strategies, evidence-based treatments and practical approaches to patient care. By offering a comprehensive guide, this book aims to equip healthcare professionals with the knowledge and tools necessary to improve patient outcomes and navigate the often-confusing landscape of urticaria management. The book will be of practical importance for dermatologists but will be of great benefit to all undergraduate and postgraduate students, internists, and family practitioners practicing not only in India but worldwide too.

We thank all contributors for finishing this herculean task in time. It has been a pleasure and a vast learning experience with an excellent team of editorial board members and authors. I would also like to thank our patients and students who directly and indirectly motivated us to accept this challenge.

We would be failing in our duties if we did not pay special thanks to my resident Dr Aditi Dabhra and undergraduates Aanya Bedi and Gauri Thukral for their tiring, selfless, sincere, and dedicated efforts in this project. We also thank our family who supported, motivated and tolerated us for stealing their precious family time.

The work would not have been possible without the support of Shri Jitendar P Vij (Group Chairman), Mr Ankit Vij (Managing Director), Ms Chetna Malhotra (Senior Director—Professional Publishing, Marketing, and Business Development) and Somoshri Banerji (Development Editor).

Happy reading!

Sanjeev Gupta
Rohit Batra
Shikha Gupta

Contents

1. **History of Urticaria and Angioedema** — 1
   Sanjeev Gupta, Aditi Dabhra

2. **Etiopathogenesis of Urticaria** — 10
   Sanjeev Gupta, Aditi Dabhra

3. **Etiopathogenesis of Angioedema** — 27
   Sanjeev Gupta, Aditi Dabhra, Namya Gupta

4. **Types of Urticaria: An Overview** — 34
   Shikha Gupta, Sanjeev Gupta, Himanshu Gupta

5. **Assessment Scales in Chronic Spontaneous Urticaria and Angioedema** — 42
   Nidhi Sharma

6. **Acute Urticaria** — 51
   Shikha Gupta, Himanshu Gupta

7. **Angioedema** — 60
   Rohit Batra, Anushruti Aggarwal, Sanjeev Gupta

8. **Anaphylaxis in Acute Urticaria** — 70
   Sunita Gupta, Aditi Dabhra, Sanjeev Gupta

9. **Chronic Spontaneous Urticaria** — 83
   Neha Taneja, Gouri RP Anand

10. **Physical Urticaria** — 98
    Mansak Shishak

11. **Contact Urticaria** — 108
    Nitika Nijhara, Sanjeev Gupta, Rohit Batra

12. **Cholinergic Urticaria** — 117
    Kritika Pandey

13. **Autoimmune Urticaria** — 123
    Sanjeev Gupta, Aditi Dabhra, Gagandeep Kaur

14. **Urticaria in Children** — 134
    Shikha Gupta, Himanshu Gupta

15. **Urticaria and Pregnancy** — 142
Deepti Saxena, Sanjeev Gupta, Aditi Dabhra

16. **Urticaria in Elderly: Causes, Management and Consideration** — 154
Kalpana Pathak

17. **Urticarial Vasculitis** — 161
Neha Rani, Sanjeev Gupta, Aneet Mahendra

18. **Urticaria Mimickers: A Comprehensive Guide to Differential Diagnosis** — 171
Rohit Batra, Anushruti Aggarwal, Sanjeev Gupta

19. **Mast Cell Disorders** — 180
Rohit Batra, Anushruti Aggarwal, Sanjeev Gupta

20. **Skin Prick Test in Urticaria** — 191
Neeraj Gupta

21. **Patch Test in Urticaria** — 198
Sanjeev Gupta, Aditi Dabhra, Saurabh Swaroop Gupta

22. **Oral Challenge Test** — 208
Payal Chauhan, Ria Sharma

23. **Autologous Serum Skin Test** — 219
Neha Rani, Sanjeev Gupta, Aditi Dabhra

24. **Autologous Blood/Serum Therapy in Urticaria** — 228
Neha Rani, Sanjeev Gupta

25. **Diet in Urticaria** — 235
Manju Keshari

26. **Antihistamines in Urticaria** — 244
Sunil Kumar Gupta

27. **Systemic Therapies in Urticaria** — 252
Aanchal Bansal, Geeti Khullar

28. **Biologicals in Urticaria** — 270
Priyadarshini Sahu, Sanjeev Gupta

29. **Quality of Life in Urticaria** — 287
Anjali Bagrodia, Riti Bhatia, Naveen K Kansal

30. **H2 Blockers in the Management of Urticaria** — 293
Rohit Batra, Anushruti Aggarwal, Aditi Dabhra

31. **Artificial Intelligence in Urticaria** — 296
Rohit Batra, Anushruti Aggarwal, Aditi Dabhra

Index — 299

CHAPTER 1

History of Urticaria and Angioedema

Sanjeev Gupta, Aditi Dabhra

HISTORY OF URTICARIA

INTRODUCTION

The history of urticaria dates back to ancient times, with references found in medical scriptures from ancient Greece and Rome. Throughout history, its understanding has evolved significantly, from early misconceptions and folk remedies to modern medical insights into its immunological basis. Different nomenclatures that have been used for the disease are summarized in **Figure 1**.

HISTORICAL MILESTONES OF URTICARIAL ERUPTIONS IN DIFFERENT GEOGRAPHICAL BOUNDARIES

- *China*: The earliest known mention of the disease, now known as urticaria, can be found in "The Yellow Emperor's Inner Classic," Huangdi Neijing, written sometime between in the era of 1000–1200 BC. In Chapter 64 of

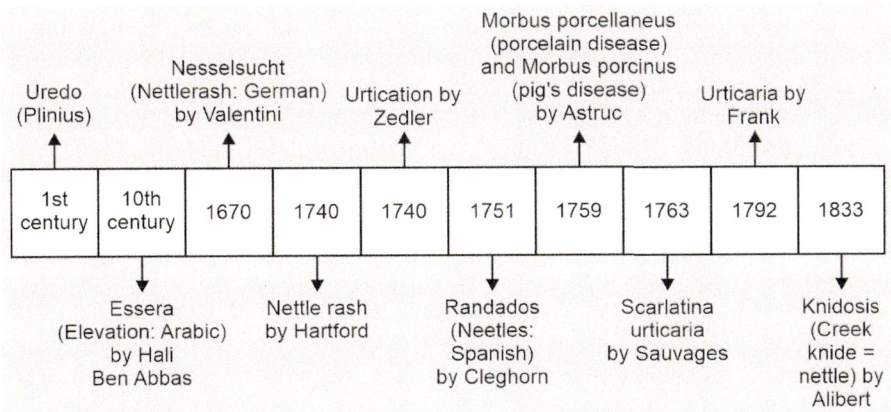

FIG. 1: History of nomenclature of urticaria.

basic inquiries (Sin Wen), urticaria is referred to as "Feng Yin Zheng," denoting a disguised rash of wind type. The term "urticaria" in Chinese still refers to a condition believed to be caused by an excess of the weaker Yin energy, leading to fluid blockage in the skin.

- *Greece*: Hippocrates documented the presence of raised, itchy skin lesions caused by nettles and mosquitoes. He referred to this condition as *"knidosis,"* derived from the Greek word for nettle, "knido." In addition, he notes that wheals can manifest in patients with gastrointestinal problems, though typically with reduced pruritus.
- *Paris*: In 1833, Jean-Louis Alibert reintroduced the same name in his book on skin diseases, which was published in Paris. Hebra employed the term "knidosis" to refer to the persistent form of urticaria, whereas in the 1963 textbook by Andrew and Domonko, it is used consistently with urticaria.
- *Latin*: Plinius (AD 32–79) coined the term *"uredo,"* which signifies burning. The phrase was employed by Latin-speaking physicians, including Carl von Linne, to describe "red, evanescent, pruritic eruptions".
- *England*: In the book "King Richard III," Thomas More provides a detailed description of a particular state or situation, but he does not explicitly label it. Nevertheless, it is noteworthy as it represents the initial instance of urticaria documented to result in death. Prior to the coronation of King Richard in 1480, the lords sought to appease him by presenting him with a cup of strawberries. After a few hours, he promptly gathered the lords and showed his chest, revealing red, raised, and pruritic spots. He lodged an accusation against one of the nobles, alleging an attempt to poison him, and promptly ordered his assassination.
- *Germany*: In his "Grosses vollständiges Universal-Lexicon" published from 1734 to 1740, Zedler replaced the term "uredo" with "urticatio". The term urticaria was initially coined by William Cullen in 1769 in his book "Synopsia Nosalogiae Methodicae". It was also included in the initial publication of Encyclopædia Britannica (1771) created by a pseudonymous group known as "A society of Gentlemen in Scotland". Peter Frank in Vienna and other medical centers later acknowledged and adopted the term *urticaria*.
- *Edinburgh*: Cullen, a professor practicing medicine at Edinburgh, began categorizing skin problems in a manner similar to Linne's classification of plants. In 1777, Robert Willan commenced his medical studies in Edinburgh and was much influenced by Cullen's thoughts on the categorization of skin diseases. Willan returned to London in 1783 and his particular focus was on skin conditions, where he refined the categorization of cutaneous diseases by examining the physical characteristics of the lesions. Although he had perused a book authored by Joseph Plenck on the topic, which was released in 1776, he chose not to reference it due to the mixture of several factors such as lesion type, location, and etiology. Willan's discoveries brought organization to the current classification system and were published in separate instalments from 1798 to 1808. In 1801, he encountered Thomas Bateman. He accompanied him in the dispensary. Bateman quickly

understood Willan's methodology and completed the work after Willan's demise, which was an influential masterpiece titled "A Practical Synopsis of Cutaneous Diseases." It was published in 1813 and translated into other languages. This document provides descriptions of several forms of urticaria:

- *Urticaria febrilis* is a condition characterized by the presence of fever and abdominal pain that precede the development of skin lesions. This form of urticaria often persists for a duration of 1 week.
- *Urticaria evanida* is a condition characterized by the appearance of new lesions over a prolonged period of months or even years and mostly cause itching at night. Therefore, it corresponds to the condition of chronic urticaria.
- *Urticaria perstans* is a condition characterized by the presence of a single central wheal that persists for many days and has a hard feel. The initial erythema surrounding the wheal subsides quickly. The description is indicative of urticarial vasculitis.
- *Lichen urticatus or papular urticaria*: Batemen also defined these in children, distinguishing it from other types of urticarias.

Nevertheless, their system was not universally accepted. One notable scholar during this time period was Jean Louis Alibert, a prominent dermatologist based in Paris. As previously stated, he favored the use of the Greek term "knidosis" to refer to urticaria and sought a new classification system due to the fact that Willan's study included only outpatients without a follow-up of a possible etiology.

Alibert's study on skin diseases garnered admiration from King Ludvig XVIII. Following King Ludvig's demise, King Charles X appointed him as his personal physician and bestowed upon him the prestigious title of Baron as a token of appreciation. Consequently, he departed from his department for an extended period of time. Laurent Biett, the most accomplished student of his, took his responsibility at work. In 1816, he paid a visit to Bateman and reintroduced the Willan–Bateman system in Paris. Upon his return to St Louis in 1829, Baron Alibert attempted to propose his innovative concept of a tree with dermatosis-infected branches. However, his endeavor proved unsuccessful due to its excessive complexity and lack of practicality.

ETYMOLOGY OF URTICARIA

The nomenclature of the illness has undergone multiple revisions throughout the centuries; however, it has consistently been determined by its presentation. In the first century, Plinius focused specifically on the perception of burning and referred to it as "uredo" in Latin. Zedler (1740) noted the resemblance between the skin lesion and the lesions caused by contact with stinging nettles, leading to its designation as "urticatio". Following other appellations such as "randados" (Spanish: nettles), Morbus porcellaneus (porcelain illness) (white discoloration), or Scarlatina urticaria, the term "urticaria" was coined in 1769 by William Cullen and subsequently embraced in 1792 by Johann Peter Frank.

HISTORY OF PATHOGENETIC THEORIES (FIG. 2)

- Hippocrates had previously observed a connection between urticaria, nettles, insect stings, and the gastrointestinal tract. Certain information can be found again in the works of the 16th century, where it was suggested that strawberries and mussels were responsible for creating urticaria.
- During this period, Libavius provided an initial description of the primary clinical characteristics of urticaria. These include its sudden onset, formation of wheals, redness, and itching, along with the transient nature of the process (*cessante per aliquot dies*). This is particularly remarkable considering that after hundred years, Sydenham (1624-1689) mentioned nettle fever as a component of erysipelas.
- During the 18th century, a scholar named Behrens, who had an allergy to shellfish, contended that the urticarial lesion must be caused by a peculiar characteristic of the patient. His rationale was founded on the straightforward observation that although many individuals were exposed to the same substances, only a select few had a reaction to them.
- Around that time, in 1703, Chemniz attempted to elucidate the waxing and waning of wheals by proposing the *humoral theory*. The occurrence was explained by other mechanisms using the *stasis theory*, which involves the blocking of the flow of humors (stasis theory). The idea of sympathies proposed a potential rationale for the connection between the stomach (consumption of food) and the skin (urtication).
- In the 18th century, Chalmers introduced his *toxins theory*, which was debated by T Caspar Gilchrist in 1908, a dermatology professor at the Johns Hopkins University. Toxins were believed to be contained in foods like nettles, or it was believed that the body converted the meal into a hazardous substance. The poisons would then cause localized stasis and urticarial lesions.
- Eulenburg, a proponent of the *nerve theory*, proposed that specific compounds present in food could impact the neural system of individuals who are susceptible.

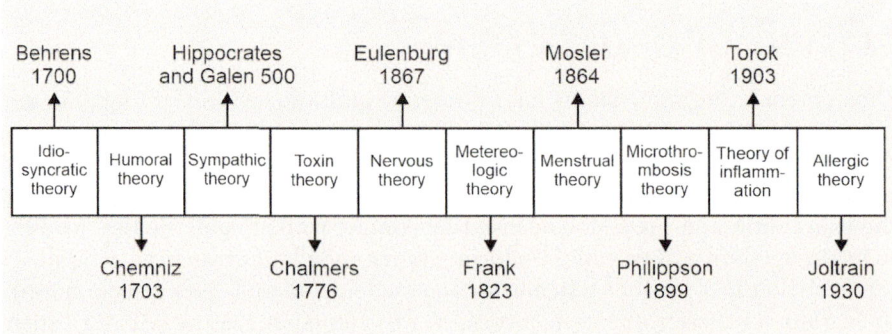

FIG. 2: Summary of theories related to the etiology of the urticarial eruptions.

- Neisser (1901) extended this perspective to the *angioneurotic theory* and regarded urticaria as a secretory neurosis characterized by vasodilation.
- The *meteorological theory* proposed by Frank (1823) posits that allergies are influenced by the specific arrangement of celestial bodies at the time of an individual's birth. This notion is currently under review due to the possibility that exposure to the allergens during pregnancy may increase the likelihood of developing allergic diseases.
- The *menstruation theory*, proposed in 1864, is grounded in the enduring fact that certain females who experience urticaria have a heightened sensitivity to their own endogenous hormones.
- The *microthrombosis theory* proposed by Philipson in 1899 offers an intriguing explanation for the migratory nature of wheals through the formation of microthrombi. Philipson challenged the angioneurotic idea by demonstrating that urticaria can occur in areas of the body that lack nerve supply.
- Gilchrist in the year 1908 and Torok in the year 1928 proposed the *hypothesis of inflammation* in the early years of the 20th century. This theory garnered substantial endorsement from the discovery and biological functions of histamine.
- In 1907, Windaus and Vogt successfully *synthesized histamine*, a substance that was later discovered by Laidlaw and Dale (1910) to produce the contraction of smooth muscles. In 1913, Eppinger found that histamine also caused whealing, erythema, and discomfort when injected into the skin.
- Histamine, derived from the Greek word "histos" meaning tissue, has been found in many tissues and has been proven to replicate all the characteristics of immediate allergic reactions, also including the well-known *triple response of Lewis*.
- Concurrent with the development of the notion of inflammation, there is mounting data suggesting that urticaria also has an allergic foundation. Given the frequent occurrence of urticaria alongside serum sickness, it was hypothesized that protein hypersensitivity was the root cause. In the seminal studies, Prausnitz and Kustner in the year 1921 transplanted an allergic individual's serum into the skin of a nonallergic individual and subsequently induced localized swelling by exposing the subject to the allergen through ingestion. They presented evidence that both a humoral component and an allergen are required for the formation of cutaneous wheal.
- The humoral factor or "reaginic antibody" found in allergic individuals was identified as a distinct class of immunoglobulins known as IgE by its discoverers, Ishizaka et al. and Johansson and Bennich.

HISTORY OF SUBTYPES OF URTICARIA (FIG. 3)

1. *Solar urticaria*: Several types of physical urticarias were early mentioned including solar urticaria which was initially documented by Borsch (1799), but it was not until 1887 that Veiel conclusively demonstrated that it is just the sun rays, and not the heat emitted by a stove or candle, that triggers this condition.

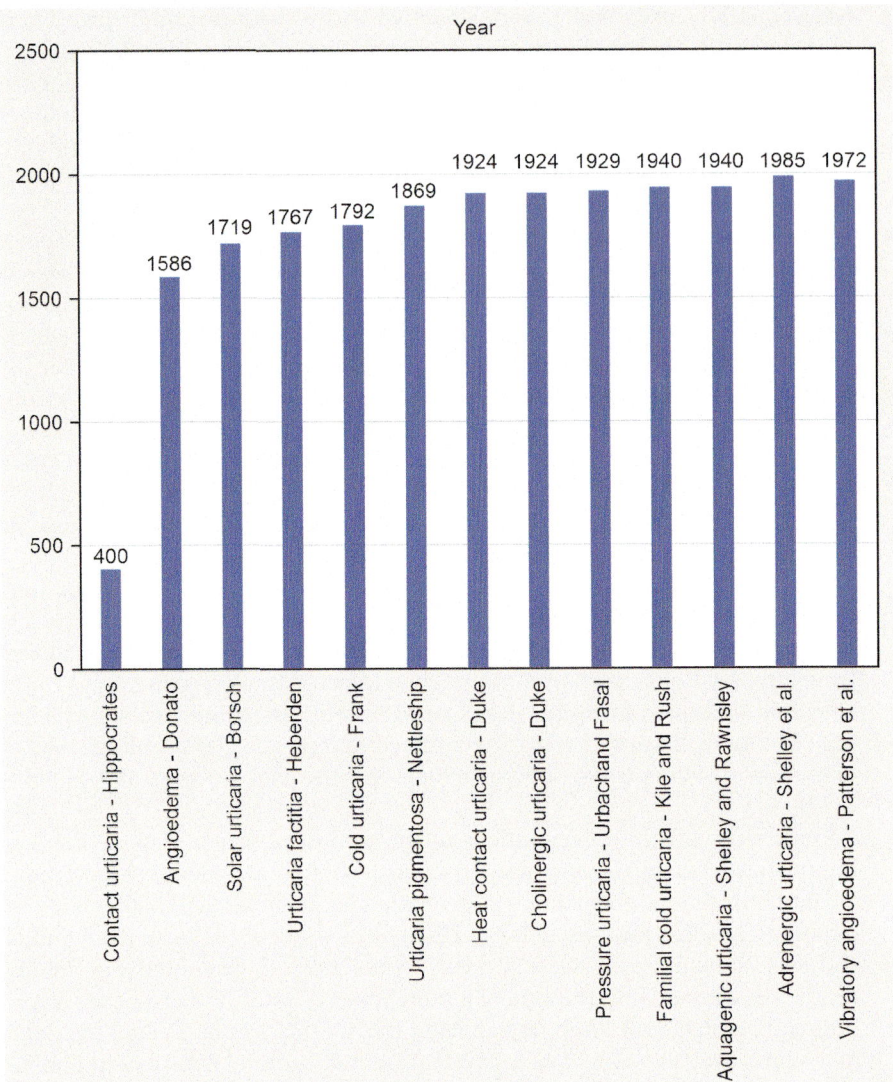

FIG. 3: Nomenclature history for subtype of urticaria.

2. *Factitial urticaria*: It was initially recorded during the medieval period, as those afflicted with this ailment were subjected to beheading or immolation because of the belief that they were associated with the devil. Heberden first documented it in the medical literature in 1767, and Gull gave it the name "factitious urticaria" in 1859.
3. *Cold urticaria*: It was first documented by Frank in the year 1792.
4. *Heat urticaria*: The article "Urticaria induced by heat and mental or physical exertion" was published in 1924 in the Journal of the American Medical Association (JAMA) by Duke.

5. *Pressure urticaria*: Urbach and Fasal first documented the occurrence of pressure urticaria in 1929.
6. *Aquagenic and adrenergic urticaria*: Shelley and Rawnsley initially reported aquagenic urticaria in 1964, whereas Shelley and Shelley described adrenergic urticaria in 1985.
7. *Urticaria pigmentosa*: It was initially described by Edward Nettleship in 1869. He referred to it as chronic urticaria, which resulted in the formation of dark spots. Sangster coined the term urticaria pigmentosa, whereas Unna identified the presence of mast cells within the lesions. Furthermore, a multitude of alternative terms have been employed to refer to the disease. The diverse clinical presentation of the illness is emphasized, as described by George Henry Fox as xanthelasmoidea in 1895; Louis Duhring called it xanthomoidea in 1898; Morrow named it papular erythema in 1899; Pick labeled it as urticaria perstans hemorrhagica in 1881; Klotz called it urticaria neviformis in 1907; Torok mentioned it as nevus pigmentosus urticans in 1928; Weber and Hellenschmied labeled it as telangiectasia macularis eruptiva perstans in 1930; Sezary called it mast cell reticulosis in 1952; and Drennan and Beare labeled it as solitary mast cell nevus in 1964 **(Fig. 4)**.

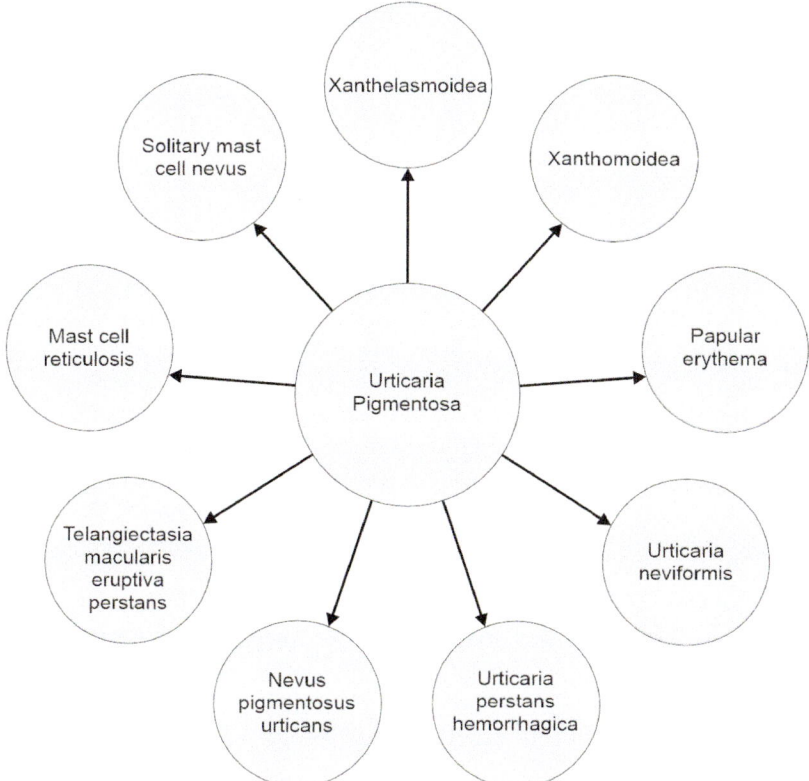

FIG. 4: Diverse clinical presentation of urticaria pigmentosa.

Subsequently, a range of factors have been linked to the prevalence of urticaria, including hormonal imbalances and the astrological signs of the individuals affected. The present understanding of the disorder is rooted in the identification of the mast cell by renowned Paul Ehrlich in 1879, the discovery of the messenger substance histamine by Adolf Windaus in 1907, and the recognition of immunoglobulin E (IgE), an antibody produced by the body's immune system, by the research teams led by Ishizaka and Johansson between 1965 and 1967.

HISTORY OF ANGIOEDEMA

Marcello Donati first documented angioedema in 1586 in a young nobleman who exhibited sensitivity to eggs. Quincke, the person whose name is associated with the sickness, released his renowned publication on the condition of sudden localized swelling of the skin in 1882.

Osler documented the occurrence of hereditary angioedema in 1888.

The case was fatal as a result of asphyxiation, which was a frequently observed cause of death within the family. In Sweden, the church has historically been responsible for registering the reason of death. In 1966, Arnoldsson et al. were able to trace a family's lineage back to the 17th century. In 1963, Donaldson and Evans discovered that these patients exhibited reduced levels of the C1 esterase inhibitor, leading to the occurrence of edema.

HISTORY OF THE TREATMENT OF URTICARIA AND ANGIOEDEMA

It is noteworthy to encounter discussions regarding the management of urticaria in the latter part of the nineteenth century, in which Fox asserts that any treatment for this ailment should be founded on the identification of its underlying causes. This remains true even in the present day. Fox also stated, "There is rarely an infection of skin for which many drugs and topicals have been studied, tested and discarded." He concluded that the difficulty in treating a disease is directly proportional to the amplitude of cures that are suggested for its treatment.

The acute urticaria caused by food was earlier treated using emetics or by administering rhubarb, castor oil, or magnesia. Topical use of vinegar, cologne, chloroform, or benzoic acid was used to alleviate the irritation. Occasionally, consuming bismuth, colchicine, sodium bicarbonate, diluted fluoric acid, or following a dyspeptic diet had proven to be beneficial.

Quinines were observed to have the ability to both treat and induce urticaria. A similar principle was applied to sodium salicylate. Ergot, arsenic, nettle tea, and strychnine were other medicines commonly utilized.

The identification of sympathomimetics during the late 19th and early 20th centuries offered a significant means for effectively managing potentially fatal allergic reactions like anaphylaxis. In the 1920s, the use of calcium injections and autohemotherapy (injections of the patient's own blood) was popular. This coincided with the practice of more advanced methods, such as desensitization with potential allergens.

Corticosteroids, discovered in 1930 by Swingler et al., provided an additional potent therapy option for acute urticaria. However, its application in chronic urticaria was rejected because of the possible hazards associated with prolonged usage. In the year 1940, the first antihistamines, which were H1 receptor antagonists, were developed. In 1942, the ethylenediamine derivative mepyramine (also known as pyrilamine) was introduced as one of the earliest antihistamines used in clinical practice. These drugs were effective in reducing symptoms but often caused significant sedation. In 1985, cetirizine, a metabolite of hydroxyzine, was developed, offering effective relief with minimal sedation.

The history of biologics in the treatment of urticaria (hives) represents a significant advancement in the management of urticaria. Urticaria was primarily managed with antihistamines and, in refractory cases, corticosteroids were the mainstay of treatment. However, these treatments were not always effective for chronic urticaria, and long-term corticosteroid use posed significant side effects. Omalizumab (monoclonal antibody against IgE), originally approved for asthma, was approved in 2014 by the Food and Drug Administration (FDA) for the treatment of chronic spontaneous urticaria in patients who remained symptomatic despite antihistamine treatment. Ongoing clinical trials and research are investigating other potential biologics for urticaria. These include ligelizumab (a next-generation anti-IgE antibody) and dupilumab (an IL-4 receptor alpha antagonist), among others.

CONCLUSION

These historical studies demonstrate that our comprehension of the pathophysiology and management of urticaria has made significant progress in recent decades. However, the underlying causes of most chronic urticarias, as well as the fundamental elements of angioedema and mast cell proliferative disease, remain largely unknown. Furthermore, the primary objective of treatment is to alleviate symptoms rather than eliminate the underlying cause. It is hoped that further advancements in the study of this disease in the next decades will aid in filling the gaps in our understanding of its development and enable more efficient therapy based on its underlying causes.

SUGGESTED READINGS

1. Hui SD, Fen WX, Wang N. Manual of Dermatology in Chinese Medicine. Seattle: Eastland Press; 1995. pp. 204-13.
2. More T. The History of King Richard III. In: Campbell WE, et al. (Eds). The English Works of Sir Thomas More. London: The Dial Press; 1931. p. 426.
3. Bateman T. A Practical Synopsis of Cutaneous Diseases. London: Longman, Hurst, Rees, Orme & Brown; 1813.
4. Shelley WB, Shelley ED. Adrenergic urticaria: A new form of stress-induced hives. Lancet. 1985;2:1031.
5. Osler W. Hereditary angioneurotic edema. Am J Med Sci. 1888;95:362.

CHAPTER 2

Etiopathogenesis of Urticaria

Sanjeev Gupta, Aditi Dabhra

INTRODUCTION

Urticaria is a prevalent condition that affects approximately 15–25% of adults at some stage in their lives. The condition is marked by recurring, itchy, raised wheals with a pale, swollen center and redness of the surrounding skin, which can occur on any area of the body. These lesions can vary in size, ranging from a few millimeters to several centimeters in diameter. They are typically transitory and usually disappear within approximately 24 hours without leaving any scars or any mark. However, in some cases, the lesions may persist for up to 48 hours. While urticaria is characterized by swelling involving the epidermis, angioedema which affects 40% of people with urticaria is characterized by the presence of swelling that is specifically limited to the subcutaneous and submucosal tissues. The pathogenesis of urticaria is multifaceted and encompasses mast cells (MC), interactions between immune cells, and other mediators.

ACUTE URTICARIA

Acute urticaria (AU) is a condition that is marked by the abrupt onset of hives or wheals on the skin. Although AU is common, there is still limited understanding of its underlying pathophysiology. Three main pathways have been linked to its development **(Flowchart 1)**.

1. *Type 1 hypersensitivity reaction*: The presence of sudden and spontaneous urticaria and swelling (angioedema) in persons experiencing a severe allergic reaction (anaphylaxis) is strongly associated with type I hypersensitivity reactions. This type of allergic reactions are immediate responses that occur when allergens (also called exoallergens) engage with pre-existing immunoglobulin E (IgE) antibodies that are already attached to high-affinity receptors (FcεRI) found on MC and basophils (BS). This contact initiates the activation and degranulation of these cells, leading to the secretion of histamine and other inflammatory substances. This mechanism results in the rapid occurrence of hives and other allergic symptoms. Typical causes of type I hypersensitivity reactions that lead to AU encompass a broad spectrum of factors, including foods, drugs, and diverse allergens.

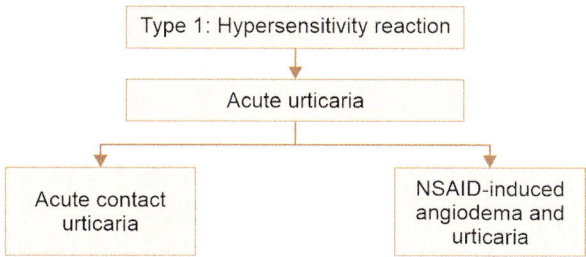

FLOWCHART 1: Three main pathways linked with the development of acute urticaria.
(NSAID: nonsteroidal anti-inflammatory drug)

2. *NSAID-induced angioedema and urticaria*: Urticaria and/or angioedema caused by nonsteroidal anti-inflammatory drugs (NSAIDs) may occur due to multiple factors, such as IgE-mediated routes, T cell-mediated reactions, or the inhibition of cyclooxygenase 1 (COX1) by NSAIDs. When the enzyme COX1 gets blocked, it might cause a rise in cysteinyl leukotrienes (LTs), which are responsible for the development of urticarial symptoms.
3. *Acute contact urticaria*: This can occur when allergens come into contact directly with the skin, as a result of either earlier sensitization or without prior sensitization. Sensitized individuals may develop urticaria on contact with allergens they were sensitized to. Occasionally, exposure to compounds that can cause urticaria can result in skin reactions even without prior sensitization. For instance, coming into contact with stinging nettles might induce acute contact urticaria in those who have not previously developed sensitivity to it.

CHRONIC URTICARIA

Chronic urticaria can be inducible (chronic inducible urticaria) or spontaneous. Chronic inducible urticaria can be because of many factors, e.g., by physical stimulus, heat, cold, pressure vibration, etc. The details of the same are dealt with in separate respective chapters.

Chronic spontaneous urticaria (CSU) may be due to some known or unknown causes, e.g., autoantibodies.

The pathophysiology of urticaria refers to the underlying mechanisms and processes that lead to the development of this condition.

Stimulation of MC and BS in individuals with CSU can occur due to:
- IgE antibodies targeting autoantigens
- IgG antibodies targeting FcεRI
- IgE antibodies targeting IgE itself
- Complement activation

Furthermore, the activation of MC and BS can be induced by chemicals that are released by other immune cells or neurons. Upon activation, both MC and BS release a variety of preformed mediators, including histamine and tryptase, as well as newly synthesized mediators, such as prostaglandins (PGs) and LTs. These mediators contribute to the process of inflammation, increased vascular permeability, vasodilation, and neuronal stimulation. The aforementioned consequences manifest as edema and pruritus. The release of cytokines by MC and BS induces the movement of other immune cells toward the surface, hence promoting skin inflammation **(Fig. 1)**.

In chronic urticaria, there are a few key players that have a major impact on the disease **(Fig. 2)**. These include MC and histamine, inflammatory mediators and cytokines, autoimmune factors, and neurogenic mechanisms.

Mast Cells and Histamine

Mast Cells

- There are different mediators secreted by MC which are involved in anaphylactic reactions. These mediators primarily cause the symptoms of IgE-mediated hypersensitivity, with histamine being a major contributor.
  The mediators secreted by MC fall into three categories:
  1. Preformed substances (such as histamine, serotonin, and heparin)
  2. Newly generated lipid mediators (such as thromboxane, PGD2, and LT C4)
  3. Cytokines [such as interleukin-4 (IL-4) and tumor necrosis factor-α (TNF-α)]
- Symptoms including hypotension, bronchospasm, and urticaria are among them. It is crucial to understand that IgE crosslinking is not the only factor that causes mast cell degranulation.
- On their surfaces, MC have a range of receptors that can trigger degranulation via several pathways. These receptors include:
  - Opioid receptors
  - Complement receptors (like C5a)
  - IgG receptors
  - Toll-like receptors (TLRs)
  - Protease-activated receptors (PARs)
  - T-cell receptors
- Although all human mast cell types are activated by FcεRI, a subset of MC found in the gut and lungs that express only tryptase is insensitive to complement components C3a, C5a, and compound 48/80 (a polymer that initiates mast cell degranulation).
- TLR-mediated activation induces the release of cytokines, chemokines, and lipid mediators but does not itself cause degranulation. It is interesting to note that infections that activate TLRs may reduce the threshold needed for degranulation brought on by different stimuli.
- There is ongoing research regarding MC function as antigen-presenting cells. NSAIDs, opiates, iodinated contrast media, vancomycin, local anesthetics, and neuromuscular blocking agents (NMBAs) are among the medicines that may activate most cells; hence, it is best to avoid using them in people who have systemic mastocytosis or chronic urticaria.
- Exacerbations may be caused by several cofactors. Simply said, mast cell degranulation may not occur with a single cofactor. However, several cofactors may cause symptoms by increasing histamine release.

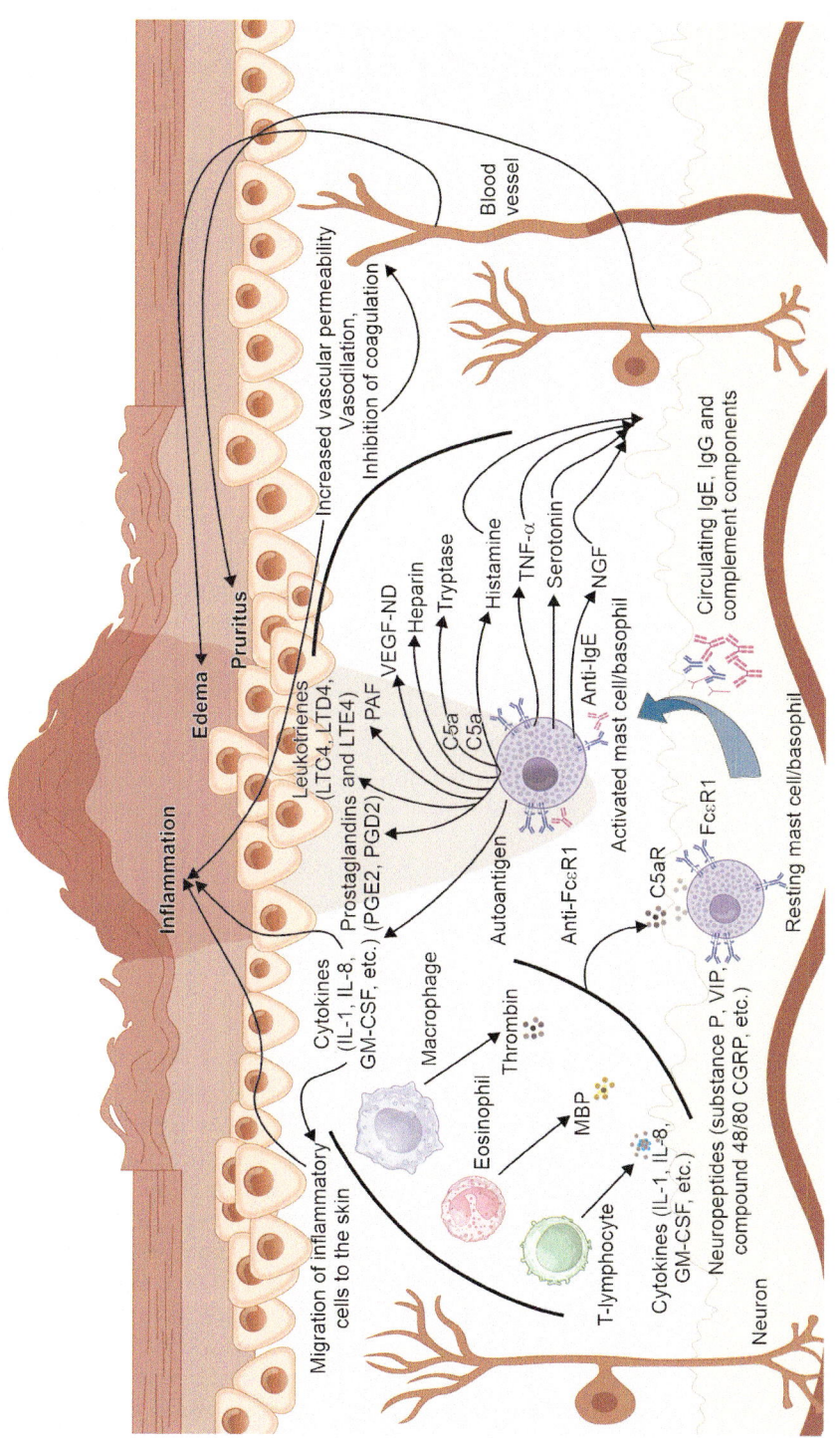

FIG. 1: Pathophysiological mechanisms of chronic spontaneous urticaria (CSU).

(CGRP: calcitonin gene-related peptide; GM–CSF: granulocyte-macrophage colony-stimulating factor; Ig: immunoglobulins; IL: interleukin; LT: leukotriene; MBP: myelin basic protein; NGF: nerve growth factor; PAF: platelet-activating factor; PG: prostaglandin; TNF: tumor necrosis factor; VEGF: vascular endothelial growth factor; VIP: vasoactive intestinal peptide)

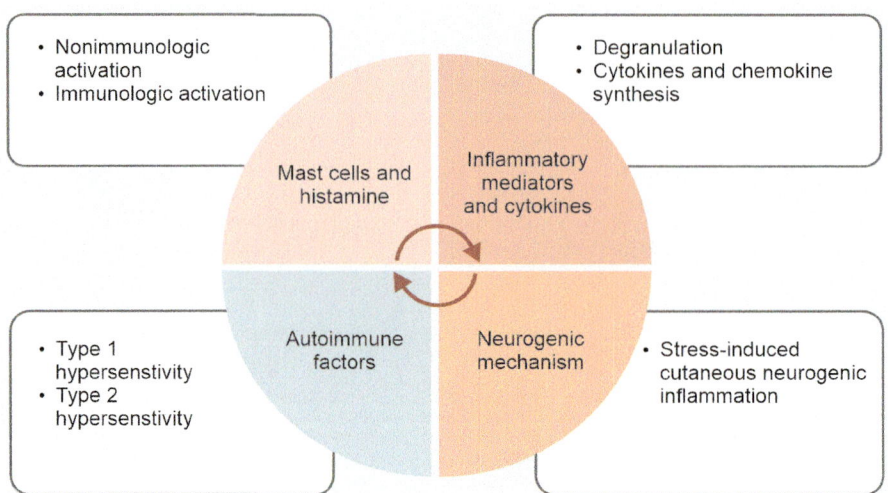

FIG. 2: Key players in chronic urticaria.

- It is crucial to highlight that the processes responsible for these reactions do not involve adaptive immunity, indicating that sensitization is not necessary for their occurrence.
- Similarly, the activation of mast cell degranulation through the MRGPRX2 receptor could be considered as an additional contributing component. This effect may depend on the simultaneous existence of additional cofactors in order to be clinically evident. This observation may provide an explanation for the limited response of just a minority of patients to neuromuscular blocking medications.
- Considering the vital significance of MC in the formation of urticaria, it is essential to recognize both the interplay between MC and other immune cells as well as the interactions between B lymphocytes and different immune cells **(Fig. 3; Table 1)**.

Histamine

The binding of histamine with the histamine receptors on the cutaneous microvasculature permits vasodilatation and hence vasopermeation. This results in the formation of a wheal. Histamine also stimulates itch by stimulating local C-fiber networks through an antidromic mechanism. The production of the flare is caused by the release of substance P from nerve terminals in the skin, rather than histamine. Activation of the H1 receptor causes a decrease in blood pressure and the accumulation of fluid in the body tissues, therefore contributing to itch, flare, erythema and wheal formation. Activation of peripheral H2 receptors elicits identical responses in the skin but without itch or flare. H2 receptors are also found in the gastric mucosa, so many people with urticaria have varying levels of acidity. H3 receptors are mostly found in the central nervous system as inhibitory autoreceptors; therefore, their activation leads to decreased synthesis of histamine, whereas H4 receptors are present on granulocytes and MC and its stimulation leads to itch in mice **(Table 2)**.

CHAPTER 2: Etiopathogenesis of Urticaria

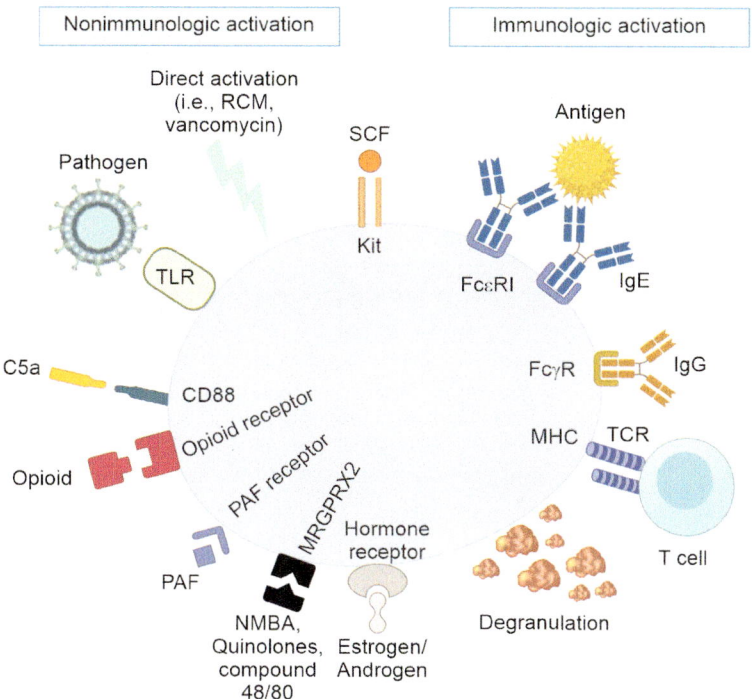

FIG. 3: Mast cell degranulation.
(FcεRI: high affinity IgE receptor; FcγR: Fc-gamma receptors; MHC: major histocompatibility complex; NMBA: neuromuscular blocking agent; PAF: platelet activation factor; RCM: radiocontrast media; SCF: stem cell factor; TCR: T-cell receptor; TLR: Toll-like receptor)

TABLE 1: Possible interaction between MC and other immune cells involved in CSU.	
Interaction of MC with other immune cells	**Impact**
Eosinophil and mast cell	• Pivotal effectors in CSU • Physical interaction between these cells during chronic and late stages of allergic inflammation • Paracrine signaling leads to mast cell-induced eosinophil migration • Eosinophils increase the release of mediators from MC at their baseline level by interaction with CD48-24 and also stimulate MC that have been activated by IgE • Eosinophils exhibit increased levels of intercellular adhesion molecule expression • Eosinophils lower the threshold for IgE response in MC by incorporating co-stimulatory signals into the pathways mediated by IgE • Long-term allergic reactions demonstrate an elevation in the release of TNF-α from eosinophils

Continued

Continued

Interaction of MC with other immune cells	Impact
Basophil and mast cell	• MC and BS are essential in initiating allergic inflammation from CD34+ hematopoietic stem cells located in the bone marrow • The activation of these BS and cutaneous MC induces the secretion of histamine and other proinflammatory mediators • This release of the mediators leads to the vasodilatation found in the afflicted skin of chronic CSU
Neutrophil and mast cell	• MC initiate the early stage of neutrophil recruitment by releasing GM-CSF, a chemical stimulant • Neutrophil lifespan is considerably prolonged by GM-CSF when activated through IgE cross-linking • It has been shown that MC release IL-1b, which stimulates the migration of neutrophils and causes leakage in blood vessels
T cells and MC	• The inflammatory site experiences intricate interplay between MC and activated T lymphocytes • T cell-derived microvesicles serve as triggers for mast cell activation, allowing for a response at the site of inflammation without direct interaction with T cells • Activated MC release inflammatory mediators, impacting extracellular matrix breakdown in T cell-mediated inflammation
Monocytes and MC	• Monocytes from CSU patients had higher chemokine expression of CCL2 and CXCL8 and CCL2 activates MC, particularly BS • When activated, monocytes release MCP-1, a potent histamine-releasing factor for MC and BS
Macrophages and MC	• Following FcεRI aggregation, macrophages release IL-6, which promotes mast cell proliferation, maturation, and response • IFN-11 can be produced by many skin cells, including MC, eosinophils, B cells, neutrophils, and macrophages which holds significance in pathogenesis of CSU
Innate lymphoid cells and mast cell	• Chronic urticaria patients had a higher number of NK cells in their peripheral blood, suggesting that innate immune pathways may play a role in wound healing. • ILC2s play an important role in type 2 inflammation by releasing IL-5 and IL-13 regardless of antigens and also influence mast cell function
Crosstalk among B lymphocytes and other immune cells	• T cells interact with B cells via cytokine production • Basophil-derived IL-4 and IL-6 affect B cells by increasing their survival, proliferation, and humoral immunity • CSU patients have lower amounts of IL-21, which corresponds inversely with total IgE levels

(BS: basophils; CSU: chronic spontaneous urticaria; GM-CSF: granulocyte-macrophage colony-stimulating factor; IFN-11: interferon 11; MC: mass cells; MCP-1: monocyte chemoattractant protein-1; NK: natural killer; TNF-α: tumor necrosis factor-α)

TABLE 2: Histamine receptors and their effects.

Histamine receptor	Site	Effect
H1	Smooth muscle, endothelial cells, central nervous system	Itch, flare, erythema, wheals
H2	Gastric parietal cells	Erythema, wheals
H3	Central nervous system	Inhibitory effect on histamine
H4	MC, eosinophils, T cells, dendritic cells	Itch

(MC: mast cells)

Inflammatory Mediators and Cytokines

Urticaria has long been linked to the rapid release of the histamine during degranulation of mast cell, which is significantly inhibited by histamine receptor antagonists (anti-H1). However, recent insights into mast cell activation processes via the IgE–FcεRI complex have revealed a more complex picture, demonstrating the participation of several enzymatic pathways upon receptor stimulation. This activation produces three unique metabolic effects:

1. *Degranulation*: MC degranulation results in the immediate release of mediators that quickly cause vasodilation and the influx of plasma into the dermis. These rapid releases include histamine, TNF-α, serotonin, proteases, and proteoglycans. These mediators, whether through direct or indirect means, play a significant role in the formation of hives, serving as an essential component of the urticaria cascade.
2. *Cytokines and chemokine synthesis*: MC, when stimulated by the IgE–FcεRI complex, release several cytokines and chemokines within a time frame of 6–24 hours after stimulation. Cytokines, such as IL-1 and TNF-α, which are often present during the initial stage of inflammation, stimulate endothelial cells, facilitating leukocytes to be recruited and for other cell types to produce cytokines. Additional molecules such as IL-3, IL-4, IL-5, IL-6, IL-8, IL-9, and IL-13, along with transforming growth factor-B, stem cell factor, granulocyte-macrophage colony-stimulating factor (GM-CSF), macrophage inflammatory protein-1a (MIP-1a), interferon-inducible protein-10, and monocyte chemoattractant protein-1 have a role in attracting leukocytes, particularly eosinophils, to the dermis. This leads to the late-phase reaction, which is clinically characterized as indurated erythema **(Table 3)**.
3. *Leukotrienes and prostaglandin synthesis*:
   - The production of LTs and PGs is aided by two enzyme systems, namely cyclooxygenases and lipoxygenases, which act on arachidonic acid after activation of mast cell. While the exact methods by which they contribute to the urticarial wheals are still uncertain, new research has emphasized the strong chemotactic activity of LTB4, which is produced by MC, in the early and specific recruitment of leukocytes.
   - Mediators play a crucial role in cases of chronic urticaria, as demonstrated by the effect of LT inhibitors and nonsteroidal anti-inflammatory medicines on the disease's chronic nature.

TABLE 3: Role of cytokines with immune cells in the pathogenesis of CSU.

Cytokines	Source	Target	Receptors	Functions	Serum level
Interleukin-1β	MC	Polymorphs	IL-1 type 2	Vascular leak by polymorphs' induction and migration	↑↑
Interleukin-2	CD4 and CD8 cells and activated T cells	T cells (CD4 and CD8), B cells	IL-2R	• Proliferate effector T and B lymphocytes • Stimulation of B cells for antibody formation	↓↓
Interleukin-3	Macrophages, MC, T cells, eosinophils, natural killer cells	BS, eosinophils	IL-3α+β c ((CD131)	Activate eosinophils and BS	↑↑
Interleukin-4	Th2 cells, MC, BS,	T and B cells, monocytes, and MC	IL-4R types I, II	Activation of T and B lymphocytes, BS, eosinophils, and monocytes	↑↑
Interleukin-5	MC, activated, eosinophils and Th2 cells	BS and eosinophils	IL-5R	Stimulates chemotactic activity of eosinophils	↑↑
Interleukin-6	T cells, MC, BS, macrophages	B cells, MC	IL-6R (sIL-6R) gp130	Differentiation of B cells, production of IgG, M, A, proliferation and maturation of MC	↑↑
Interleukin-8	Eosinophils and MC	Polymorphs, NK cells, T cells, BS, and eosinophils	CXCR1 and CXCR2	Increases chemotaxis of polymorphs, eosinophils, BS, etc.	↑↑
Interleukin-9	T cells, eosinophils, and MC	T and B lymphocytes and MC	IL-9R	Inhibition of cytokines, proliferates CD8+ cells and MC	↑↑
Interleukin-10	T lymphocytes	T and B lymphocytes	IL-10R1/IL-10R2 complex	Activates B cells for Ab production, and inhibition of Th1 response	↑↑
Interleukin-13	T, NKT, MC, BS, and eosinophils	MC, B cells, and eosinophils	IL-13R1a1 and IL-13R1a2	Eosinophils and MC activation	↑↑
Interleukin-17	Th17 cells	T and B lymphocytes, Monocytes, and macrophages	IL-17R	Activates neutrophils and causes recruitment of chemokines and cytokines	↑↑
Interleukin-18	Macrophages	Macrophages, natural killer cells	IL-18R	Stimulates IFN-γ, Th1 and Th2 response and natural killer cells cytotoxicity	↑↑

Continued

Continued

Cytokines	Source	Target	Receptors	Functions	Serum level
Interleukin-21	T cells	T cells (CD4 and CD8), B cells, macrophages, and dendritic cells	IL-21R	Inhibits B cells' proliferation and causes Ag specific apoptosis of B cells	↓↓
Interleukin-23	Macrophages	Natural killer cells, macrophages, T cells (Th17), eosinophils, and monocytes	IL-23R	Production of IL-17, stimulation of Th17 cells	↑↑
Interleukin-24	T cells, monocytes and B cells	MC	IL-20R1/IL-20R2 and IL-22R1/IL-20R2	Works as autoantigen in CSU	↑↑
Interleukin-25	T cells, MC, eosinophils, and BS	BS, Th2 memory cells, macrophages, natural killer cells	IL-17RA and IL-17RB	Stimulation of Th2, inhibition of Th1 and Th17 responses, stimulation of IgG1, E and IL-4, -5, -13 production	↑↑
Interleukin-31	T cells, MC, and BS	BS, eosinophils, and MC	IL-31RA/OSM Rβ	Stimulation of IL-6, 8, CXCL1 and 8, CCL2 and 8, production in eosinophils	↑↑
Interleukin-33	Th2 cells, macrophages, MC, eosinophils, and BS	MC, BS, eosinophils, macrophages, dendritic cells, natural killer cells, T and B lymphocytes	ST2	Increased integrin expression in eosinophils and BS, stimulate synthesis of IL-31	↑↑
Interleukin-35	Treg cells and monocytes	Activated T cells and natural killer cells	IL-12Rβ2/gp130, IL-12Rβ2/IL 12Rβ2, gp130/gp1 30	Inhibition of proliferation of effector T cells, increases production of IL-10	↓↓
TNF-α	T cells, MC, and BS	Eosinophils	TNFR1 (p55/60, CD120a) and TNFR2 (p75/80, CD120b)	Increases expression of eosinophils ICAM-1	↑↑
IFN-γ	T cells, MC, and macrophages	Polymorphs, lymphocytes, eosinophils, MC, and macrophages	IFNGR1/IF NGR2	Aggregation of polymorphs, MC, macrophages, lymphocytes and eosinophils	↓↓
IFN-λ1	T cells, macrophages, and MC	Polymorphs, lymphocytes, eosinophils, MC, and macrophages	IFNLR1 IL-10R2	Regulate Th1 and Th2 responses	↑↑ (in the plasma)
TGF-β	Eosinophils, macrophages, and Treg cells	Polymorphs, eosinophils, monocytes, MC, and macrophage, natural killer cells, T cells	TβR-I and TβR-II	Inhibition of MC, regulate and differentiate subsets of Th cells	↑↑

(Ag: antigen; BS: basophils; CSU: chronic spontaneous urticaria; IFN: interferon; MC: mast cell; TGF: transforming growth factor)

- MC activation can result in diverse physiologic reactions, which vary in magnitude depending on the specific stimuli. Therefore, mast cell activation can lead to any combination of the three mentioned events or even a partial manifestation of them, rather than a consistent and identical reaction. Therefore, it is possible to stimulate the production of cytokines without necessarily causing mast cell degranulation.
- The findings indicate a thought-provoking viewpoint: Urticaria may not always be directly linked to histamine release or solely associated with mast cell degranulation.

Autoimmune Factors in Urticaria

It is worth mentioning that CSU is often caused by autoimmune mechanisms that activate cutaneous MC. The autoimmunity in CSU can be classified into two primary categories: Types I and IIb. In type I, the presence of IgE antibodies against autoallergens [such as thyroid peroxidase (TPO) and IL-24] triggers the activation of dermal mast cells (MCs) and the subsequent release of mediators like histamine. This process leads to cellular infiltration and contributes to the formation of wheals. In IIb, IgG autoantibodies against IgE and its receptor FcεRI activate dermal MCs, resulting in a similar release of mediators and the development of wheals **(Fig. 4)**. Therefore, CSU's genesis can be understood as a complicated interaction of hypersensitivity reactions, autoallergy, and antibody-mediated processes that trigger mast cell activation.

- *Type 1 hypersensitivity: Autoallergy*
    - In type 1 hypersensitivity, self-antigens crosslink the IgE antibodies existing on MC and BS, causing the release of vasoactive mediators **(Fig. 4)**.
    - Rorsman first proposed the concept of autoallergy in 1962 to explain urticaria-associated basopenia, a condition in which antigens activate mast degranulation cells.
    - In 1999, IgE antibodies against thyroid microsomal antigen were found in the serum of a female CSU patient, providing supporting evidence.
- *Type 2 hypersensitivity: Antibody-mediated*
    - This type of hypersensitivity occurs when antibodies, usually IgG or IgM, attach to antigens on target cells **(Fig. 4)**.
    - The concept of type II reaction gained popularity after IgG autoantibodies against IgE were detected in three out of six patients with CSU.
    - The autoantibodies were confirmed using autologous serum skin tests (ASSTs), in which the patient's sera caused wheal and flare responses when injected intradermally.
    - Later on, it was shown that some patients with chronic CSU have IgG-anti-FcεRI autoantibodies. These autoantibodies target the high affinity receptor for IgE found on MC and BS.
    - Another possible approach involves the presence of IgG-anti-FcεRII/CD23 autoantibodies in the sera of patients with CSU. These autoantibodies have the potential to activate eosinophils, which in turn can cause mast cell degranulation. This process leads to the production of substances that stimulate MC.

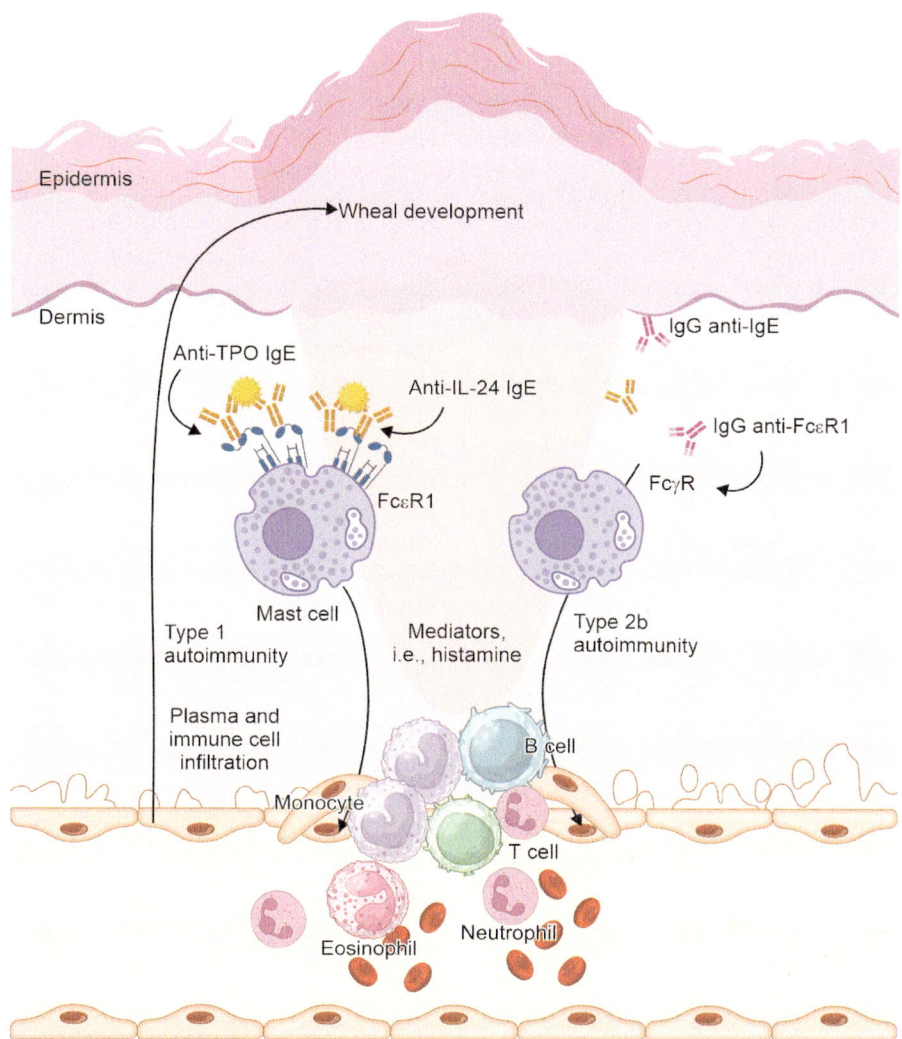

FIG. 4: A schematic depiction of autoimmune mechanisms in chronic spontaneous urticaria (CSU).

(Anti-TPO: anti-thyroid peroxidase; FcγR: Fc-gamma receptors; IL: interleukin)

Breakthroughs in unravelling autoimmune urticaria mechanisms:
- *Gruber et al.* discovered autoantibodies and suggested they may cause persistent urticaria or angioedema. They found IgG and IgM autoantibodies targeting IgE in these patients. Cold urticaria patients had 55% IgG antibodies against IgE and 22% IgM antibodies. IgG anti-IgE antibodies were 50% in chronic urticaria and urticarial vasculitis patients.
- *Fiebiger et al.* later found that 32% of Western blots from chronic urticaria patients had an FcεRI response. Further testing showed that 69% of chronic urticaria patients exhibited FcεRI and IgE and IgG autoantibodies. Compared to controls and atopic dermatitis patients, these autoantibodies were specific to chronic urticaria patients.

Neurogenic Mechanisms

- Without a doubt, dermal MCs and the many mediators they release are the primary factors responsible for the development of wheals and the progression of urticaria in all its forms. The stimulation of cutaneous MC initiates an instantaneous process of degranulation, releasing preexisting mediators that are contained in granules **(Fig. 5)**.
- FcεRIα/IgE includes substances such as histamine, serotonin, heparin, chymase, tryptase, nerve growth factor (NGF), and tumor necrosis factor-β (TNF-β).
- Furthermore, when MC are activated, they produce arachidonic acid metabolites such as LTs, PGs, and platelet activation factor (PAF), which are then released into the surrounding tissue.
- This activation also triggers the release of numerous cytokines and chemotactic agents, including ILs such as IL-1, IL-4, IL-5, IL-6, IL-8, IL-10, IL-31, IL-33, MIP-1, GM-CSF, transforming growth factor β (TGF-β), vascular endothelial growth factor (VEGF), fibroblast growth factor (FGF), TNF-α, and C-C chemokine ligands 2 and 5 (CCL2 and CCL5).
- The vasoactive features of mast cell mediators cause increased vasodilation, higher expression of adhesion molecules, enhanced vascular permeability, and leakage of plasma from blood vessels. As a result, there is a noticeable buildup of cells and proteins that cause inflammation in the affected skin. Specifically, substances such as substance P (SP), NGF, and vasoactive intestinal peptide (VIP) have the ability to interact with nerve endings in the peripheral nervous system, thereby stimulating sensory nerves.
- The interaction between MCs (MC) and neural tissue is the fundamental mechanism behind stress-induced cutaneous neurogenic inflammation.
- Urticarial wheals exhibit an elevated abundance of neutrophils, eosinophils, BS, CD4+ cells, and monocytes. Furthermore, discrepancies in the distribution and functions of T-cell subtypes have been noted in the serum of patients with CSU in comparison to people unaffected by the illness.
- These imbalances consist of increased amounts of proinflammatory Th17 cells and changes in Treg cells. Analysis of skin biopsies has revealed increased levels of some cytokines in both urticarial wheals and unaffected skin areas.
- These cytokines are IL-4, IL-5, IL-25, IL-33, and thymic stromal lymphopoietin (TSLP). These cytokines can stimulate a Th2-related immune response, which enhances chronic inflammation and angiogenesis.
- Interestingly, the presence of increased interferon-γ (IFN-γ) expression in afflicted skin indicates a combination of Th1- and Th2-skewed polarization of the skin's immune response in CSU.

Steps Involved in Neurogenic Mechanism (Fig. 5)

1. The central and peripheral axes of the hypothalamic–pituitary–adrenal (HPA) system are responsible for regulating the skin's barrier function and inflammatory responses.

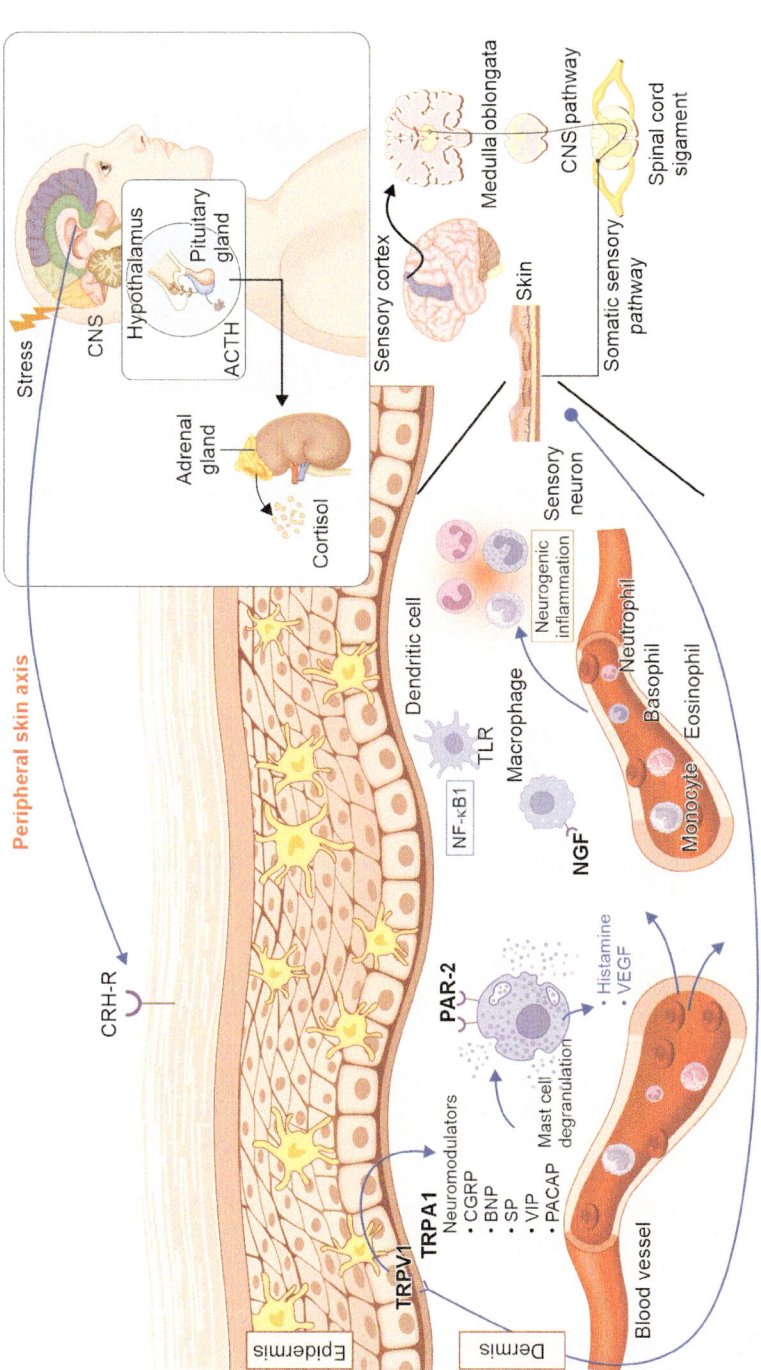

FIG. 5: Pathophysiology of the neurogenic mechanism of chronic spontaneous urticaria (CSU).

(ACTH: adrenocorticotropic hormone; BNP: brain natriuretic peptide; CGRP: calcitonin gene-related peptide; CNS: central nervous system; NGF: nerve growth factor; PACAP: pituitary adenylate cyclase activating polypeptide; PAR: proteinase-activated receptor; SP: substance P; TRPA1: transient receptor potential ankyrin 1; VEGF: vascular endothelial growth factor; VIP: vasoactive intestinal peptide)

2. Various stressors activate the release of neuromediators (CRF) from the hypothalamus and other areas of the central nervous system. These neuromediators can stimulate the release of norepinephrine and cortisol from the adrenal glands, as well as the release of leukocytes in the circulatory system through CRF and MC receptors. This activation helps modulate immune responses during inflammation and immunity.
3. Cytokines and neuropeptides produced by immune cells regulate inflammatory reactions in the skin.
4. The activation of PAR2 on the plasma membrane of sensory nerve endings occurs when tryptase is released from degranulated MC (MCs). This activation then leads to the release of calcitonin gene-related peptide and tachykinins from the sensory nerve terminals.
5. Vasoactive sensory nerve peptides are secreted in response to mediators generated by MC and other inflammatory cells. Proliferation of intracellular calcium ions by PAR2 at the spinal cord level triggers the release of calcitonin gene-related peptde (CGRP) and SP from central nerve endings.
6. Neurotransmitters that are released upon activation by sensory nerves regulate cutaneous inflammation, pain, and also itching.

Immunohistological Studies in Chronic Urticaria (Table 4)

Due to a rigorous immunohistologic study, the molecular immunopathogenesis and complicated effector mechanisms of chronic urticaria have been better understood. The investigations studied invading cell immunophenotypes, cytokines, chemokines/chemokine receptors, and adhesion molecules These studies generally used successive urticarial wheal biopsies. The findings are as follows:

- The urticarial wheal is typically characterized by vasodilation, dermal edema, and the presence of a non-necrotizing infiltrate around blood vessels, primarily consisting of mononuclear cells. The main constituents of this composition are primarily CD+ lymphocytes, along with varied amounts of monocytes, neutrophils, eosinophils, and BS.
- Approximately 60 minutes following the development of a wheal, a noticeable increase in the number of neutrophils in the skin occurs, with neutrophils being the most abundant type of cells present. Significantly, the number of MC remains unaltered, matching the counts seen in normal skin and healthy individuals.
- Regarding the cytokine profile, there is an increase in the levels of IL-4, IL-5 and IFN-γ RNA, indicating a combined Th1/Th2 immune response. The influx of cytokines is accompanied by increased levels of chemokines and enhanced expression of adhesion molecules.
- The healthy skin reflects the same levels of preregulated soluble mediators and adhesion molecules as the afflicted skin. In addition, there is a notable increase in T-cell counts in unaffected skin, while the presence of neutrophils is only found in healed skin.

TABLE 4: Pattern of infiltrating cell seen in urticarial wheal as compared to uninvolved site and control.

Type of cell	Wheals (urticaria)	Uninvolved site	Healthy control
Eosinophil	High in number	Not significant	Not significant
Mast cell	Normal	Normal	Normal
Basophil	Increased in number specially after 30 minutes of wheal formation	Less in number	Not significant
Lymphocyte	T-cell count increased	Increased T cell as compared to lesional site	Low T-cell count
Neutrophil	Major cell infiltrate seen after 1 hour of urticarial wheal formation	Less infiltrate	Low T-cell count
CXCR3/CCR3 (chemokines)	Expression is similar to the control	Expression is high	Expression is similar to lesional skin and healthy control
Interleukin 4 (IL-4)	Expression is high	Low expression	Not seen
Interleukin 5 (IL-5)	Expression is high	Low expression	Not seen
Interleukin 8 (IL-8)	Expression is moderate	Expression is moderate	Not seen
Interferon-γ (IFN-γ)	Expression is high	Low expression	Not seen
Adhesion molecule	Expression is high	Expression is intense	Expression is significant

- Chronic urticaria begins when MC in the dermal layer of the skin are activated and they degranulate. This initial event is crucial in the underlying pathophysiology, especially in the early stages. The chemicals secreted by these activated MC establish the foundation for the earliest stage of inflammation. Subsequently, this inflammation involves an intricate interaction between several substances that promote inflammation, such as proinflammatory mediators, cytokines, chemokine receptors, chemokines, and adhesion molecules.
- The precise coordination of these factors controls the regulation of the blood vessel activity and the unique dynamics of cellular infiltration, ultimately resulting in a hypersensitive reaction driven by lymphocytes and granulocytes. The manifestation of this reaction is observed as the distinctive urticarial wheals.
- Additionally, the inflammatory cells that enter the damaged area have a crucial function in maintaining this sequence of events. They accomplish this by generating supplementary proinflammatory mediators, which subsequently attract and stimulate other types of cells. This enhances and prolongs the immunological response within host. The observed rise in inflammatory compounds, virtually equal levels of adhesion molecules and chemokines,

along with elevated T-cell counts in unaffected skin, emphasize the significant activation of the immune system.
- This indicates the presence of a mild, ongoing inflammatory condition in skin that appears to be unaffected, confirming the concept of hidden, minimum inflammation. This predisposes the MC to lower trigger thresholds which makes them more susceptible to urticaria even when the symptoms are not present.

CONCLUSION

- Chronic urticaria (CU) is a complex and multifaceted condition that extends beyond its physical symptoms, significantly affecting patients' mental health, quality of life, and socioeconomic stability.
- Its chronic and unpredictable nature demands a comprehensive approach to management, emphasizing timely diagnosis, accurate identification of triggers, and individualized treatment plans.
- Advances in understanding the pathophysiology of CU, particularly the role of mast cells, histamine, and autoimmune mechanisms, have paved the way for targeted therapies, offering hope to refractory cases.

SUGGESTED READINGS

1. Grattan CE. Autoimmune urticaria. Review. Immunol Allergy Clin North Am. 2004;24:163-81.
2. Ying S, Kikuchi Y, Meng Q, Barry Kay A, Kaplan AP. TH1/TH2 cytokines and inflammatory cells in skin biopsy specimens from patients with chronic idiopathic urticaria: comparison with the allergen-induced late-phase cutaneous reaction. J Allergy Clin Immunol. 2002;109: 694-700.
3. Puccetti A, Bason C, Simeoni S, Milo E, Tinazzi E, Beri R, et al. In chronic idiopathic urticaria autoantibodies against Fc epsilonRII/CD23 induce histamine via eosinophil activation. Clin Exp Allergy. 2005;35:1599-607.
4. Grattan CE, Francis DM, Hide M, Greaves MW. Detection of circulating histamine releasing autoantibodies with functional properties of anti-IgE in chronic urticaria. Clin Exp Allergy. 1991;21:695-704.
5. Niimi N, Francis DM, Kermani F, O'Donnell BF, Hide M, Kobza-Black A, et al. Dermal mast cell activation by autoantibodies against the high affinity IgE receptor in chronic urticaria. J Invest Dermatol. 1996;106:1001-6.
6. Hennino A, Bérard F, Guillot I, Saad N, Rozières A, Nicolas JF. Pathophysiology of urticaria. Clin Rev Allergy Immunol. 2006;30(1):3-11.

CHAPTER 3

Etiopathogenesis of Angioedema

Sanjeev Gupta, Aditi Dabhra, Namya Gupta

INTRODUCTION

Angioedema (AE) is a medical condition that involves the abrupt and localized swelling of the skin and mucosal membranes in a specific area. It poses a complex clinical problem. While isolated angioedema can occur, it is commonly linked to urticarial disorders, for example, acute urticaria as well as chronic spontaneous urticaria (CSU), especially in cases of bradykinin-induced angioedema.

Angioedema is primarily classified into two types:
1. Histamine-mediated angioedema
2. Bradykinin-mediated angioedema

Comprehending the fundamental distinctions in the pathophysiology of these various types is crucial for developing precise diagnostic and treatment approaches.

Angioedema predominantly occurs as a result of histamine-mediated mechanisms. It typically manifests as a rapid type I hypersensitivity reaction, affecting the face, tongue, lips, and throat, and may be followed by urticaria or hives. Angioedema caused by histamine usually shows a positive response to conventional allergy treatments, including antihistamines, corticosteroids, and epinephrine.

On the other hand, angioedema caused by bradykinin can occur due to stress, trauma, or specific drugs, sometimes without any obvious triggers. Bradykinin-mediated angioedema is a medical disorder characterized by the extravasation of fluid caused by the vasodilatation and increased permeability of blood vessels. This is triggered by bradykinin, a powerful substance that causes vasodilatation. The pathophysiology of this condition is primarily influenced by the intricate interaction among high-molecular-weight kininogen (HMWK), bradykinin, and kallikrein. Imbalance in this equilibrium results in distinct symptoms such as nonpruritic, nonpitting, asymmetrical, and a localized swelling of the skin and/or mucosa. Involvement of the gastrointestinal mucosa, for example, can cause stomach pain, nausea, vomiting, or diarrhea. The etiology, pathophysiology, and clinical symptoms of angioedema mediated by bradykinin are not yet fully understood, and improper care can result in fatal outcomes.

HISTAMINE-MEDIATED ANGIOEDEMA

Angioedema caused by histamine is frequently seen in emergency departments, making up approximately 40–50% of all angioedema cases.

While this response is generally restricted on its own, the involvement of the larynx in acute severe reactions like anaphylaxis may be extremely dangerous because it can lead to asphyxia.

- *Type I hypersensitivity reaction*: This mechanism is the most well-known process of angioedema caused by histamine. It comprises two phases: Initial-phase reaction and late-phase reaction.
  i. *Initial-phase reaction*:
     - During the sensitization phase of type I hypersensitivity reaction, presence of the allergens, particularly food allergens such as wheat or milk, stimulates an elevated production of antigen specific immunoglobulin E (IgE) molecules by the plasma cells.
     - During this asymptomatic response, IgE attaches to high-affinity FcεRI receptor that is constantly present on the mast cells and also on the basophils.
     - When a person is exposed to the same allergen again, the IgEs in their body bind to the allergen, causing basophils and mast cells to degranulate, thus indicating the initial stage of a type I hypersensitivity reaction.
     - Biogenic amines (e.g., histamine) and serine proteases (e.g., tryptase and chymase) are released as inflammatory mediators. This leads to disturbed vascular integrity through the dilatation and opening of the endothelial cell junctions.
     - This vasodilation and increased capillary permeability lead to the buildup of fluid in the gaps between cells, resulting in nonpitting edema. This condition primarily affects the face, tongue, lips, neck, genitalia, hands, and feet.
  ii. *Late-phase reaction*:
     - The "late-phase" response, however, does not necessarily rely on IgEs. Unlike the initial-stage reactions, the cutaneous symptoms of a delayed-phase reaction entail the buildup and infiltration of the eosinophils, neutrophils, CD4+ T cells, and basophils.
     - Late-phase reactions exhibit a slower pace compared to initial-phase reactions, usually manifesting hours instead of minutes after being exposed to the antigen again.
- *Direct activation of mast cells and basophils*: In addition to type I hypersensitivity reactions, histamine-mediated angioedema can develop as a result of the direct activation of the mast cells or basophils, which triggers the release of many inflammatory mediators. Direct activation can be triggered by either internal or external stimuli. Anaphylatoxins, which include complement pieces C3a, C4a, and also C5a, are natural substances that directly activate mast cells and cause them to release their contents. This activation occurs when the anaphylatoxins attach to the receptors on the cell membrane of mast cells that are not the FcεRI receptors. Iodine- and gadolinium-based

contrast agents are exogenous substances that directly induce degranulation of the mast cells and the basophils by acting on their cell membranes.
- *Nonsteroidal anti-inflammatory drug (NSAID)-induced angioedema*: Interference with the arachidonic-acid pathway can result in histamine-induced angioedema. An obvious instance is the development of urticaria/angioedema caused by NSAIDs, commonly referred to as NSAID-induced urticaria/angioedema (NIUA). NSAIDs exert a potent inhibitory effect on cyclooxygenase-1 (COX-1) enzymes, hence modifying the arachidonic-acid pathway. This disturbance results in an increase in the number of eosinophils, mast cells, and proinflammatory mediators. Consequently, there is an amplified production of cysteinyl leukotrienes, a class of lipid mediators recognized for their inflammatory characteristics. Cysteinyl leukotrienes enhance vascular permeability. In laboratory investigations, it has been observed that cysteinyl leukotrienes can stimulate histamine hyper-responsiveness by upregulating expression of the histamine receptors. Overall, angioedema occurs.

BRADYKININ-MEDIATED ANGIOEDEMA

The development of bradykinin-mediated angioedema was once thought to rely on a lack of C1 inhibitor (C1-INH) and also the activation of the complement system. The suggested etiology of angioedema is attributed to a peptide known as "C2-kinin" which originates from C2. Further examination found that this peptide could not be produced from its pure elements. It was determined that the bradykinin was the sole vasoactive peptide present in plasma of individuals with hereditary angioedema (HAE). Angioedema attacks in HAE patients were confirmed to be caused by elevated levels of bradykinin, which serves as a mediator of swelling.

> The primary enzymes responsible for the production of bradykinin are activated factor XII and also plasma kallikrein. Both of these enzymes are regulated by C1-INH, which inhibits their activity.

- *C1-INH*: It possesses many roles that are pertinent to the synthesis of bradykinin, such as:
  - The suppression of plasma kallikrein, factor XIIa, and coagulation factor XIa.
  - Furthermore, it has a role in controlling the activation of complement system.
  - Without C1-INH, there is an excessive synthesis of bradykinin caused by unregulated action of these enzymes **(Fig. 1)**.
- *Factor XII*: It possesses a limited enzymatic capacity that is adequate for triggering the bradykinin-forming cascade upon contact with macromolecules that have a negative charge. Upon activation, factor XIIa has the ability to activate factor XI, thus initiating the intrinsic coagulation cascade. Additionally, it can also convert plasma prekallikrein into kallikrein which enzymatically breaks down HMWK in order to liberate bradykinin.

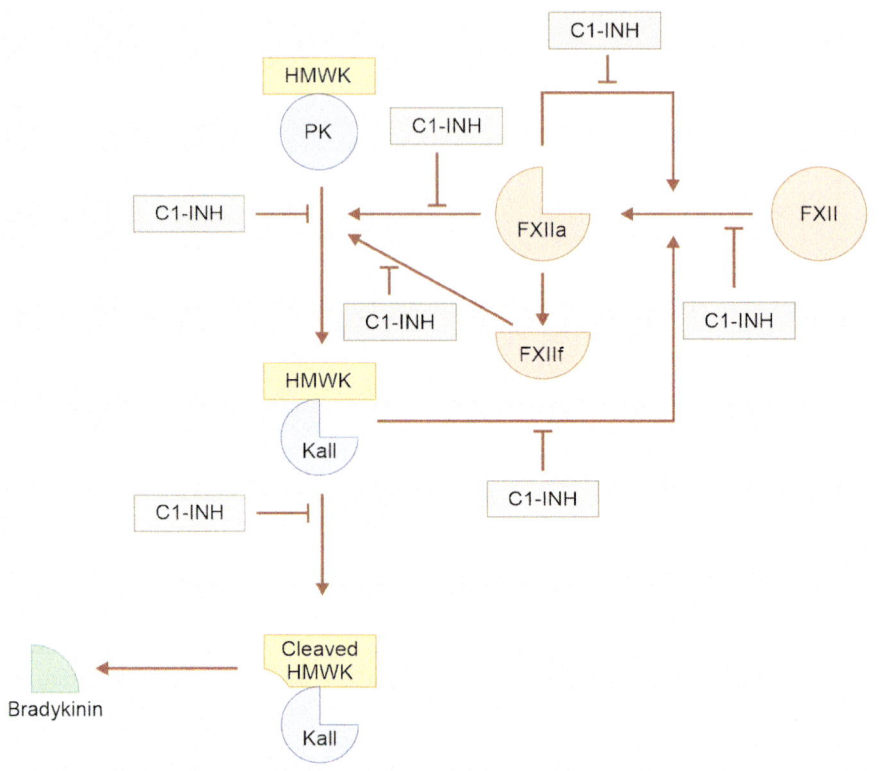

FIG. 1: Plasma kallikrein–kinin and the contact activation systems.
(C1-INH: C1 inhibitor; HMWK: high-molecular-weight kininogen; PK: prekallikrein; Kall-kallikrein)

- *Plasma kallikrein*: Positive feedback loop occurs where plasma kallikrein quickly converts the factor XII to factor XIIa, hence enhancing the activation of cascade.
- *Fibrinolytic route*: In addition, there is a fibrinolytic route where plasminogen is converted to plasmin via factor XIa, factor XIIa, and kallikrein. This route is highly significant in bradykinin-mediated angioedema, particularly HAE with normal C1-INH activity. The plasmin has the ability to cleave and activate factor XII, which in turn contributes to bradykinin forming cascade.
- *Endothelial role*: The attachment of all parts of bradykinin-producing process to the endothelial cells implies that endothelium might have a role in starting angioedema episodes. Endothelial cells secrete heat shock protein 90 (HSP-90) and prolylcarboxypeptidase, which can lead to activation of the HMWK–prekallikrein complex and can also contribute to the production of bradykinin.

The plasma kallikrein–kinin and the complement activation systems consist of a sequence of processes in which factor XII and also the plasma prekallikrein undergo autoactivation to produce the factor XIIa and plasma kallikrein, respectively. These elements can mutually stimulate one another, hence intensifying the route. In addition, XIIa generates XIIf, which has the ability to transform prekallikrein into kallikrein. The sequence of events results in the generation of the bradykinin from HMWK, which is controlled by C1 esterase inhibitor **(Fig. 1)**.

It is crucial to take into account the bradykinin-mediated angioedema as a potential alternative diagnosis. HAE and specific drug-induced angioedemas, such as angiotensin-converting enzyme (ACE) inhibitor-induced angioedema, should be evaluated as possible causes. HAE is distinguished by diminished activity of the C1-INH, which can be attributed to either a shortage (type I) or malfunction (type II) of C1-INH protein. Additionally, there are types of HAE that exhibit normal C1-INH function but are linked to abnormalities in different genes, such as factor XII.

Role of Drugs in Pathogenesis of Bradykinin-mediated Angioedema

Aside from HAE, bradykinin-mediated angioedema can also result from specific drugs, such as ACE inhibitors and dipeptidyl peptidase-4 inhibitors (gliptins). These medications inhibit degradation of the bradykinin, resulting in its buildup and the subsequent occurrence of angioedema. To distinguish between these reasons, it may be necessary to do genetic testing and assess the individual's family history.

> To summarize, the development of C1-INH deficit mainly involves unregulated activation of bradykinin-forming cascade, resulting in increased levels of the bradykinin. Factors such as plasma kallikrein, factor XII, and endothelial cell components are significant contributors to this process. Gaining a comprehensive understanding of the fundamental mechanisms behind bradykinin-mediated angioedema is essential for accurately diagnosing and effectively managing those who are affected by it.

DISTINGUISHING BRADYKININ- VERSUS HISTAMINE-MEDIATED ANGIOEDEMA: NAVIGATING SYMPTOM OVERLAP

- Distinguishing between the bradykinin-mediated angioedema and the histamine-mediated angioedema is difficult because the symptoms of the two conditions sometimes overlap. However, specific variations in clinical characteristics can help clinicians determine the accurate underlying pathophysiology.
- Pruritus, or itching, is a significant distinguishing element in histamine-mediated angioedema. It occurs when histamine excites certain histamine-sensitive unmyelinated C fibers. The bradykinin-mediated angioedema, in contrast, is usually not associated with itching.
- It is uncommon for people with histamine-mediated angioedema to experience gastrointestinal symptoms. For example, symptoms such as vomiting and diarrhea, though they can be seen especially in young children, may occur in patients with the bradykinin-mediated angioedema more often.

TABLE 1: Distinguishing features of bradykinin-mediated angioedema and histamine-mediated angioedema.

Characteristic	Bradykinin-mediated angioedema	Histamine-mediated angioedema
Presence of pruritus (itching)	Absent	Present
Gastrointestinal symptoms (e.g., vomiting, diarrhea)	May be present	Rarely present
Response to antihistamines, corticosteroids, or epinephrine	No response	Positive response
Diagnostic indicators	Elevated concentrations of the cleaved high-molecular-weight kininogen (HMWK), threshold-stimulated kallikrein activity	No specific indicators mentioned

- In addition, individuals with histamine-mediated angioedema exhibit a positive response to the treatment with antihistamines, epinephrine, or corticosteroids. However, patients with the bradykinin-mediated angioedema do not respond to these treatments.
- Distinguishing between the bradykinin-mediated angioedema and the histamine-mediated angioedema is difficult because there are no definitive and dependable diagnostic indicators available. But there are few diagnostic indicators which can help us reach a diagnosis; e.g., elevated concentrations of cleaved HMWK in blood plasma can also be used to detect type I HAE.
- Additionally, threshold-stimulated kallikrein activity tests can help distinguish between angioedemas caused by histamine and those caused by bradykinin. This investigation is of utmost importance, not only as a scholarly endeavor but also as a critical milestone in the development of efficient therapeutic and control approaches for these disorders **(Table 1)**.

CONCLUSION

- Angioedema is defined by the presence of swelling that is specifically limited to subcutaneous and also submucosal tissues. This chapter offers a comprehensive examination of angioedema, encompassing several classifications, stimuli, and fundamental pathophysiologic principles.
- Hereditary and acquired angioedema result from the deregulation of the kinin and complement pathways. On the other hand, allergic and drug-induced angioedema occur when our immune system is activated and vasoactive mediators are released.
- Advancements in comprehending the underlying mechanisms of angioedema have resulted in the creation of specific treatments, including monoclonal antibodies, complement inhibitors, and bradykinin receptor antagonists.
- These therapies show potential in enhancing the overall medical outcomes for patients with this complex condition. A thorough understanding of the complex and varied pathophysiology of angioedema is essential for accurately diagnosing and efficiently treating this condition.

SUGGESTED READINGS

1. Kanani A, Betschel SD, Warrington R. Urticaria and angioedema. Allergy Asthma Clin Immunol. 2018;14(Suppl 2):59.
2. Zuberbier T, Aberer W, Asero R, Abdul Latiff AH, Baker D, Ballmer-Weber B, et al. The EAACI/GA(2)LEN/EDF/WAO guideline for the definition, classification, diagnosis and management of urticaria. Allergy. 2018;73(7):1393-414.
3. Kaplan AP, Joseph K. Pathogenesis of hereditary angioedema: the role of the bradykinin-forming cascade. Immunol Allergy Clin North Am. 2017;37(3):513-25.
4. Zuraw BL. Clinical practice. Hereditary angioedema. N Engl J Med. 2008;359(10):1027-36.
5. James C, Bernstein JA. Current and future therapies for the treatment of histamine-induced angioedema. Expert Opin Pharmacother. 2017;18(3):253-62.

CHAPTER 4

Types of Urticaria: An Overview

Shikha Gupta, Sanjeev Gupta, Himanshu Gupta

INTRODUCTION

Urticaria is a very commonly encountered mast cell-derived disease that presents clinically with wheals or angioedema or both wheals and angioedema. The exact mechanisms by which mast cells are stimulated are still not completely understood and many theories have been postulated to explain this phenomenon, including autoimmune processes.

This condition has to be differentiated from the other disorders presenting with wheals/angioedema or both—like anaphylaxis, urticarial vasculitis, hereditary angioedema, autoinflammatory syndromes, and bullous pemphigoid to name a few.

BURDEN OF URTICARIA

Chronic urticaria affects around 1% of the global population across all ages. However, a systematic analysis has observed the burden is slightly higher among women and younger populations. It usually persists for >1 year in 25–75% of cases. More than a quarter of cases are resistant to first-line therapy (antihistamines), and among the resistant ones, one-third are not controlled adequately by any form of therapy. Chronic urticaria and angioedema have both been found to impair Dermatology Life Quality Index (DLQI) and health-related quality of life (HRQoL) independently.

DEFINITIONS

Urticaria is clinically characterized by wheals or angioedema or both. It is imperative to understand the clinical presentation of these two as they may be difficult to differentiate in certain areas with loose connective tissue such as the eyelids.

Wheal

A wheal is a well-defined, superficial cutaneous swelling that typically has the following features:
- A sharply circumscribed superficial central swelling of variable size and shape
- Generally surrounded by reflex erythema
- Accompanied usually by itching sensation or sometimes burning
- Transient, and usually within 30 minutes to 24 hours, the skin returns to its normal appearance

Wheals can be of various sizes and shapes (round/oval/arciform/annular/serpiginous) and larger wheals generally indicate a more difficult prognosis. A dark red/violaceous color usually implies an underlying cutaneous vascular damage.

Angioedema

Angioedema is characterized by the development of:
- Sudden, erythematous or skin-colored deep swelling in the lower dermis and subcutis or mucous membranes
- Symptoms include tingling, burning, feeling of tightness, and sometimes pain (rather than itch)
- Slow resolution; sometimes, angioedema takes up to 72 hours to resolve

Since the swelling is deeper, it presents in certain areas such as eyelids, lips, or tongue.

PATHOPHYSIOLOGY OF URTICARIA

- The pathophysiology of urticaria, commonly known as hives can be classified into immunologic (IgE-dependent) and nonimmunologic (non-IgE-dependent) types.
- *Immunologic urticaria* involves a type I hypersensitivity reaction where an allergen binds to IgE receptors on the surface of mast cells or basophils **(Fig. 1)**. Urticaria can also be caused by autoimmune mechanisms that activate cutaneous mast cells. The autoimmunity in CSU can be classified into two primary categories: Types I and IIb (refer to Chapter 2 for more details).
- This leads to activation and degranulation of mast cells, causing an inflammatory response and release of histamine along with other inflammatory mediators such as tumor necrosis factor alpha (TNF-α), serotonin, proteases, and proteoglycans.
- The histamine then binds to H1 receptors on smooth muscle cells, endothelial cells, and central nervous system (CNS) neurons, H1 and H4 receptors on peripheral C nerve fibers, and H2 receptors.
- This results in the triple response of Lewis, characterized by vasodilation (leading to local erythema), vasopermeability (resulting in wheals), and the axon reflex in the CNS (causing pruritus).

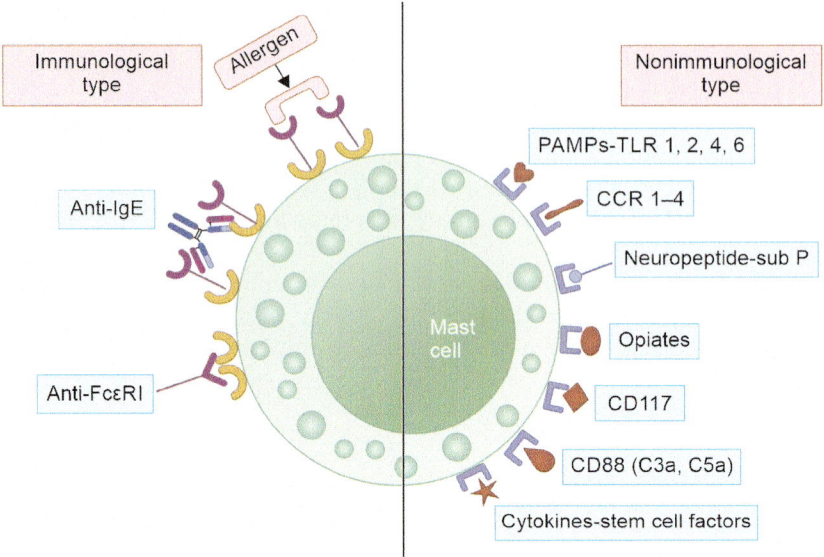

FIG. 1: Different mast cell receptors involved in immunological and nonimmunological mechanisms of urticaria.

(FcεRI: Fc epsilon RI; Ig: immunoglobulin; PAMPs: pathogen-associated molecular patterns; TLRs: toll-like receptors)

- *Nonimmunologic urticaria*, on the other hand, involves the activation of specific receptors without prior sensitization. It can be triggered by the activation of membrane receptors involved in innate immunity (e.g., complement, cytokines, chemokines), direct toxin stimulation [e.g., opiates, aspirin, nonsteroidal anti-inflammatory drugs (NSAIDs)], emotional stressors, and physical stimuli such as aquagenic (water), solar (UV, visible light), cholinergic (heat, sweating, cold) factors **(Fig. 1)**.
- Similar to immunologic urticaria, the activation of these receptors leads to the degranulation of mast cells and subsequent release of histamine and other inflammatory mediators, resulting in vasodilation and local erythema.

CLASSIFICATION OF URTICARIA

The 2022 International EAACI/GA²LEN/EuroGuiDerm/APAAACI urticaria guidelines recommend classifying urticaria **(Box 1)**.
- On the basis of duration
- On the basis of its triggers

It should be kept in mind that there occurs a varied presentation of different subtypes of urticaria. Also, two or more subtypes of urticaria can coexist in a particular patient. Therefore, let us discuss the classification of urticaria in details.

On the basis of duration:
- *Acute urticaria*: It encompasses the occurrence of wheals/angioedema or both for a duration of 6 weeks or less.

> **Box 1: Classification of urticaria on the basis of underlying triggers and duration.**
>
> *Duration:*
> - Acute urticaria (lasting <6 weeks)
> - Chronic urticaria (persisting for >6 weeks)
>
> *Underlying triggers:*
> - Spontaneous urticaria (no definite trigger is responsible for inducing symptoms)
> - Inducible urticaria (specific triggers are responsible for producing symptoms)

- *Chronic urticaria*: It can have symptoms occurring with a daily/near-daily frequency or in an intermittent/recurrent pattern. It is not uncommon in a patient of chronic spontaneous urticaria (CSU), the recurrence of symptoms after months or years of complete remission.

On the basis of underlying trigger:
- *Spontaneous urticaria* implies that there are no definite triggers consistently producing the symptoms of urticaria. Some patients can have their disease activity aggravated by some triggers; however, those triggers do not always produce symptoms and the symptoms can also occur even without their presence.
- *Inducible urticaria*: It is characterized by the definite triggers (which are specific to the subtype) producing wheals and/or angioedema. These triggers are definite as the symptoms always and never occur in the presence and absence of a trigger, respectively. For instance, pressure urticaria occurs only in response to pressure applied over the body by tight clothing or otherwise. Rarely, the combined presence of two specific triggers is required for symptom elicitation, for instance, cold-induced cholinergic urticaria. The prevalence of the inducible urticaria in the general population is around 0.5%.

Flowchart 1 describes the classification of urticaria into various subtypes.

The most commonly seen types of inducible urticaria are dermographism > cholinergic urticaria > delayed-pressure urticaria. It is important to understand the various subtypes of inducible urticaria and their triggers for appropriate management.

It is also worthwhile to note that the various subtypes of chronic inducible urticaria can be grouped as *physical urticarias* and *nonphysical urticarias* **(Box 2)**.

The *physical urticaria group* includes dermographism, delayed-pressure urticaria, exercise-induced urticaria, cold urticaria, heat urticaria, solar urticaria, and vibratory urticaria. A new term "follicular traction urticaria" also has been described in a few patients who develop follicular wheals after certain epilatory procedures such as waxing. The *nonphysical urticaria group* includes cholinergic urticaria, contact urticaria, and aquagenic urticaria.

Physical urticarias are usually more commonly encountered cases and occur in around 10–50% of chronic urticaria patients and in up to 5% of the general population. It is imperative to understand the underlying trigger for the urticarial rash by taking a thorough clinical history and performing a meticulous

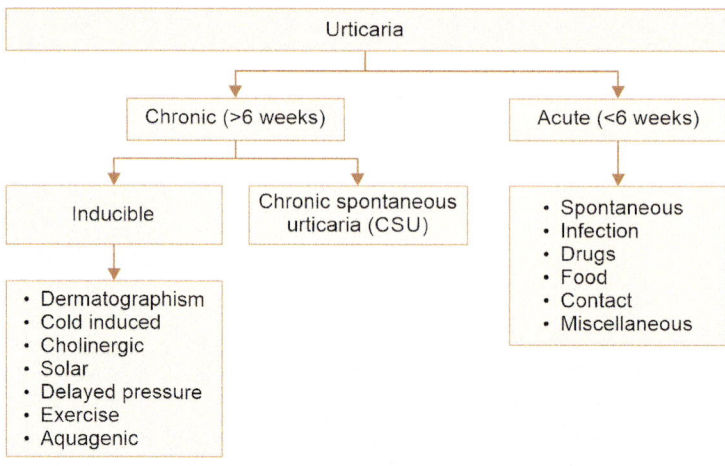

FLOWCHART 1: Classification of urticaria into various subtypes.

Box 2: Classification of chronic inducible urticaria.

Physical urticarias:
- Dermographism
- Delayed-pressure urticaria
- Exercise-induced urticaria
- Cold urticaria
- Heat urticaria
- Solar urticaria
- Vibratory urticaria

Nonphysical urticarias:
- Cholinergic urticaria
- Contact urticaria
- Aquagenic urticaria

examination of the patient, because in many cases, trigger can be avoided, at least to some extent.

Table 1 provides us an overview of various subtypes of chronic inducible urticaria.

It should be kept in mind that while diagnosing the patients presenting with wheals and/or angioedema, certain medical conditions which present similarly must be ruled out.

Some important clinical mimickers of urticaria are described in brief in the following text:
- *Urticaria pigmentosa*: Usually occurs in children; postinflammatory hyperpigmentation usually present; bullous lesions also sometimes seen
- *Urticaria vasculitis*: Wheals persist for >24 hours; Burning typically felt rather than itching; petechial spots may be present; skin biopsy diagnostic

TABLE 1: An overview of various subtypes of chronic inducible urticaria.

Type of chronic inducible urticaria	Subtype	Trigger	Clinical characteristic	Treatment
Physical urticaria	Dermographism (Simple and symptomatic)	Shear force on skin	• Wheal-and-flare response occurs within 5 minutes and fades after 30 minutes • Pruritus only in symptomatic dermographism	• Avoidance of triggers • H1 and H2 antihistamines (only in symptomatic dermographism)
	Delayed-pressure urticaria	Sustained pressure to the skin	Erythema + swelling 4–6 hours after pressure application	• Avoidance of tight clothing • Antihistamines • Dapsone • Chloroquine • Sulfasalazine • Omalizumab
	Cold urticaria	Exposure to cold objects, cold air/wind	• Wheals develop within minutes of exposure • Limited to exposed areas	• Avoid cold exposure • H1 antihistamines • Omalizumab • Danazol • Etanercept • Anakinra
	Heat urticaria	Exposure to heat	Wheals develop on exposed area only; within minutes	Antihistamines; oral cromolyn
	Solar urticaria	Exposure to sunlight (UVA, visible light)	Wheals develop within 5–10 minutes over sun-exposed areas	• H1 antihistamines • Omalizumab • Desensitization • Ciclosporine

Continued

CHAPTER 4: Types of Urticaria: An Overview

Continued

Type of chronic inducible urticaria	Subtype	Trigger	Clinical characteristic	Treatment
Physical urticaria	Exercise-induced urticaria	Exercise	Wheals are larger than those encountered in cholinergic urticaria	Antihistamines
	Vibratory urticaria	Exposure to vibration	• Usually hands are involved • Wheals occur within a few minutes, peak in 4–6 hours and resolve by 24 hours	• Avoidance of trigger • H1 antihistamines
Nonphysical urticaria	Cholinergic urticaria	Due to increased core body temperature	Numerous small, punctate wheals (1–3 mm) surrounded by large flares (which may coalesce to form large areas of erythema)	• Avoiding triggers • H1 antihistamines • Omalizumab • Anticholinergic scopolamine • Danazol
	Contact urticaria	Triggered by contact with offending agent	Wheal developing within minutes over the site of contact	• Avoidance of known trigger • H1 antihistamines
	Aquagenic urticaria	Triggered by contact with water, usually seen after bathing	• Around 1–3 mm wheals over body, especially on neck, upper trunk and arms • Within 30 minutes of exposure to water; can last upto 2 hours	• Cutting down of water-based activities • H1 antihistamines

- *Hereditary angioedema*: Only angioedema is seen; no pruritus or wheals; recurrent; bradykinin is the chief mediator
- *Autoinflammatory syndromes*: Urticarial wheals associated with recurrent episodes of fever, arthralgia/arthritis, eye inflammation, headache, elevated C-reactive protein (CRP), leukocytosis along with negative serologic tests for connective tissue diseases
- *Schnitzler's syndrome*: It is characterized by the recurrent urticarial type rash, monoclonal gammopathy, recurrent episodes of fever, arthralgia/arthritis, and lymphadenopathy; the diagnostic test is serum protein electrophoresis
- *Wells syndrome*: Eosinophilic granulomatous dermatitis/eosinophilic cellulitis
- *Bullous pemphigoid*: The precursor to bullae is often pruritus with or without urticarial wheals

CONCLUSION

It is important to understand the type and subtype of urticaria while managing the patient as the treatment options vary among different subtypes. A thorough history taking is essential to ascertain duration and any triggers responsible for development of the lesions. Triggers, if identified, need to be avoided as much as possible.

SUGGESTED READINGS

1. Zuberbier T, Abdul Latiff AH, Abuzakouk M, Latiff AHA, Baker D, Ballmer-Weber B, et al. The international EAACI/GA^{2}LEN/EuroGuiDerm/APAAACI guideline for the definition, classification, diagnosis, and management of urticaria. Allergy. 2022;77(3):734-66.
2. Gonçalo M, Gimenéz-Arnau A, Al-Ahmad M, Ben-Shoshan M, Bernstein JA, Ensina LF, et al. The global burden of chronic urticaria for the patient and society. Br J Dermatol. 2021;184(2):226-36.
3. Liu X, Cao Y, Wang W. Burden of and trends in urticaria globally, regionally, and nationally from 1990 to 2019: Systematic analysis. JMIR Public Health Surveill. 2023;9:e50114.
4. Pozderac I, Lugović-Mihić L, Artuković M, Stipić-Marković A, Kuna M, Ferček I. Chronic inducible urticaria: classification and prominent features of physical and non-physical types. Acta Dermato venerol Alp Pannonica Adriat. 2020;29(3):141-8.
5. Duman H, Topal IO, Kocaturk E. Follicular traction urticaria. A Bras Dermatol. 2016;91 (5 Suppl 1):64-5.

CHAPTER 5

Assessment Scales in Chronic Spontaneous Urticaria and Angioedema

Nidhi Sharma

INTRODUCTION

Chronic urticaria is a common and debilitating skin dermatosis. Symptoms of urticaria frequently vary greatly from day to day. The symptoms of chronic spontaneous urticaria (CSU), formerly known as chronic idiopathic urticaria (CIU), include wheals/hives, angioedema, or both, and they must persist for at least 6 weeks without a known cause. Around 0.5–1% of the general population is affected by chronic urticaria, out of which two-third cases have CSU.

Patients with chronic urticaria are highly affected by this disease in their daily activities and work, with disturbance in their sleep and emotional and psychological well-being.

Hence, one needs to establish the degree, extent, and regulation of the illness during subsequent checkups. Validated survey instruments [patient-reported outcome measures (PROMs)] include **(Table 1)**: Urticaria activity score (UAS), weekly urticaria activity score (UAS7), angioedema activity score (AAS), chronic urticaria quality of life questionnaire (CU-Q2oL), angioedema quality of life questionnaire (AE-QoL), urticaria control test (UCT), and angioedema control test (AECT). These questionnaires can be accessed in a variety of languages.

TABLE 1: Patient-reported outcome measures for assessment of disease activity/control and quality of life in chronic urticaria.

Measurement	Itch and hives	Angioedema
Disease activity	Weekly urticaria activity score (UAS7)	Angioedema activity score (AAS)
Quality of life	Chronic urticaria quality of life questionnaire (CU-Q2oL)	Angioedema quality of life questionnaire (AE-QoL)
Disease activity, quality of life, and treatment effectiveness	• Urticaria control test (UCT) • Angioedema control test (ACT)	

URTICARIA ACTIVITY SCORE/ANGIOEDEMA ACTIVITY SCORE

UAS7 can be used in clinical practice and research settings for patients of CSU developing wheals.

UAS7 is a simple unified scoring system which uses key symptoms of hives (wheals, pruritus), which are documented by patients themselves, making it particularly valuable. As urticaria activity often fluctuates, it is measured by self-evaluation by the patient recording their daily scores over several days. UAS7 is used in routine clinical practice by calculating the sum score for 7 consecutive days to assess disease severity and determine the treatment response of patients with CSU. The use of the UAS7 also makes it possible to compare results obtained from different research trial centers. For patients with CSU who develop angioedema, whether with or without wheals, it is recommended to utilize the AAS to evaluate the severity of the disease activity. When CSU patients have both wheals and angioedema, the UAS7 score should be used together with AAS. **Table 2** briefly describes UAS7 and AAS.

TABLE 2: Urticaria activity score (UAS) and angioedema activity score (AAS) for assessment of disease activity in chronic spontaneous urticaria (CSU).

UAS		
Score	Wheals	Pruritus
0	None	None
1	Mild (<20 wheals/24 hours)	Mild (present but not annoying or troublesome)
2	Moderate (20–50 wheals/24 hours)	Moderate (troublesome but does not interfere with normal daily activity or sleep)
3	Intense (>50 wheals/24 hours or large confluent areas of wheals)	Intense (severe pruritus, which is sufficiently troublesome to interfere with normal daily activity or sleep)
AAS		
Score	Dimension	Answer Options
–	Have you had a swelling episode in the last 24 hours?	No, yes
0–3	At what time(s) of day was this swelling episode(s) present? (please select all applicable times)	Midnight–8 AM, 8 AM to 4 PM, 4 PM to midnight
0–3	How severe is/was the physical discomfort caused by this swelling episode(s)? (e.g., pain, burning, itching?)	No discomfort, slight discomfort, moderate discomfort, severe discomfort
0–3	Are/were you able to perform your daily activities during this swelling episode(s)?	No restriction, slight restriction, severe restriction, no activities possible

Continued

Continued

AAS		
Score	Dimension	Answer Options
0–3	Do/did you feel your appearance is/was adversely affected by this swelling episode(s)?	No slightly, moderately, severely
0–3	How would you rate the overall severity of this swelling episode?	Negligible, mild, moderate, severe

- For the UAS7, the sum of the score (0–3 for wheals plus 0–3 for pruritus) for each day is summarized over 1 week (7 days) for a maximum of 42.
- For the AAS, scores are aggregated up to an AAS day sum score (0–15), 7 AAS day sum scores to an AAS week sum score (AAS7, 0–105), and 4 ASS week sum scores may be summed up to an AAS 4-week sum score (AAS28, 0–420).

Copyright for UAS: GA^{2}LEN; copyright for AAS (UK version): MOXIE GmbH (www.moxie-gmbh.de).

Source: Armstrong AW, Soong W, Bernstein JA. Chronic Spontaneous Urticaria: How to Measure It and the Need to Define Treatment Success. Dermatol Ther (Heidelb). 2023;13(8):1629-46.

Urticaria activity score has been regarded as a gold standard for evaluating disease activity in patients of CSU but has the following limitations:
- As it is a prospective tool, it cannot be used to measure disease activity during the patient's first visit.
- It does not cover angioedema which is frequently observed in patients of CSU.
- If a patient misses recording the values on even a single day, it becomes incomplete.
- Also, it covers only patients suffering from CSU and not CIU (e.g., dermatographism, cholinergic urticaria, etc.)
- Lastly, it does not calculate the disease control in the patient.

URTICARIA CONTROL TEST AND ANGIOEDEMA CONTROL TEST

Apart from the disease activity, we must consider how well the disease is controlled in both clinical practice and during trials. Disease control must also be assessed among patients with CSU. UCT can be used for this purpose in patients of CSU who present with wheals with or without angioedema **(Fig. 1A)**. AECT should be employed for those patients suffering from CSU experiencing episodes of angioedema either with or lacking urticarial lesions **(Fig. 1B)**. Both UCT and AECT ought to be used for individuals suffering from hives and angioedema. These tests were developed and also validated to establish the level of disease control across all forms of CU including CIU.

Urticaria control test was developed in 2014 for chronic urticaria and angioedema to measure the quality of life of patients. It incorporates four questions, each one of which evaluates the extent of impairment in the past 4 weeks, with 5 column points for answers that range from "not at all" to "very much".

The first parameter takes information about the frequency of all symptoms such as itching/hives/swelling, the second parameter asks about an overall impact on the quality of life of patient, the third question includes the effectiveness of treatment in controlling the symptoms, and the last question asks how effectively the disease has been controlled. Answers to the questions are scored from 0 to 4 (the total score will range from 0 to 16), with higher scores representing milder and better-controlled urticaria and angioedema.

However, there are few limitations of UCT too:
- It has a recall period of 4 weeks which is quite long for its practical use, as the efficacy or results of antihistamines start in a much shorter time. So, to overcome this limitation, a new version called UCT7 is recommended which has a recall period of 7 days.

Urticaria Control Test

Patient name: _____ Date: (dd mm yyyy): ___ ___ ___

Date of birth (dd mm yyyy): ___ ___ ___

Instructions: You have urticaria. The following questions should help us understand your present health situation. Please read through each question carefully and choose an answer from the five options that *best fits* your situation. Please limit yourself to the *last four weeks*. *Please don't think about the questions for a long time*, and do remember to answer *all questions* and to provide *only one answer to each question*.

1. How much have you suffered from the **physical symptoms of the urticaria [itch, hives (welts) and/or swelling]** in the last four weeks?
   O very much   O much   O somewhat   O a little   O not at all

2. How much was your **quality of life** affected by the urticaria in the last 4 weeks?
   O very much   O much   O somewhat   O a little   O not at all

3. How often was the **treatment** for your urticaria in the last 4 weeks **not enough** to control your urticaria symptoms?
   O very often   O often   O sometimes   O seldom   O not at all

4. **Overall**, how well have you had your urticaria **under control** in the last 4 weeks?
   O not at all   O a little   O somewhat   O well   O very well

A

FIGS. 1A AND B: *Continued*

Continued

**Angioedema Control Test
(AECT)**

Patient name: _____ Date: (dd mm yyyy): ____ ____ ____

Date of birth (dd mm yyyy): ____ ____ ____

Instructions: You have recurrent swelling referred to as angioedema. Angioedema is a temporary swelling of the skin or mucous membranes which can occur in any part of the body but most commonly involves the lips, eyes, tongue, hands and feet and which can last from hours to days. Some patients develop abdominal angioedema, which is often not visible but painful. Some forms of swelling can also be associated with hives also known as urticaria.

The following four questions assess your current state of health. For each question, please choose the answer from the five options that *best fits your situation*. Please answer *all questions* and please provide *only one answer to each question*.

1. In the last 4 weeks, how often have you had angioedema?
   ○ very often   ○ often   ○ sometimes   ○ seldom   ○ not at all

2. In the last 4 weeks, how much has your quality of life been affected by angioedema?
   ○ very much   ○ much   ○ somewhat   ○ a little   ○ not at all

3. In the last 4 weeks, how much has the unpredictability of your angioedema bothered you?
   ○ very much   ○ much   ○ somewhat   ○ a little   ○ not at all

4. In the last 4 weeks, how well has your angioedema been controlled by your therapy?
   ○ not at all   ○ a little   ○ somewhat   ○ well   ○ very well

B

FIGS. 1A AND B: (A) Urticaria control test (UCT); and (B) Angioedema control test (AECT).
Source: MOXIE GmbH, Berlin, Germany (www.moxie-gmbh.de).

CHRONIC URTICARIA QUALITY OF LIFE QUESTIONNAIRE/ANGIOEDEMA QUALITY OF LIFE QUESTIONNAIRE

The CU-Q2oL **(Fig. 2)** should be applied to determine QoL impairment in CSU patients with wheals. For CSU patients who have angioedema without or with wheals, AE-QoL should be used. In cases where both wheals and angioedema are seen in CSU patients, using both CU-Q2oL and AE-QoL would be appropriate.

CHAPTER 5: Assessment Scales in Chronic Spontaneous Urticaria and Angioedema

The original German version of the AE-QoL comprises 17 questions across four domains (functioning, fatigue/mood, fear/shame, and food), which collectively assess the extent of recurrent angioedema (RAE) dependent QoL impairment over the previous 4 weeks **(Fig. 3)**. Each question offers five response options scored from 1 to 5, where lower scores indicate less adverse impact and higher scores indicate more adverse effects. The total score is converted to a linear scale ranging from 0 to 100, with 100 representing the worst level of impairment in health-related quality of life (HRQoL).

Chronic Urticaria Quality of Life Questionnaire (CU-Q2oL)

In the past 14 days how much were you troubled by the following symptoms?

	Not at all	A little	Rather	A lot	Very much
1. Itching					
2. Wheals					
3. Swelling of your eyes					
4. Swelling of your lips					

Indicate how often you were limited by your hives (urticaria) in the past 14 days in the following areas of daily life

	Never	Rarely	Sometimes	Often	Very often
5. Work					
6. Physical activities					
7. Sleep					
6. Free time					
7. Sleep					
8. Free time					
9. Social relationships					
10. Eating					

In the following questions, we would like to know more about the difficulties and problems that could be related to your hives (urticaria) (regarding the past 14 days)

	Never	Rarely	Sometimes	Often	Very often
11. Do you have difficulties falling asleep?					
12. Do you wake up at night?					
13. Are you tired during the day because you did not sleep well at night?					
14. Do you have difficulties concentrating?					
15. Do you feel nervous?					
16. Do you feel miserable?					
17. Do you have to limit your food choices?					
18. Are you bothered by the symptoms of hives (urticaria) that appear on your body?					
19. Are you embarrassed to go to public places?					
20. Is it a problem for you to use cosmetics (e.g. perfumes, creams, lotions, bubblebath, make up)?					
21. Do you have to limit your clothing choices?					
22. Are your sports activities limited because of your hives (urticaria)?					
23. Do you suffer side-effects from the medications you take for hives (urticaria)?					

FIG. 2: The CU-Q2oL.

Source: MOXIE GmbH, Berlin, Germany (www.moxie-gmbh.de).

AE-QoL
Quality of Life Questionnaire for Patients with Recurrent Swelling Episodes

Patient name: _____

Date questionnaire completed (dd mm yyyy): _____ _____ _____

Instructions: This questionnaire asks a number of questions. Please read each question carefully and choose from the five answers the one that fits best for you. Please do not think too long about the questions; be sure to answer all of the questions and to give only one answer to each question, i.e., to check only one box for each question.

Indicate how often within the **last 4 weeks** you have been restricted in the areas of your daily life listed below because of swelling episodes (angioedema). (regardless of whether or not you have actually experienced swelling episodes during that time period)	Never	Rarely	Occasionally	Often	Very often
1. Work	☐	☐	☐	☐	☐
2. Physical activity	☐	☐	☐	☐	☐
3. Leisure time	☐	☐	☐	☐	☐
4. Social relations	☐	☐	☐	☐	☐
5. Eating and drinking	☐	☐	☐	☐	☐
In the following questions we would like to get more details about the difficulties and problems that may be associated with your recurrent swelling episodes (angioedema) (during the **last 4 weeks**)	Never	Rarely	Occasionally	Often	Very often
6. Do you have difficulty falling asleep?	☐	☐	☐	☐	☐
7. Do you wake up during the night?	☐	☐	☐	☐	☐
8. Are you tired during the day because you are not sleeping well at night?	☐	☐	☐	☐	☐
9. Do you have trouble concentrating?	☐	☐	☐	☐	☐

A

FIGS. 3A AND B: *Continued*

Continued

In the following questions we would like to get more details about the difficulties and problems that may be associated with your recurrent swelling episodes (angioedema) (during the last 4 weeks)	Never	Rarely	Occasionally	Often	Very often
10. Do you feel depressed?	☐	☐	☐	☐	☐
11. Do you have to limit your choices of food or beverages?	☐	☐	☐	☐	☐
12. Do the swelling episodes place a burden on you?	☐	☐	☐	☐	☐
13. Are you afraid that a swelling episode could occur suddenly?	☐	☐	☐	☐	☐
14. Are you afraid that the frequency of the swelling episodes might increase?	☐	☐	☐	☐	☐
15. Are you ashamed to go out in public because of the swelling episodes?	☐	☐	☐	☐	☐
16. Do the swelling episodes make you embarrassed or self-conscious?	☐	☐	☐	☐	☐
17. Are you afraid that the treatment of the swelling episodes could have negative long-term effects for you?	☐	☐	☐	☐	☐

B

FIGS. 3A AND B: The AE-Q2oL.

Source: MOXIE GmbH, Berlin, Germany (www.moxie-gmbh.de).

CONCLUSION

PROMs are extensive and are mainly used for detailed research assessment. However, in the absence of clinical biomarkers in allergic and inflammatory diseases like chronic spontaneous urticaria and angioedema, the routine use of PROMs in clinical practice may play an important role in measuring the minimally important difference (MID) in a patient's disease activity, severity, and response to therapy.

SUGGESTED READINGS

1. Ghadersohi S, Price CPE, Jensen SE, Beaumont JL, Kern RC, Conley DB, et al. Development and preliminary validation of a new patient-reported outcome measure for chronic rhinosinusitis (CRS-PRO). J Allergy Clin Immunol Pract. 2020;8:2341-50.
2. Weller K, Zuberbier T, Maurer M. Clinically relevant outcome measures for assessing disease activity, disease control and quality of life impairment in patients with chronic spontaneous urticaria and recurrent angioedema. Curr Opin Allergy Clin Immunol. 2015;15(3):220-6.

3. Mlynek A, Zalewska-Janowska A, Martus P, Staubach P, Zuberbier T, Maurer M. How to assess disease activity in patients with chronic urticaria? Allergy. 2008;63(6):777-80.
4. Zuberbier T, Latiff AHA, Abuzakouk M, Aquilina S, Asero R, Baker D, et al. The international EAACI/GA^{2}LEN/EuroGuiDerm/APAAACI guideline for the definition, classification, diagnosis, and management of urticaria. Allergy. 2022;77(3):734-66.
5. Maurer M, Eyerich K, Eyerich S, Ferrer M, Gutermuth J, Hartmann K, et al. Urticaria: Collegium Internationale Allergologicum (CIA) update 2020. Int Arch Allergy Immunol. 2020;181(5): 321-33.
6. Hawro T, Ohanyan T, Schoepke N, Metz M, Peveling-Oberhag A, Staubach P, et al. Comparison and interpretability of the available urticaria activity scores. Allergy. 2017;73(1):251-5.
7. Weller KG, Magerl M, Tohme M, Martus P, Krause K, Metz M, et al. Development, validation and initial results of the angioedema activity score. Allergy. 2013;68(9):1185-92.
8. Weller K, Donoso T, Magerl M, Aygören-Pürsün E, Staubach P, Martinez-Saguer I, et al. Validation of the Angioedema Control Test (AECT)-A Patient-Reported Outcome Instrument for Assessing Angioedema Control. J Allergy Clin Immunol Pract. 2020;8(6):2050-7.
9. Avila PC. Patient-reported outcome measures for urticaria and angioedema. J Allergy Clin Immunol 2023;152:1090-1.
10. Baiardini I, Pasquali M, Braido F, Fumagalli F, Guerra L, Compalati E, et al. A new tool to evaluate the impact of chronic urticaria on quality of life: chronic urticaria quality of life questionnaire (CU-QoL). Allergy. 2005;60:1073-8.
11. Weller K, Magerl M, Peveling-Oberhag A, Martus P, Staunch P, Maurer M. The Angioedema Quality of Life Questionnaire (AE-QoL) - assessment of sensitivity to change and minimal clinically important difference. Allergy. 2016;71(8):1203-9.

CHAPTER 6

Acute Urticaria

Shikha Gupta, Himanshu Gupta

INTRODUCTION

Urticaria is a condition characterized clinically by the development of wheals (hives), angioedema, or both. It can be classified as acute or chronic on the basis of its duration. When urticarial lesions occur for <6 weeks, the disease is termed as *acute urticaria*. Clinically, *wheals* are evanescent, edematous, erythematous papules or plaques, which are associated with marked itching. On the other hand, *angioedema* is characterized by edematous, nonpitting swelling over the face, larynx, and genitalia and may be associated with burning/tightness or sometimes pain. **Table 1** enlists clinical features differentiating these two entities.

It is important to differentiate acute urticaria from *anaphylaxis*, which is potentially life-threatening. When wheals and/or angioedema are associated with systemic symptoms, like cough, wheezing, vomiting, diarrhea, dizziness, fainting, and changes in blood pressure or heart rate, it points toward anaphylaxis. If it is not possible to rule out anaphylaxis, epinephrine should be administered.

Acute urticaria is usually caused by mast cell and basophil activation, from various triggers which include both IgE-mediated and non-IgE-mediated mechanisms. This condition is commonly seen across all age groups. Probably, since it is characterized by transient wheals, it remains an underdiagnosed entity.

TABLE 1: Clinical differences between wheal and angioedema.

Wheal	Angioedema
Superficial swelling, so sharply circumscribed	Deep swelling, so less well-defined
Usually surrounded by erythema	May be skin-colored or erythematous
Itching/burning sensation +	Tingling/burning/tightness/pain
Fleeting, so resolves within 30 minutes to 24 hours	May persist up to 72 hours

DEFINITION

According to the latest GA²LEN/EDF/EAACI/WAO (Global Allergy and Asthma European Network/European Dermatology Forum/European Academy of Allergology and Clinical Immunology/World Allergy Organization) guidelines published in 2023, acute urticaria is defined as the occurrence of wheals, angioedema, or both, for 6 weeks or less. It may be spontaneous or inducible.

Inducible urticaria implies that wheals/angioedema/both have certain specific triggers for their development. The causal relationship between triggers and the onset of clinical features is definite, in the sense that the lesions occur only after trigger exposure and do not occur otherwise. Cold urticaria and drug-induced urticaria are a few examples. Rarely, the combined presence of two specific triggers is required for producing clinical features, for instance, cold-induced cholinergic urticaria. On the other hand, *spontaneous urticaria* occurs without any specific triggers.

PREVALENCE

Acute urticaria is commonly seen among adults and children. In fact, it is one of the most common dermatological conditions encountered in emergency departments. It has been found that 12–22% of the population suffers from at least one subtype of urticaria at some point with the prevalence of 0.11–0.6%. The females are slightly more affected (60%) in some studies.

In children < 2 years presenting with urticaria, 85% had acute urticaria. In older children, the distribution of acute and chronic urticaria is similar to that seen in adults.

CAUSES

Acute urticaria has been found to be *idiopathic* in 30–50% of cases. In rest of the cases, it may be triggered by drugs, infections, or food. **Box 1** enlists the commonly encountered causes of acute urticaria.

It is important to note that in children, *infections*, particularly respiratory infections, are the leading cause of acute urticaria (40–50%). Among the viral infections, Epstein–Barr virus (EBV), herpes simplex virus (HSV), and hepatitis virus are more commonly seen to be causative. This may also explain the seasonal incidence of acute urticaria cases in children. Furthermore, streptococcal infection is also responsible for around 15–20% of cases of acute urticaria in children.

Drugs are frequently encountered cause of acute urticaria, particularly in elderly patients. In fact, the most commonly seen manifestation (10–15%) of drug-induced rash is urticaria/angioedema. Among drugs, penicillin, cephalosporins, and nonsteroidal anti-inflammatory drugs (NSAIDs) are commonly found associated with acute urticaria. Drug reactions also may lead to anaphylaxis. It is also difficult to ascertain whether urticaria is triggered by the infection itself or the drug/antibiotic used to treat it. In many cases, especially in children, the

> **Box 1: Causes of acute urticaria.**
>
> *Viral infections:*
> - Adenovirus
> - EBV, CMV
> - Hepatitis A,B,C
> - HSV
> - Influenza virus
> - VZV
> - SARS-CoV-2
>
> *Bacterial infections:*
> - Hemophilus influenzae
> - Group A beta-hemolytic *Streptococcus*
> - *Staphylococcus aureus*
>
> *Drugs:*
> - ACE Inhibitors
> - Aspirin, other NSAIDs
> - Cephalosporins, beta-lactams
> - Isotretinoin
> - Paracetamol
>
> - Vaccination
> - Blood products
>
> *Food products:*
> - Cow milk
> - Egg
> - Fish and seafood
> - Nuts
> - Fruits—banana, peach
> - Vegetables—tomato
> - Wheat
>
> *Others:*
> - Idiopathic
> - Scabies
> - *Mycoplasma*
> - Malaria
> - Insect bites/stings
> - Latex
> - Cow urine (Gomutra) gargle
>
> (ACE: angiotensin-converting enzyme; CMV: cytomegalovirus; EBV: Epstein–Barr virus; HSV: herpes simplex virus; NSAIDs: nonsteroidal anti-inflammatory drugs; VZV: varicella zoster virus; SARS-CoV-2: severe acute respiratory syndrome coronavirus 2)

trigger is not the antibiotic per se, but the excipients present in the drug solution. However, it is important to note that drug reactions are urticarial more commonly in children than adults.

Food has been associated with 0–18% of acute urticaria in various studies in children as well as adults. In cases of children < 6 months, cow's milk allergy may be important. Food urticaria generally occurs either immediately or within 60 minutes of food intake. Skin prick test and specific IgE test may not be useful because of direct histamine release by some foods such as tomato, cheese, strawberry, and lobster, which is non-IgE mediated. It is important to note that to avoid dietary deficiency, blanket restriction of food items is not advised, especially in children.

Immunological Mechanisms

There are multiple underlying mechanisms that lead to acute urticaria. Despite being quite common, the pathomechanisms of mast cell degranulation in acute urticaria are underexplored. The following pathways are usually involved in mast cell degranulation, leading to development of acute urticaria:
- *Type 1 hypersensitivity reaction*: These reactions involve interactions between allergens and preexisting IgE antibodies already bound to high-affinity receptors (FcεRI) located on mast cells and basophils. This results

in activation and degranulation of these cells releasing inflammatory mediators such as histamine. Thus, the wheals and other symptoms of allergy are swiftly produced by the trigger, which may be a certain food (peanuts or tomatoes), medication such as antibiotics, latex, insect stings, and so on.
- *NSAID-induced urticaria and angioedema*: NSAIDs can produce acute urticaria and/or angioedema by different mechanisms including IgE-mediated pathways, T-cell mediated reactions or inhibition of COX-1-producing inhibition of prostaglandin synthesis and increase in leukotriene levels. It is also hypothesized that there may be a genetic susceptibility to develop sensitivity to aspirin in patients. The reason for this assumption is that there have been various genetic polymorphisms identified in genes of enzymes metabolizing aspirin, like *TBXA2R* (*thromboxane receptor A2* gene) and in genes involved in arachidonic acid pathway. Also, promoter polymorphisms in genes, such as tumor necrosis factor-alpha (TNFα), interleukin-10 (IL-10), and IL-18 have been found in aspirin sensitivity.
- *Acute contact urticaria*: Acute contact urticaria can develop after direct contact with allergen, with or without prior sensitization, for instance, contact with stinging nettle can trigger acute urticaria without prior sensitization.

CLINICAL FEATURES

Wheals are itchy and are variable in size, number and extent of body surface area involved. More than 50% of the body may also be involved. Along with wheals, angioedema may or may not be present. It is seen in around 15–30% of acute urticaria cases.

Dermographism may be reproduced by stroking an area with a blunt object with development of wheal and erythema around 5–15 minutes later. Simple dermographism can also be seen in 5% of normal population.

Systemic symptoms are seen in 15–25% patients and include wheezing, breathlessness, nasal discharge, dizziness, flushing, gut symptoms (nausea/vomiting, diarrhea, and pain abdomen), tachycardia, fever, and joint pains. It is important to note that these symptoms may be indicative of anaphylaxis, especially if they are rapid in onset.

DIAGNOSIS

The diagnosis of acute urticaria is established in the presence of episodes of transient wheals, lasting for <24 hours, with or without accompanying angioedema and does not require any diagnostic workup routinely since this condition self-resolves in most cases.

The only indications of skin prick tests or radioallergosorbent tests (RAST) include cases where type 1 food allergy or drug hypersensitivity is suspected.

The following steps describe clinical assessment in detail.

Step 1: History-taking

The first step in the diagnosis of any urticaria patient is detailed history-taking. History-taking should include eliciting the following information:
- Duration of disease
- Type of lesions, shape/size, and distribution of lesions, symptoms with lesions including pain/itching or burning, frequency of occurrence of wheals
- Associated angioedema (swelling around eyes, lips, difficulty breathing/hoarseness of voice)
- Family or personal history of urticaria
- Any previous or current allergies, infections and systemic diseases
- History of drug intake (NSAIDs, homeopathic/ayurvedic medicines, immunization) or insect bite
- Any relationship of disease severity with sun exposure/exercise/cold/pressure/vibration/menstrual cycle/food (milk, eggs, nuts, or fish)
- Previous treatment and its response
- Impact on quality of life (QOL)

Step 2: Physical Examination

The next step is a thorough physical examination. Vital signs (pulse, heart, and respiratory rates, and blood pressure) should be recorded.

On cutaneous examination, it is important to differentiate wheals from angioedema, which can be very difficult in area around the eyes. It is also important to look for residual purpura to exclude urticarial vasculitis.

Step 3: Ruling Out Other Differentials

Urticaria needs to be differentiated from other medical conditions where wheals, angioedema, or both can occur as clinical features, for instance, *anaphylaxis* (characterized by dyspnea, wheals, swelling, abdominal cramps, nausea, diarrhea, tachycardia, hypotension, dizziness), *autoinflammatory syndromes* (history of fever and joint pains positive), *urticarial vasculitis* (characterized by burning rather than itching, purpuric lesions lasting more than 24 hours), or bradykinin-mediated angioedema including *hereditary angioedema (HAE)* (recurrent episodes of angioedema without wheals or itching).

HISTOPATHOLOGY

Most cases of acute urticaria are diagnosed clinically; however, rarely one has to resort to taking skin biopsy in order to differentiate from urticarial vasculitis and other differentials.

Urticaria is characterized by a mixed cellular perivascular infiltrate and acute urticaria has abundance of neutrophils. Angioedema is characterized by inflammation in the reticular dermis and subcutaneous tissue. Vascular damage is not seen and if present, indicates toward urticarial vasculitis.

ASSESSMENT OF DISEASE ACTIVITY

Patient should ideally be assessed for disease activity and impact on day-to-day life on first visit as well as on each subsequent visit. There are a few validated patient-reported outcome measures (PROMs) for this purpose including the Urticaria Activity Score (UAS), angioedema activity score (AAS), weekly activity score (UAS7), urticaria control test (UCT), angioedema control test (AECT) and angioedema quality of life questionnaire (AE-QoL). These PROMs have been validated in various languages and are widely available for use. **Tables 2 and 3** delineate the UAS and AAS, respectively in brief.

MANAGEMENT

- *Basic goal of therapy*: Complete symptom control should be aimed for managing acute urticaria patients, keeping in mind safety profile of drugs and QoL of the patient. The patient should also be made aware of the nature of this condition and possible risk, if any, of anaphylaxis and should be explained the steps to follow in case the condition deteriorates.

  If anaphylaxis is suspected, then the patient requires intramuscular epinephrine, intravenous antihistamines, intravenous corticosteroids, oxygen support, fluid replacement, and salbutamol according to the examination findings.

- *Establishing and eliminating underlying causes*: It is imperative to establish any underlying cause, if present, by a thorough history and physical examination.
  - *Drugs*: It is essential to discontinue the causative drugs and substitute with another class preferably.
  - *Infections*: If a patient presents with sore throat, testing for *Streptococcus* or *Mycoplasma* and treating accordingly with an antibiotic is necessary.
  - *Food*: Avoiding a food item which has been repeatedly shown to trigger episodes of acute urticaria is helpful in cases of food allergy.
- *Pharmacological treatment*: The guidelines on urticaria available in literature including the recent 2021 international EAACI/GA²LEN/EuroGuiDerm/

TABLE 2: Urticaria activity score (UAS).

Score	Wheals in past 24 hours	Pruritus
0	None	None
1	Mild (<20)	Mild (not troublesome)
2	Moderate (20–50)	Moderate (troublesome but no effect on sleep or daily activity)
3	Intense (>50 or large confluent areas of wheals)	Severe (interferes with sleep or daily activity)

UAS7 score: Measures the disease activity during past 1 week. The sum of scores of wheals and pruritus for each day is obtained for past 7 days and added to obtain the UAS7 score (maximum 42).

TABLE 3: Angioedema activity score (AAS).		
Score	Dimension/Question	Answer options
–	Swelling episode in past 24 hours?	Yes, No
0–3	At what time(s), swelling episodes present?	Midnight to 8 AM, 8 AM to 4 PM, 4 PM to midnight
0–3	How severe was physical discomfort with swelling (pain/itching/burning, etc.)?	No discomfort, slight discomfort, moderate discomfort, severe discomfort
0–3	Were you able to perform daily activities during this swelling episode(s)?	No restriction, slight restriction, severe restriction, no activities possible
0–3	Do you feel your appearance is adversely affected by this swelling episode(s)?	No, slightly, moderately, severely
0–3	How would you rate the overall severity of this swelling episode?	Negligible, mild, moderate, severe

AAS score: The AAS day sum score can range from 0 to 15 and provides an idea about the severity and discomfort experienced by the patient.

AAS7 score/AAS week sum score: The AAS7 score can be calculated by adding each day score for a week. It can range from 0 to 105.

APAAACI (Asia Pacific Association of Allergy, Asthma, and Clinical Immunology) guideline are focused more on chronic urticaria, probably because acute urticaria is self-resolving in many patients, especially after elimination of the underlying trigger. Let us now discuss the systemic therapy in detail.

First-line Treatment

H1 Receptor Antagonists

The first step in the management of acute urticaria involves administering H1 receptor antagonists, which cause improvement in majority of patients. The low-sedating second-generation antihistamines such as levocetirizine, desloratadine, and fexofenadine are preferred because of fewer central nervous system (CNS) side effects such as dizziness and sedation than the first-generation antihistamines. The reason is lesser penetration of the blood–brain barrier by the former. It has also been observed that levocetirizine and loratadine possess anti-inflammatory properties too in therapeutic dose by interfering with mast cell release of cytokines, thus potentially producing better results than sedating antihistamines.

The treatment is usually started with once-a-day therapy with low-sedating antihistamine such as levocetirizine or loratadine.

In case the symptoms are not improving within 2 days, updosing of antihistamines (to up to two to four times the initial dose) and/or prescribing sedating antihistamines (first-generation), such as hydroxyzine is recommended. The sedating antihistamine is started in low dose and at night to minimize sedation. Patient's age and job requirements must be taken into consideration while prescribing a sedating antihistamine, for instance, they should be used judiciously in an elderly patient or a person who drives for long hours. Infrequently, an H2 receptor antagonist such as montelukast may be added to obtain symptom control.

The treatment goal is complete suppression of symptoms. *It is important to note that the antihistamine therapy should be administered daily to prevent the formation of new wheals/angioedema*, rather than on SOS basis. The reason is that these antihistamines have an inverse agonist effect on H1 receptor and thus stabilize its inactive state. Furthermore, safety data for most antihistamines is available for continuous use over many years. Therefore, an antihistamine regimen, which controls symptoms effectively, is continued for 4 weeks and then gradually tapered off and discontinued.

Second-line Treatment

The second-line and third-line treatment algorithms in various guidelines on urticaria specifically pertain to chronic spontaneous urticaria (CSU) patients patients. There is a paucity of literature exploring the use of other modalities of treatment in acute urticaria not responding to antihistamines, probably because most antihistamine-nonresponder cases respond to short-term therapy with corticosteroids.

Systemic Corticosteroids

Oral corticosteroids (prednisolone 1 mg/kg/day) are indicated in severe episodes of urticaria for a short period (3–5 days), especially if symptoms do not fade in 2 days despite treatment or are accompanied by angioedema or in the presence of prominent systemic symptoms. It is advised to avoid prolonged use of systemic corticosteroids. If patient is at a high risk to develop anaphylaxis, he/she should be asked to keep epinephrine autoinjectors beforehand.

Omalizumab

Although omalizumab has been extensively studied in CSU patients, there is a relative paucity of literature exploring its use in acute urticaria. The drug has been licensed for use in patients of CSU not responding to antihistamines. Therefore, the recent EAACI/GA^{2}LEN/EuroGuiDerm/APAAACI guidelines put omalizumab as the next step of treatment when a CSU patient is not responding to antihistamines. The recommended dose in such a patient is 300 mg subcutaneously every 4 weeks.

There are few case reports of use of this drug in acute urticaria not responding to antihistamines with good results.

CONCLUSION

Acute urticaria usually has good prognosis, especially if the underlying cause is treated/eliminated. It is a self-limiting condition, which usually resolves in <6 weeks, though usually, it resolves in 2–3 weeks only. Around 25% of cases last >6 weeks and then identified as chronic.

The condition may recur, especially if the underlying causes are not eliminated. According to a study, 20–30% of children can develop chronic or recurrent episodes in 2 years. There are not many studies exploring the rates of conversion of acute urticaria into chronic urticaria.

It is important to note that in certain patients, it may be accompanied by acute angioedema, which implies a rare risk of severe airway obstruction.

The mainstay of treatment is with second-generation antihistamines, and the dose increased to 2–4 times if there is an inadequate response.

SUGGESTED READINGS

1. Zuberbier T, Abdul Latiff AH, Abuzakouk M, Aquilina S, Asero R, Baker D, et al. The international EAACI/GA²LEN/EuroGuiDerm/APAAACI guideline for the definition, classification, diagnosis, and management of urticaria. Allergy. 2022;77(3):734-66.
2. Schaefer P. Acute and chronic urticaria: Evaluation and treatment. Am Fam Physician. 2017;95(11):717-24.
3. Sabroe RA. Acute urticaria. Immunol Allergy Clin North Am. 2014;34(1):11-21.
4. Huang SW. Acute urticaria in children. Pediatr Neonatol. 2009;50(3):85-7.
5. Wang S, Chen X, Bai J, Sun Q, Qiao J, Fang H. Omalizumab for the treatment of refractory acute urticaria. Am J Ther. 2024;31(4):e487-e9.

CHAPTER
7

Angioedema

Rohit Batra, Anushruti Aggarwal, Sanjeev Gupta

INTRODUCTION

Angioedema is swelling of the deep dermis, subcutaneous, or submucosal tissue due to vascular leakage. Acute episodes often involve the lip, eyes, and face; however, angioedema may affect other body parts, including respiratory and gastrointestinal (GI) mucosa. This condition can be acute or chronic and life-threatening if it involves the airway. Unlike urticaria, which affects the superficial dermis, angioedema involves the deeper dermis and subcutaneous tissues, leading to more pronounced swelling.

HISTORICAL PERSPECTIVE

The term "angioedema" was coined by Heinrich Quincke in 1882, who described cases of recurrent, nonpitting edema of the skin and mucous membranes.

EPIDEMIOLOGY

While hereditary angioedema (HAE) is a rare genetic disorder, the more commonly seen subtypes are acquired and drug-induced forms. Angioedema can occur at any age, but hereditary forms often present in childhood or adolescence. Also, HAE is reported to be more common in females.

PATHOPHYSIOLOGY

Angioedema is due to a sudden increase in local vascular permeability in subcutaneous or submucosal tissue. Histamine and bradykinin are the most commonly involved vasoactive mediators. Bradykinin-mediated angioedema is primarily seen in hereditary and angiotensin-converting enzyme (ACE) inhibitor-induced forms, while histamine-mediated angioedema is typically related to allergic reactions. Other mechanisms, including prostaglandins, leukotrienes, and the complement system, also play a role in certain types of

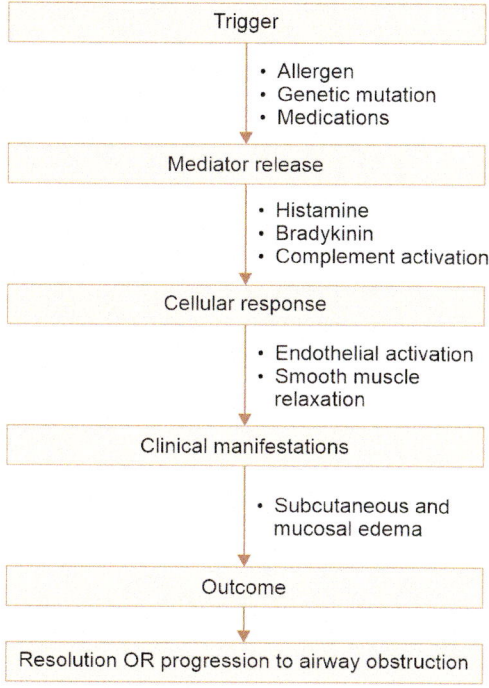

FLOWCHART 1: Pathophysiology of angioedema.

angioedema. Understanding these mechanisms is crucial for effective diagnosis and management **(Flowchart 1)**. Let us discuss these mechanisms one by one.

Mast Cell-mediated Angioedema

Mast cell-mediated angioedema is usually associated with allergic reactions where histamine is released from mast cells and basophils in response to an allergen, leading to vasodilation and increased vascular permeability. It is the most common type of angioedema. Stress can be a trigger for this type.

Bradykinin-mediated Angioedema

Bradykinin-mediated angioedema results from the excessive production or impaired degradation of bradykinin, a potent vasodilator. Bradykinin increases vascular permeability and leads to fluid leakage into surrounding tissues, causing swelling. C1-inhibitor is a regulator of the complement pathway. If there is a deficiency of the C1-inhibitor, it leads to uncontrolled production of kallikrein leading to proteolysis of high molecular weight kininogen and bradykinin, leading to edema by increased vascular permeability.

Hereditary Angioedema

Hereditary angioedema is a genetic disorder characterized by recurrent episodes of severe swelling. It is further classified into three types. Type I HAE is due to a deficiency in C1 inhibitor (C1-INH), a protein that regulates the complement and contact systems. The mutated gene is the *SERPING1* gene. In type 2 HAE, the C1-INH levels are normal or elevated but the protein secreted is dysfunctional. Type 3 HAE often affects women and is influenced by estrogen levels. It is associated with mutations in the *F12* gene, which affects the factor XII protein involved in the production of bradykinin.

Acquired Angioedema

Acquired angioedema (AAE) develops later in life, often associated with other conditions. Type I is due to consumption of C1-INH by autoantibodies or associated with malignancies such as lymphoproliferative disorders. Type II AAE is associated with the production of autoantibodies against C1-INH.

Drug-induced Angioedema

Angioedema can be triggered by medications, particularly those affecting the bradykinin pathway.
- *ACE inhibitors*: They reduce the breakdown of bradykinin and blood and tissue levels of bradykinin rise. It presents with swelling of eyelids, lips, tongue, and airway can also be involved.
- *Nonsteroidal anti-inflammatory drugs* (*NSAIDs*): They can trigger angioedema through various mechanisms, including shifting the arachidonic acid pathway toward leukotriene production, which can cause mast cell degranulation. Angioedema typically involves the face, lips, and eyelids, often with urticaria.

Idiopathic Angioedema

Angioedema is said to be idiopathic only after ruling out all other causes by thorough evaluation. No allergic etiology is present, complement levels are normal and family history is mostly absent. It presents with recurrent episodes of angioedema without identifiable triggers.

Other Mechanisms

Other less common mechanisms include involvement of the prostaglandins, leukotrienes, and complement pathway. Prostaglandins and leukotrienes can increase vascular permeability and contribute to angioedema. Activation of the complement pathway can lead to the release of anaphylatoxins (C3a, C5a) that increase vascular permeability. Research shows that complement activation can play a role in some cases of idiopathic and autoimmune-related angioedema.

CLINICAL PRESENTATION OF ANGIOEDEMA

The hallmark of angioedema is localized swelling of the deeper dermis and subcutaneous tissue. Episodes of swelling usually develop over minutes to hours and can last for 24-72 hours. The clinical presentation can vary depending on the type and underlying cause of the angioedema.

Specific Clinical Features by Type of Angioedema

- *HAE*:
  - Recurrent episodes of swelling involving the skin and mucous membrane, occur often without an identifiable trigger. Gastrointestinal symptoms such as abdominal pain, nausea, vomiting, and diarrhea may be associated due to swelling of the intestinal walls.
  - Laryngeal edema can occur causing potentially life-threatening airway obstruction. Episodes may occur spontaneously or be triggered by trauma, stress, hormonal changes, or certain medications.
- *AAE*: It involves recurrent episodes affecting the skin, gastrointestinal tract, and respiratory system. It can be associated with autoimmune disorders or lymphoproliferative diseases. Age of onset is late as compared to hereditary angioedema.
- *Drug-induced angioedema*:
  - *ACE inhibitors*: Swelling typically affects the face, lips, tongue, and airway. It can occur at any time during treatment, even after years of use of the drug. Prompt recognition is important.
  - *NSAIDs*: Swelling may be associated with urticaria and often involves the face, lips, and extremities.
  - *Clinical course*: Symptoms usually resolve upon discontinuation of the offending drug. Treatment with epinephrine, antihistamines, or corticosteroids might be required in the management of drug-induced angioedema.
- *Idiopathic angioedema*:
  - *Presentation*: Recurrent episodes of angioedema without a known cause. Affected areas include the face, extremities, and genitals.
  - *Duration*: Episodes can vary in frequency and severity, often lasting for several days.
- *Allergic angioedema*:
  - *Symptoms*: Often occur with urticarial and can be triggered by allergens such as foods, insect stings, medications, and environmental factors.
  - In severe cases, it can be part of an anaphylactic reaction, characterized by systemic symptoms such as hypotension, bronchospasm, and shock.
  - *Management*: Immediate treatment with antihistamines, corticosteroids, and epinephrine is essential.

Special Considerations

As with other disorders, management of angioedema needs specific considerations in special groups like children, pregnancy, and elderly.
- *Pediatric angioedema:*
  - Clinical features are similar as in adult angioedema.
  - Infections, vaccinations, and trauma are common triggers in children.
  - Avoiding known triggers and close monitoring during episodes is required.

- *Angioedema in pregnancy:*
  - *Hormonal influence:* Pregnancy can exacerbate hereditary angioedema due to hormonal changes.
  - *Treatment considerations:* Certain treatments may be contraindicated during pregnancy, necessitating careful management.
- *Angioedema in the elderly*:
  - *Age-related factors*: Comorbidities and polypharmacy can complicate diagnosis and management.
  - *Presentation*: Similar to younger adults, but with increased risk of drug-induced angioedema.

Comparison of Types of Angioedema
See **Table 1**.

Differential Diagnosis of Angioedema
See **Table 2**.

TABLE 1: Types of angioedema.

Type	Cause	Clinical features	Laboratory findings	Treatment
Allergic angioedema	Allergens (food, drugs, insect stings)	Urticaria, rapid onset swelling	Normal C4, elevated tryptase	Antihistamines, corticosteroids, epinephrine
Hereditary angioedema	Genetic mutation (C1-INH deficiency)	Recurrent, non-pruritic swelling, no urticaria	Low C4, low C1-INH levels	C1-INH replacement, bradykinin inhibitors
Angiotensin-converting enzyme (ACE) inhibitor-induced	ACE inhibitors	Facial swelling, no urticaria	Normal C4, normal C1-INH	Discontinuation of ACE inhibitor, bradykinin inhibitors
Idiopathic	Unknown	Recurrent, episodic swelling	Normal C4, normal C1-INH, normal tryptase	Antihistamines, corticosteroids

TABLE 2: Differential diagnosis of angioedema.

Condition	Morphology of lesion	Distinguishing features
Angioedema	Swelling without redness, affects deep layers	Often asymmetric, can involve airway
Urticaria	Raised, red, itchy wheals, affects superficial skin	Transient wheals
Cellulitis	Red, warm, tender swelling, often with fever	Involves infection, spreads over time
Dermatitis	Itchy, red, inflamed skin, may blister	Often related to contact or irritant exposure
Lymphatic obstruction	Chronic, nonpitting swelling	Often due to cancer or infection

DIAGNOSTIC APPROACH TO ANGIOEDEMA

Clinical History and Examination

- Detailed history of the symptoms, frequency and duration of episodes need to be taken. The sites affected including face, lips, tongue, throat, extremities, and gastrointestinal tract need to be noted. Any associated symptoms such as abdominal pain, difficulty breathing, urticaria, itching, or systemic reactions need to be taken into consideration.
- Triggering factors such as foods, medications, physical trauma, stress, hormonal changes, or recent infections need to be asked. Check for a family history of angioedema or related conditions to assess for hereditary forms.
- History of medicines, especially ACE inhibitors, NSAIDs, and estrogens. Consider underlying conditions such as autoimmune diseases, infections, or malignancies.

While performing clinical examination, assessment of affected areas for the extent, consistency, and presence of urticaria should be carried out. It is important to check for signs of airway compromise, such as stridor, hoarseness, or difficulty breathing. Any signs of gastrointestinal involvement, such as tenderness or distension, should be evaluated. Also, it is necessary to rule out any signs of systemic illness or malignancy.

Laboratory Investigations

Basic Tests

- *Complete blood count (CBC)*: To identify signs of infection or hematologic abnormalities
- *Electrolytes and liver function tests*: Important to rule out systemic causes
- *Thyroid function tests*: To check for thyroid abnormalities

Specific Tests for Angioedema

- *C1 esterase inhibitor (C1-INH) levels and function:*
    - *Type I HAE*: Low C1-INH levels and low C4 levels
    - *Type II HAE*: Normal or elevated C1-INH levels with dysfunctional protein and low C4 levels
- *C4 levels*: Typically low during and between attacks in HAE
- *C1q levels*: Decreased in acquired angioedema due to lymphoproliferative disorders
- *Bradykinin levels*: Elevated in bradykinin-mediated angioedema
- *C1-INH autoantibodies*: Present in acquired angioedema due to autoimmune mechanisms

Allergy Testing

- *Skin prick tests or serum-specific IgE*: To identify allergen triggers in cases of suspected allergic angioedema
- *Oral challenge tests*: Performed under medical supervision to confirm specific food or drug triggers

Imaging Studies
Ultrasound or CT Scan
- *Abdominal imaging*: Useful in patients with gastrointestinal symptoms to assess for bowel wall edema
- *Airway imaging*: To evaluate the extent of laryngeal or pharyngeal involvement in severe cases

Genetic Testing
Genetic Analysis
- *SERPING1 gene mutations:* To confirm hereditary angioedema types I and II
- *F12 gene mutations*: To identify type III hereditary angioedema

Functional Tests
Bradykinin Pathway Assessment
- *Kallikrein activity*: To measure the activity of kallikrein, which is involved in bradykinin production
- *Bradykinin receptor function*: To assess the responsiveness of bradykinin receptors

Differential Diagnosis
Exclude Other Causes
- *Urticaria*: Differentiate between angioedema and urticaria by assessing the depth and nature of swelling.
- *Cellulitis*: Consider bacterial infection presenting as localized swelling and erythema.
- *Thrombophlebitis*: Assess for venous thrombosis presenting as unilateral limb swelling.
- *Lymphatic obstruction*: Rule out causes such as malignancy or infection leading to localized edema.

Provocative Tests
Provocation with Known Triggers
- *Physical triggers:* Cold, pressure, or vibration tests to identify physical urticarias that may present with angioedema
- *Medication withdrawal and rechallenge:* To confirm drug-induced angioedema under controlled conditions

MANAGEMENT OF ANGIOEDEMA

The management of angioedema depends on the underlying cause, the severity of the symptoms, and whether the condition is acute or chronic.

General Principles
Initial assessment includes evaluating the severity of symptoms, especially if there are signs of airway compromise. Conduct a thorough history and physical examination to identify potential triggers and underlying causes.

Immediate Management
- *Airway management*: Ensure the airway is patent. In cases of laryngeal edema, intubation or tracheostomy may be needed.
- *Symptomatic relief*: Provide symptomatic relief for pain and swelling.

Specific Management based on Type of Angioedema
Hereditary Angioedema
Acute Attacks

In HAE types I and II, the treatment of choice in acute attacks consists of infusion of C1-INH concentrate (20U/kg) or ecallantide. Another option is icatibant.
- *C1 Inhibitor concentrate*: C1-INH concentrates are available which are derived from pooled plasma (Berinert, Cinryze) and recombinant C1 INH (Ruconest). It is approved for the treatment of acute HAE attacks. The dose is 20 U/kg body weight intravenously. Side effects such as infections and dysgeusia can occur. Cinryze can be given every 3–4 days in a dose of 1,000 units.
- *Bradykinin receptor antagonist (icatibant)*: It is a selective bradykinin 2 receptor antagonist, approved by the Food and Drug Administration (FDA) for use in patients 18 years and more. A 30-mg dose is given subcutaneously, which can be repeated after 6 hours. Maximum it can be given up to three times in 24 hours. Few side effects such as nausea, rash, headache, and fever can occur.
- *Kallikrein inhibitor (ecallantide)*: Use to reduce bradykinin production. It can be given to patients 12 years or older. Three subcutaneous injections of 10 mg each are given. It should only be given by healthcare professionals as risk of anaphylactoid reaction is present. The side effect profile is similar to icatibant.

Long-term Prophylaxis
- *C1-INH concentrate*: Regular prophylactic administration in patients with frequent or severe attacks
- *Androgens (danazol)*: Used in low doses (200 mg oral danazol) to increase hepatic synthesis of C1-INH, though their use is decreasing due to side effects
- *Antifibrinolytics (tranexamic acid)*: Consider in patients who cannot tolerate C1-INH or androgens

Acquired Angioedema related to Angiotensin-converting Enzyme Inhibitor
Treatment is with antihistamines, epinephrine, and glucocorticoids. Care should be taken to stop the offending ACE inhibitor, and the patient should be not rechallenged with any of the ACE inhibitors in the future.

Acquired C1 Inhibitor Deficiency Angioedema

Majority of cases are asymptomatic and respond to immunochemotherapy. Treatment of acute attacks with icatibant and plasma-derived C1 inhibitor concentrate, and prophylaxis is with rituximab with or without chemotherapy and splenectomy.

CONCLUSION

Angioedema is a complex condition marked by episodic swelling of deeper skin and mucosal tissues, requiring precise diagnosis and tailored treatment. With varied pathophysiology involving mast cell degranulation, bradykinin production, or autoimmune processes, hereditary, drug-induced, and idiopathic types each need distinct management. Early recognition and prompt treatment are critical, especially for cases affecting the airway.

Advances in understanding molecular pathways have led to targeted therapies, enhancing patient outcomes. Continued research is necessary to clarify uncommon mechanisms and develop improved treatments. Clinicians should remain vigilant in assessing recurrent swelling, particularly when conventional treatments fail.

Overall, effective management of angioedema relies on patient education, trigger evaluation, and appropriate diagnostics, integrating research insights with clinical expertise for personalized care.

SUGGESTED READINGS

1. Kaplan AP, Greaves M. Pathogenesis of chronic urticaria. Clin Exp Allergy. 2009;39(6):777-87.
2. Zuraw BL. Hereditary angioedema: A current state-of-the-art review, IV: Mechanisms of pathophysiology. Ann Allergy Asthma Immunol. 2008;100(1);S7-12.
3. Cicardi M, Zanichelli A. Acquired angioedema. Allergy Asthma Clin Immunol. 2010;6(1):14.
4. Varga L, Farkas H. Drug-induced angioedema. Med Clin North Am. 2008;90(5):1035-43.
5. Grigoriadou S, Longhurst HJ. Clinical immunology review series: An approach to the patient with angio-oedema. Clin Exp Immunol. 2009;155(1):1-13.
6. Maurer M, Duvillard C, Zuberbier T, et al. Diagnosis and treatment of angioedema beyond ACE inhibitor-associated angioedema. Allergy. 2018;73(4):803-16.
7. Zuraw BL, Banerji A, Bernstein JA, et al. Management of hereditary angioedema: 2020 international consensus algorithm and updated US approach. Allergy Asthma Clin Immunol. 2020;16(1):62.
8. Busse PJ, Shapiro G, Riedl MA, et al. Hereditary angioedema management: Consensus 2010. Allergy Asthma Clin Immunol. 2012;8(1):26.
9. Cicardi M, Bork K, Caballero T, Craig T, Li HH, Longhurst H, et al. Evidence-based recommendations for the therapeutic management of angioedema owing to hereditary C1 inhibitor deficiency: Consensus report of an International Working Group. Allergy. Allergy. 2012;67(2):147-57.
10. Bork K, Meng G, Staubach P, Hardt J. Hereditary angioedema: New findings concerning symptoms, affected organs, and course. Am J Med. 2006;119(3):267-74.
11. Bafunno V, Patuzzo G, Zingale L, et al. Genetic characterization of a large cohort of patients with hereditary angioedema. J Allergy Clin Immunol. 2002;119(3):662-8.
12. Frank MM. Hereditary angioedema: A current state-of-the-art review, VI: Novel therapies for hereditary angioedema. Ann Allergy Asthma Immunol. 2008;100(1):S17-22.

13. Craig T, Pursun EM, Bork K, Pawankar R, Zuraw B, Maurer M, et al. (2012). WAO guideline for the management of hereditary angioedema. World Allergy Organ J. 2012;5(12):182-99.
14. Lang DM, Aberer W, Bernstein JA, Chng HH, Grumach AS, Hide M, Maurer M, et al. (2012). International consensus on hereditary and acquired angioedema. Ann Allergy Asthma Immunol. 2012;109(6):395-402.
15. Busse PJ, Christiansen SC. Hereditary angioedema. N Engl J Med. 2020;382(12):1136-48.
16. Banerji A, Riedl MA, Bernstein JA, et al. Lanadelumab for the prevention of hereditary angioedema attacks. N Engl J Med. 2017;376(12):1131-40.
17. Moldovan D, Rojas-Hernandez C, Farkas H, et al. Berotralstat for the prevention of hereditary angioedema attacks. N Engl J Med. 2021;384(2):130-8.
18. Grumach AS, Santos A, Libério A, et al. Icatibant for the treatment of ACE inhibitor-induced angioedema. N Engl J Med. 2013;369(14):1323-30.
19. Longhurst HJ, Cicardi M, Agostoni A, et al. Self-administered subcutaneous C1-inhibitor concentrate for hereditary angioedema. N Engl J Med. 2017;376(12):1131-40.
20. Aygören-Pürsün E, Bygum A, nap Grivcheva-Panovska V, Magrel M. Oral plasma kallikrein inhibitor for prophylaxis in hereditary angioedema. N Engl J Med. 2018;379(4):352-62.

CHAPTER 8

Anaphylaxis in Acute Urticaria

Sunita Gupta, Aditi Dabhra, Sanjeev Gupta

INTRODUCTION

Anaphylaxis can present with or without urticaria and angioedema. To better understand anaphylaxis, it is essential to first understand urticaria and angioedema. Urticaria is a medical disorder that affects up to 20% of people during their lifetime. It is characterized by the appearance of raised, itchy skin lesions known as wheals, as well as swelling beneath the skin called angioedema. Acute urticaria, characterized by symptoms lasting up to 6 weeks, can either be the sole indication of a hypersensitivity reaction or might be accompanied by other systemic symptoms, suggesting an anaphylactic reaction.

Characteristics commonly associated with a wheal:
- A distinct and superficial swelling in the center, with varying sizes and forms, almost always accompanied by surrounding redness
- Pruritus or occasionally a burning sensation
- Transient in nature, with the epidermis reverting to its typical appearance, typically within a time frame of 30 minutes to 24 hours

Characteristics of angioedema:
- Angioedema is defined by the abrupt and noticeable red or skin-colored swelling that occurs in the deeper layers of the skin (lower dermis and subcutis) or mucous membranes
- Sensations of tingling, burning, tightness, and even pain instead of itchiness
- A resolution with a longer duration than wheals (may take up to 72 hours)

PATHOGENESIS (TABLE 1)

- Urticaria and anaphylaxis are frequently associated with mast cell activation caused by various triggers, such as IgE-mediated and non-IgE-mediated processes. However, it is important to note that this relationship is not always present.
- Mast cells have a significant function in both the innate and the acquired immune response. This is due to their ability to express various receptors that

TABLE 1: Key regulators in the pathogenesis of anaphylaxis.	
Mast cell activation	Urticaria and anaphylaxis often involve mast cell activation through IgE-mediated and non-IgE-mediated processes
Mast cell functions	Mast cells play roles in the innate and acquired immune responses via various receptors
Location of mast cells	Predominantly found in tissues exposed to external pathogens like skin, GI tract, and airway
Types of mast cells	• *MCT*: Positive for tryptase, negative for chymase, found in mucosal tissues, reliant on T lymphocytes, more abundant in allergic diseases • *MCTC*: Positive for both tryptase and chymase, found in epidermis and GI submucosa, 99% of dermal mast cells in CSU patients
Activation mechanisms	Both MCT and MCTC degranulate upon IgE stimulation; MCTC can also be triggered by non-IgE processes
IgE–FcεRI pathway	Activation occurs when allergen-specific IgE binds to allergens and interacts with FcεRI receptors on mast cells
Receptors on mast cells	FcεRI, IgG receptors (FcγRII/III), complement receptors (C3a/C5a), drug receptors (MRGPRX2), opioid receptors, neuropeptide receptors, nerve growth factor receptors, stem cell factor receptors, and cytokine receptors
Functions affected by receptor activation	Survival, maturation, differentiation, growth, apoptosis, and degranulation
MRGPRX2 receptor	Activated by fluoroquinolones, icatibant, and anesthetics (e.g., atracurium, rocuronium), independent of IgE–FcεRI pathway, leading to calcium release and degranulation
MRGPRX2 and CSU	Elevated MRGPRX2 protein expression in the skin of CSU patients; may contribute to neurogenic inflammation, discomfort, itch, and pruritic conditions

(CSU: chronic spontaneous urticaria; GI: gastrointestinal; MCT: mast cells positive for tryptase but negative for chymase; MCTC: mast cells positive for both tryptase and chymase)

respond to specific antigens, the circulating complement components and fragments, immune complexes that bind to IgG and IgM, cytokines, variations in blood pressure, and immunologic activation. Hence, mast cell activation in individuals suffering from urticaria and anaphylaxis is prone to transpire via many pathways, apart from IgE. Mature mast cells are predominantly located in tissues that serve as entry points for external pathogens, such as the skin, gastrointestinal tract, and airway.
- Immunological labeling of tissues has identified two distinct types of human mast cells based on their neutral protease content: Mast cells that are positive for tryptase but negative for chymase (referred to as MCT) and mast cells that are positive for both tryptase and chymase (referred to as MCTC).
- Mast cells (MCT) are commonly located in mucosal tissues, including the intestine, lung, and nose. They rely on T lymphocytes for their function and are known to be more abundant in allergic diseases.
- Unlike lymphocytes, the development of MCTC is not influenced by them. MCTCs are mainly found in the epidermis and gastrointestinal submucosa.

MCTC cells constitute about 99% of the mast cells present in the dermis of both affected and unaffected skin of patients with chronic spontaneous urticaria (CSU).
- Stimulation that depends on IgE causes degranulation of both subtypes. However, MCTC can also be triggered by processes that do not rely on IgE.

Activation of Mast Cell

- Mast cells are activated when allergen-specific IgE binds to allergen and interacts with the high-affinity IgE receptor (FcεRI) on their surfaces.
- Human mast cells express a variety of receptors, including FcεRI, IgG receptors (FcγRII/III), complement receptors (C3a/C5a), drug receptors (Mas-related G protein-coupled receptor X2 or MRGPRX2), opioid receptors, neuropeptide receptors, nerve growth factor receptors, stem cell factor receptors, and cytokine receptors.
- Activation of these receptors can modify various aspects of mast cell function, such as survival, maturation, differentiation, growth, apoptosis, and degranulation.
- Mast cells can undergo activation via the recently discovered MRGPRX2 receptor by fluoroquinolones like ciprofloxacin, icatibant, and general anesthetics such as atracurium, rocuronium, and tubocurarine. This activation occurs independent of the IgE–FcεRI pathway. Binding of these medicines and compounds expressing the THIQ (tetrahydroisoquinoline) motif directly to MRGPRX2 activates the protein kinase A and phosphoinositide 3-kinase pathway, leading to calcium release and degranulation.
- Furthermore, the stimulation of mast cells via MRGPRX2 could potentially play a role in the development of neurogenic inflammation, discomfort, itch, and pruritic skin conditions, such as CSU.
- Patients with CSU have shown elevated levels of MRGPRX2 protein expression in their skin.

TRIGGERS FOR ANAPHYLAXIS

Food

- The profile of anaphylactic triggers varies according to age and geographic location, much like urticaria. Furthermore, in approximately 35% of cases of anaphylaxis, a particular cause may not be determined at the immediate occurrence or in subsequent assessments, indicating an idiopathic presentation.
- Globally, the most common causes of allergic reactions are food, insect venom, and medications. Severe anaphylactic responses in children are most commonly triggered by food, whereas adults are commonly triggered by medications and insect venom.
- Anaphylaxis from food and medications is significantly more common in young children, leading to a higher rate of hospitalization.

- Anaphylaxis is most commonly caused by certain foods, including cow milk, eggs, peanuts, tree nuts, sesame, and wheat, in newborns and young children. Additionally, school children can experience anaphylaxis as a result of consuming nuts, cashews, and hazelnuts.
- Food dyes rarely cause food allergies. The incidence of food-induced anaphylaxis in adults differs depending on the geographical region and the type of food consumed.
- Peanuts and nuts are the primary causes of anaphylaxis in North America and Australia, whereas shellfish is most commonly linked to anaphylaxis in Asia. Peanuts, tree nuts, sesame, wheat, and shellfish are the primary food allergens linked to anaphylaxis in central Europe. Nevertheless, in the southern regions of Europe, the most common food allergens are lipid transfer proteins (pan-allergens that cause cross-reactivity between fruits, vegetables, and pollens) in conjunction with cofactors.
- Anaphylaxis is frequently triggered by sesame seed in the Middle East and by buckwheat in Korea. Further investigation should be conducted on less-prevalent allergens, such as alpha-gal, which have the potential to induce delayed anaphylactic episodes.

Medicines

- Medicines can also trigger anaphylaxis, with symptoms typically manifesting in children and teenagers attending school. They have been identified as the primary cause of anaphylaxis-related fatalities in both adults and children across several nations. However, the specific prevalence may differ based on the research methodology and database used.
- Beta-lactam antibiotics, specifically, are identified as the primary causes of drug-induced anaphylaxis in children, whereas there are limited instances of anaphylaxis to other non-beta-lactam antibiotics, like macrolides. The antibiotics that are most commonly associated with adverse effects in adults are penicillin, cephalosporins, and sulfonamides.
- Nonsteroidal anti-inflammatory drugs (NSAIDs) are the second most common cause of drug-induced anaphylaxis in children globally. Nevertheless, they remain the primary cause of adverse effects in both children and adults in Latin America. Perioperative anaphylaxis commonly involves antibiotics, NSAIDs, neuromuscular blockers, anesthetics, opioids, hypnotics, ethylene oxide, plasma expanders, and dyes such as patent blue and methylene blue.
- Latex allergies continue to be a major cause of perioperative anaphylaxis in certain areas. However, the occurrence of latex allergy has declined in numerous locations as a result of primary preventative strategies, including the utilization of powder-free latex gloves and surgical materials that are free of latex in the operating room.
- Adverse reactions to radiographic contrast media have been less common when nonionic and low osmolality contrasts are used, as compared to monomeric ionic contrasts.

- Additional triggers that can cause anaphylaxis have been found, such as immunobiological medicines, chemotherapeutics, chlorhexidine, polyethylene glycol, and methylcellulose. Medications are the primary cause of deadly anaphylaxis in both adults and children.
- In the United States, antibiotics, NSAIDs, immunomodulators, and biologic medicines are the primary causes of drug-induced anaphylaxis. In contrast, general anesthetics are commonly linked to deadly drug-induced anaphylaxis in the United Kingdom.

Insects

Anaphylaxis caused by insect venom also displays regional patterns. Bee venom is the primary cause of allergic reactions in South Korea, and it is more commonly observed in children. Within central Europe, the wasp is the bug that most commonly triggers anaphylaxis. In several other regions, including America, Asia, and certain parts of Australia, venom plays a crucial role in triggering anaphylaxis. Adults are most commonly connected with fatal cases of anaphylaxis caused by insect venom.

Exercise

- Exercise-induced anaphylaxis and anaphylaxis produced by food-dependent exercise are two infrequent yet noteworthy conditions. Engaging in activities such as yard work, walking, and running can elicit a condition known as exercise-induced anaphylaxis. Symptoms may manifest during or following physical exertion; however, accurately forecasting crises is typically difficult.
- In cases of food-dependent exercise-induced anaphylaxis, symptoms manifest when the triggering item, such as seafood, dairy products, or wheat, is consumed within minutes to several hours prior to engaging in physical activity. Patients should refrain from consuming these items during a time frame of 4–6 hours before engaging in exercise.

External Cofactors

- External cofactors and associated conditions can significantly contribute to the development of allergic reactions, including anaphylaxis. These cofactors, such as physical exercise, certain medications (such as nonsteroidal anti-inflammatory drugs and proton-pump inhibitors), acute infections, alcohol consumption, and menstruation, can either trigger allergic reactions at lower doses or lead to more severe and life-threatening symptoms.
- Additionally, there are certain associated conditions, such as unstable asthma, mast cell disorders, and cardiovascular diseases, that act as cofactors and increase the risk of complications and mortality.
- Although the exact mechanisms of action for these cofactors are not yet fully understood, potential explanations include increased bioavailability of allergens due to enhanced intestinal permeability and absorption, lowered activation threshold at the cellular level, and temporary plasma hyperosmolality.

- Allegedly, cofactors are involved in around 14–30% of anaphylactic responses. Hence, it is imperative to always take into account these additional aspects in the medical background of a patient and strive to eradicate them wherever feasible, in order to minimize the likelihood of a subsequent severe reaction.

DIAGNOSTIC APPROACH FOR ANAPHYLAXIS

One severe allergic reaction that can happen quickly and be lethal is anaphylaxis. Manifestations on the skin and mucous membranes are common but not always seen. Anaphylaxis is quite likely to occur when any one of these three conditions is met **(Table 2)**.

TABLE 2: Criteria for anaphylaxis.	
Criteria	Description
Acute onset of illness: • Respiratory compromise • Reduced blood pressure (BP) or end-organ dysfunction	Sudden onset (minutes to hours) with skin or mucosal involvement (e.g., hives, itching, flushing, swollen lips/tongue) and at least one of the following: • Difficulty breathing, wheezing, stridor, hypoxemia • Hypotension, fainting, collapse, incontinence
Rapid onset after allergen exposure: • Skin–mucosal involvement • Respiratory compromise • Reduced BP or end-organ dysfunction • Gastrointestinal symptoms	Two or more of the following symptoms occurring quickly after exposure to a likely allergen: • Hives, itching, flushing, swollen lips/tongue • Difficulty breathing, wheezing, stridor, hypoxemia • Hypotension, fainting, collapse, incontinence • Persistent vomiting, diarrhea, abdominal pain
Reduced BP after known allergen exposure: • Infants and children • Adults	Low BP occurring minutes to hours after exposure to a known allergen: • Low systolic BP (age-specific) or >30% decrease in systolic BP, low systolic BP: <70 mm Hg from 1 month to 1 year; <70 mm Hg + (2 × age) from 1 to 10 years; <90 mm Hg from 11 to 17 years • Systolic BP < 90 mm Hg or >30% decrease from baseline

TABLE 3: Key points for investigating tryptase levels in anaphylaxis.	
Serum tryptase levels	• Levels rise 30 minutes after the onset of anaphylaxis, peak at 60–90 minutes, decline after 2 hours, and normalize in 24–48 hours • Blood samples should be taken 1–4 hours after the reaction and again within 24–48 hours to determine baseline levels
Baseline tryptase levels	• Baseline levels > 8 ng/mL are considered high but do not always indicate mast cell activation • Use the formula 1.2 × baseline + 2 ng/mL to determine significant rise
Comparison of reactions	Tryptase levels are higher and more persistent in reactions to intravenous medicines and insect venom compared to oral triggers like food
Diagnostic criteria	Tryptase must rise by at least 20% over baseline plus 2 ng/mL within 4 hours of the allergic reaction for confirmation

As a result, anaphylaxis may happen without involving the skin, which could cause a delay in the diagnosis of the condition. About 80-90% of cases with anaphylaxis have cutaneous symptoms of urticaria and angioedema, which are the most common manifestations and often persist less than 24 hours. It is noteworthy that there is no direct correlation between the severity of anaphylaxis and urticaria. Instances have been reported of fatal anaphylaxis in which severe anaphylaxis manifested without urticaria.

Vasodilation and enhanced capillary permeability are two pathogenic mechanisms shared by angioedema, urticaria, and anaphylaxis. The symptoms of anaphylaxis can vary depending on the age group. For instance, older children are more prone to feeling chest tightness, dizziness, hypotension, and cardiovascular collapse, whereas younger children are more likely to experience vomiting and cough.

Distinct clinical symptoms can be caused by different elicitors. Cutaneous symptoms of perioperative anaphylaxis could be difficult to detect. Only after the surgical drapes are removed or perfusion is restored can urticaria and angioedema become noticeable. In a perioperative anaphylaxis research, 266 reports of Grades 3-5 anaphylaxis from all UK NHS hospitals were examined over a 1-year period. They discovered that tachycardia (9.8%), hypotension (46%), bronchospasm (18%), oxygen desaturation (4.7%), bradycardia (3%), and decreased or nonexistent capnography trace (2.3%) were the most common presenting symptoms.

TRYPTASE AND ITS ROLE IN INVESTIGATING ANAPHYLAXIS (TABLE 3)

- One indicator of mast cell activity is tryptase. It is a serine protease that is expressed in basophils to a lesser extent and in mast cells. Out of the four isoforms, only α and β are thought to be physiologically significant.
- Tryptase levels in serum during anaphylaxis can be seen 30 minutes after symptoms appear, peaking 60-90 minutes later, declining after 2 hours, and then returning to normal in 24-48 hours.
- Blood samples must therefore be taken 1-4 hours after the reaction. Both total (released at baseline) and mature (released only after activation) tryptase can be detected using immunoassays.
- Within 24-48 hours following anaphylaxis, another blood sample is required to determine the basal level of tryptase. Although baseline tryptase levels > 8 ng/mL are generally regarded as excessive, mast cell activation is not always indicated by these levels.
- Determining the diagnosis's cutoff point is challenging. Anaphylactic episodes are caused by mast cell activation, which cannot be confirmed at specific levels. Instead, the formula must be applied to determine each person's baseline tryptase levels. 1.2 × baseline + 2 ng/mL.
- Compared to oral triggers such as food, tryptase levels are usually greater and more persistently raised in anaphylactic reactions to intravenous medicines and insect venom. Moreover, increases and hypotension are correlated.

- However, because the sensitivity is suboptimal, normal tryptase levels do not rule out anaphylaxis. Serum tryptase levels are affected when approximately 27% of the population lacks α-tryptase genes, which explains this.
- Tryptase must rise by at least 20% over baseline plus 2 ng/mL within 4 hours of the allergic reaction, according to an equation used in a number of investigations. Patients with low baseline tryptase have considerably higher tryptase levels (≥2 ng/mL + 1.2 times baseline).
- Those with acute myelocytic leukemia, systemic mastocytosis (SM), myelodysplastic syndromes, severe renal failure, immunologic disorders (hypereosinophilic syndrome) or familial tryptasemia—a disease marked by the expression of more than two α-tryptase genes—are among the patients with differential diagnoses of elevated total tryptase levels.

CHALLENGES IN IDENTIFYING ANAPHYLACTIC TRIGGERS

- The diagnosis of anaphylaxis should rely on pertinent clinical history and a combination of accessible testing, such as skin tests, in vitro tests [including serum tryptase, specific IgE serum levels, basophil activation test (BAT), or histamine-release assays], and/or provocation tests.
- Nevertheless, the examination of precipitating factors can be difficult due to the intricate range of clinical symptoms, several simultaneous exposures, and various potential causes, as seen in cases of anaphylaxis during surgery.
- Acute serum tryptase level is a crucial component of the diagnostic assessment for anaphylaxis; however, it is not universally accessible. Furthermore, it exhibits a high level of specificity, but a low level of sensitivity, and the obtained data should be meticulously analyzed and evaluated **(Table 4)**.
- Anaphylactic reactions mediated by IgE can be evaluated using either in vivo tests, such as skin tests to foods, venom, medications, and latex, or in vitro tests, such as measuring particular IgE levels in the serum for foods, venom, and certain drugs. It is important to mention that, in the context of anaphylaxis, their identification helps in determining the specific allergen to be employed in provocation tests **(Table 4)**.
- Nevertheless, a positive skin test or high specific IgE is only valuable in confirming the cause of an allergic reaction if the clinical history is indicative; otherwise, they simply indicate sensitization.
- Although most skin tests are generally safe and quick, they are not completely devoid of systemic effects. The optimal timing for doing skin testing may vary depending on the specific allergies. Typically, it is recommended to wait for a minimum of 4 weeks following an allergic episode.
- However, for cases of anaphylaxis caused by medication, a longer interval may be necessary. It is important to evaluate each patient on an individual basis. Prior to testing, it is necessary to address comorbidities such as asthma and temporarily stop taking drugs that include antihistamines, high-dose corticosteroids, antidepressants, and antipsychotics with antihistamine effects.

TABLE 4: Various tests that aid in the diagnosis of triggers of anaphylaxis.

Test	Description	Details
Skin tests	In vivo tests to identify allergens (foods, venom, medications, latex)	Positive results confirm sensitization; safe and quick but not without systemic effects; timing varies, usually 4 weeks postreaction, longer for drug-induced cases
Serum tryptase levels	Measure tryptase, a marker of mast cell activity	High specificity, low sensitivity; crucial for diagnosing anaphylaxis; samples taken 1–4 hours postreaction and 24–48 hours for baseline; calculation formula: $1.2 \times$ baseline $+ 2$ ng/mL
Specific IgE levels	In vitro test measuring IgE levels for specific allergens (foods, venom, certain drugs)	Confirms allergen's presence if clinical history is indicative; establishing cutoff values is challenging due to variability
Provocation tests	Confirms hypersensitivity or tolerance to specific allergens (foods, medications)	Most reliable but risky due to potential anaphylaxis; decision based on clinical history, age, symptoms, and prior test results; avoided if specific IgE sensitivity is confirmed
Basophil activation test (BAT)	Assesses basophil activation in response to allergens (foods, medications, venoms, latex)	Useful for severe, high-risk anaphylaxis; mainly used in clinical research due to lack of standardized kits
Molecular allergy diagnostics	Utilizes molecular biology to improve diagnosis accuracy and differentiate between cosensitization and cross-sensitization phenomena	Most effective for identifying peanut and tree nut allergies; aids in guiding provocation tests

- One challenge encountered when doing skin testing and measuring serum specific IgE levels is establishing cutoff values that can definitively confirm a diagnosis and eliminate the need for provocation tests. Furthermore, the specificity and sensitivity of the reaction depend on the specific trigger implicated, making it impossible to reliably estimate universal values for specific IgE.
- The utilization of molecular biology-based components has facilitated progress in precision medicine by providing increased accuracy in diagnosis. This has allowed for the differentiation between discriminative cosensitization and cross-sensitization phenomena, as well as the categorization of clinical risk associated with a particular sensitization pattern. Additionally, it has improved the guidance for conducting provocation tests in cases of food-induced anaphylaxis. The use of molecular allergy diagnostics has shown the most favorable outcomes in identifying allergies to peanuts and tree nuts **(Table 4)**.
- Despite the significant scientific progress made in recent years, the provocation test is widely regarded as the most reliable method for identifying

hypersensitivity to both foods and medications, regardless of the specific underlying physiological cause.
- These tests are employed to verify, eliminate, or establish an individual's tolerance to a specific food or substance and assess a secure substitute. One notable drawback is the potential for anaphylaxis, which greatly increases the danger associated with provocation.
- The decision on its implementation is impacted by factors such as the patient's clinical history, age, kind of symptom, time elapsed since the previous reaction, and results of skin tests and/or blood levels of particular IgE.
- Ultimately, the decision is made collaboratively by the physician and patient, carefully weighing the potential risks and benefits. Individuals who have a well-documented history of anaphylaxis caused by a particular allergen and have confirmed evidence of specific IgE sensitivity should avoid doing provocation tests.
- Additional examinations, such as the BAT using substances including food, medications, Hymenoptera venoms, and latex, provide insight into the sensitization and activation of mast cells in the tissues. The primary utilization of allergy kits is in clinical research due to the absence of standardized kits for the majority of allergens. Nevertheless, BAT should be regarded as a diagnostic instrument for specific patients, particularly those experiencing severe and high-risk anaphylaxis associated with medications **(Table 4)**.
- Additional clarification of the fundamental mechanisms of anaphylaxis is necessary in order to more accurately define the characteristics and subtypes of anaphylaxis and reduce the number of cases classified as idiopathic anaphylaxis.

TREATMENT (FLOWCHART 1)

- *Triage*: It is crucial to prioritize the assessment of any allergic reaction due to the potential for rapid deterioration and the development of anaphylaxis, especially if anaphylaxis has not already occurred.
- *Airway*: Ensuring proper airway management is of utmost importance. Conduct a comprehensive assessment of the patient to see if their airway is clear and if there are any signs that suggest they may soon experience a blocked airway. Perioral edema, stridor, and angioedema are extremely dangerous, and it is absolutely necessary to secure an airway. Procrastination can decrease the likelihood of a successful intubation as swelling persists, hence increasing the risk of needing a surgical airway.
- *Decontamination*: Once the airway is properly secured, the immediate focus should be on decontaminating any known harmful substances in order to minimize further exposure and worsening of the patient's condition. Extract any stingers, if present. Avoid performing stomach lavage in situations of ingestion, as it may not be efficacious and can impede timely treatment.
- *Epinephrine*: It is administered via intramuscular injection at a dosage of 0.3–0.5 mL of a 1:1,000 concentration of epinephrine. The recommended dosage for pediatric patients is 0.01 mg/kg of body weight, administered

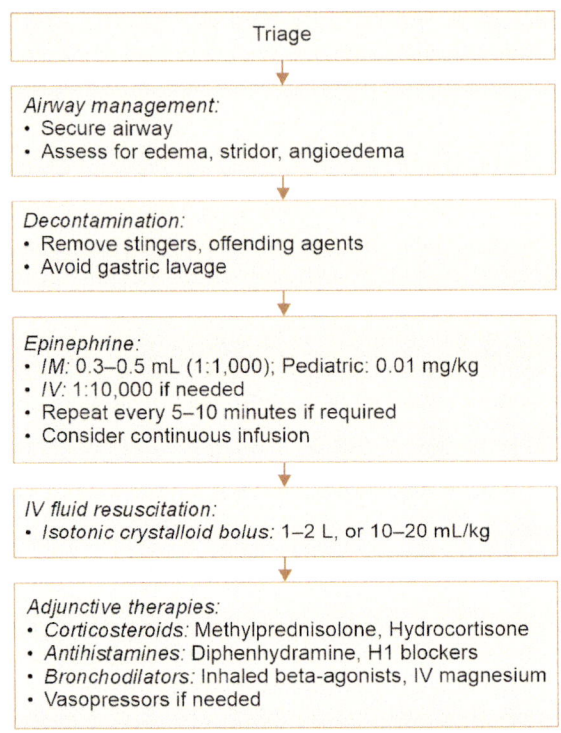

FLOWCHART 1: Treatment of anaphylaxis.

intramuscularly (IM). This dosage is specifically for the administration of epinephrine injection in pediatric patients. Intramuscular administration has demonstrated superior efficacy and faster onset of action compared to subcutaneous or intravascular routes. It is important to mention that if IV epinephrine is going to be administered, the necessary concentration is 1:10,000. When feasible, the thigh is the preferred site over the deltoid. Multiple replicated studies have consistently demonstrated that healthcare personnel frequently delay administration of epinephrine, which is the preferred treatment option. The prompt and substantial advantages of administering the medication far surpass the potential hazards associated with withholding therapy. Although the majority of patients only need one dose, further doses can be administered every 5–10 minutes if necessary, until symptoms improve. If patients need numerous doses, it may be appropriate to administer a continuous infusion of epinephrine. Begin by initiating an initial intravenous infusion of 0.1 mg of a 1:10,000 solution, administered over a period of 5–10 minutes. If additional amount is needed, initiate the infusion at a rate of 1 μg/min and adjust accordingly to get the desired outcome. Discontinue intravenous infusion if the patient has arrhythmia or chest discomfort. IV use of epinephrine significantly increases the likelihood of cardiovascular problems. Close blood pressure monitoring is recommended

for patients who are using beta-blockers, as there is a danger of unopposed alpha-adrenergic effects caused by epinephrine.
- *IV fluid resuscitation*: Anaphylaxis triggers a distributive shock that usually responds well to fluid resuscitation and the administration of epinephrine mentioned above. An isotonic crystalloid bolus of 1–2 L or 10–20 mL/kg should be administered in cases of observed hypotension. Albumin or hypertonic solutions are not recommended.
- *Adjunctive therapies*: Frequently, when anaphylaxis is identified, simultaneous treatment is commenced with corticosteroids, antihistamines, inhaled bronchodilators, and vasopressors. Glucagon may be employed if deemed necessary. These medications can help with difficult-to-treat initial severe allergic reactions or reduce the occurrence of subsequent reactions and two-phase reactions.
- *Corticosteroids*: The approved therapies during the acute phase include methylprednisolone (80–125 mg IV) or hydrocortisone (250–500 mg IV). After the acute phase, treatment is continued with oral prednisone (40–60 mg daily or divided twice per day) for 3–5 days. If the source of the condition is uncertain or if there is a concern about a protracted period before seeing a doctor, a steroid taper of up to 2 weeks may be prescribed. Fluid retention is caused by mineralocorticoid activity. In individuals who are at risk, dexamethasone and methylprednisolone are the preferable drugs since they have the least mineralocorticoid effect.
- *Antihistamines*: These are often and regularly administered, with the most frequently utilized being H1 blockers, specifically diphenhydramine, given intravenously or intramuscularly at a dosage of 25–50 mg. Although there is no conclusive evidence of its effectiveness in treating anaphylaxis, its usefulness is clearly demonstrated in less-severe allergic reactions. In severe instances, H1 blockers like ranitidine (administered intravenously at a dosage of 50 mg over a period of 5 minutes) or cimetidine (administered intravenously at a dosage of 300 mg) may be employed with H-blockers. This is because there is evidence indicating that histamine exhibits crossover selectivity of receptors. It is important to be aware that cimetidine has several precautions that need to be taken into consideration for individuals who are at risk, such as patients with impaired kidney or liver function, or those who are using beta-blockers. Although IV administration is the primary method used for stabilizing patients, once the patient's condition has improved, oral administration may be used for ongoing therapy if desired.
- *Bronchodilators*: These are beneficial additional treatments for people with bronchospasm. Individuals who have already experienced respiratory conditions, particularly asthma, are at the greatest risk. Inhaled beta-agonists, such as albuterol alone or in combination with ipratropium bromide, are the preferred initial treatment for wheezing. In cases with persistent wheeze that does not respond to treatment, intravenous administration of magnesium is recommended. The dosage and treatment protocol for this should be identical to those used for severe asthma exacerbations.

- *Vasopressors*: If a patient experiences adverse effects such as arrhythmia or chest pain from the intravenous infusion of epinephrine, vasopressors might be used as an alternative when the patient needs additional doses of epinephrine. If there is no specific second-line pressor discovered in a particular case, the treatment instructions for a patient in hypotensive shock would be the same as those for any other patient.

CONCLUSION

Anaphylaxis is a serious, potentially fatal complication of acute urticaria that requires swift recognition and treatment.

Effective management hinges on early identification, immediate intervention, and planning for future risks, particularly in patients with recurrent reactions.
Patients at risk of anaphylaxis should know early warning signs like swelling around lips. eyelids, wheezing shortness of breath, dizziness, lightheadedness, and respond quickly.

SUGGESTED READINGS

1. Cardona V, Ansotegui IJ, Ebisawa M, El-Gamal Y, Fernandez Rivas M, Fineman S, et al. World allergy organization anaphylaxis guidance 2020. World Allergy Organ J. 2020;13:100472.
2. Nguyen SMT, Rupprecht CP, Haque A, Pattanaik D, Yusin J, Krishnaswamy G. Mechanisms Governing Anaphylaxis: Inflammatory Cells, Mediators, Endothelial Gap Junctions and Beyond. Int J Mol Sci. 2021;22:7785.
3. Peavy RD, Metcalfe DD. Understanding the mechanisms of anaphylaxis. Curr Opin Allergy Clin Immunol. 2008;8:310-5.
4. Muñoz-Cano R, Picado C, Valero A, Bartra J. Mechanisms of Anaphylaxis Beyond IgE. J Investig Allergol Clin Immunol. 2016;26:73-82.
5. Pier J, Bingemann TA. Urticaria, Angioedema, and Anaphylaxis. Pediatr Rev. 2020;41:283-92.
6. Allen KJ, Koplin JJ. The epidemiology of IgE-mediated food allergy and anaphylaxis. Immunol Allergy Clin North Am. 2012;32:35-50.

CHAPTER 9

Chronic Spontaneous Urticaria

Neha Taneja, Gouri RP Anand

INTRODUCTION

Urticaria can be categorized into two main types: spontaneous and inducible. *Spontaneous* urticaria occurs without a clear trigger, while *inducible* urticaria is caused by specific, identifiable triggers. Chronic idiopathic urticaria, also known as chronic spontaneous urticaria (CSU), is a prevalent immunological condition affecting up to 20% of the global population at some point in their lives.

Chronic spontaneous urticaria is characterized by the recurrent appearance of intensely itchy hives, angioedema, or both, lasting for more than 6 weeks. This condition arises from autoreactivity or non-specific internal factors rather than external physical stimuli. In some patients with CSU; stress, certain foods, drugs [especially nonsteroidal anti-inflammatory drugs (NSAIDs)], or infections can trigger flare-ups. NSAID hypersensitivity occurs in up to 30% of CSU cases and is referred to as NSAID-exacerbated CSU. Exacerbations usually happen within minutes or hours after taking COX1 inhibitors, while selective COX2 inhibitors are generally tolerated. This sensitivity can be confirmed through oral drug provocation testing. *Acute urticaria*, on the other hand, persists for less than 6 weeks, with most cases resolving within a week; however, 5–40% of cases can progress to a chronic form. Acute urticaria often has no identifiable cause, although infections, medications, and foods may be relevant triggers in some instances.

Angioedema involves localized, non-pitting swelling of the deeper layers of the skin, commonly affecting the face and extremities. It can be warm and painful. Both urticaria and angioedema can occur separately or together. Angioedema occurs in 40–50% of CSU patients, while 13% of patients with CSU experience angioedema without hives.

Individual *wheals* develop rapidly, can change shape, and may merge to form larger patterns (annular, serpiginous or map-like patterns, and giant wheals). They typically resolve within 24 hours, although new wheals can appear repeatedly. Angioedema usually takes between 2 days and a week to subside. CSU symptoms can appear at any time but are often more common in the evening and night. This pattern may be linked to circadian variations in mast cell activity and differences in the disease's underlying mechanisms. Notably, the occurrence of symptoms at night has been associated with an autoimmune subtype of CSU. The associated intense itching can significantly impact daily activities and sleep. Systemic symptoms occur in 25–30% of cases and may include gastrointestinal issues, flushing, headaches, joint pain, and palpitations. Rarely, CSU can be associated with life-threatening anaphylaxis.

Certain populations are at *higher risk* for urticaria, including children, middle-aged women, and those with a history of atopy or allergies. The condition has a female-to-male ratio of 2:1 and often begins between the third and fifth decades of life.

Chronic spontaneous urticaria is *unpredictable* and usually resolves on its own within 1–5 years. The estimated rates of spontaneous remission are 17% at 1 year, 45% at 5 years, and 73% at 20 years. There is no cure for CSU; treatment focuses on managing symptoms. There is ongoing research into new targeted therapies, with several promising treatments in development.

This chapter explores the epidemiology, pathophysiology, diagnosis, screening, management, and quality of life associated with CSU, as well as recent advances in understanding the disease's pathogenesis and potential treatments.

RISK FACTORS

Genetic predisposition to CSU has been linked to polymorphisms in several genes, including interferon γ (*IFN-γ*), interleukin 6 (*IL-6*), interleukin 17 receptor A (*IL-17RA*), *IL-10*, transforming growth factor beta (*TGF-β*), tumor necrosis factor (*TNF*), protein tyrosine phosphatase non-receptor type 22 (PTPN22), *IL-1*, *IL-2*, and human leukocyte antigen (HLA) class I and II alleles. Notably, some of these genes, such as *PTPN22* and HLA alleles like HLA-DR4, are also implicated in the susceptibility to various autoimmune diseases. For instance, HLA-DR4 has shown a strong association with autoimmune CSU, particularly in cases where a positive basophil histamine release assay (BHRA) is present, as well as with other autoimmune disorders like rheumatoid arthritis and type 1 diabetes mellitus.

There is an increased risk of developing *autoimmune diseases* within 10 years after being diagnosed with CSU, especially among middle-aged women with autoimmune CSU. For example, women with CSU are significantly more likely to develop hypothyroidism and rheumatoid arthritis, being 23 and 20 times more likely, respectively, compared to controls. Around 80% of patients received a CSU diagnosis before being diagnosed with autoimmune diseases such as rheumatoid arthritis, systemic lupus erythematosus, type 1 diabetes mellitus, and celiac disease, while about 20% were diagnosed with CSU afterward. Patients, particularly women, with autoimmune thyroid diseases face a higher risk of developing CSU. Additionally, up to 25% of CSU patients, especially those with markers of autoimmune urticaria, report a family history of CSU. Female patients with conditions such as peptic ulcer disease and abnormal uterine bleeding are also at a higher risk of developing CSU.

PATHOPHYSIOLOGY

Chronic spontaneous urticaria arises from the *activation and degranulation of mast cells* in the skin, which subsequently release histamine and other mediators. This process triggers sensory nerve activation, vasodilation, plasma leakage, and the recruitment of immune cells **(Fig. 1)**.

Chronic spontaneous urticaria is primarily caused by *two mechanisms*:
1. Autoallergy (type I autoimmunity), involving IgE autoantibodies
2. Type IIb autoimmunity, involving IgG autoantibodies

These autoantibodies, along with immune cell infiltration, coagulation and complement system activation, are believed to play a central role in the development and progression of CSU.

Role of mast cells: Mast cells in the skin are crucial in the pathogenesis of urticaria. Their activation leads to the release of both pre-formed *mediators* (such as histamine, tryptase, and cytokines) and *newly synthesized mediators* (including leukotrienes, prostaglandin D2, and platelet-activating factor). This release results in vasodilation, increased vascular permeability, and stimulation of sensory nerve endings. Mast cell progenitors typically express the *c-Kit receptor and the high-affinity IgE receptor (FcεRI)* on their surface, which are essential for their survival and function. Various *cytokines, chemokines, and adhesion molecules*, such as IL-4, IL-5, IL-6, IL-15, IL-13, IL-17, IL-31, IL-33, IL-25, TNF-α, CCL-2, thymic stromal lymphopoietin (TSLP), and vascular cell adhesion molecule-1 (VCAM-1) derived from the tissue microenvironment, regulate the growth, migration, and maturation of mast cell precursors. However, the binding of *stem cell factor* (SCF) produced by fibroblasts, endothelial cells, and mast cells to the c-Kit receptor provides the most potent signal for their differentiation, migration, proliferation, and survival and apoptosis.

In some patients with CSU, an immunologic mechanism involving histamine-releasing *IgG autoantibodies* directed against the α subunit of FcεRI has been identified. These IgG autoantibodies can also target IgE/FcεRI complexes on the mast cell surface, leading to FcεRI cross-linking and activation of downstream signaling pathways, resulting in the release of both preformed and newly synthesized mediators. The anaphylatoxin C5a, produced during this process, may play a significant role. When FcεRI is activated by IgG-anti-FcεRI, C5a is generated and acts on its receptor, which is upregulated on skin mast cells in CSU. This type of immune response, involving IgG autoantibodies, is classified as type IIb autoimmune CSU. Patients with this form of CSU are at a higher risk of developing other autoimmune diseases, such as Hashimoto's thyroiditis or vitiligo. It is also characterized by elevated levels of IgG against thyroid peroxidase (TPO), low levels of IgE, a positive BHRA, reduced counts of basophils and eosinophils (basopenia and eosinopenia), and a positive autologous serum skin test (ASST). Traditionally, autoimmune CSU is typically diagnosed using a set of three criteria: Presence of IgG autoantibodies detected by immunoassay, the functional activity of these autoantibodies confirmed through basophil tests (basophil activation test and/or BHRA), and skin autoreactivity demonstrated by

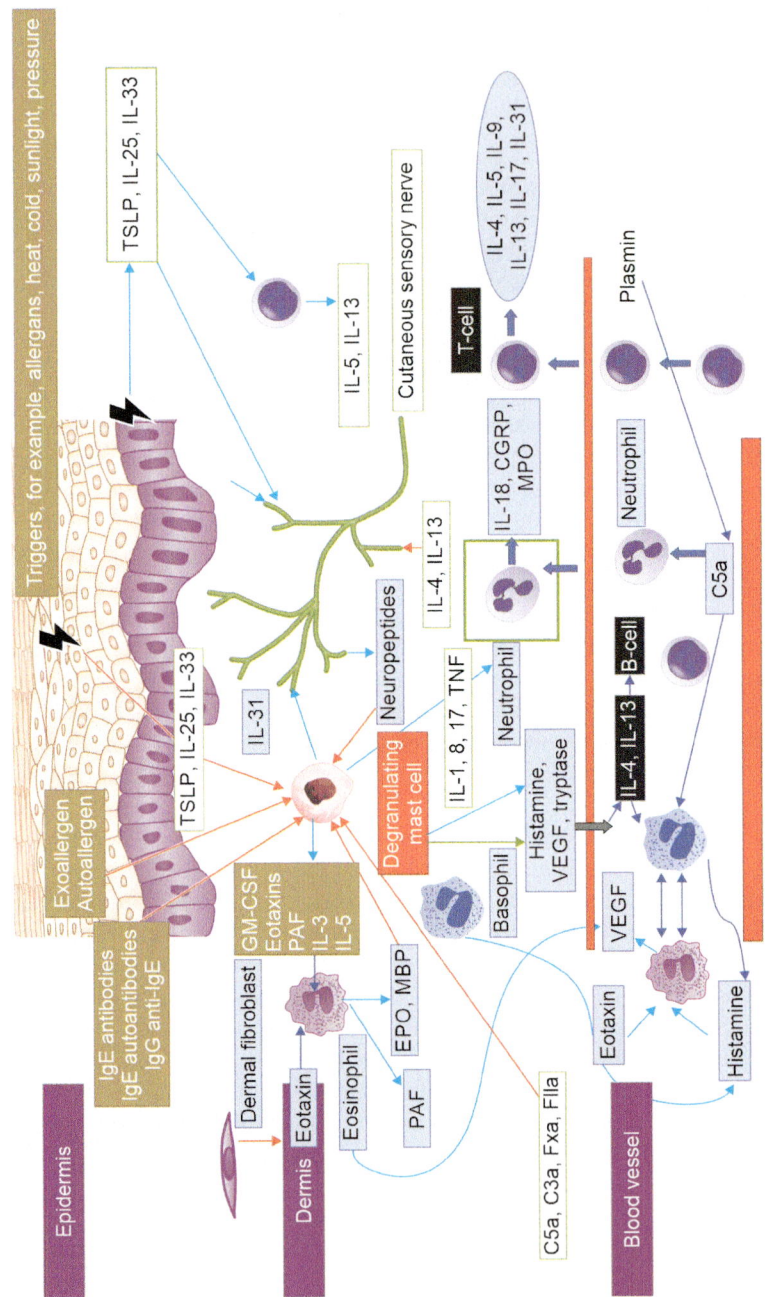

FIG. 1: Mechanisms and pathophysiology of chronic spontaneous urticaria.

a positive ASST. Although when these stringent criteria are used, only about 8% of CSU patients are classified as having autoimmune CSU.

The type I autoimmune endotype is defined by the presence of *IgE autoantibodies* targeting thyroid antigens, such as TPO, eosinophil peroxidase (EPO), and other autoallergens like tissue factor, thyroglobulin, double-stranded DNA, eosinophil cationic protein (ECP), and IL-24. These IgE autoantibodies can trigger mast cell degranulation by cross-linking the FcεRI receptor.

In addition to FcεRI, mast cells can be activated by several other receptors on their surface. These include the *Mas-related G-protein-coupled receptor-X2 (MRGPRX2)*, which can be triggered by substances such as major basic protein (MBP), EPO, substance P, cortistatin, vasoactive intestinal peptide (VIP), host defense peptides, certain small molecule drugs, opioids, antibiotics, and iodinated contrast media. Another important receptor is the *C5a receptor*, which is activated by the anaphylatoxin C5a. Mast cells also express *protease-activated receptors (PAR1 and PAR2)*, which respond to proteases like trypsin, tryptase, thrombin, and coagulation factors FVIIa and FXa, as well as tissue factor. Additionally, mast cells can be activated by the *chemoattractant receptor-homologous molecule expressed on Th2 cells (CRTh2)* and various cytokine receptors.

The activation of FcεRI involves several cytoplasmic signaling proteins, including *LYN, spleen tyrosine kinase (SYK), and Bruton's tyrosine kinase (BTK)*. These proteins phosphorylate downstream targets, leading to mast cell activation and degranulation. The signaling process begins with the phosphorylation of the FcεRI β-chain and γ-chain by LYN, which then activates SYK and BTK. BTK, a cytosolic tyrosine kinase, is a key positive regulator in this pathway, promoting mast cell activation and cytokine production. Additionally, BTK is essential for signaling through the B-cell receptor (BCR).

Recent in-vitro and ex-vivo studies have significantly advanced our understanding of the signal transduction pathways in human mast cells, particularly highlighting the roles of *SYK and BTK*. These kinases have emerged as potential targets for inhibiting mast cell activity in CSU, due to their involvement in early signaling processes. For instance, the SYK inhibitor GSK2646264 has been shown to inhibit histamine release from skin mast cells in ex vivo dermal tissue studies. Moreover, research involving BTK-null mice and patients with BTK deficiency has demonstrated the importance of BTK signaling in the activation of mast cells and basophils via FcεRI cross-linking. The absence of BTK in these models results in a reduced release of histamine and inflammatory cytokines from mast cells and basophils. Thus, targeting BTK signaling could potentially disrupt MC activation through FcεRI and hinder autoantibody production by B cells via BCR signaling. Recent clinical trials evaluating BTK inhibitors for CSU have yielded promising results regarding their efficacy and safety.

Role of cytokines, chemokines, endothelium, and coagulation systems: Chemokine signaling plays a major role in regulating the migration of inflammatory cells into the skin. Key chemokines, including *CCL2/monocyte chemoattractant protein (MCP)-1, CCL8/MCP-2, CCL7/MCP-3, and CCL13/MCP-4, along with CCL3/eotaxin-1, CCL24/eotaxin-2, CCL26/eotaxin-3, and CCL5/Regulated upon Activation, Normal T Cell Expressed and Secreted (RANTES)*, are mainly responsible for recruiting monocytes, eosinophils, basophils, neutrophils, and lymphocytes to urticarial lesions. Other chemotactic factors include *IL-5, C3a, C5a, TNF, IL-17, and platelet activating factor (PAF)*. These chemoattractants are released by mast cells, activated endothelial cells, TH2 cells, and dermal fibroblasts. *CCL5/RANTES* can also promote the migration, differentiation, and activation of progenitor mast cells in the dermal tissue. Since CCL5/RANTES is produced by mast cells and other inflammatory cells in the skin and circulation, its effects in CSU could persist over time, contributing to chronic inflammation.

This complex network of chemokines regulates cellular trafficking in inflamed tissues, working alongside the endothelium, which plays a crucial role in controlling fluid passage into tissues and influencing cellular infiltration in the dermis. Increased biomarkers of endothelial dysfunction, such as *soluble VCAM-1 and intercellular adhesion molecule-1 (ICAM-1)*, in the circulation and lesional skin of CSU patients indicate a proinflammatory state of the endothelium.

Additionally, the coagulation cascade, involving both extrinsic and intrinsic pathways, is activated in about 50% of CSU patients, evidenced by *elevated levels of mean platelet volume, factor VIIa, prothrombin fragment 1+2, D-dimer, fibrin, and fibrinogen degradation products*. The interplay between the endothelium and coagulation systems is significant. After endothelial activation, tissue factors are released, activating the extrinsic pathway, leading to the production of activated coagulation factors, such as factors Xa (FXa) and FIIa (thrombin) and promoting fibrinolysis. Thrombin, once produced, can directly affect the endothelium by increasing vascular permeability and vasodilation, thus amplifying inflammation. Plasma D-dimer levels, often elevated in severe CSU cases, tend to decrease following anti-IgE therapy, highlighting the connection between circulating autoantibodies, coagulation cascade activation, and fibrin degradation in severe cases of the disease.

Coagulation factors, histamine, VEGF, bradykinin, PAF, and other molecules can cause the formation of gaps between *vascular endothelial cells* through PAR1, other specific receptors, or direct action on endothelial cells. This process leads to the leakage of plasma-containing autoantibodies to IgE or FcεRI and/or autoantigens for specific IgE bound to mast cells in the skin, resulting in mast cell activation and the formation of wheals and flares. Additionally, thrombin and FXa can induce mast cell degranulation via action on PAR1 and PAR2, respectively. The complement component *C5a* is believed to be produced following the activation of the extrinsic coagulation pathway, fibrinolysis, or binding of IgG anti-FcεRI to FcεRI on mast cells and basophils. Activated coagulation factors (FXa and FIIa) and plasmin can generate C5a and C5b from C5, and/or C3a and C3b from C3. C3a and C5a in leaked plasma can activate mast cells and basophils via C3aR and C5aR, respectively. Moreover, specific IgE antibodies targeting tissue factor have been shown to release leukotriene C4 from tissue factor-stimulated peripheral basophils.

In patients with CSU, elevated levels of C-reactive protein (CRP) have been found to correlate with increased levels of *D-dimer, IL-6, C3, and C4*, as well as with CSU activity and positive ASST results. This suggests a strong connection between autoimmunity, inflammation, and the activation of complement and coagulation pathways in the pathogenesis of CSU, potentially contributing to the persistence and amplification of urticarial inflammation.

Neurogenic inflammation: In CSU, neurogenic inflammation involves a complex interaction between mast cells, immune cells, and sensory nerves. This interaction is mediated by the release of histamine, IL-31, neuropeptides, and other substances, leading to symptoms like vasodilation, plasma leakage, pruritus, and other urticarial symptoms. The MRGPRX2 is crucial in this process, as it mediates mast cell activation independent of IgE. Exogenous and endogenous substances, including MBP and EPO, can trigger histamine release via MRGPRX2. Elevated levels of the neuropeptide substance P, an MRGPRX2 agonist, have been observed in CSU, correlating with disease activity and increased skin reactivity. Additionally, the number of mast cells expressing MRGPRX2 is increased in patients with CSU.

Other cellular infiltrates: In approximately 10–15% of patients with CSU, blood basopenia and eosinopenia may indicate the migration of these cells into the skin. These conditions are linked to disease activity, the presence of autoantibodies, and a poor response to H1 antihistamines and omalizumab. *Eosinophils and neutrophils* were observed around blood vessels in wheals 30 minutes after the intradermal injection of autologous serum, with numbers increasing along with T lymphocytes over the following 2 hours, and then decreasing after 48 hours for neutrophils and later for eosinophils and *lymphocytes*. Both blood and skin-migrated *basophils* may contribute to CSU pathogenesis by releasing histamine, leukotrienes, and cytokines via activation of FcεRI and C5aR.

In the wheals of CSU patients, eosinophil granule proteins such as MBP have been detected. MBP can induce mast cell activation and degranulation, indicating a potential interaction between eosinophils and mast cells in CSU. Eosinophils can be activated by mast cell mediators like IL-5, TNF, PAF, eotaxin, and IgG autoantibodies targeting the low-affinity IgE receptor. Activated eosinophils can also release SCF, a growth factor for mast cells. Eosinophils may also play a significant role in activating the coagulation cascade and the MRGPRX2 on mast cells by expressing tissue factor and releasing MRGPRX2 agonists.

Th2 cells are the predominant lymphocytes found in CSU skin biopsy samples, although Th1 and Th17 cells are also present. Th2 cells play a major role in allergic diseases by releasing various cytokines, stimulating IgE production, and activating mast cells, basophils, and eosinophils. In CSU patients, increased levels, or expression of cytokines such as IFN-γ, TNF, TGF-β, IL-1β, IL-3, IL-4, IL-5, IL-6, IL-13, IL-17, IL-23, IL-24, IL-31, and IL-33 have been noted in the blood and/or lesional skin. These cytokines correlate with disease activity, including TNF, IL-6, IL-17, IL-23, and IL-24, as well as ASST positivity, particularly IL-17.

Table 1 enlists some of the biomarkers used in CSU as indicators of disease activity/severity.

TABLE 1: Biomarkers in chronic spontaneous urticaria (CSU).

Biomarkers	Marker of disease activity/severity
Anti-IL-24 IgE	Active disease
Anti-TPO or IgE and/or IgG	Active disease
IgG- anti-FcεRI	Active disease and poor treatment response
C5a	Active disease
D-dimer	Active disease and poor treatment responses to antihistamines
• IL-6, CRP, • IL-33, 35 (lesional) • Thymic stromal lymphopoietin (TSLP)	• Active disease • Increased CRP is associated with poor treatment responses
IL-17	Recurrent flares
IgE	• Low level in type 2b CSU • Low levels associated with lower chances of response to omalizumab and vice versa
FcεRI	• Low levels in type 2b CSU • Low level associated with lower chances of responses to omalizumab
Basopenia and eosinopenia	• Both are markers of type 2b CSU • Basopenia associated with increased disease severity • Eosinopenia associated with active disease • Both are indicators of poor treatment responses

DIAGNOSIS AND EVALUATION

The 7C concept for comprehensive workup of CSU include (The International EAACI/GA²LEN/EuroGuiDerm/APAAACI guidelines, 2022):
- *Confirming* diagnosis; exclude differential diagnoses like dermatoses mimicking urticaria and pseudourticaria
- Checking for any underlying *causes*; excludes physical urticarias by skin challenge testing and checking for markers of autoimmune urticaria
- Check for any triggers (*cofactors*) that may modify disease activity
- Looking for any *comorbidities* (autoimmune disorder, mental health disorders)
- Checking for the *consequences* of disease (sleep disturbance, distress, impaired sexual health, and social performance)
- Assessing the predictors (*components*) of disease course and response to treatment
- Monitoring disease activity and control (*course*)

Guidelines recommend minimal laboratory investigations for CSU. Key steps include *clinical history, physical examination*, and review of prior images of wheals and angioedema. The lesions in CSU are noninducible, and provocation/challenge tests typically yield negative results. Routine laboratory tests such as *complete and differential blood count, CRP level, and/or erythrocyte sedimentation rate (ESR)* are suggested. A high ratio of *IgG-anti-TPO* to *total IgE* may indicate autoimmune CSU, particularly in patients who do not respond to H1 antihistamines. This can help identify the presence of antibodies against IgE, FcɛRI, or FcɛRII or other histamine-releasing factors and predict treatment outcomes with omalizumab or immunosuppressants like cyclosporin, although these biomarkers are not routinely tested. *ASST* may also be used to diagnose an autoreactive form of the disease, although it has limited predictive value.

ASSOCIATED CONDITIONS WITH CHRONIC SPONTANEOUS URTICARIA

Chronic inducible urticaria (CIndU) is a common comorbidity of CSU, with studies showing that over 10% of CSU patients also have CIndU.

Autoimmune diseases, particularly autoimmune thyroid diseases like Hashimoto's thyroiditis, are found in approximately 28% of CSU patients. Other autoimmune conditions include vitiligo, rheumatoid arthritis, autoimmune gastritis, and diabetes mellitus.

Bacterial infections, including *Helicobacter pylori* and focal infections like dental issues, have been reported in up to 77% of CSU patients, although the evidence linking these infections to CSU is inconclusive. The impact of *viral infections* (such as viral hepatitis and HIV) and fungal infections on CSU is still unclear and likely minimal. During the COVID-19 pandemic, chronic urticaria did not alter the course of the virus, though *COVID-19* exacerbated CSU symptoms in about one-third of patients, particularly those with severe cases. There is some evidence that treating *helminth or protozoal infections* with antiparasitic drugs can improve CSU symptoms, though the connection between CSU and parasitic infections is not well established.

Patients with CSU are significantly more likely to have *allergic conditions* compared to the general population. Type I hypersensitivity to allergens should be excluded as a cause of CSU, especially in patients with intermittent symptoms, temporal correlation with a specific allergen, or symptoms related to other allergic conditions like asthma.

Malignancy, primarily non-hematologic, has been reported in about 0.1–9% of patients with CSU. Some cases showed resolution of CSU following cancer remission. The development of CSU in cancer patients may be linked to immune dysregulation caused by cancer, such as activation of the complement and coagulation cascades.

Mental health disorders, including depression and anxiety, are present in up to 60% of CSU patients, significantly impairing their quality of life.

Additionally, the prevalence of *metabolic syndrome*—central obesity, dyslipidemia, hyperglycemia, and hypertension—is notably higher in patients with CSU.

TABLE 2: 7-Day Urticaria Activity Score for assessing disease activity in chronic spontaneous urticaria (CSU).		
Score	Wheals	Pruritus
0	None	None
1	Mild (<20 wheals per 24 hours)	Mild (not annoying/troublesome)
2	Moderate (20–50 wheals per 24 hours)	Moderate (troublesome but does not interfere normal activity/sleep)
3	Intense (>50 wheals per 24 hours) or large confluent wheals	Intense (severe pruritus interfere with daily normal activity/sleep)

ASSESSMENT OF DISEASE ACTIVITY AND CONTROL IN CHRONIC SPONTANEOUS URTICARIA

The impact of CSU on patients is significant, affecting quality of life, sleep, physical and emotional well-being, and performance at work or school. The *7-Day Urticaria Activity Score (UAS7)* is a gold standard score for assessing disease activity and treatment response. For patients with angioedema, with or without wheals, the *Angioedema Activity Score* should also be used, alongside UAS7. Quality of life (QoL) can be measured using the *Chronic Urticaria Quality of Life (CU-Q2oL)* questionnaire for patients with wheals and the *Angioedema Urticaria Quality of Life questionnaire* for those with angioedema.

The goal of treatment is to achieve and maintain symptom control (UAS7 ≤ 6) or remission (UAS7 = 0 and UCT = 16). **Table 2** provides a brief outline of the UAS7 for assessing disease activity in CSU.

Urticaria control test (UCT) is a validated tool used to measure disease control in CSU. It consists of four questions with five answer options, with a score of 12 or above indicating well-controlled disease. The questions assess the frequency of physical symptoms (itching, wheals, swelling), quality of life over the past month, adequacy of treatment in controlling symptoms, and overall disease control.

The *Angioedema Control Test (AECT)* is used to measure disease control in patients with CSU and angioedema, as well as those with other forms of recurrent angioedema. It has two versions: One with a 4-week recall period and another with a 3-month recall period. A score of 10 or above indicates well-controlled disease.

Both UCT and AECT scores help guide treatment decisions.

Remission is defined as the total absence of disease signs or symptoms without treatment for 2 weeks with standard H1-antihistamines (H1-AH), 4 weeks with up-dosed H1-AH, and 3–6 months with biological therapy. *Recurrence* is defined as the return of symptoms at least 6 months after stopping controller therapy and the resolution of previous chronic urticaria symptoms. These definitions are not yet standardized.

DIFFERENTIAL DIAGNOSIS IN CHRONIC SPONTANEOUS URTICARIA

For patients with wheals without angioedema, consider differential diagnoses like *autoinflammatory disorders* such as Schnitzler syndrome or cryopyrin-associated periodic syndromes. Wheals in these conditions are often resistant to antihistamines and may present as neutrophilic urticarial dermatosis.

In *urticarial vasculitis*, both long-lasting wheals (>24 hours) with pain/burning and angioedema can occur. Diagnosis involves histological criteria including leukocytoclasia, fibrin deposits in vessel wall, and extravasated red blood cells (RBCs).

For patients with recurrent angioedema without wheals, exclude *bradykinin-mediated angioedema*, including those induced by angiotensin-converting enzyme inhibitors and hereditary angioedema.

TREATMENT OF CHRONIC SPONTANEOUS URTICARIA

*The 3A management approach—assess, act, and adjust—*acknowledges the significance of various comorbidities linked to urticaria. It also recognizes the fluctuating severity of the disease over time, emphasizing the need to escalate or de-escalate therapies to achieve complete disease control while minimizing costs and adverse effects.

Assess:
- *Diagnosis*: Exclude mimics
- *Comorbidities and special populations*: Children or pregnancy
- *Severity assessment*: Patient-reported outcome measures
- Patient preferences
- Adverse effects expected

Act:
- Start treatment **(Flowchart 1)** and treat comorbidities.
- Look at nonpharmacological interventions.
- Patient education

Adjust:
- Step up if inadequate control **(Flowchart 1)**
- Change if adverse effects occur
- Step down if symptom free for 3-6 months

Second-generation H1 antihistamines are first-line treatments for CSU, although no single drug stands out as the most effective. Instead of blocking histamine binding, second-generation H1 antihistamines function as inverse agonists, producing an opposite effect on the receptor compared to histamine and thus shifting the equilibrium toward the inactive state. About 61% of CSU patients do not respond to standard doses of H1 antihistamines, so the EAACI/

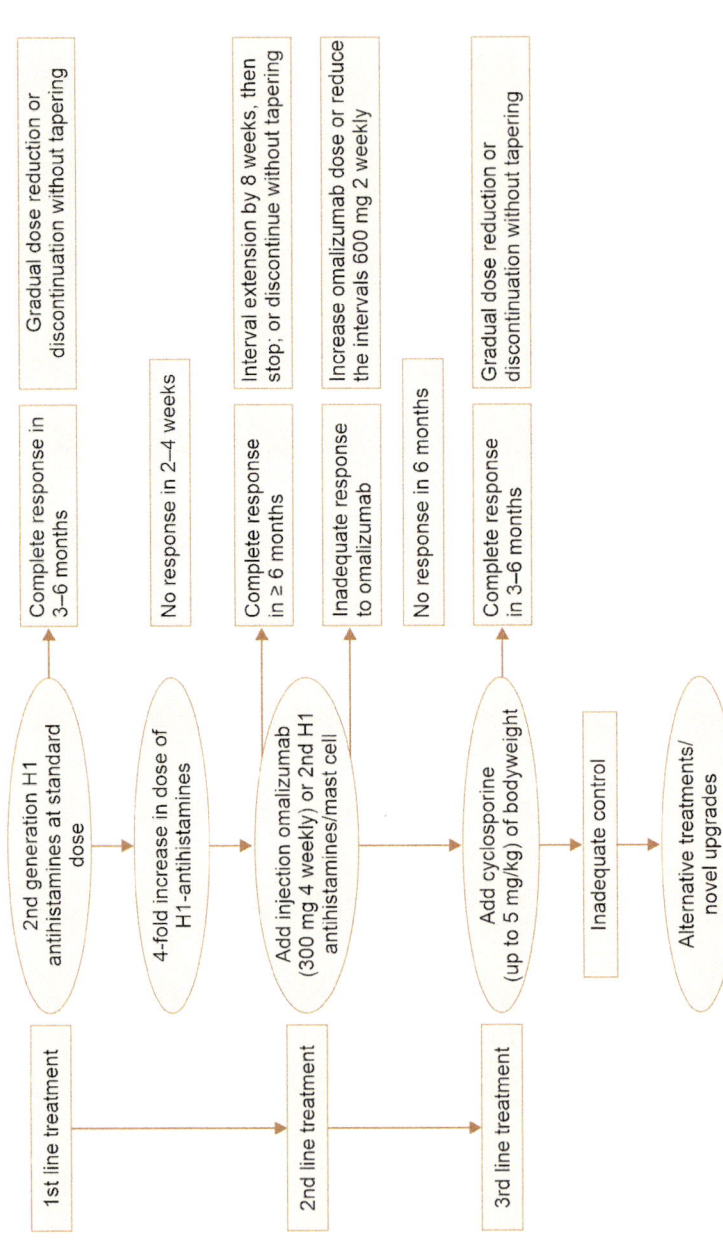

FLOWCHART 1: Treatment guidelines for chronic spontaneous urticaria.

GA²LEN/EuroGuiDerm/APAAAC International Urticaria guidelines recommend adjusting treatment (stepping up and stepping down) based on disease control. Considering the half-life of antihistamines, a 2-week period is typically adequate to observe the effects of changes in treatment for CSU. For patients not responding to standard doses of second-generation H1 antihistamines or UCT score of 12 or lesser, a four-fold increase in dosage is advised, which usually leads to complete remission in around 50–60% of the patients. After achieving complete control for at least 3 consecutive months, stepping-down treatment is advised. If the control is lost during treatment step-down, revert to the last effective dose. It has also been demonstrated in studies that while only 10% of children may be unresponsive to maximally updosed second-generation H1 antihistamines, unresponsiveness might be seen in up to 50% of adults.

Omalizumab, an anti-IgE antibody, approved by the Food and Drug Administration (FDA) since 2014 for patients over 12 years of age, is given at a dose of 300 mg every 4 weeks, with adjustments possible up to 600 mg every 14 days. Also, a maximum of up to 6 months should be allowed for response assessment. It is considered as the second-line therapy as an add-on to second-generation H1 antihistamines and is indicated in patients with CSU who do not respond to four-fold doses of antihistamines. It binds to and reduces free IgE levels, leading to the downregulation of FcεRI on basophils and mast cells. This reduction in FcεRI expression decreases the cells' susceptibility to activation by IgE and IgG anti-FcεRI, thereby preventing histamine release and inflammation. It has been shown to have a rapid and effective response in patients with IgE autoantibodies against allergens such as TPO (Type 1 CSU). A poor or slow response to omalizumab has been associated with various markers and characteristics of autoimmune CSU, such as BHRA positivity and low total IgE levels. The response to omalizumab can be as rapid as 1 week to within 4 weeks or delayed as 4 weeks to within 24 weeks. It has demonstrated effectiveness in several studies, with response rates between 26% and 83%. However, around 30% of patients may not respond to a 6-month course. Discontinuation of omalizumab is done after 6–12 months of treatment in cases of adequate response and relapses are usually observed after 24 weeks of stopping therapy. The risk–benefit profile of high-dose omalizumab is superior to that of cyclosporine, which should be considered for the treatment of patients who do not respond to higher than standard doses of omalizumab. Local side effects include skin inflammation at the injection site, while systemic reactions can involve anaphylaxis. There is limited long-term data on the use of omalizumab for CSU.

Long-term treatment with *cyclosporine* (third-line treatment agent) is generally safe and effective, although blood pressure and renal function (blood urea nitrogen and creatinine levels) should be monitored every 6 weeks. It is an immunosuppressive agent targeting T cells that also inhibits the release of mediators from basophils and mast cells. A network meta-analysis indicated that combining cyclosporine with antihistamines leads to better improvement in UAS7 for CSU patients compared to *methotrexate and azathioprine*, with an overall response rate of 54–73% with cyclosporine.

Systemic corticosteroids are only recommended for acute flares for a rapid control. Experts and guidelines suggest that oral steroid therapy should be limited to a maximum of 10 days, using the lowest effective dose.

Other treatments include *leukotriene receptor antagonists (montelukast), mast cell stabilizers, first-generation antihistamines, doxepin, and H2 antihistamines (ranitidine)*, with combined therapy offering benefits. *Dapsone, colchicine, sulfasalazine, along with other immunosuppressants like mycophenolate mofetil (MMF), interferons, and phototherapy* can be tried for resistant cases.

Ligelizumab (second-generation humanized anti-IgE monoclonal antibody), with 40-fold higher IgE affinity and a slower offloading time, showed better results than placebo but was not superior to omalizumab in phase III trials (PEARL1 and PEARL2 trials).

Dupilumab (anti-IL-4Rα mAb) was also ineffective in omalizumab-resistant cases.

Anti-IL-5 (*mepolizumab*) and anti-IL-5R (*benralizumab*) monoclonal antibodies have shown promising early results, while *canakinumab* (anti-IL-1b) did not prove effective in clinical trials.

New therapies such as *fenebrutinib and remibrutinib (BTK inhibitors), barzolvolimab (anti-KIT mAb), tezepelumab, lirentelimab (anti-Siglec-8 mAb), secukinumab (anti-IL-17 mAb), and CDX-0159* are in clinical trials, and *plasmapheresis and intravenous immunoglobulin* may be occasionally effective.

CONCLUSION

The landscape of urticaria pathogenesis and treatment is rapidly evolving. In the coming years, significant advancements in chronic urticaria therapy are expected as new small molecules and biologics become available, addressing many of the current unmet needs. These emerging targeted treatments will facilitate a personalized therapeutic approach for patients and aid in endotype characterization and biomarker development, ultimately aiming for disease modification and remission. Additionally, their use will enhance the understanding of disease mechanisms, including the roles of mast cells, basophils, B cells, and other inflammatory cells in urticaria.

SUGGESTED READINGS

1. Zuberbier T, Bernstein JA, Maurer M. Chronic spontaneous urticaria guidelines: What is new? J Allergy Clin Immunol. 2022;150(6):1249-55.
2. GlobeNewswire.com. (2021). Novartis provides an update on phase III ligelizumab (QGE031) studies in chronic spontaneous urticaria (CSU). [online] Available from https://www.globenewswire.com/news-release/2021/12/20/2354923/0/en/Novartis-provides-an-update-on-Phase-III-ligelizumab-QGE031-studies-in-chronic-spontaneous-urticaria-CSU.html [Last accessed November, 2024].
3. Kolkhir P, Giménez-Arnau AM, Kulthanan K, Peter J, Metz M, Maurer M. Urticaria. Nat Rev Dis Primers. 2022;8(1):61.
4. Church MK, Kolkhir P, Metz M, Maurer M. The role and relevance of mast cells in urticaria. Immunol Rev. 2018;282(1):232-47.

5. Kaplan A, Lebwohl M, Giménez-Arnau AM, Hide M, Armstrong AW, Maurer M. Chronic spontaneous urticaria: Focus on pathophysiology to unlock treatment advances. Allergy. 2023;78(2):389-401.
6. Greaves M. Autoimmune urticaria. Clin Rev Allergy Immunol. 2002;23(2):171-83.
7. Armstrong AW, Soong W, Bernstein JA. Chronic Spontaneous Urticaria: How to Measure It and the Need to Define Treatment Success. Dermatol Ther (Heidelb). 2023;13(8):1629-46.
8. Giménez-Arnau AM, Jáuregui I, Silvestre-Salvador JF, Valero A, Ferrer M, Sastre J, et al. Consensus on the definition of disease control and response assessment in chronic urticaria. J Investig Allergol Clin Immunol. 2022;32:261-9.
9. Kim JK, Har D, Brown LS, Khan DA. Recurrence of chronic urticaria: incidence and associated factors. J Allergy Clin Immunol Pract. 2018;6:582-5.
10. Guillen-Aguinaga S, Jáuregui Presa I, Aguinaga-Ontoso E, Guillen-Grima F, Ferrer M. Updosing nonsedating antihistamines in patients with chronic spontaneous urticaria: a systematic review and meta-analysis. Br J Dermatol. 2016;175(6):1153-65.
11. Yosipovitch G, Biazus Soares G, Mahmoud O. Current and Emerging Therapies for Chronic Spontaneous Urticaria: A Narrative Review. Dermatol Ther (Heidelb). 2023;13(8):1647-60.
12. Terhorst-Molawi D, Fox L, Siebenhaar F, Metz M, Maurer M. Stepping Down Treatment in Chronic Spontaneous Urticaria: What We Know and What We Don't Know. Am J Clin Dermatol. 2023;24(3):397-404.
13. Gabrielli S, Le M, Netchiporouk E, Miedzybrodzki B, Baum S, Greenberger S, et al. Chronic urticaria in children can be controlled effectively with updosing second-generation antihistamines. J Am Acad Dermatol. 2020;82:1535-7.
14. Sarti L, Barni S, Giovannini M, Liccioli G, Novembre E, Mori F, et al. Efficacy and tolerability of the updosing of second-generation non-sedating H1 antihistamines in children with chronic spontaneous urticaria. Pediatr Allergy Immunol. 2021;32:153-60.
15. Casale TB, Gimenez-Arnau AM, Bernstein JA, Holden M, Zuberbier T, Maurer M. Omalizumab for Patients with Chronic Spontaneous Urticaria: A Narrative Review of Current Status. Dermatol Ther (Heidelb). 2023;13(11):2573-88.
16. Kolkhir P, Muñoz M, Asero R, Ferrer M, Kocatürk E, Metz M, et al. Autoimmune chronic spontaneous urticaria. J Allergy Clin Immunol. 2022;149(6):1819-31.
17. Bei W, Qian J, Zilu Q, Kai C, Ruili J, Feng H, Liuqing C. Comparing four immunosuppressive agents for chronic spontaneous urticaria-A network meta-analysis. Int Immunopharmacol. 2023;123:110577.
18. Kulthanan K, Chaweekulrat P, Komoltri C, Hunnangkul S, Tuchinda P, Chularojanamontri L, et al. Cyclosporine for Chronic Spontaneous Urticaria: A Meta-Analysis and Systematic Review. J Allergy Clin Immunol Pract. 2018;6(2):586-99.
19. de Silva NL, Damayanthi H, Rajapakse AC, Rodrigo C, Rajapakse S. Leukotriene receptor antagonists for chronic urticaria: a systematic review. Allergy Asthma Clin Immunol. 2014;10(1):24.
20. Khan S, Chopra C, Mitchell A, Nakonechna A, Yong P, Karim MY. Resistant Chronic Spontaneous Urticaria - A Case Series Narrative Review of Treatment Options. Allergy Rhinol (Providence). 2022;13:21526575221144951.

CHAPTER 10

Physical Urticaria

Mansak Shishak

INTRODUCTION

Physical urticaria is a group of inducible urticarial conditions where lesions appear following an exogenous contact or trigger. Some of these include cold contact urticaria, dermographism, heat contact urticaria, delayed pressure urticaria, and vibratory urticaria/angioedema. Physical urticarias are induced by environmental stimuli acting on the skin, including thermal (cold, heat), electromagnetic radiation (solar radiation), and mechanical triggers (friction, pressure, vibration).

Physical urticarias are frequently associated with chronic urticarial symptoms and constitute up to 17% of chronic urticarias.

It is important to distinguish physical urticaria from spontaneous urticaria as well as other inducible forms of urticaria. The types of physical urticaria are elucidated in **Box 1**. Though cholinergic urticaria is mentioned as a form of physical urticaria, strictly speaking, it is not a true type as its symptoms are induced by an increase in the core body temperature and not due to external physical stimuli.

DERMOGRAPHISM

Dermographism is also known as dermatographism, meaning "to write on the skin." Firm stroking of the skin produces an initial red linear rash (capillary

---

Box 1: Types of physical urticaria.

- Dermographism
- Solar urticaria
- Aquagenic urticaria
- Cholinergic urticaria
- Cold urticaria
- Pressure urticaria
- Vibratory urticaria
- Exercise-induced anaphylaxis

dilation), followed by an axon reflex flare with broadening/spread of the erythema and formation of wheal (edema stage). Simple dermatographism is characterized by stroking of the skin with moderate pressure resulting in a wheal and flare reaction without pruritus. As it has no itch symptom, it is considered asymptomatic. It typically takes 6–7 minutes to observe the response and 15–30 minutes for lesions to subside. Whereas in symptomatic dermographism, there is earlier onset formation of linear, pruritic wheals (within 2–5 minutes of applied friction) and can last from 1/2 to 3 hours. It is accompanied by symptoms such as mild-to-moderate itch.

Symptoms often appear at sites of mild pressure, for example, around neck collars and wristbands or watches, or areas of pressure around elasticated garments and ankles where the socks pull over. It is estimated to affect around 2–5% of the general population. Commonly, the lesions resolve quickly within 10–20 minutes and generally within 1 hour.

Dermographism may also be classified into intermediate and delayed forms (delayed-pressure urticaria). The delayed types develop more slowly and can last many hours to several days. It differs from common symptomatic dermographism in that it presents with additional symptoms such as burning and pain. The wheals are typically known to be painful, with stinging or burning sensation, as opposed to being pruritic and may have a slight local rise in temperature on palpation.

Delayed pressure urticaria is one of the rarest subtypes and can occur simultaneously with chronic idiopathic urticaria in up to 40% of cases. It is important to identify a pressure as a triggering factor of new lesions. Lesions commonly present as deep-seated swellings, resembling vasculitides, and can occur anywhere after prolonged pressure has been exerted to the skin. Stimuli include sitting, use of hand tools, holding objects tight against the body, or on close contact clothing or accessories, such as belts, or shoes. Wheals frequently develop few hours following a stimulus and can last up to 3 days.

Associated conditions are hypereosinophilic syndrome where up to 75% patients have been found to have dermographism. Stress and psychological factors may be associated triggers though a clear link is not proven.

Pathogenesis

Trauma following scratching may release an antigen that interacts with membrane-bound IgE of mast cells. This releases inflammatory mediators such as histamine into the tissues. Other mediators include kallikrein, leukotrienes, heparin, bradykinin, and substance P. Symptomatic dermographism may be triggered by insect bite and *Helicobacter pylori* infection. Cases triggered by coral reef as well as dermographism as a manifestation of dermatomyositis have been reported.

Diagnosis

Asymptomatic or simple dermographism is the most common variant and is well controlled. Associations with thyroid disorder are not well-established. Mechanically agitating the skin by rubbing can elicit symptoms. the appearance of wheals is influenced by stressors including mental stress. In clinical settings, it can be demonstrated by scratching the skin with tools such as keys, or pen; following which wheal and flare reaction is often observed, with varying intensities within minutes. By using a dermographometer, well-defined pressure is exerted on the subject's skin where the response in simple dermatographism is obtained at 4,900 g/cm^2, while in symptomatic dermatographism the threshold is 3,200–3,600 g/cm^2.

DIFFERENTIAL DIAGNOSIS

- Systemic mastocytosis
- Urticaria pigmentosa

TYPES OF DERMOGRAPHISM

- *White dermographism*: Blanching response, following scratch due to vasoconstriction and is observed in atopics
- *Black dermographism*: A dark discoloration, which is not true dermographism and occurs due to direct contact with metallic objects
- *Yellow dermographism*: Bile pigment deposits on skin may mimic a similar vascular response.
- *Red derrmographism*: As seen in Urticaria

Treatment

Simple or asymptomatic dermographism rarely requires active treatment but can be distressing. In symptomatic dermographism, avoidance of known/established triggers is helpful. Antihistaminic agents such as H1 antihistamines are the initial drugs of choice. Combination of two antihistamines is required in some cases. Omalizumab, a recombinant monoclonal antibody against immunoglobulin E (IgE), has been used in some cases and shown to improve quality of life (QoL) following symptom control. Phototherapy with ultraviolet B (UVB) light and PUVA may give temporary relief of symptoms.

SOLAR URTICARIA

First described by Merklen in 1904, solar urticaria refers to the induction of recurrent episodes of pruritus, erythema, and wheal formation after brief exposure of the skin to sunlight. It may also follow exposure to an artificial light source of specific wavelengths. It is considered as a chronic acquired photosensitivity disorder. Little is known about it; it may cause extreme distress, thus severely reducing the QoL of affected individuals. The radiation spectrum of action for solar urticaria ranges from ultraviolet B to visible light (wavelength of 300–500 nm) and is variable from one patient to another. It is an uncommon subset of physical urticaria, and most literature is limited to case reports and series. In a review of 2,310 cases of urticaria over three decades, it was found that only 0.4% were classified as solar urticaria. It accounts for only 0.5% of chronic urticaria worldwide. There appears to be a predilection for a slightly higher incidence in females, with a mean age of initial presentation at 35 years.

Pathogenesis

Following sun exposure, it is postulated that the UV radiation activates an endogenous substance (chromophore) present in the serum and/or the dermis. This converts it into an immunologically active agent with photoallergen potential, which later induces the degranulation of mast cells. Clinically, patients present with urticarial wheals which may be localized to sites of exposure or generalized affecting widespread areas.

An intradermal injection test using a patient's serum irradiated with UV light when positive confirms the hypothesis of a circulating chromophore as the causative culprit in solar urticaria. This also strongly hints at an IgE-mediated hypersensitivity reaction.

Drug-induced Solar Urticaria

Certain drugs have been implicated in causing solar urticarial wheals. These include tetracyclines, atorvastatin, chlorpromazine, and oral contraceptives.

Diagnosis

Solar urticaria is diagnosed by patient history. In addition, clinical phototesting may aid its confirmation; it is of two types:
1. *Anamnesis*: It refers to the development of transient urticarial lesions occurring a few minutes after exposure to sunlight and is a direct correlation strongly suggestive of solar urticaria. In the absence of solar trigger/sun exposure, physical examination is normal.
2. *Photopatch test*: This has theoretical value in ruling out other photosensitive conditions such as photocontact dermatitis.

DIFFERENTIAL DIAGNOSIS

- Polymorphous light eruption (PMLE)
- Lupus erythematosus (LE) and its variants
- Drug-induced photosensitivity, including chemotherapeutic agents
- Photocontact dermatitis/photoallergic dermatitis
- Porphyria cutanea tarda (PCT)

Treatment

The management involves ruling out differentials of solar urticaria. Prevention of episodes after implication of UV radiation/sun exposure as trigger is key. However, this is barely feasible and leads to a very impaired QoL. Photoprotection with broad-spectrum sunscreens is vital, with adequate frequency of application.

First-line drug therapy includes second-generation antihistamine H1 receptor antagonists: Loratadine, fexofenadine, and cetirizine. It involves increased frequency of dosing, and erythema does not settle fully despite higher doses. This shows the chronicity of condition, where spontaneous remission is less likely.

Second-line therapy involves phototherapy. Use of UVA, UVB, visible light, and photochemotherapy (PUVA) gradually induces tolerance to sunlight and enables a decrease in the severity of symptoms.

Other agents: In severe or refractory cases, intravenous immunoglobulin, plasma exchange, cyclosporine, and omalizumab have been tried and found to be of moderate benefit. There is always the possibility of concurrent photoaggravating dermatosis, which can delay response to treatment. In such cases, combination treatments may be more helpful to attain clinical relief and remission. The therapeutic role of oral steroids and oral antioxidants such as beta-carotene, antimalarials, and prostaglandin inhibitors is doubtful.

Patient counseling is difficult, and prognosis remains challenging due to many being restricted to living a life indoors and away from light triggers.

AQUAGENIC URTICARIA

Aquagenic urticaria, as the name suggests, is urticaria arising from direct skin contact with water. It is vital to distinguish it from aquagenic pruritus and other physical urticarias, particularly cholinergic and cold-induced urticaria. It is a rare condition and first described by Shelley and Rawnsley. There is a slight female preponderance, with an age of onset slightly at or after puberty. A strong family history has been recorded.

Pathogenesis

Shelley and Rawnsley postulated that water alone was not responsible but its interaction with sebum to form a substance capable of mast cell degranulation, resulting in histamine release. Chalamidas' study on patch testing with a patient's sweat produced only erythema, whereas testing with sweat and sebum produced marked urticaria, seemingly confirming Shelly's hypothesis. Sibbald et al. showed that complete removal of the stratum corneum layer of the skin worsened the lesions. Pretreatment with organic solvents enhanced the ability of water to penetrate stratum corneum and increased the chances of aquagenic wheals.

Clinical Features

Temporary urticarial wheals appear rapidly (20–30 minutes) after direct contact with any source of water (i.e., distilled, tap, or saline). They are small, punctate (1 –3 mm), perifollicular lesions that can be generalized over the body, usually sparing the palms and soles. Lesions are not influenced by temperature or pH of water, and last up to 1 hour. These may be associated with systemic symptoms.

Differential Diagnosis
- Cholinergic urticaria
- Aquagenic pruritus

Treatment
The response to antihistamines is variable. Narrowband UVB (NB-UVB) light treatment and PUVA have been tried. In a patient with HIV, response to the anabolic steroid stanozolol was dramatic and effective but lesions recurred on stopping of treatment.

COLD URTICARIA

Cold urticaria is a type of chronic inducible urticaria characterized by the development of wheals, angioedema, or both in response to cold stimulus and limited to the site of cold contact, whether on skin and/or mucosa.

Cold urticaria can be classified into typical or atypical types, wherein typical cold urticaria refers to development of wheals post cold contact, resolving within an hour. This is clinically reproducible with "ice cube test" with generation of wheals soon after ice contact. Atypical cold urticaria is more complex and less defined. Here, lesions do not respond but appear typically following ice cube stimulation. Furthermore, cold urticaria may be subdivided into systemic atypical, localized cold urticaria, localized cold reflex urticaria, delayed and cold-induced cholinergic urticaria, and cold-dependent dermographism.

Pathogenesis
There may be de novo formation of autoantigens capable of inducing an IgE response and, in sensitized individuals, IgE-dependent mast cell degranulation.

Clinical Features
There may be associated systemic features along with wheal development such as fever, nausea, hypotension, dizziness, pain abdomen, syncope, and angioedema.

There are varied temperature responses to label or identify the temperature threshold responsible for the trigger. Individual critical temperature thresholds vary from below 4°C to higher than 27°C.

Treatment
Identification of cold triggers and avoidance of cold stimulation prevent the episodes of cold urticarias. This is especially important in cases of oropharyngeal symptoms on consumption of cold foods and beverages. Second-generation antihistamines such as desloratadine and bilastine have been tried and found to be useful. Other agents include off-label and alternative options such as doxepin,

ciclosporin, azathioprine, omalizumab, mycophenolate mofetil, etanercept, dupilumab, and reslizumab.

Differential Diagnosis
- Cryoglobulinemic vasculitis
- Mastocytosis
- Cold panniculitis
- Chilblain lupus erythematosus

VIBRATORY URTICARIA

Vibratory angioedema refers to the development of pruritus and swelling after the application of a vibratory stimulus to the skin. Patterson et al. first described four members of a family with vibration-induced edema, which was of autosomal-dominant inheritance.

Pathogenesis

A missense variant in *ADGRE2* gene is the basis of autosomal-dominant vibratory urticaria, notably a rare variant, and is clinically and pathophysiologically an entity distinct from dermatographism and other physical urticarias.

Clinical Features

Vibratory triggers for urticaria include riding a motorcycle or horse, handling a jackhammer, mowing the lawn, and clapping and occupational triggers involving carpentry and machinists.

Treatment

Avoidance of specific vibratory stimuli is the first line of therapy once diagnosis is established. Oral terfenadine taken before a vibratory stimulus may delay symptom onset and reduce the overall severity of the attack.

EXERCISE-INDUCED ANAPHYLAXIS

It may be considered a subtype of physical urticaria where anaphylaxis develops following physical activity. Prior to anaphylaxis itself, diffuse warmth, erythema, sweating and pruritus (most common) occur followed by the development of typical urticarial lesions and angioedema. Endorphin release during exercise, which are known to be mast cell secretagogues, are responsible though the exact mechanism is unknown. Physical activities such as jogging, cycling, sudden exertion, and other sports can incite anaphylaxis. Prevention of episodes and access to prompt resuscitation measures are vital.

CONCLUSION

Different types of physical urticarias cause varying degrees of distress to patients, and symptom relief remains less predictable even with treatment. Unlike other forms of urticaria that respond fairly well with oral antihistamines, the treatment of physical urticarias is difficult, and no guidelines exist. Due to its variability in presentation, it poses diagnostic dilemma, especially in cases such as solar urticaria. Treatment is generally avoidance of identifiable triggers and use of antihistamines for symptom relief, inducing remission and for prophylaxis. Other modalities are occasionally effective. It can occasionally present with acute flares that can be life-threatening. Most physical urticarias lead to impaired QoL, and this remains a therapeutic challenge.

SUGGESTED READINGS

1. Metzger WJ. Urticaria, angioedema, and hereditary angioedema. In: Patterson R, Grammer LC, Greenberger PA (Eds). Allergic Diseases: Diagnosis and Management, 5th edition. Philadelphia: Lippincott Raven Publishers; 1997. pp. 265-83.
2. Zuberbier T, Bindslev-Jensen C, Canonica W, et al. EAACI/GA2 LEN/EDF guideline: definition, classification and diagnosis of urticaria. Allergy. 2006;61:316-20.
3. Holgate ST, Church MK. Urticaria-Pathophysiology. Allergy. London: Mosby-Year Book Europe Limited; 1993:21.1-12.
4. Kirby JD, Matthews CN, James J, Duncan EH, Warin RP. The incidence and other aspects of factitious whealing (dermographism). Br J Dermatol. 1971;85(4):331-5.
5. Kennedy MS. Comprehensive care in the allergy/asthma office: Evaluation of chronic eczema and urticaria and angioedema. Immunol Allergy Clin North Am. 1999;19:20-33.
6. Kontou-Fili K, Borici-Mazi R, Kapp A, Matjevic LJ, Mitchel FB. Physical urticaria: Classification and diagnostic guidelines. An EAACI position paper. Allergy. 1997;52:504-13.
7. Kobza-Black A. Delayed pressure urticaria. J Invest Dermatol Symp Proc. 2001;6:148-9.
8. Dice JP. Physical urticaria. Immunol Allergy Clin North Am. 2004;24(2):225-46.
9. Greaves M. Chronic urticaria. J Allergy Clin Immunol. 2000;105(4):664-72.
10. Taskapan O, Harmanyeri Y. Evaluation of patients with symptomatic dermographism. J Eur Acad Dermatol Venereol. 2006;20(1):58-62.
11. Wallergren J, Isaksson A. Urticarial Dermographism: Clinical features and response to psychosocial stress. Acta Derm Venereol. 2007;87:493-8.
12. Wu JJ, Huang DB, Murase JE, Weinstein GD. Dermographism secondary to trauma from a coral reef. J Eur Acad Dermatol Venereol. 2006;20:1337-8.
13. Rahim KF, Dawe RS. Dermatomyositis presenting with symptomatic dermographism and raised troponin T: a case report. J Med Case Rep. 2009;3:7319.
14. Breathnach SM, Allen R, Ward AM, Greaves MW. Symptomatic dermographism: natural history, clinical features, laboratory investigations and response to therapy. Clin Exp Dermatol. 1983;8(5):463-76.
15. Schoepke N, Mlynek A, Weller K, Church MK, Maurer M. Symptomatic dermographism: an inadequately described disease. J Eur Acad Dermatol Venereol. 2015;29(4):708-12.
16. Sharpe GR, Shuster S. In dermographic urticaria H2 receptor antagonists have a small but therapeutically irrelevant additional effect compared with H1 antagonists alone. Br J Dermatol. 1993;129(5):575-9.

17. Maurer M, Schuetz A, Weller K, Schoepke N, Peveling-Oberhag A, Staubach P, et al. Omalizumab is effective in symptomatic dermographism-results of a randomised placebo-controlled trial. J Allergy Clin Immunol. 2017;140:870-3.
18. Juhlin L, De Vos C, Rihoux JP. Inhibiting effect of cetirizine on histamine-induced and 48/80-induced wheals and flares, experimental dermographism and cold-induced urticaria. J Allergy Clin Immunol. 1987;80:599-602.
19. Johnsson M, Flak ES, Volden G. UV-B treatment of factitious urticaria. Photodermatol. 1987;4:302-4.
20. Merklen P. Urticaria. In: Besnier E, Brocq L, Jacquet L (Eds). La pratique dermatologique: trait de dermatologie applique´e. Paris: Masson et Cie; 1904. pp. 728-71.
21. Snyder M, Turrentine JE, Cruz PD. Photocontact dermatitis and its clinical mimics: an overview for the allergist. Clin Rev Allergy Immunol. 2019;56(1):32-40.
22. Champion RH. Urticaria: then and now. Br J Dermatol. 1988;119(4):427-36.
23. Harris BW, Crane JS, Schlessinger J. Solar Urticaria. 2023 Jun 28. Treasure Island (FL): StatPearls Publishing; 2024.
24. Uetsu N, Miyauchi-Hasimoto H, Okamoto H, Horio T. The clinical and photobiological characteristics of solar urticaria in 40 patients. Br J Dermatol. 2000;142(1):32-8.
25. Ryckaert S, Roelandts R. Solar urticaria: A report of 25 cases and difficulties in phototesting. Arch Dermatol. 1998;134(1):71-4.
26. Griffin LL, Haylett AK, Rhodes LE. Evaluating patient responses to omalizumab in solar urticaria. Photodermatol Photoimmunol Photomed. 2019;35(1):57-65
27. Chicharro P, Rodríguez-Jiménez P, Capusan TM, Herrero-Moyano M, de Argila D. Induction of Light Tolerance Using Narrowband UV-B in Solar Urticaria. Actas Dermosifiliogr (Engl Ed). 2018;109(10):888-92.
28. Farr PM. Erythropoietic protoporphyria and solar urticaria. Br J Dermatol. 2018;179(2):542.
29. Harris BW, Crane JS, Schlessinger J. Solar urticaria. Treasure Island (FL): StatPearls Publishing; Jan 2024.
30. Maurer M, Fluhr JW, Khan DA. How to Approach Chronic Inducible Urticaria. J Allergy Clin Immunol Pract. 2018;6(4):1119-30.
31. Snast I, Kremer N, Lapidoth M, Enk CD, Tal Y, Rosman Y, et al. Omalizumab for the Treatment of Solar Urticaria: Case Series and Systematic Review of the Literature. J Allergy Clin Immunol Pract. 2018;6(4):1198-204.e3.
32. Morgado-Carrasco D, Fustà-Novell X, Podlipnik S, Combalia A, Aguilera P. Clinical and photobiological response in eight patients with solar urticaria under treatment with omalizumab, and review of the literature. Photodermatol Photoimmunol Photomed. 2018;34(3):194-9.
33. Shelley WB, Rawnsley HM. Aquagenic urticaria contact sensitivity reaction to water. JAMA, 1964;189:895-8.
34. Treudler R, Tebbe B, Steinhoff M, Orfanos CE. Familial aquagenic urticaria associated with familial lactose intolerance. J Am Acad Dermatol. 2002;47(4):611-3.
35. Chalamidas SL, Charles CR. Aquagenic urticaria. Arch Dermatol. 1971;104:541-6.
36. Sibbald RG, Kobza Black A, Eady RAJ, James M, Greaves MW. Aquagenic urticaria: evidence of cholinergic and histaminergic basis. Br J Dermatol. 1981;105:297-302.
37. Fearfield LA, Gazzard B, Bunker CB. Aquagenic urticaria and human immunodeficiency virus infection: treatment with stanozolol. Br J Dermatol. 1997;137:620-2.
38. Magerl M, Altrichter S, Borzova E, Giménez-Arnau A, Grattan CEH, Lawlor F, et al. The definition, diagnostic testing, and management of chronic inducible urticarias – The EAACI/GA2LEN/EDF/UNEV consensus recommendations 2016 update and revision. Allergy. 2016;71:780-802.
39. Kurtz AS, Kaplan AP. Regional expression of cold urticaria. J Allergy Clin Immunol. 1990;86(2):272-3.
40. Mathelier-Fusade P, Leynadier F. Localized cold urticaria. Br J Dermatol. 1995;132:666-7.

41. Czarnetzli BM, Frosch PJ, Sprekeler R. Localized cold reflex urticaria. Br J Dermatol. 1981;104:83-7.
42. Mlynek A, Magerl M, Siebenhaar F, et al. Results and relevance of critical temperature threshold testing in patients with acquired cold urticaria. Br J Dermatol. 2010;162:198-200.
43. Maltseva N, Borzova E, Fomina D, Bizjak M, Terhorst-Molawi D, Košnik M, et al. Cold urticaria—what we know and what we do not know. Allergy. 2021;76(4):1077-94.
44. Patterson R, Mellies CJ, Blankenship ML, Pruzansky JJ. Vibratory angioedema: a hereditary type of physical hypersensitivity. J Allergy Clin Immunol. 1972;50(3):174-82.
45. Boyden SE, Desai A, Glenn C, Young ML, Bolan HC, Scott LM, et al. Vibratory Urticaria Associated with a Missense Variant in ADGRE2. N Engl J Med. 2016;374:656-63.
46. Wener MH, Metzger WJ, Simon RA. Occupationally acquired vibratory angioedema with secondary carpal tunnel syndrome. Ann Intern Med. 1983;98(1):44-6.
47. Keahey T, Indrisano R, Lavker R, Kaliner MA. Delayed vibratory angioedema: insights into pathophysiologic mechanisms. J Allergy Clin Immunol. 1987;80(6):831-8.
48. Lawlor F, Black AK, Breathnach AS, Greaves MW. Vibratory angioedema: lesion induction, clinical features, laboratory and ultrastructural findings and response to therapy. Br J Dermatol. 1989;120(1):93-9.
49. Sheffer AL, Austen KF. Exercise-induced anaphylaxis. J Allergy Clin Immunol. 1980;6:106-11.
50. Casale TB, Bowman S, Kaliner M. Induction of human cutaneous mast cell degranulation by opiates and endogenous opioid peptides: evidence for opiate and nonopiate receptor participation. J Allergy Clin Immunol. 1984;73:775-81.

CHAPTER 11

Contact Urticaria

Nitika Nijhara, Sanjeev Gupta, Rohit Batra

INTRODUCTION

Contact urticaria (CU) is characterized by a transient wheal-and-flare reaction that occurs within 10–60 minutes at the site of contact with the allergen or irritant and completely resolves within 24 hours. This phenomenon has long been recognized, although this term was introduced by Fischer in 1973.

While CU is not usually life-threatening, it can significantly impact an individual's quality of life due to discomfort and cosmetic concerns.

Common triggers include certain foods, latex, cosmetics, medications, and environmental factors such as heat or cold.

Symptoms typically develop within minutes to hours after contact and may persist for variable durations.

Management of CU involves identifying and avoiding the triggering substances, as well as using antihistamines or topical corticosteroids to relieve symptoms. In severe cases, allergen immunotherapy may be considered to desensitize the individual to specific allergens.

Understanding the triggers and implementing appropriate preventive measures are crucial in managing CU effectively. Patients should seek medical evaluation and guidance for proper diagnosis and management.

CONTACT URTICARIA SYNDROME

Contact urticaria syndrome (CUS) is a condition characterized by the development of urticaria and other allergic reactions upon contact with specific allergens or stimuli. This syndrome encompasses both immediate and delayed hypersensitivity reactions.

Contact urticaria syndrome is an inflammatory skin response to various agents that trigger different immediate contact skin reactions (ICSR). Systemic involvement can also be seen in CUS, manifesting as asthma, rhinitis, conjunctivitis, difficulty in swallowing, lip swelling, and even anaphylaxis.

Contact urticaria syndrome can involve both conditions—CU and PCD (protein contact dermatitis), manifesting as wheals in CU and eczema in PCD cases.

Protein contact dermatitis is a relatively uncommon form of contact dermatitis that occurs when the skin comes into contact with proteins found in certain substances.

As described by Hjorth and Roed–Peterson in 1976, PCD is an immediate dermatitis induced after contact with proteins. While PCD shares some similarities with other types of contact dermatitis, such as irritant contact dermatitis and allergic contact dermatitis, its distinct triggers and symptoms warrant special attention.

Thirty-three food caterers who had increased itching followed by erythema and vesicles soon after coming into contact with fish, meat, and vegetables have been reported. When the relevant items were applied to the affected skin, urticaria or eczema developed.

Staging of Contact Urticaria Syndrome

A localized wheal and flare is the typical reaction of CU, while additional reactions include nonspecific symptoms (itching, tingling, burning), anaphylaxis, and widespread urticaria **(Table 1)**.

It is important to note that the staging of CUS may vary depending on the classification system used and individual patient characteristics **(Table 1)**.

PATIENT HISTORY

To determine the cause of CU, a thorough medical history is necessary. Symptoms of CU typically arise 1 hour after coming into contact with the agent that triggered the reaction, and the patient would be able to link these symptoms to a particular exposure.

It is necessary to determine the degree of extracutaneous involvement.

The patient might be able to pinpoint precisely what they were doing when the symptoms first appeared enabling the doctor to narrow down the possibilities. It is also important to find out about a patient's occupation because several occupational factors contribute to CU.

Staging of CUS	Clinical Features
Localized urticaria	Redness and swelling, or with some nonspecific symptoms like itching, burning/ tingling sensations
Generalized urticaria	Extensive urticarial lesions
Extracutaneous reactions	Pulmonary, oropharyngeal/laryngeal, and GIT symptoms like bronchial asthma, wheezing, rhinitis, conjunctivitis, epiphora, swollen lips, hoarseness, abdominal cramps, diarrhea, vomiting, nausea, etc. difficulty swallowing
Generalized anaphylaxis	Anaphylaxis or shock

TABLE 1: Different stages of contact urticaria.

(CUS: contact urticaria syndrome; GIT: gastrointestinal tract)

MECHANISM OF ACTION

The mechanisms underlying ICSR are of two different types, namely immunologic and nonimmunologic.

Immunological contact urticaria (ICU) is an immunoglobulin E (IgE)-mediated reaction that requires prior sensitization. Proteins or hapten-forming molecules are the main cause of this reaction, which can develop into systemic symptoms or even spread beyond the area of contact as generalized urticaria.

Nonimmunological contact urticaria (NICU) can develop at the first encounter with the eliciting agent, such as stinging nettles, jellyfish, or compounds like cinnamon aldehyde, and does not require prior sensitization. Lesions are restricted to the regions where the eliciting agent comes into close contact with the skin.

Nonimmunological Contact Urticaria

Natural History of NICU

The most prevalent kind of immediate CU is known as NICU, which does not require prior sensitization. After coming into contact with the provoking agent, redness may persist for up to 6 hours, although NICU reactions often manifest within a few minutes to 1 hour and the edema goes away after 1 hour. The agent, vehicle, concentration, mode, and exposure site all affect NICU symptoms. The symptoms typically appear and remain limited to the area of contact.

Talking about the vulnerability to NICU agents, the face is the most sensitive anatomic region, followed by the volar forearm, upper back, upper arm, antecubital fossa, and lower back, in a decreasing order.

Mechanism of Action

The mechanism of NICU is not completely understood.

Vasogenic mediators like prostaglandins are known to be the primary cause of NICU.

Urticariogens can behave in a variety of ways:
- Certain plants, like nettles, or animals, such as caterpillars and jellyfish, may directly inject vasoactive substances, resulting in this type of CU.
- Exposure to food additives like sorbic acid or benzoic acid in foods like tomato ketchup, or cosmetics like cinnamic aldehyde and balsam of Peru is a more prevalent kind.
- Ammonium persulfate exposure at work in the hairdressing industry.

This suggests that prostaglandin is the main mediator of NICU reactions rather than histamine. It is also believed that the source of prostaglandins lies in the epidermis.

Antihistamines have no impact on reactivity to common NICU agents like methyl nicotinate, benzoic acid, cinnamic acid, or cinnamic aldehyde. However, acetylsalicylic acid (ASA) and nonsteroidal anti-inflammatory medications (NSAIDs) can inhibit these common NICU agents both topically and orally, indicating the role of prostaglandins.

Agents Causing NICU

A list of various substances that are identified as nonimmunologic causes of CU is as follows:
- Medicaments such as chloroform, benzocaine, methyl salicylate, camphor, tincture of benzoin, black mustard, alcohol, tar extracts, thyme oil, capsaicin, Friar's balsam, dimethylsulfoxide (DMSO), nicotinic acid esters, and witch hazel
- Foods such as fish, cayenne pepper (capsicum) and thyme
- Animals such as arthropods, jellyfish, moths, roe deer, stinging insects, and caterpillars
- Flavorings and fragrances such as cinnamic acid, balsam of Peru, cassia (cinnamon) oil, menthol, vanilla, and benzaldehyde
- Plants such as coral, nettles, and chrysanthemums
- Preservatives and germicidal agents such as sorbic acid, benzoic acid, sodium benzoate, formaldehyde, and chlorocresol
- Miscellaneous such as acetic acid, cobalt chloride, resorcinol, ammonium persulfate, naphtha 21/99, sulfur, pine oil, turpentine, benzophenone, and butyric acid

Immunological Contact Urticaria

Natural History of ICU

The ICU is an IgE-mediated reaction requiring previous sensitization. While chemicals with a low molecular weight (<1,000) act like a hapten and bind to carrier protein such as albumin to cause ICU, proteins with high molecular weight (>10,000) lead to sensitization directly.

A special feature of ICU is that it is not only related to skin but can be generalized with respiratory and gastrointestinal system involvement and anaphylaxis leading to systemic symptoms.

The most common allergen responsible for ICU is natural rubber latex. Gloves, tourniquets, catheters, masks, stethoscopes, condoms, etc., contain latex. Health workers and even the general population are at a risk of developing ICU.

Mechanism of Action

Immunological contact urticaria is a type I hypersensitivity response, involving mast cell degranulation with histamine release, and is triggered by the percutaneous or mucosal penetration of an allergen to which the individual has already developed specific IgE. This results in an immediate, localized outbreak that resolves in 2 hours, generalized urticaria, or even anaphylaxis if the individual is extremely hypersensitive.

A common observation in many ICU reactions is cross-allergy. A patient may become sensitized to a particular protein and experience allergic reactions to other proteins containing the same or a chemically related protein. In the 1970s, it was discovered that birch pollen, fruits, and vegetables form one of the greatest cross-allergy families, which was followed by reports of pollen and spice allergies.

Agents Causing Immunological Contact Urticaria (Boxes 1 to 3)

Metals responsible for ICU: Nickel, cobalt, copper, mercury, zinc, gold, platinum, tin.

Hair care products responsible for ICU: Henna, paraphenylenediamine, basic blue 99 (amino ketone dye).

Preservatives and disinfectants responsible for ICU: Benzyl alcohol, ammonia, chlorhexidine, benzoic acid, formaldehyde, parabens, polysorbates, gentian violet, chloramine, sodium hypochlorite, hexamidine, phenylmercuric propionate.

Fragrances and flavorings responsible for ICU: Cinnamic aldehyde, balsam of Peru, menthol, vanillin, and benzoic acid.

Enzymes responsible for ICU: α-Amylase, xylanases, cellulases.

Miscellaneous agents responsible for ICU: Acrylic acid, acetyl acetone, acrylic monomer, seminal fluid, sodium silicate, sodium sulfide, sulfur dioxide, plastic, carbonless copy paper, ammonium persulfate, ammonium chloride, benzophenone, epoxy resin, polypropylene, polyethylene, polyethylene glycol, perlon, nylon, tinofix, tobacco, xylene, textile finish, and zinc diethyldithiocarbamate.

TESTING

The diagnosis of CU is made using the patient's past medical history, skin prick tests, description of skin symptoms, and, if feasible, blood analysis of specific IgE.

Box 1: List of various natural derivatives of animals and plants causing immunological contact urticaria (ICU).

Animal derivatives:
- Amniotic fluid
- Blood
- Dander
- Cockroaches
- Gut (pig)
- Brucella abortus
- Gelatine
- Liver
- Locust
- Mealworm
- Saliva
- Serum
- Wool
- Silk
- Spider mite
- Urine

Plant derivatives:
- Abietic acid
- Algae
- Birch
- Henna
- *Bougainvillea*
- *Chrysanthemum*
- Fennel
- Garlic
- Mahogany
- Mulberry
- Mustard
- Cornstarch
- Lily
- Latex rubber
- Hops
- Colophony

> **Box 2: List of drugs responsible for immunological contact urticaria (ICU).**
>
> - *Antibiotics*: Ampicillin, Cephalosporins, Penicillin, Streptomycin, Gentamycin, Neomycin, Bacitracin, Rifamycin, Chloramphenicol
> - Benzoyl peroxide
> - Acetylsalicylic acid
> - Hydrocortisone
> - Fumaric acid derivatives
> - Lindane
> - Clobetasol 17-propionate

> **Box 3: List of foods responsible for immunological contact urticaria (ICU).**
>
> - Meats
> - Seafood
> - *Dairy*: Milk, eggs, cheese
> - *Vegetables*: Beans, cabbage, onion, potato, tomato, soybean, cucumber, celery, lettuce, garlic, carrot, chives
> - *Fruits*: Banana, kiwi, apple, strawberry, apricot, mango, orange, peach, plum, watermelon
> - *Nuts*: Peanuts, sesame seed, sunflower seed
> - *Grains*: Buckwheat, rice, wheat, maize

For both ICU and NICU, the open test, prick test, scratch test, and scratch-chamber test are commonly used in vivo skin testing.

It is imperative to perform positive (histamine @ 1 mg/mL) and negative (normal saline) controls in any of these tests.

In vitro radioallergosorbent test (RAST) can also be used to diagnose ICU patients in addition to in vivo techniques.

The patient's serum is used in this technique to identify antigen-specific IgE molecules, which is rarely required for ICU diagnosis.

Let us discuss these in vivo techniques in detail.

Open Test

0.1 mL of the testing substance is taken in a vehicle (such as petrolatum, ethanol water) and spread on the desired site over a 3 × 3 cm area. The test sites are then read at 20, 40, and 60 minutes. To see the maximal response, ICU reactions usually appear within 15–20 minutes, while NICU reactions can be delayed up to 45–60 minutes following application.

Prick Test

When the open test yields a negative result, the prick test is frequently a recommended course of action. The allergen in the vehicle is placed on the volar aspect of the forearm, where it is punctured with a lancet into the skin. Since prick testing introduces a very little amount of allergen into the skin, it theoretically has the lowest risk of causing anaphylaxis. Usually, test sites are read in 30 minutes or less.

A positive result shows a wheal of at least 3 mm in diameter and at least half the size of the histamine control in the absence of such a reaction in the vehicle control.

Scratch Test

A superficial (5–10 mm) scratch is formed with a lancet and the test substance is then applied to the scratch. Evaluation is done after 5–20 minutes. Interpretation of the result is difficult because it is an unstandardized procedure. Positive result appears as an edematous reaction at least as wide as the histamine control positive in the absence of such reaction in the vehicle control.

Chamber Test

The test substance is applied in aluminum containers and then attached to the skin via a porous tape. The results are read at 20, 40, and 60 minutes.

INTERPRETATION OF RESULTS

Contact urticaria can be graded by the degree of edema and erythema on a simple scale:
- *Scale to score edema*:
  - Score of 1 signifies slight edema, which is barely visible or palpable.
  - Score of 2 is given for an easily palpable wheal.
  - Score of 3 is a solid, tense wheal.
  - Lastly, score of 4 signifies a tense wheal, extending further away from the test area.
- *Scale to score erythema*:
  - Score of 1+ means slight erythema, which is either spotty or diffuse.
  - Score of 2+ signifies moderate uniform erythema.
  - Score of 3+ is intense redness.
  - Lastly, score of 4+ is given to fiery redness with edema.

TREATMENT AND PROGNOSIS

The ability of the patient to avoid contact with the eliciting chemical is the only factor that determines the prognosis of CU. When individuals actively refrain from using the substance, their prognosis is typically favorable.

In case of contact with allergens, management can be divided into first-, second-, and third-line therapies.

First-line Therapy

First-line therapy primarily includes educating the patient and then using H1 receptor antihistamines. H1 receptor antihistamines have been well studied to suppress the wheal-and-flare response in urticaria.

H2 receptor antagonists, namely cimetidine, ranitidine, famotidine, and nizatidine, are usually used in combination with H1 receptor antihistamines in the treatment of urticaria in general. But in the case of CU, as preventing further exposure remains the ideal approach, these agents should infrequently be needed.

Second-line Therapy

Second-line therapies are only taken into consideration if antihistamines fail.

These include the use of UV radiation, photochemotherapy, tricyclic antidepressants, corticosteroids, and leukotriene receptor antagonists.

- *UV radiation and photochemotherapy*: By induction of T-lymphocyte apoptosis and encouraging mast cells and Langerhans cells decrease in the dermis, UVA and UVB light may be able to control flares. By preventing mast cells and basophils from releasing histamine, radiation also lessens pruritus.
- *Tricyclic antidepressants*: Doxepin is a molecule having both H1 and H2 receptor antagonist activity and can be used in conjunction with H1 antihistamines.
- Systemic steroids are preferred when rapid control is needed. Steroids are usually given for short-term relief, and corticosteroid-sparing immunosuppressive modalities are added to the treatment regimen if steroids need to be given for a prolonged period.
- Leukotriene receptor antagonists, like montelukast, have also proven to be effective in the treatment of CU.

Third-line Therapy

Immunomodulatory agents like cyclosporine and methotrexate are used as third-line therapy in CU.

In a study of 100 patients by Kessel and Toubi with severe urticaria, treated with 2–3 mg/kg cyclosporine, 40% of the patients showed disappearance of urticaria, while 30% displayed great improvement.

These drugs are not preferred for long-term use due to severe side effects such as liver toxicity, kidney toxicity, and hypertension.

CONCLUSION

Contact urticaria can result from a variety of chemicals that are frequently encountered in daily life. Numerous and ever-changing factors can cause CU. There are still a lot of case reports of CU brought on by different substances.

Since prevention is the main treatment for CU, it is crucial to determine the substance that triggers the reaction. Patients who refrain from using the inciting substance typically have a good prognosis.

SUGGESTED READINGS

1. Fisher AA. Contact Dermatitis, 2nd edition. Philadelphia: Lea & Febiger; 1973. pp. 283-6.
2. Aquino M, Mawhirt S, Fonacier L. Review of contact urticaria syndrome—evaluation to treatment. Curr Treat Options Allergy. 2015;2:365.

3. Bhatia R, Sharma VK. Occupational dermatoses: An Asian perspective. Indian J Dermatol Venereol Leprol. 2017;83:525-35.
4. Hjorth N, Roed-Petersen J. Occupational protein contact dermatitis in food handlers. Contact Dermatitis. 1976;2:28-42.
5. Magerl M, Altrichter S, Borzova E, Giménez-Arnau A, Grattan CEH, Lawlor F, et al. The definition, diagnostic testing, and management of chronic inducible urticarias—The EAACI/GA(2) LEN/EDF/UNEV consensus recommendations 2016 update and revision. Allergy. 2016;71(6):780-802.
6. Hannuksela M. Mechanisms in contact urticaria. Clin Dermatol. 1997;15:619-22.
7. Maibach HI, Johnson HI. Contact urticaria syndrome: contact urticaria to diethyltoluamide (immediate-type hypersensitivity). Arch Dermatol. 1975;111:726-30.
8. Gollhausen R, Kligman AM. Human assay for identifying substances which induce non-allergic contact urticaria: the NICU test. Contact Dermatitis. 1985;13:98-106.
9. Lahti A. Terfenadine (H1-antagonist) does not inhibit nonimmunologic contact urticaria. Contact Dermatitis. 1987;16:220.
10. Lahti A, Oikarinen A, Viinkka L, Ylikorkala O, Hannuksela M, et al. Prostaglandins in contact urticaria induced by benzoic acid. Acta Derm Venereol. 1983;63:425-7.
11. Lahti A, Vaananen A, Kokkonen E-L, Hannuksela M. Acetylsalicylic acid inhibits non-immunologic contact urticaria. Contact Dermatitis. 1987;16:133-5.
12. Johansson J, Lahti A. topical non-steroidal anti-inflammatory drugs inhibit non-immunologic immediate contact reactions. Contact Dermatitis. 1988;19:161-5.
13. Warner MR, Taylor JS, Leow Y. Agents causing contact urticaria. Clin Dermatol. 1997;15:623-35.
14. Bourrain JL. Occupational contact urticaria. Clin Rev Allergy Immunol. 2006;30(1):39-46.
15. Wakelin SH. Contact urticaria. Clin Exp Dermatol. 2001;26(2):132-6.
16. Lachapelle J-M, Maibach HI (Eds). Methodology of open (non-prick) testing, prick testing, and its variants. In: Patch Testing and Prick Testing: A Practical Guide. Berlin: Springer Verlag; 2009. pp. 141-52.
17. Amaro C, Goossens A. Immunological occupational contact urticarial and contact dermatitis from proteins: a review. Contact Dermatitis. 2008;58:67-75.
18. Hannuksela M, Lahti A. Immediate reactions to fruits and vegetables. Contact Dermatitis. 1977;3:79-84.
19. Niinimaki A, Hannuksela M. Immediate skin test reactions to spices. Allergy. 1981;26:487-93.
20. Amin S, Maibach HI. Nonimmunologic contact urticaria; Immunologic contact urticaria definition. In: Amin S, Lahti A, Maibach HI (Eds). Contact Urticaria Syndrome. Toronto: eRC Press; 1997.
21. Gillard M, Benedetti MS, Chatelain P, Baltes E. Histamine H1 receptor occupancy and pharmacodynamics of second generation H1-antihistamines. Inflamm Res. 2005;54:367-9.
22. Kozel MM, Sabroe RA. Chronic urticaria: Aetiology, management and current and future treatment options. Drugs. 2004;64:2515-36.
23. Kaplan AP. Clinical practice: Chronic urticaria and angioedema. N Engl J Med. 2002;346:175-9.
24. Kessel A, Toubi E. Low-dose cyclosporine is a good option for severe chronic urticaria. J Allergy Clin Immunol. 2009;123:970; author reply-1.

CHAPTER 12

Cholinergic Urticaria

Kritika Pandey

INTRODUCTION

Cholinergic urticaria (CholU) is marked by pinpoint, highly itchy, or often painful erythematous wheals. It is a rare type of chronic inducible urticaria triggered by an increase in core body temperature. It can be induced by exercise, hot bath, high environmental temperature, hot and spicy food, or emotional stress.

Multiple mechanisms contribute to the occurrence of CholU. Release of histamine, allergy with sweat, cholinergic-related substance intake, and hypohidrosis (reduced sweating) or anhidrosis (absence of sweating) are the most common factors associated with it.

It mostly appears as pinpoint urticarial eruptions with severe itching. Lesions are mostly localized to the abdomen, chest, back, and limbs. Urticarial wheals in CholU usually disappear rapidly on their own within a few hours. In rare cases, systemic involvement with a wheal-flare reaction may develop resulting in difficulty in breathing, wheezing, or abdominal pain.

Patients with CholU have reported high scores on Dermatological Life Quality Index (DLQI). Many aspects of the disease remain poorly understood.

PREVALENCE

The prevalence of CholU in temperate zone countries has been reported from 0.023 to 11.2%. Studies from India found prevalence of CholU to be 1.7% and 4.16% while a German study found it to be a 11.2%. A study from Thailand found that 14% of physical urticaria patients had CholU.

PATHOPHYSIOLOGY (FIG. 1)

The terminology of "cholinergic urticaria" is taken from the finding that lesions similar to those of CholU can be produced in skin tests using cholinergic agonists like methacholine and acetylcholine. The pathomechanisms of CholU are poorly understood and several different theories have been proposed.

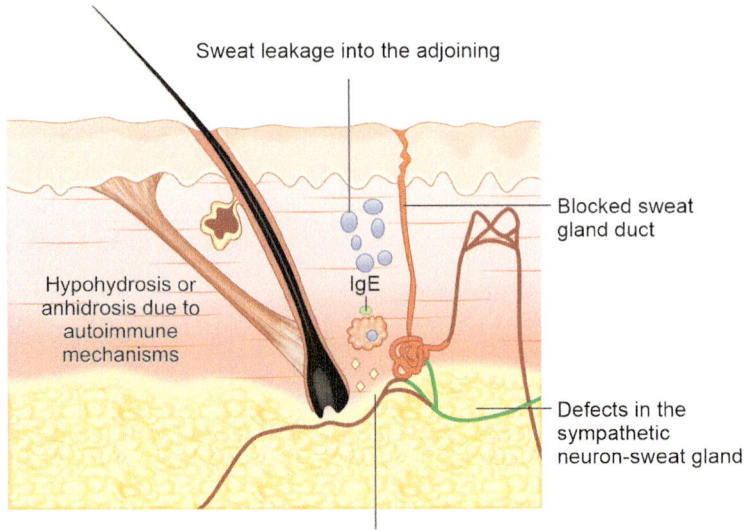

FIG. 1: Pathophysiology of cholinergic urticaria.

- Blocked sweat gland duct
- Hypohydrosis or anhidrosis due to autoimmune mechanisms
- Sweat leakage into the adjoining cells
- Sweat antigen-induced IgE-mediated mast cell activation
- Defects in the sympathetic neuron–sweat gland conduction

CLINICAL FEATURES

CholU is identified by itching, redness, stinging pain, and papular or pinpoint wheals. Rarely, it may be associated with angioedema (AE) or anaphylaxis. It can be induced by an increase in core body temperature caused by exercise and passive warming. Emotional stress and hot or spicy foods may also induce CholU in some patients.

A typical cutaneous lesion of CholU is the development of punctate wheals of 1–3 mm for a short duration (10–15 minutes). The most commonly affected part of the body is the chest, abdomen, back, arms, and legs **(Figs. 2A to D)**. It generally spares the palms, soles, and axillae. In rare instances, CholU may become associated with serious symptoms such as AE, dyspnea, severe pain, and anaphylaxis. Studies are being conducted to differentiate food-independent exercise-induced anaphylaxis (EIA) and CholU with anaphylaxis.

CholU mostly affects patients with onset of symptoms during the second or third decade.

The exacerbation of symptoms is generally seen in hot and humid weather. However, in patients having CholU with anhidrosis, the worsening may be seen even during the colder seasons.

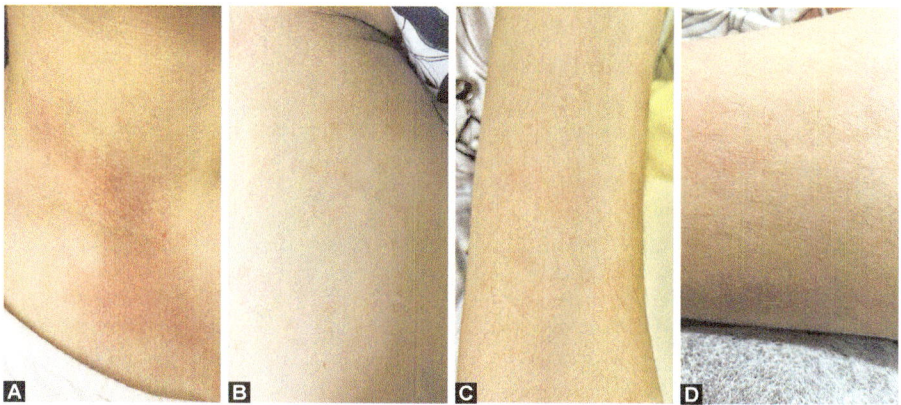

FIGS. 2A TO D: Clinical features of cholinergic urticaria. (A) Redness over upper chest. Papular wheals over (B) abdomen, (C) arm and (D) leg.

SUBTYPES OF CHOLINERGIC URTICARIA

The subtypes of CholU have been described on the basis of etiology, pathogenesis, and clinical features.
- *Type 1 allergy type* (allergy to the patient's own sweat):
  - Conventional sweat allergy-type CholU
  - CholU with palpebral AE (CholU-PA)
- *Follicular-type CholU*: CholU with a positive autologous serum skin test (ASST)
- *CholU with in anhidrosis and/or hypohidrosis (CholU-Anhd)*: Often classified as acquired idiopathic generalized anhidrosis (AIGA)

The causes, pathophysiology, and therapeutic approach of each subtype are distinct; therefore, it is very important to examine and evaluate the patients for various possible etiologies with awareness of the subtypes of CholU.

DIAGNOSIS

The diagnosis of CholU is made by clinical history and use of provocation tests that are appropriate considering the patient's age and general condition.

Heavy exercise machine test, passive warming test, metacholine skin test (release of acetylcholine), thermoregulatory sweat test, and drug-induced sweat test have been utilized to confirm the diagnosis of CholU **(Table 1)**.

CholU is diagnosed by the appearance of wheal and flare reaction that develops immediately or within a few minutes after an increase in core body temperature due to heavy exercise or passive warming. The lesions commonly vanish within 15–60 minutes.

The severity of CholU is measured by the Cholinergic Urticaria Severity Index. It is a sum of score that measures the frequency of CholU symptoms, triggering factors, duration of skin lesions, and symptoms-like itching. The Cholinergic Urticaria Severity Index score ranges from 0 to 21 points.

TABLE 1: Diagnosis of cholinergic urticaria.

Test	Method of testing	Observation	Result
Exercise machine test	Patient rides static bicycle or treadmill (the cutoff is increase in pulse rate of 3 beats/min	Doctor monitors the sign and symptoms of CholU	The positive result shows pinpoint-sized wheals
Passive warming test	Patient stays in a chamber with temperature set at 42°C for 15 minutes	Physician monitors body temperature	The positive result shows pinpoint-sized wheals with surrounding erythema
Methacholine skin test	100 μg of methacholine in 0.1 mL of saline solution is given intradermally	Wheal-flare reaction that occurs within 1 minute of the injection	Wheal-flare reaction that occurs within 1 minute of the injection
• Thermoregulatory sweat test • Drug-induced sweat test	• Thermography Quantitative sweat test	Evaluate the presence or absence of abnormal sweating function	Decreased or absent sweat

DIFFERENTIAL DIAGNOSIS OF CHOLINERGIC URTICARIA

- *Exercise-induced urticaria*: Heavy exercise may provoke both EIA and CholU, whereas passive warming induces only CholU and not EIA. The wheals are typically small pinpoint sized in CholU, whereas in EIA they are large and may even present as diffuse erythema.
- *Heat urticaria*: This is a rare type of physical inducible urticaria. Itchy erythematous and well-demarcated wheals appear soon after heat exposure. Lesions of heat urticaria appear only at the site of heat exposure.
- *Aquagenic urticaria*: It is a rare form of chronic inducible urticaria in which contact with water, regardless of its temperature or pH, results in small pinpoint wheals surrounded by erythema.
- *Adrenergic urticaria*: This subtype can be differentiated from CholU by the presence of a white halo of vasoconstriction surrounding the small red or pink wheals. An intradermal injection of adrenaline or noradrenaline can induce the characteristic rash of adrenaline urticaria.

TREATMENT

Treatment of CholU focuses on the control of symptoms and avoidance of conditions that trigger them, i.e., heat or increase in core body temperature change.

The latest EAACI/GA^{2}LEN/EDF/UNEV consensus suggests nsAH1 (nonsedative H1 receptor antihistamine) as the first choice of treatment for CholU.

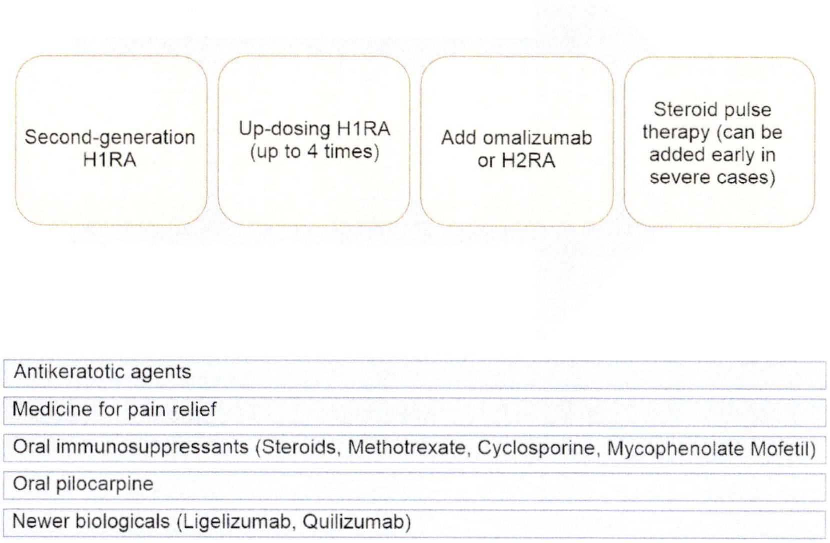

```
┌─────────────────┐  ┌─────────────────┐  ┌─────────────────┐  ┌─────────────────┐
│ Second-generation│ │ Up-dosing H1RA  │  │ Add omalizumab  │  │ Steroid pulse   │
│      H1RA        │ │  (up to 4 times)│  │   or H2RA       │  │ therapy (can be │
│                  │ │                 │  │                 │  │  added early in │
│                  │ │                 │  │                 │  │  severe cases)  │
└─────────────────┘  └─────────────────┘  └─────────────────┘  └─────────────────┘
```

Antikeratotic agents
Medicine for pain relief
Oral immunosuppressants (Steroids, Methotrexate, Cyclosporine, Mycophenolate Mofetil)
Oral pilocarpine
Newer biologicals (Ligelizumab, Quilizumab)

FIG. 3: Treatment of cholinergic urticaria.
(H1RA: H1-receptor antagonist; H2RA: H2-receptor antagonist)

Up-dosing of nsAH1 up to four-fold is advised if the standard dose fails to give results. A short course of steroid can be given in severe cases **(Fig. 3)**.

IgE-specific monoclonal antibody omalizumab is the second-line treatment to be added with nsAH1 in resistant and recalcitrant patients.

Currently, newer biologics like Ligelizumab and Quilizumab are being studied as upcoming therapies for CholU. Ligelizumab is a humanized IgG1 monoclonal antibody that attaches to the Cε3 domain of IgE whereas Quilizumab, a humanized IgG1, binds the M1 prime segment of membrane-expressed IgE. They contribute to inhibiting the interaction with the FCεRI domain on the surface of mast cells and basophils, thereby decreasing the IgE levels.

Desensitization therapy has been described in various studies. It can be achieved with regular physical exercise and/or bathing. Exercise with regular sweating is effective in reducing the symptoms of CholU with or without hypohidrosis. Treatment with autologous sweat subcutaneous injections can be done in patients with sweat allergy subtypes of CholU.

CONCLUSION

Cholinergic urticaria is a unique, temperature sensitive condition that significantly impacts patients' quality of life. While its exact mechanisms remain unclear, advances in understanding subtypes and triggers have paved the way for better diagnostic tools and targeted treatments. Early diagnosis and management, including antihistamines, steroids, newer molecules like biologicals and desensitization techniques, can effectively control symptoms and improve outcomes. Recognizing the distinct clinical features and subtypes are essential for personalized care and reducing the burden of this challenging condition.

SUGGESTED READINGS

1. Zuberbier T, Abdul Latiff AH, Abuzakouk M, Aquilina S, Asero R, Baker D, et al. The international EAACI/GA^{2}LEN/EuroGuiDerm/APAAACI guideline for the definition, classification, diagnosis, and management of urticaria. Allergy. 2022;77(3):734-66.
2. Kim JH, Park HS, Ye YM, Shin YS, Kang HR, Chung SJ, et al. Omalizumab Treatment in Patients with Cholinergic Urticaria: A Real-World Retrospective Study in Korea. Allergy Asthma Immunol Res. 2020;12(5):894-6.
3. Ritzel D, Altrichter S. Chronic inducible urticaria. Immunol Allergy Clin North Am. 2024;44(3):439-52.
4. Fukunaga A, Oda Y, Imamura S, Mizuno M, Fukumoto T, Washio K. Cholinergic Urticaria: Subtype Classification and Clinical Approach. Am J Clin Dermatol. 2023;24(1):41-54.
5. Rujitharanawong C, Tuchinda P, Chularojanamontri L, Chanchaemsri N, Kulthanan K. Cholinergic Urticaria: Clinical Presentation and Natural History in a Tropical Country. Biomed Res Int. 2020;2020:7301652.
6. Antolín-Amérigo D, Vlaicu PC, De La Hoz Caballer B, Cano MS. Anaphylaxis like cholinergic urticaria. Can Fam Physician. 2013;59(7):745-6.
7. Altrichter S, Mellerowicz E, Terhorst-Molawi D, Grekowitz E, Weller K, Maurer M. Disease Impact, Diagnostic Delay, and Unmet Medical Needs of Patients with Cholinergic Urticaria in German-Speaking Countries. Front Allergy. 2022;3:867227.
8. Godse K, Farooqui S, Nadkarni N, Patil S. Prevalence of cholinergic urticaria in Indian adults. Indian Dermatol Online J. 2013;4(1):62-3.
9. Wang Y, Scheffel J, Vera CA, Liu W, Günzel D, Terhorst-Molawi D, et al. Impaired sweating in patients with cholinergic urticaria is linked to low expression of acetylcholine receptor CHRM3 and acetylcholine esterase in sweat glands. Front Immunol. 2022;13:955161.
10. Tokura Y. 2016. New etiology of cholinergic urticaria. In: Katayama I, Murota H, Yokozeki H (Eds). Current Problems in Dermatology: Perspiration Research. Berlin: Karger Publishers; 2016.
11. Borzova EY, Popova CY, Kurowski M, Rukhadze MT, Darlenski R, Zaborova VA, et al. Cholinergic urticaria: novel aspects of pathogenesis, diagnosis and management. Russian J Skin Venereal Dis. 2021;24(3):211-26.
12. Commens CA, Greaves MW. Tests to establish the diagnosis in cholinergic urticaria. Br J Dermatol. 1978;98(1):47-51.
13. Altrichter S, Salow J, Ardelean E, Church MK, Werner A, Maurer M. Development of a standardized pulse-controlled ergometry test for diagnosing and investigating cholinergic urticaria. J Dermatol Sci. 2014;75(2):88-93.
14. Hosey RG, Carek PJ, Goo A. Exercise-induced anaphylaxis and urticaria. Am Fam Physician. 2001;64(8):1367-72.
15. Rothbaum R, McGee JS. Aquagenic urticaria: diagnostic and management challenges. J Asthma Allergy. 2016;9:209-13.
16. Pezzolo E, Peroni A, Gisondi P, Girolomoni G. Heat urticaria: a revision of published cases with an update on classification and management. Br J Dermatol. 2016;175(3):473-8.
17. Hogan SR, Mandrell J, Eilers D. Adrenergic urticaria: review of the literature and proposed mechanism. J Am Acad Dermatol. 2014;70(4):763-6.
18. Trischler J, Bottoli I, Janocha R, Heusser C, Jaumont X, Lowe P, et al. Asthma: learnings from the clinical development programme. Clin Transl Immunol. 2021;10(3):e1255.
19. Kozaru T, Fukunaga A, Taguchi K, Ogura K, Nagano T, Oka M, et al. Rapid desensitization with autologous sweat in cholinergic urticaria. Allergology. 2011;60:277-81.

CHAPTER 13

Autoimmune Urticaria

Sanjeev Gupta, Aditi Dabhra, Gagandeep Kaur

INTRODUCTION

Chronic spontaneous urticaria (CSU) is characterized by recurrent wheals and severe itching, often lasting for years. CSU impacts both children and adults, with a significant female predominance in the latter group. Both symptoms arise from cutaneous mast cell activation and the release of mediators, leading to inflammatory cell involvement, including T cells, basophils, and eosinophils. Autoimmune chronic spontaneous urticaria (aiCSU) is a type of CSU. Two autoimmune endotypes, type I and type IIb, are recognized in CSU, each involving distinct autoantibodies that target self-antigens and activate mast cells. Type I aiCSU, or autoallergic CSU, involves IgE autoantibodies, while type IIb aiCSU involves IgG autoantibodies.

Because type I hypersensitivity is characterized by the aberrant production of IgE antibodies, patients harboring IgE autoantibodies have been classified into the type I autoimmune endotype of CSU (type I aiCSU), also called autoallergic CSU. Now referring to the intriguing part of why there is type IIB autoimmune urticaria and missing type IIA autoimmune urticaria. Type IIA immunity involves the destruction of cells via mechanisms like complement activation or antibody-dependent cytotoxicity and type IIB immunity which is characterized by autoantibodies stimulating cells to create pathogenic states. Therefore, autoimmune urticaria aligns more with type IIB immunity due to the role of stimulating autoantibodies, rather than type IIA, which involves cell lysis or destruction. Although they share similar symptoms, including wheals and angioedema, these type I and type IIb aiCSU endotypes have differences in treatment response and prevalence.

TYPE I AUTOIMMUNE CHRONIC SPONTANEOUS URTICARIA (AUTOALLERGIC CHRONIC SPONTANEOUS URTICARIA)

Introduction

Evidence in the final decade of the previous century indicated an involvement of immunoglobulin E (IgE) autoantibodies in CSU. Based on these findings, omalizumab, an anti-IgE antibody, was the subject of the first randomized controlled clinical trial in patients with CSU and IgE autoantibodies to thyroid peroxidase (TPO), a prevalent CSU autoallergen. The name of this study was The Xolair in Chronic Urticaria Induced by Serum IgE Targeting Endoallergens [X-CUISITE] experiment. Administering omalizumab to these individuals led to a rapid response and a high percentage of complete response, 70%, surpassing the figures reported in several later trials on omalizumab in CSU. Further investigation into the frequency, function, significance, and specific targets of IgE autoantibodies in individuals with CSU, together with the findings from X-CUISITE and other omalizumab trials in CSU, confirmed the presence of type I aiCSU endotype.

Prevalence and Pathogenesis

- In 1999, the discovery of IgE autoantibodies against TPO in patients of CSU suggested autoallergy as a proposed mechanism.
- Altrichter et al. reported increased levels of IgE-anti-TPO in 54% and 61% of CSU patients, but other studies found lower rates (0–34%).
- Some studies showed higher IgE-anti-TPO levels in CSU patients compared to those with autoimmune thyroid disease and healthy controls.
- Elevated IgE-anti-TPO in CSU patients correlated with increased rates of positive skin tests to TPO.
- Passive IgE-anti-TPO transfer studies demonstrated skin reactions to TPO, but caution is needed as specific IgE to allergens can occur without clinical disease.
- Recent findings also reported IgE autoantibodies against eosinophil peroxidase (EP) and also against eosinophilic cationic protein (ECP), suggesting cross-reactivity between TPO and EP.
- Patients with CSU have IgE against various autoantigens, including double-stranded DNA, interleukin 24 (IL-24), tissue factor, ECP, and thyroglobulin, with functional relevance confirmed for some in vitro.
- Overall, patients with CSU have IgE to more than 200 autoantigens, more than healthy controls; however, this needs further confirmation as some autoantibodies are also found in healthy individuals.
- Increased IL-24 mRNA expression was observed in lesional skin of CSU patients, potentially explaining the localized autoallergen interaction and mast cell activation in the skin.

Demographic Patterns of Autoallergic Chronic Spontaneous Urticaria

- Limited information is available about the demographic characteristics of patients with autoallergic CSU.
- However, recent studies suggest that specific demographic factors may be associated with this condition, particularly in relation to IgE autoantibody presence. A possible demographic association was highlighted by a study involving 1,100 adult Chinese Han patients, which found that IgE-anti-TPO is an independent predictor of antihistamine-refractory CSU.

Clinical Features of Autoallergic Chronic Spontaneous Urticaria

- Clinically, patients with autoallergic CSU, particularly those with IgE-anti-TPO, tend to have significantly increased total IgE levels and a higher prevalence of comorbid allergic diseases compared to those without these autoantibodies.
- Some patients also show correlations between IgE-anti-IL-24 levels and disease activity, including basopenia.
- Additionally, machine-learning analyses of CSU subtypes have identified clusters where the highest total IgE levels are associated with the highest rates of comorbid atopic dermatitis, lower anti-nucleic antibody rates, and IgG-anti-TPO positivity.

Laboratory Features of Autoallergic Chronic Spontaneous Urticaria

- Laboratory findings in autoallergic CSU reveal elevated total IgE levels in patients with IgE-anti-TPO.
- Interestingly, while some studies report no significant differences in total IgE levels between CSU patients and healthy individuals, the proportion of autoreactive IgE in CSU patients is substantially higher, with a 1,000-fold increase compared to healthy controls.
- The lipophilic character of this autoreactive IgE has also been observed.
- In addition, treatment with omalizumab in cases of severe CSU has been linked to a decrease in IgE-antitissue factor and IgE-antithyroglobulin, which is consistent with the therapeutic response to the medication.

Diagnosing Type I Autoimmune Chronic Spontaneous Urticaria

- IgE autoantibodies must be tested in order to diagnose type I autoimmune disease, also known as autoallergic CSU. Unfortunately, there are not any commercially accessible or standardized tests for these antibodies at the moment.

- Although tests for IgE autoantibodies, such as IgE-anti-TPO or IgE-anti-IL-24, have been developed by a few urticaria centers of reference and excellence, they are not yet a standard component of clinical treatment.
- In many CSU patients, IgE-anti-TPO is accompanied by IgG-anti-TPO, which can interfere with IgE-anti-TPO detection and lead to discrepancies in positive rates across different assays and patient populations.
- There is an urgent need for standardized, widely accessible tests for IgE autoantibodies relevant to CSU.
- Additionally, the complete range of autoantigens targeted by IgE autoantibodies in CSU patients must be thoroughly characterized.
- Research is needed to understand the prevalence, cross-reactivity, and functional relevance of these IgE autoantibodies, including their potential to form circulating immune complexes.
- It remains unclear how various IgE autoantibodies contribute to a shared pathogenic mechanism in CSU.

TYPE IIB AUTOIMMUNE CHRONIC SPONTANEOUS URTICARIA

Introduction

Mast cell targeted IgG autoantibodies to IgE or its receptor FcεRI have been linked to CSU for over 30 years. The first report in 1988 identified histamine-releasing IgG autoantibodies against IgE, leading to the development of the autologous serum skin test (ASST) and the discovery that IgG-anti-FcεRI autoantibodies activate mast cells **(Table 1)**. This condition, known as type IIb aiCSU, has been challenging to characterize due to limited immunoassays and the fact that not all autoantibodies are functionally active. The three defining aspects of type IIb aiCSU were assessed for the first time utilizing the International Profiling Urticaria for the Identification of Subtypes (PURIST) study which included basophil tests, IgG-anti-FcεRI or IgG-anti-IgE immunoassays, and ASST. Less than 10% of CSU patients, in this study, had type IIb aiCSU, which is linked to a more severe form of the disease, low levels of total IgE, and high levels of TPO autoantibodies. Recent findings also suggest that IgM and/or IgA autoantibodies against FcεRI may play a role, and new markers such as nocturnal symptoms, eosinopenia, and low total IgA have been identified. Type IIb aiCSU often shows poor or slow responses to antihistamines and omalizumab.

Prevalence and Pathogenesis

- Type IIb aiCSU results from activating autoantibodies that target mast cells.
- IgE autoantibodies targeting autoallergens (type I autoallergy) or IgG-anti-IgE or IgG-anti-FcεRI autoantibodies (type IIb autoimmunity) activate mast cells. IgG-anti-FcεRI interacts with FcεRI present on mast cells and basophils, leading to complement activation and histamine release via C5aR. Mast cells, basophils, and eosinophils are activated, and IgE production is stimulated by

TABLE 1: Timeline highlighting key advances in the research on autoimmune chronic spontaneous urticaria (aiCSU).

Year	Study finding	Author
1983	Autoreactivity in CSU identified via the ASST	Grattan et al.
1986	Association of CSU with thyroid autoimmunity discovered	Leznoff et al.
1988	Detection of IgG antibodies against IgE in CSU patients	Gruber et al.
1991	Histamine release assay finds functional IgG-anti-IgE in CSU sera	Grattan et al.
1993	Detection of functional IgG-anti-FcεRI antibodies in CSU patients	Hide et al.
1999	Familial history of urticaria correlates with ASST positivity	Asero et al.
2002	First detection of IgE-anti- TPO antibodies in a CSU patient	Bar-Sela et al.
2011	BHRA and ASST positivity found to predict a slower response to omalizumab	Gericke et al.
2017	Detection of IgE-anti-IL-24 in CSU patients	Schmetzer et al.
2018	Research reveals a CSU subset with autoimmune diseases through the PURIST study	Schoepke et al.
2019	Identification of IgE-anti-EP and IgE-anti-ECP in severe CSU	Sánchez et al.
2020	Passive transfer of IgE-anti-TPO in CSU patients demonstrated through control skin experiments	Sánchez et al.
2021	Identification of new aiCSU markers, including eosinopenia, high IgG-anti-TPO, low IgE, low IgA, and nocturnal symptoms	Kolkhir et al., Marcelino et al.
2022	Recent studies highlight an overlap between type I and type IIb autoimmunity in CSU	Asero et al., Zhang et al.

(aiCSU: autoimmune chronic spontaneous urticaria; ASST: autologous serum skin test; BHRA: basophil histamine release assay; TPO: thyroid peroxidase; ECP: eosinophil cationic protein; EP: eosinophil peroxidase)

TH2 cytokines such as IL-4, IL-5, and IL-13. Multiple molecular targets, such as IgE, IL-4Ra, Siglec-8, C5aR, KIT, MRGPRX2, CD20, IL-5R, thymic stromal lymphopoietin (TSLP), IL-17, IL-5, and bruton tyrosine kinase (BTK), are under consideration for the treatment of CSU both currently and in future research **(Fig. 1)**.

- CSU patients can have IgG, IgA, and/or IgM autoantibodies to IgE or its high affinity receptor FcεRI.
- It is unknown if CSU patients have mast cell activating autoantibodies against other receptors like MRGPRX2 or C5aR.
- Rates of IgG-anti-FcεRI and/or IgG-anti-IgE in CSU patients range from 0% to 69%, with most studies showing 20–50%.
- Recent studies found 24%, 60%, and 57% of CSU patients with elevated IgG-, IgM-, and IgA-anti-FcεRI levels, respectively.
- 26% of CSU patients had both IgG-anti-FcεRI and positive basophil histamine release assay (BHRA), 25% had positive ASST plus BHRA, and 32% had BHRA alone.

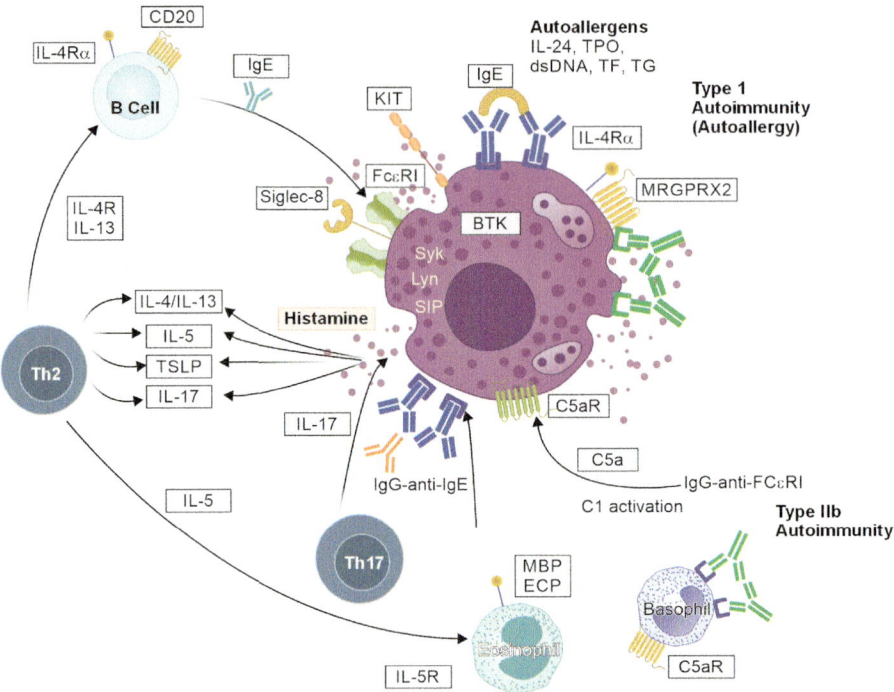

FIG. 1: The pathophysiology, endotypes, and potential therapeutic targets of CSU. Tissue factor (TF), eosinophil cationic protein (ECP), major basic protein (MBP), bruton tyrosine kinase (BTK), and thyroglobulin (TG).

- The PURIST study, using all three markers (ASST, basophil tests, and IgG autoantibodies immunoassay), found less than 10% with type IIb aiCSU.
- Older studies used fewer markers, but the strict criteria of the PURIST study do not exclude patients with only one or two positive biomarkers from having a type IIb response.
- In vitro studies indicate that IgG autoantibodies targeting FcεRI or IgE are associated with mast cell activation and its mediator release; however, 15% of CSU patients possess anti-FcεRI autoantibodies that do not exhibit histamine-releasing activity.
- Mast cell activation correlates with complement-fixing IgG subclasses 1 and 3, and to a lesser degree, IgG4, while IgG2 shows no association.
- IgG autoantibodies targeting FcεRI and/or IgE are present in healthy individuals and various disease states, yet their role in CSU remains ambiguous.
- Low serum IgE in type IIb aiCSU might reduce IgE occupancy on FcεRI, making natural anti-FcεRI autoantibodies pathogenic.

Demographic Features

- A typical patient with type IIb aiCSU is an adult female exhibiting high disease activity alongside associated autoimmune conditions, primarily autoimmune thyroiditis and/or vitiligo.

- There is often a family history present of autoimmune disorders.
- Studies, including the PURIST study, highlight a higher prevalence of type IIb aiCSU among females, with a significant proportion of patients having first-degree relatives with urticaria.

Clinical Features

- Type IIb aiCSU is linked with higher disease activity, as evidenced by associations with CD63/203c and/or BHRA positivity.
- Patients with IgG-anti-TPO, a marker for autoimmune thyroid disease, often experience higher rates of CSU recurrence after remission.
- Additional markers include angioedema, nocturnal symptoms, and symptoms lasting more than 5 days per week.
- The high prevalence of aiCSU among females is also supported by associations between female sex, positive ASST results, and thyroid autoimmunity.

Laboratory Features

- Emerging laboratory markers for type IIb aiCSU include low levels of total IgE and IgA, basopenia, eosinopenia, and poor response to conventional treatments.
- Elevated levels of IgM-anti-FcεRI, but not IgG- or IgA-anti-FcεRI, are associated with low blood basophil and eosinophil counts.
- The presence of these autoantibodies is linked to the activation of mast cells and disease characteristics.

Diagnosis of Type IIb Autoimmune Chronic Spontaneous Urticaria

- *Standard diagnostic criteria*: The "criterion standard" for diagnosing type IIb aiCSU includes positive ASST, positive functional bioassay [basophil tests like BHRA or basophil activation test (BAT)], and the detection of IgG-anti-FcεRI or IgG-anti-IgE via immunoassay.
- *Basophil tests versus ASST*: Basophil tests (BHRA or BAT) are the best single tests for the diagnosis of type IIb aiCSU, correlating better with other markers and treatment response compared to ASST or immunoassays. ASST alone has low predictive value and can be influenced by nonautoantibody factors like coagulation factors.
- *ASST limitations and use*: ASST has limited predictive value for type IIb aiCSU and may produce false positives. It is useful as a screening tool when combined with other markers, such as angioedema, elevated thyroid autoantibodies, and low total IgE levels. A negative ASST result is a reliable indicator for excluding functional circulating autoantibodies.
- *Diagnostic markers*: Hashimoto's thyroiditis is commonly associated with type IIb aiCSU, but detection of IgG-anti-TPO alone is not very specific. The combination of high IgG-anti-TPO and low total IgE levels is a useful diagnostic marker for type IIb aiCSU. Current guidelines recommend assessing these levels before starting omalizumab treatment.

OVERLAP OF TYPE I AND TYPE IIB AUTOIMMUNE CHRONIC SPONTANEOUS URTICARIA

- Not all CSU patients fit strictly into autoallergic or type IIb autoimmune endotypes based solely on IgE or IgA/IgM/IgG autoantibodies.
- Overlap rates between different autoantibodies are unknown because many studies did not exclude patients with mixed endotypes or assess co-expression of IgE and other autoantibodies.
- Recent research found that over 50% of patients had both IgE and IgG autoantibodies to various antigens, with 25% having IgE-anti-FcεRI.
- Both type IIb aiCSU markers (e.g., basophil tests) and autoallergic CSU markers (e.g., IgE-anti–IL-24) correlate with disease activity and basopenia.
- IgE-anti-TPO and IgG-anti-TPO are reported to be coexpressed in some CSU patients.
- Correlation between the IgG and IgE autoantibodies has been noted in various other autoimmune diseases; some CSU patients with low total IgE may still have IgE autoantibodies.
- Patients with elevated IgE-anti-TPO levels often have lower IgA and/or IgE levels.
- Late responders to the drug omalizumab have high levels of both antitissue factors IgE and IgG compared to early responders.
- Further studies are needed to understand the coexistence of autoallergic and autoimmune mechanisms in CSU and how the overlap of IgE and IgG autoantibodies affects treatment efficacy.

TREATMENT OF PATIENTS WITH AUTOIMMUNE CHRONIC SPONTANEOUS URTICARIA

Available Treatments

- *Standard treatment for CSU*:
    - First-line: Second-generation anti H1 antihistamines
    - If unresponsive, increase the dose up to four times.
    - Only 38.6% respond to standard doses of second-generation anti-H1.
- *Omalizumab (anti-IgE antibody)*:
    - Used in antihistamine-refractory cases
    - Blocks IgE from binding to its receptors, reducing mast cell activation
    - Shows 70% efficacy in antihistamine-resistant CSU patients with IgE-anti-TPO autoantibodies
    - Response types: Early responders (before 4 weeks) and late responders (up to 24 weeks)
- *Omalizumab nonresponders*:
    - Linked to factors like BHRA/BAT positivity, low IgE, high IgG-anti-TPO levels, eosinopenia, and basopenia
    - Higher ratio of IgG-anti-TPO to IgE associated with poor omalizumab response

- *Cyclosporine (immunosuppressant)*:
  - Used as third-line treatment when omalizumab fails
  - Response rates: 54–73%
  - Best responders: Patients with low total IgE and positive basophil tests
  - More effective in type IIb aiCSU patients, potentially leading to longer remissions
- *Alternative treatments*:
  - Plasmapheresis, rituximab (anti-CD20), intravenous immunoglobulin (IVIG), methotrexate, cyclophosphamide, and mycophenolate mofetil have shown efficacy in small case studies for antihistamine-resistant CSU with autoimmune markers.

NOVEL TREATMENTS UNDER DEVELOPMENT

- *Ligelizumab (anti-IgE antibody)*:
  - Higher affinity to IgE and greater efficacy compared to omalizumab
  - In phase 2b trials, more patients achieved complete control of CSU symptoms with ligelizumab than omalizumab
- *Anti-C5 and anti-C5aR therapies*:
  - Target complement factor C5a, which induces mast cell activation
  - Expected to work across CSU endotypes, particularly effective in type IIb aiCSU
- *BTK inhibitors (e.g., Fenebrutinib, Rilzabrutinib, Remibrutinib)*:
  - Block mast cell and basophil activation via FcεRI signaling
  - Fenebrutinib shows faster response in type IIb aiCSU.
  - Remibrutinib shows dose–response improvement in CSU symptoms.
- *IL-17 and IL-23 inhibitors*:
  - Serum levels of IL-17 and IL-23 are higher in CSU patients, especially in type IIb aiCSU.
  - Secukinumab (anti–IL-17A) is effective, but response onset is slow.
- *Dupilumab (anti-IL-4Ra antibody)*:
  - Targets IL-4 and IL-13 and reduces CSU symptoms
  - Expected to be more effective in type I aiCSU
  - Shows efficacy in omalizumab-naive and antihistamine-resistant patients
- *Lirentelimab (anti-Siglec-8 antibody)*:
  - Targets mast cells and eosinophils and shows efficacy in antihistamine-resistant patients
  - Disease activity drop noted in both omalizumab-naive and omalizumab-refractory patients.
- *CDX-0159 (anti-KIT antibody)*:
  - Depletes skin mast cells and reduces CSU symptoms, especially in antihistamine-refractory cases
- *Benralizumab and Mepolizumab (anti–IL-5 receptor)*:
  - Target eosinophils and show potential in reducing CSU symptoms
  - Ongoing studies for efficacy in antihistamine-resistant CSU

TABLE 2: Differences between type I (autoallergic) and type IIb aiCSU.

Feature	Type I aiCSU (autoallergic)	Type IIb aiCSU
Autoantibodies	IgE autoantibodies to autoantigens (e.g., TPO, IL-24, EP)	IgG/IgM/IgA autoantibodies targeting FcεRI or IgE
Prevalence	Accounts for a subset of CSU patients, higher IgE-anti-TPO positivity (varies in studies)	Less than 10% of CSU patients (PURIST study)
Pathogenesis	IgE binds to autoantigens and activates mast cells	IgG/IgA/IgM autoantibodies activate mast cells via FcεRI, etc.
Key diagnostic markers	IgE-anti-TPO, IgE-anti-IL-24, elevated total IgE, comorbid allergic diseases	Positive ASST, IgG-anti-FcεRI, low IgE, basophil activation
Skin test results	Positive skin reactions to specific autoantigens (TPO)	Positive ASST or BAT/BHRA
Demographics	Limited information but IgE autoantibodies (e.g., IgE-anti-TPO) more common in some populations	Predominantly adult females with autoimmune comorbidities (e.g., Hashimoto's thyroiditis)
Comorbidities	Higher prevalence of allergic diseases (e.g., atopic dermatitis, allergic rhinitis)	Higher prevalence of autoimmune diseases (e.g., Hashimoto's thyroiditis, vitiligo)
Disease severity	Variable disease severity, correlations with higher total IgE	Higher disease activity, often more severe and refractory
Angioedema	Present but less associated with severity markers	Common (62–76%), often associated with nocturnal symptoms and higher disease activity
Total IgE levels	Elevated total IgE levels; some patients with higher autoreactive IgE	Low total IgE levels; often associated with poor treatment response
Basophil/eosinophil counts	Variable; some associations with basopenia in IgE-anti-IL-24 positive patients	Lower basophil and eosinophil counts (basopenia and eosinopenia)
Treatment response	Better response to omalizumab, especially early responders	Poorer or slower response to omalizumab; better response to cyclosporine
Response to antihistamines	Moderate-to-good response in some cases	Poor response to antihistamines, requiring higher doses or alternative treatments
Laboratory findings	High total IgE, positive skin tests for specific autoantigens, elevated IgE autoantibodies	Low total IgE, positive basophil tests, IgG-anti-FcεRI, or IgG-anti-IgE
Overlap with other endotypes	Significant overlap with type IIb aiCSU in some patients	Overlap with type I aiCSU; some patients have both IgE and IgG autoantibodies
Treatment of nonresponders	Omalizumab or cyclosporine for severe cases	Cyclosporine, plasmapheresis, or rituximab for nonresponders

(aiCSU: autoimmune chronic spontaneous urticaria; ASST: autologous serum skin test; BAT: basophil activation test; BHRA: basophil histamine release assay; TPO: thyroid peroxidase; EP: eosinophil peroxidase)

- *MRGPRX2 and Alarmins (e.g., TSLP, IL-33, IL-25)*:
  - MRGPRX2 involved in IgE-independent mast cell activation, being targeted by antagonists in preclinical stages.
  - Tezepelumab (anti-TSLP mAb) is under investigation for CSU treatment.

Table 2 highlights the differences between type I (autoallergic) and type IIb aiCSU, showing the distinct diagnostic markers, treatment responses, and associated clinical features for both.

CONCLUSION

Urticaria can be classified based on its etiology into different types, such as acute and chronic urticaria, with the latter lasting more than 6 weeks. Chronic urticaria is further divided into CSU and chronic inducible urticaria (CIU), with CSU occurring without obvious triggers. While diagnosing urticaria itself is usually straightforward, identifying the underlying cause can be quite challenging, especially in chronic cases. CSU is often idiopathic, but recent advances have suggested that autoimmune mechanisms may play a significant role in a subset of patients. Various tests, such as the ASST, BAT, and antithyroid antibody testing, have been developed to help identify autoimmune urticaria. These tests are valuable for guiding treatment in cases where conventional approaches fail to identify an external trigger.

SUGGESTED READINGS

1. Gruber BL, Baeza ML, Marchese MJ, Agnello V, Kaplan AP. Prevalence and functional role of anti-IgE autoantibodies in urticarial syndromes. J Invest Dermatol. 1988;90:213-7.
2. Grattan CE, Wallington TB, Warin RP, Kennedy CT, Bradfield JW. A serological mediator in chronic idiopathic urticaria–a clinical, immunological and histological evaluation. Br J Dermatol. 1986;114:583-90.
3. Ertas R, Ozyurt K, Atasoy M, Hawro T, Maurer M. The clinical response to omalizumab in chronic spontaneous urticaria patients is linked to and predicted by IgE levels and their change. Allergy. 2018;73:705-12.
4. Soundararajan S, Kikuchi Y, Joseph K, Kaplan AP. Functional assessment of pathogenic IgG subclasses in chronic autoimmune urticaria. J Allergy Clin Immunol. 2005;115:815-21.
5. Attar MHZ, Merk HF, Kotliar K, Wurpts G, Röseler S, Moll-Slodowy S, et al. The CD63 basophil activation test as a diagnostic tool for assessing autoimmunity in patients with chronic spontaneous urticaria. Eur J Dermatol. 2019;29:614-8.

CHAPTER 14

Urticaria in Children

Shikha Gupta, Himanshu Gupta

INTRODUCTION

Urticaria is a disease, characterized by wheals and/or angioedema that presents across all age groups, including infancy and childhood. Although the presentation is similar in many ways to adults, there are important management concerns unique to this age group that necessitates a detailed discussion of this topic.

Like adults, urticaria is classified in the pediatric age group as acute (<6 weeks' duration) and chronic (>6 weeks' duration). In chronic spontaneous urticaria (CSU), which includes around 80% of chronic urticaria (CU) cases found in the pediatric age group, the clinical symptoms (wheal and/or angioedema) appear without a clear discernible etiology; however, in chronic inducible urticaria (CIU), specific stimuli are responsible for triggering the clinical symptoms.

The prevalence of CU in children is lesser than that of adults (0.1–0.5% in children vs. 1–1.8% in adults) and most cases are observed between 6 and 11 years of age. The prognosis appears to be better in children, with one-third cases of CSU remitting spontaneously within 1 year and one half within 3 years.

However, while managing the patient in this age group, the clinician needs to keep quality of life impairment particularly in mind, since the disease as well as the sedative drugs might interfere with child's school performance, sleep, and his social behavior/play. There are a number of guidelines focusing on the management of adult urticaria; however, there is a paucity of research on clinical features and management options in the pediatric age group. In this chapter, we will attempt to summarize the available evidence and focus on the management concerns in children.

FACTORS TRIGGERING URTICARIA IN PEDIATRIC AGE GROUP

There are distinct triggers for acute and chronic urticaria in childhood **(Table 1)**. Let us discuss in brief about them.

Triggers of acute urticaria in children:
- *Infections*: It is important to note that infections, particularly respiratory infections, are the leading cause of acute urticaria in children (40–50%). Among

TABLE 1: Common triggers for urticaria in childhood.	
Triggers of acute urticaria	**Triggers of chronic urticaria**
Infections: • *Viral*: EBV, HSV, hepatitis B • *Bacterial*: Group A β-hemolytic streptococci, *Mycoplasma pneumoniae*	*Infections:* • *Viral*: Adenovirus, rotavirus, enterovirus, HHV-6, herpesvirus, respiratory syncytial virus • Parasitic (*Blastocystis hominis, Giardia lamblia, Fasciola hepatica, Toxocara canis, Ascaris lumbricoides, Anisakis*) • *Bacterial*: *Staphylococcus aureus, Helicobacter pylori*, oral flora (*Veillonella species*)
Drugs: • Penicillin • Cephalosporin • NSAIDs	*Inducible*: • Physical urticaria (cold, pressure, vibration, solar) • Nonphysical types (cholinergic, aquagenic, contact)
Food	Autoimmune
	Food (uncommon)

(EBV: Epstein–Barr virus; HSV: herpes simplex virus; HHV-6: human herpesvirus-6; NSAIDs: nonsteroidal anti-inflammatory drugs)

the viral infections, Epstein–Barr virus (EBV), herpes simplex virus (HSV), and hepatitis virus are more often causative. This may also explain the seasonal incidence of acute urticaria cases in children. Another common infection associated with acute urticaria in children is *Mycoplasma pneumoniae*.

Furthermore, streptococcal infection is also responsible for around 15–20% of cases of acute urticaria in children. These children usually recover after an antibiotic course.

- *Drugs*: Among drugs, penicillin, cephalosporins, and NSAIDs are commonly found to be associated with acute urticaria. Drug reactions also may lead to anaphylaxis. It is also difficult to ascertain in many cases, whether urticaria is triggered by the infection itself or by the drug/antibiotic used to treat it. To make the matter more complicated, in many cases, especially in children, the trigger is not the antibiotic per se, but the excipients present in the drug solution. However, it is important to note that drug reactions in the pediatric population tend to be urticarial more often than in adults.
- *Food*: Food has been associated with 0–18% of acute urticaria studies in various studies in children as well adults. In children, ingestion of foods such as eggs, nuts, milk, seafood, soy, peanuts, or wheat may trigger acute urticaria, especially more frequently than adults.

    Particularly in infants < 6 months, cow's milk allergy may be important. Food urticaria generally occurs either immediately or within 60 minutes of food intake. Skin prick test and specific IgE test may not be useful in the diagnosis because of direct histamine release (non-IgE mediated) by some foods such as tomato, cheese, strawberry, and lobster. It is important to note that blanket restriction of food items cannot be advised in children to avoid dietary deficiency, which may impair their growth.

Triggers of chronic urticaria in children:
- *Infections*: It is generally seen that in children, new episodes of infections are accompanied by triggering of urticarial episodes (reappearance/aggravation), causing CSU. The prevalence of this association with infection tends to decrease with age. The most common infections associated with triggering CU in children are upper respiratory tract infections, such as adenovirus, rotavirus, enterovirus, and respiratory syncytial virus. There is recent data emerging that also associates human herpesvirus-6 (HHV-6) and other herpesvirus with CU in this age group.

    Parasitic infections such as *Blastocystis hominis, Giardia lamblia, Fasciola hepatica, Toxocara canis, Ascaris lumbricoides,* and *Anisakis* also constitute an important cause of urticaria in the pediatric age group, especially in the regions where these infections are endemic.

    Among bacterial infections, *Helicobacter pylori* is a frequently mentioned cause of urticaria in literature, however, its prevalence in children (2–18%) has been observed to be lower than that found in adults. Moreover, it has been observed that successful eradication of *H. pylori* is not a foolproof method of recovery from this disease.

    Children with CU have been observed to have a higher prevalence of nasal carriage of *Staphylococcus aureus*.

    It is also recommended to check the condition of oral cavity in children with CU as lipopolysaccharides of certain microorganisms in oral flora can lead to histamine release by mast cells in the presence of odontogenic infections.
- *Food*: Food allergy is an uncommon cause of CU. Food additives and natural salicylates (tomato, orange, raspberry, and others) may exacerbate the symptoms of CU but are rarely the only cause of the disease.
- *Autoimmune*: In 2013, the European Academy of Allergy and Clinical Immunology (EAACI) published the criteria for the diagnosis of autoimmune urticaria: (a) positive biological tests in vitro demonstrating functional activities of autoantibodies (basophil histamine-release test) or detection of CD63 and CD203 activation markers on the basophil surface with the method of flow cytometry, (b) positive autologous serum skin test (ASST), (c) detection of autoantibodies to FcεR1α.

    However, in everyday practice, only ASST is available to diagnose autoimmune urticaria with a sensitivity of around 70% and a specificity of around 80%. The frequency of a positive ASST in CU is similar in children and adults.

    The diagnosis is important as many children can have other autoimmune pathologies, including thyroiditis and systemic lupus erythematosus.

    Also, it has been observed that in children with CU have been found to have a greater frequency of celiac disease than controls. Symptoms resolved after a 2-week gluten-free diet in most of these children.
- *Inducible urticaria*: About 20% of CU cases in children are inducible, i.e., occur in response to a specific trigger. Inducible urticaria in children, such as adults, is of two subtypes: (i) physical urticaria and (ii) nonphysical subtype.

1. *Physical urticaria* includes a group of disorders where wheals are induced by physical stimuli—cold, heat, pressure, vibration, and UV rays, and is commonly seen in children and adults.
   - Cold-induced urticaria here deserves particular mention since it may be associated with severe anaphylactic reactions. It may be triggered by cold air, fluids or objects. Cold-induced urticaria in children may be primary, or secondary to infections (herpesvirus, bacterial, or helminthic), autoimmune disorders, or cryoglobulinemia.
   - Delayed-pressure urticaria and solar urticaria are uncommonly seen in this age group.
2. *Nonphysical types of urticaria* present with the development of wheals in response to core body temperature elevation (cholinergic), contact with water (aquagenic), or contact with chemical agents such as latex (contact), all of which are quite uncommon in the pediatric age group.

CLINICAL FEATURES

Wheals are itchy and are variable in size, number, and extent of body surface area involved. The appearance/presentation is similar to adults in most instances. More than 50% of the body may also be involved. Along with wheals, angioedema may or may not be present. In children, accompanying angioedema is seen in 30–45% of cases of acute urticaria. Food-induced urticaria usually presents immediately or within a few hours after the food intake.

Cholinergic urticaria is characterized by pinpoint-sized/small wheals whereas pressure urticaria is usually seen over sites of tight clothing.

Systemic symptoms include wheezing, breathlessness, nasal discharge, dizziness, flushing, gut symptoms (nausea/vomiting, diarrhea, and pain abdomen), tachycardia, fever, and joint pains. It is important to note that these symptoms may be indicative of anaphylaxis, especially if they are rapid in onset.

PROGNOSIS

Chronic urticaria in children has a better prognosis with cases self-resolving earlier than that seen in adults. In various available studies in the pediatric population, remission rates after 1 year were 16–37%, and after 5 years were 50–67.5%. It has also been found out that after 7 years, 96% of children were symptom-free, in contrast to adults, 20% of whom remain symptomatic even after 10 years.

COEXISTENT DISEASES

A few studies have shown an association between CSU occurring in the pediatric age group and diseases associated with atopy, including allergic rhinitis, asthma, atopic dermatitis, and food allergy in as many as 30–50% of cases. Food allergy was found in one study to be associated with CSU in 15% of cases.

Moreover, CSU has also been observed to be associated with autoimmune diseases such as celiac disease, thyroiditis, and systemic lupus erythematosus.

DIFFERENTIAL DIAGNOSES

Urticaria needs to be differentiated from other medical conditions where wheals, angioedema, or both can occur as clinical features, for instance, *anaphylaxis* which is characterized by dyspnea, wheals, swelling, abdominal cramps, nausea, diarrhea, tachycardia, hypotension, and dizziness.

Among other differentials in this age group, of particular mention are the *autoinflammatory syndromes*, which have in common a few features—history of recurrent fever, joint pains and the wheals not responding to antihistamines. Cryopyrin-associated periodic syndromes (CAPS) is a group of autosomal dominant inherited disorders with a defect in the cryopyrin-encoding gene and include familial cold autoinflammatory syndrome (FCAS), Muckle–Wells syndrome (MWS) and neonatal-onset multisystem inflammatory disease (NOMID). Presentation of CAPS usually occurs in the neonatal period or early infancy. Symptoms of FCAS include fever and pruritic urticarial rash with burning and joint pains and develop after cold exposure. MWS is not cold-exposure dependent and also is characterized by sensorineural deafness. Another autoinflammatory disease worth describing here is *systemic-onset juvenile idiopathic arthritis*, which is seen in children < 16 years of age and clinical features include arthritis present for >6 weeks and fever of at least 2-week duration. The rash in this condition is usually pruritic and urticarial, and may be associated with linear dermographism.

Urticaria multiforme presents in children between 4 months and 4 years with polycyclic or annular plaques resembling urticaria wheals, but with bruising. It may be preceded by fever and a viral illness and lesions respond favorably to antihistamines.

Urticarial vasculitis is characterized by burning rather than itching; purpuric lesions lasting > 24 hours and is usually associated with fever and joint pains, whereas bradykinin-mediated angioedema including *hereditary angioedema (HAE)* presents with recurrent episodes of angioedema without wheals or itching.

DIAGNOSIS

The diagnosis is based on clinical signs and symptoms. A detailed history will identify the need for skin testing if a specific trigger like drug or food is suspected. Dermographism should be evaluated. Skin biopsy is rarely required.

Routine laboratory assessment is not recommended for acute urticaria. In cases of CSU, a differential blood count, erythrocyte sedimentation rate (ESR) and/or C-reactive protein are tested. Further assessment is carried out on the basis of suspected causes/triggers as detailed in **Table 2**.

MANAGEMENT

The evaluation tools used in adult urticaria must also be applied in this age group to assess the disease activity because it plays a role in the effective management of the disease, though there are no validated, disease-specific assessment tools are available for use in children.

TABLE 2: Assessment of chronic urticaria (CU) in children.	
Criteria	**Urticarial rash > 6-week duration**
Subtypes	• Spontaneous • Inducible
Exacerbating factors	Infections, drugs (NSAIDs, penicillin), inconsistent treatment, autoimmune
Initial laboratory investigations	• Differential leukocyte counts • ESR and/or CRP
Specific laboratory investigations	• *Inducible urticaria*: Cold, pressure, heat, sunlight, exercise challenge • *Possible drug/ food trigger*: Skin prick tests with drug/food; specific IgE antibody measurement • *Suspected infection*: Eosinophilia, leukocytosis, ASLO titer, stool examination, urine, blood culture • *Suspected systemic/autoimmune disease*: ASST, antithyroid antibodies, ANA, anti-tTG

(ANA: antinuclear antibody; Anti-tTG: anti-tissue transglutaminase; ASLO: antistreptolysin o; ASST: autologous serum skin test; CRP: C-reactive protein; ESR: erythrocyte sedimentation rate; IgE: immunoglobulin E; NSAIDs: nonsteroidal anti-inflammatory drugs)

All efforts should be made to identify the triggers for exacerbations and if necessary, similar tests for provocation and trigger thresholds may be conducted, taking into consideration the child's age and ability to cooperate with the assessments.

The goal of treatment is to efficiently manage the condition, until complete resolution is achieved, aiming for a restoration of normal quality of life. The treatment should be adjusted according to the symptoms, and should be continuous, rather than on an SOS basis.

Thus, the cornerstones of the management of urticaria in this age group, not unlike those in adults, are:
- Identification, and if possible, elimination of underlying causes:
  ○ Antibiotics, antiparasitic therapy, and thyroid hormone replacement can be done as and when required
- Avoidance of factors responsible for triggering the disease/worsening the disease activity
- Induction of tolerance, whenever feasible, to reduce disease activity
- Pharmacological treatment for symptomatic control

Guideline Recommendations

The updated GA²LEN/EDF/WAO (Global Allergy and Asthma European Network/European Dermatology Forum/World Allergy Organization) guidelines support the use of nonsedating second-generation antihistamines as the mainstay of treatment for the management of CU in children as well as adults.

Many authors have reported a better response in children with standard doses of antihistamines **(Table 3)** as compared to adults, in whom an updosing is required more often. It should be kept in mind that there may be a risk of respiratory depression in infants with the updosing of sedating antihistamines.

TABLE 3: Doses of antihistamines in pediatric age group.

Drug	Dosage
Hydroxyzine	2 mg/kg/day in three divided doses
Diphenhydramine	0.5 mg/kg/dose Q6–8 hourly
Cetirizine	*2–5 years*—2.5 mg OD, *6–11 years*—5 mg OD, *>12 years*—10 mg OD
Levocetirizine	*2–5 years*—1.25 mg OD, *6–11 years*—2.5 mg OD, *>12 years*—5 mg OD
Fexofenadine	*6–11 years*—30 mg BD, *>12 years*—60 mg BD
Loratadine	*2–5 years*—5 mg OD, *>6 years*—10 mg OD
Bilastine	*>6 years*—10 mg/day

Also, there may be sedation and even paradoxical hyperactivity in children with the administration of first-generation antihistamines. Therefore, first-generation antihistamines are not recommended as first-line therapy for urticaria in children.

Levocetirizine and cetirizine may be safely used in children > 1 year of age. It is worthwhile to mention here that the pharmacokinetics of levocetirizine in children up to 6 years of age differs from older children and adults. Younger children eliminate levocetirizine rapidly, therefore, in children <7 years age, levocetirizine needs to be administered in higher dose twice a day.

Other second-generation antihistamines studied in the pediatric population for urticaria include bilastine (may be used in children >6 years of age in the dose of 10 mg/day), desloratadine, fexofenadine, loratadine, and rupatadine. The choice of which antihistamine is to be selected for a child mainly depends upon the age of child and the drug availability as a dispersible tablet/syrup (for younger children).

The updated GA^{2}LEN/EDF/WAO guidelines using the same treatment algorithm in children as adults, with weight-adjusted dosage and recommend updosing of these antihistamines to up to two to four times if there is no improvement after 2–4 weeks (as opposed to using different antihistamines at the same time); however, safety studies for updosing are required for most of these antihistamines in children.

According to these guidelines, if there is still no improvement, oral steroid (strictly short-term and as a very restricted measure), cyclosporine or omalizumab may be added.

Omalizumab is a humanized antibody against IgE, which has been approved to treat chronic urticaria—spontaneous and inducible—in children over 12 years of age. It appears to be safe with minimal side effects; however, there is a paucity of data evaluating its use in children so far. The recommended initial dose in CSU is 300 mg every 4 weeks. Dosing is independent of total serum IgE.

Ciclosporin is off-label for use in urticaria and is only recommended in diseases not responding to antihistamines and omalizumab. However, in practice, in resource-limited settings and in children < 12 years age, where omalizumab cannot be afforded, it may be started as a second-line therapy. It is administered in the dose of 3.5–5 mg/kg/day and has a far better risk/benefit ratio than systemic steroids.

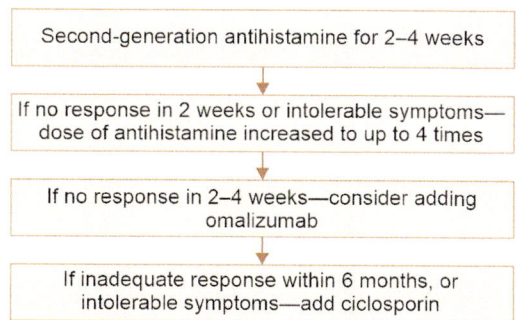

FLOWCHART 1: Management of chronic urticaria in children [Indian Academy of Pediatrics (IAP), 2022].

Flowchart 1 gives an overview of the 2022 Indian Academy of Pediatrics (IAP) guidelines for the management of chronic urticaria in children.

There is no evidence to support the role of pseudoallergen-free/preservative-free diet in urticaria in children. Moreover, the clinical recommendations by an Italian multidisciplinary panel recommend against using such a diet in children with urticaria.

CONCLUSION

There is a need to have more standardized studies exploring the epidemiology of urticaria, its clinical features, and treatment response in children. Currently, second-generation antihistamines form the mainstay of treatment of urticaria in the pediatric age group, however, newer antihistamines are still not studied extensively in children.

Above all, it is imperative to understand the unique requirements of this age group since the dermatologist should not only aim to attain adequate symptom control but also must choose the therapeutic options that allow for optimum social performance during school and in the playground.

SUGGESTED READINGS

1. Zuberbier T, Abdul Latiff AH, Abuzakouk M, Aquilina S, Asero R, Baker D, et al. The international EAACI/GA²LEN/EuroGuiDerm/APAAACI guideline for the definition, classification, diagnosis, and management of urticaria. Allergy. 2022;77(3):734-66.
2. Kudryavtseva AV, Neskorodova KA, Staubach P. Urticaria in children and adolescents: An updated review of the pathogenesis and management. Pediatr Allergy Immunol. 2019;30(1):17-24.
3. Caffarelli C, Paravati F, El Hachem M, Duse M, Bergamini M, Simeone G, et al. Management of chronic urticaria in children: a clinical guideline. Ital J Pediatr. 2019;45(1):101.
4. Papadopoulos NG, Zuberbier T. The safety and tolerability profile of bilastine for chronic urticaria in children. Clin Transl Allergy. 2019;9:55.
5. Simons FE; Early prevention of asthma in atopic children study group. H1-antihistamine treatment in young atopic children: effect on urticaria. Ann Allergy Asthma Immunol. 2007;99(3):261-6.

CHAPTER
15

Urticaria and Pregnancy

Deepti Saxena, Sanjeev Gupta, Aditi Dabhra

INTRODUCTION

Urticaria appears as elevated, well-demarcated areas of redness and swelling accompanied by itching. In classic urticaria, lesions can appear on any part of the body and disappear on their own without leaving any marks. About 10–20% of the population usually have symptoms of urticaria due to an allergic reaction, infection, or drug induced.

The lifetime prevalence of acute urticaria is reported to be up to 20% in general population. The prevalence of chronic urticaria, on the other hand, is reported to be 0.5–5% and women are affected twice as often as men. Currently, there is a lack of published data on the prevalence of urticaria during pregnancy. However, considering that it commonly affects young women, it is anticipated that the prevalence of urticaria in pregnancy is either equal to or possibly higher than that in the general population.

CLASSIFICATION OF URTICARIA

Urticaria is called chronic if lesions remain for >6 weeks and acute if the duration is <6 weeks **(Flowchart 1)**.

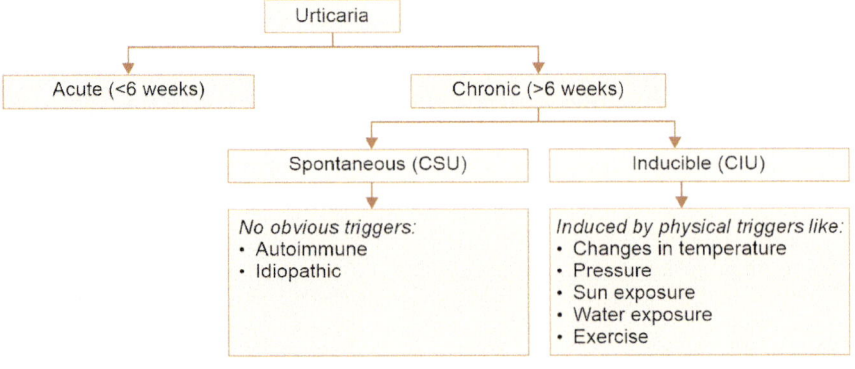

FLOWCHART 1: Classification of urticaria.
(CIU: chronic idiopathic urticaria; CSU: chronic spontaneous urticaria)

VARIOUS CHANGES DURING PREGNANCY

Hormonal and Immunological Changes

Pregnancy is a distinct physiological condition characterized by significant alterations in hormonal and immunological factors and their intricate interaction. The hormonal fluctuations that occur during pregnancy have a significant impact on the immune system, playing a crucial role in maintaining the pregnancy and preventing the mother's body from rejecting the fetus, which is considered "foreign" to her immune system. Several of these modifications impact the progression of immune-mediated illnesses, such as urticaria.

The immunological changes that occur during pregnancy are not merely suppressive but rather dynamic and sensitive, depending on the specific stage of pregnancy **(Table 1)**.

Various hormonal and immunological changes which influence chronic urticaria in pregnancy are given in **Table 2** and **Figure 1**.

TABLE 1: Changes in immunological milieu on different trimesters of pregnancy.

Trimester	Immune status	Physiological function
First trimester	Proinflammatory	Helps implantation and placental growth
Second trimester	Anti-inflammatory	Helps growth of fetus
Third trimester	Proinflammatory	For labor/delivery preparation

TABLE 2: Hormonal and immunological changes in pregnancy.

Human chorionic gonadotrophin (hCG)	A glycoprotein secreted by the placenta that peaks during the first trimester and then slowly declines until delivery. It also maintains the secretion of progesterone from the corpus luteum
Progesterone	A steroid hormone crucial for maintaining pregnancy. Initially secreted by the ovarian corpus luteum, and by 10–12 weeks of pregnancy, the placenta takes over. Levels rise as pregnancy progresses and drop after delivery
Estrogens	Steroid hormones of three types: Estradiol, estriol, and estrone. Estradiol is the most potent and predominant estrogen in reproductive-age females, secreted by the ovaries. Estriol is the main estrogen during pregnancy, secreted by the placenta. Levels increase over trimesters and drop at delivery
Cortisol	Levels increase by the end of the first trimester and peak in the third trimester. Its primary source is the adrenal cortex, with the placenta contributing by secreting corticotropic hormone toward the end of the third trimester, triggering labor. It exhibits significant anti-inflammatory effects
Prolactin	Prolactin concentration increases during gestation and stimulates and activates the immune system and is associated with several autoimmune disorders

Cytokines

Cytokines are peptide molecules released by different immune cells that have a crucial function in intercellular communication. Typically, there exists a delicate equilibrium between proinflammatory and anti-inflammatory cytokines. The equilibrium tilts toward the proinflammatory aspect throughout early pregnancy and toward the final stages of pregnancy to facilitate implantation and labor, respectively. Throughout the remainder of the pregnancy, it undergoes a shift toward the anti-inflammatory/tolerogenic side **(Figs. 2 and 3)**.

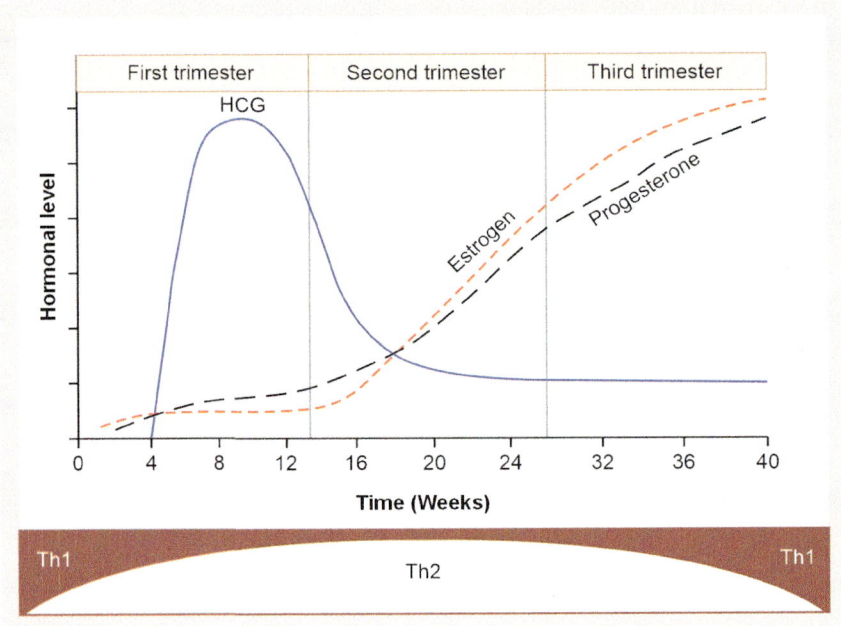

FIG. 1: Changes in hormone levels and adaptive immunity in pregnancy.

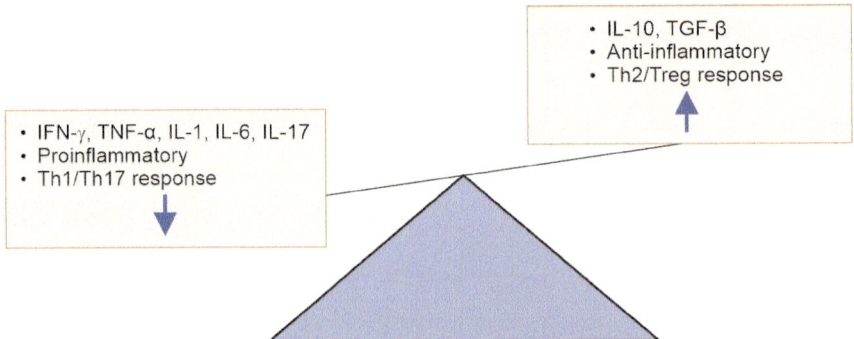

FIG. 2: Alteration of adaptive immunity during pregnancy (except very early and very late pregnancy).
(IL: interleukin; IFN-γ: interferon gamma; TGF: transforming growth factor; TNF-α: tumor necrosis factor alpha)

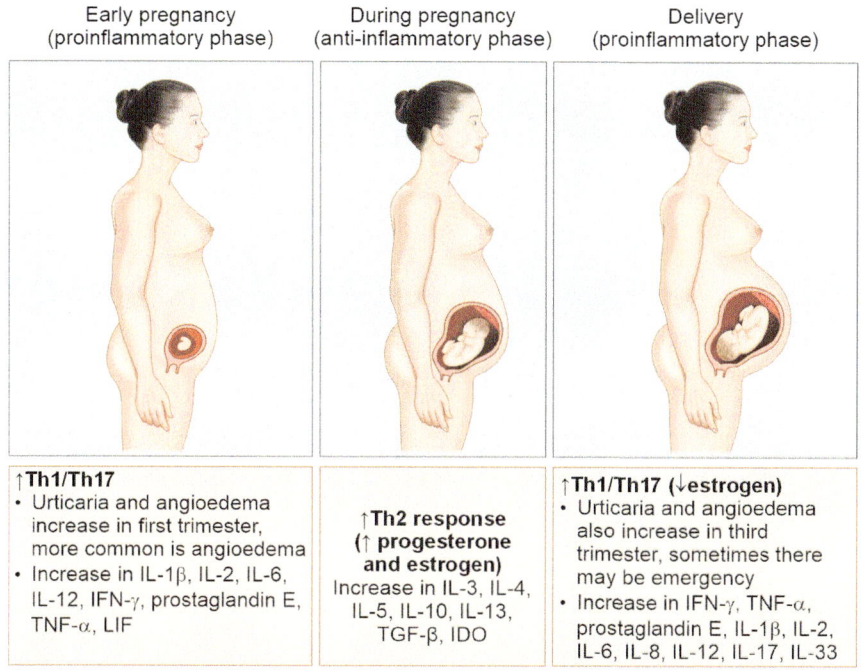

FIG. 3: Immunological changes that occur during various stages of pregnancy.
(IDO: indoleamine 2, 3-dioxygenase; IL: interleukin; IFN-γ: interferon gamma; TGF: transforming growth factor; TNF-α: tumor necrosis factor alpha)

EFFECT OF PREGNANCY ON THE COURSE OF URTICARIA

- Pregnancy often leads to alterations in chronic inflammatory diseases due to changes in the immune response, characterized by a decrease in Th1/Th17 type cytokines and an increase in Th2 type cytokines.
- Furthermore, there is a rise in the Treg (T-regulatory) cytokines such as interleukin (IL)-10 and transforming growth factor β (TGF-β), which effectively inhibit all T helper cell responses.
- As a result, autoimmune disorders that are influenced by the Th1/Th17 pathway, such as rheumatoid arthritis and psoriasis, tend to improve during pregnancy.
- Conversely, autoimmune diseases that are influenced by the Th2 route, such as systemic lupus erythematosus or atopic dermatitis, tend to worsen.
- The course of chronic urticaria in pregnancy does not follow a uniform pattern. While the condition improves in some patients, it flares up in others. This phenomenon can be ascribed to the perplexing impact of many hormones.

A recent study conducted by PREG-CU examined 288 patients with chronic urticaria from 21 centers across 13 nations. They actively engaged by completing a questionnaire pertaining to the progression of the illness throughout pregnancy. Approximately 51% of patients had disease improvement, while 29% reported

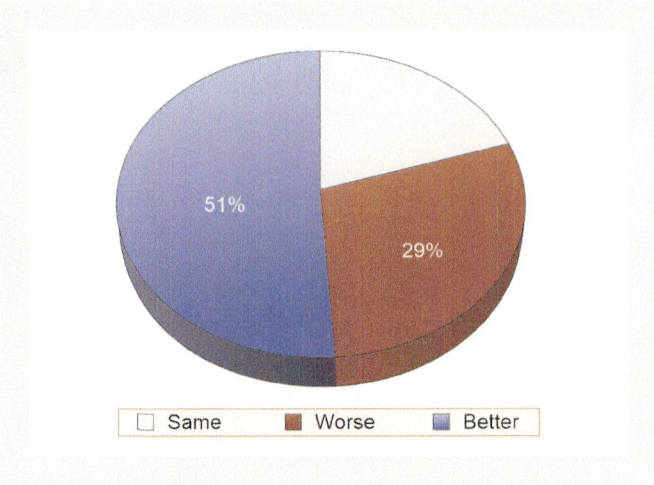

FIG. 4: PREG-CU study: The course of chronic urticaria in pregnancy.

disease deterioration. The remaining 20% of patients stated that their disease remained stable. Exacerbations of chronic urticaria primarily occurred during the third trimester or the first trimester due to the prevalence of Th1 immune responses and proinflammatory signals during these periods. Out of the patients who showed improvement during pregnancy, 50% of them saw a deterioration in the postpartum period, while the remaining patients reported no change **(Fig. 4)**.

EFFECT OF URTICARIA ON THE OUTCOME OF PREGNANCY

- Given its benign nature, urticaria is unlikely to have any impact on the progression or outcome of pregnancy.
- The new PREG-CU study found no significant impact on pregnancy outcomes for patients with chronic urticaria, when compared to the general population.
- Both groups experienced a comparable frequency of difficulties such as premature birth or neonatal medical issues. This is regardless of the recommended therapies.
- A total of 60% of the pregnant females who participated in this trial maintained their urticaria treatment throughout their pregnancy. The prescribed drugs consisted of both regular and higher doses of first- and second-generation antihistamines, as well as omalizumab.
- While urticaria and its regularly prescribed therapies may not have a direct impact on pregnancy, some medical conditions connected with urticaria and certain treatments may potentially influence the outcome of pregnancy.
- Anxiety, depression, and sleep difficulties linked to urticaria can heighten maternal stress levels, potentially leading to adverse effects on pregnancy outcomes, such as an increased risk of low birthweight infants and premature

deliveries. Therefore, it is imperative to evaluate the influence of urticaria on the patient's quality of life and appropriately address the condition.
- Furthermore, the indiscriminate usage of systemic therapies such as glucocorticoids or cyclosporine can lead to problems such as hypertension, nephrotoxicity, gestational diabetes, preeclampsia, and macrosomia. This necessitates prudent administration of drugs during pregnancy while closely monitoring for any negative consequences.

CLINICAL FEATURES AND MANIFESTATIONS

Urticaria in pregnancy presents as raised, well-circumscribed, erythematous, and swelled-up lesions on the skin that are accompanied by intense itching. These lesions may vary in size and shape and may appear and disappear within hours at different sites.

Some patients can also present with angioedema, which involves swelling of deeper layers of the skin, mainly around the eyes, lips, and throat.

Urticaria in pregnancy disturbs quality of life of the mother as the itching and swelling lead to physical discomfort, sleep disturbances, anxiety, and stress.

Types of Urticarial Dermatoses in Pregnancy
- Progesterone urticaria
- Chronic urticaria during pregnancy
- *Hereditary angioedema in pregnancy*:
  - Type I
  - Type II
  - Type III
- *Specific urticarial-like dermatoses of pregnancy*:
  - Pruritic urticarial papules and plaques in pregnancy (PUPPP)
  - Pemphigoid gestationis

Progesterone urticaria: This is an autoimmune disease which presents as angioedema, erythema multiforme-like lesions, papulovesicular eruptions, and fixed drug eruptions associated with progesterone. It presents as aggravation of symptoms during the luteal phase of the menstrual cycle and decrease in symptoms with the onset of menstruation. Lesions are mostly present on the trunk and extremities, sparing the face or genitalia. Diagnosis is confirmed by the cyclic nature of the appearance of lesions and positive skin tests for progesterone. It is observed that the females treated with progesterone before and during pregnancy for placental insufficiency are more prone to developing progesterone dermatitis or presents with aggravation of their existing lesions during pregnancy. Progesterone dermatitis in pregnancy is reported very less, because of the remission of disease in pregnancy, as the levels of progesterone are raised during pregnancy in contrast to the cyclic rise and fall during the menstrual cycle.

Chronic urticaria during pregnancy: Patients with chronic urticaria mostly have autoimmunity, and there are increased chances of autoimmune thyroid diseases and the occurrence of IgG antibodies-directed IgE receptor on mast cells and basophils. The high prevalence of chronic urticaria in females is possibly due to correlation between sex hormones and the autoimmunity. The pattern of chronic urticaria is not well defined during pregnancy. Some patients present with flare-up of urticaria, while some may show improvement.

Hereditary angioedema in pregnancy:
- *Hereditary angioedema types I and II*: Hereditary angioedema is an uncommon disease which presents as edema of the skin and mucous membranes. The duration of symptoms varies from 2 to 5 days and resolves spontaneously, except in some cases where there is involvement of the oral cavity, which leads to obstruction of airways and may lead to death. The most common site of appearance of lesions is the abdomen. *Pathogenesis*: In type I hereditary angioedema there is deficiency of C1 esterase inhibitor while in type II there is malfunction of the enzyme C1 esterase inhibitor. In patients with hereditary angioedema, overactivation of kallikrein leads to accumulation of bradykinin in the blood and tissues of patients and there is vasodilatory effect leading to edema. Type I hereditary angioedema is more common and occurs in 85% of cases and type II occurs in only 15%. The episode starts with tissue damage, which further triggers the activation of the coagulation, complement, and contact systems. For example, dental repair leads to perioral swelling, whereas an upper respiratory tract infection results in laryngeal edema. It has been observed that the rapid increase in estrogen levels at the starting and at the end of pregnancy is responsible for the symptoms, whereas the balance between estrogen and progesterone in the second trimester decreases the chance of occurrence of symptoms. During pregnancy, attack presents as uterine contractions and surgical emergencies because trigger starts most commonly in the abdomen. In some case reports, a higher attack rate was observed during puerperium. Delivery did not lead to angioedema but may lead to local swelling of the genitalia.
- *Type III hereditary angioedema*: This is a type of familial angioedema which mostly presents in women. In this variant, the level and function of C1E1 are normal. Typically, the disease manifests after the second decade of life with infrequent attacks, which usually involve the face, tongue, and larynx. Pregnancy influences the course of hereditary angioedema type III presenting as the trigger for the first attack or attacks that become more frequent and severe; in some cases, pregnant women bearing the mutation develop severe complications, which may also lead to fetal death.

Specific urticarial-like dermatoses of pregnancy: These dermatoses present with urticarial-like rashes but are not typical urticarias.
- *PUPPP*: This is a common, self-limited disease that usually occurs in the last trimester of pregnancy; it presents with urticarial papules and plaques, accompanied by intense pruritus. It is the most common dermatosis of pregnancy, occurring in 1 in 160 pregnancies, usually in the primigravidas, and more often in twin/triplet pregnancies and in obese patients. The

eruption usually begins on the abdomen, classically within striae, and shows periumbilical sparing. There is rapid spread to the extremities, where it may become confluent with urticarial plaques. Involvement of the palms, soles, or face is uncommon. Although the pathogenesis is unknown, it is related to factors such as stretching of the abdomen, increased maternal–fetal weight gain, or maternal exposure to fetal antigens. Progesterone also plays an important role by aggravating inflammation at the tissue level. There is increased reactivity of progesterone receptors in skin lesions of PUPPP. The duration of symptoms is typically brief, usually 6 weeks. The lesions and pruritus spontaneously resolve within days after delivery. The disease has no tendency to recur in subsequent pregnancies.
- *Pemphigoid gestationis*: This is a least common disease that occurs in 1 in 50,000–60,000 pregnancies. It presents during late pregnancy as intense pruritus, typically on the abdomen adjacent to umbilicus, and is followed by a papular urticarial rash with erythematous lesions on the abdomen, trunk, limbs, and back. The mucous membranes and face are spared. Later, large blisters develop after 1–2 weeks. Direct immunofluorescence is positive for C3 in the basal membrane zone and, in some cases, also positive for IgG1. Histopathology reveals a subepidermal vesicle with a perivascular infiltrate of lymphocytes and eosinophils. Recurrences are seen in women taking oral contraceptives in 20–50%, of cases and there is worsening during the premenstrual period as hormonal factors also play an essential role in the pathogenesis of the disease. Mostly, disease remits spontaneously over weeks to months following delivery. The prognosis for the mother is good, but the disease can recur in subsequent pregnancies.

MANAGEMENT

Urticaria in pregnancy is managed by:
- Nonpharmacological measures
- Pharmacological measures

Nonpharmacological measures:
- The first step in managing urticaria is to identify and avoid triggers whenever possible.
- Pregnant women should be advised to avoid known triggers, such as certain foods, medications, and environmental factors, to minimize the risk of exacerbating their symptoms.
- For mild-to-moderate cases of urticaria, nonpharmacological interventions may be sufficient to alleviate symptoms. These interventions may include applying cool compresses to affected areas, wearing loose-fitting clothing, and practicing stress-reduction techniques such as yoga or meditation.

Pharmacological measures: In cases where nonpharmacological interventions are insufficient, pharmacological treatments may be considered. Antihistamines are the mainstay of treatment for urticaria.

DRUGS USED IN PREGNANCY

Antihistamines are the main drugs that are used for the treatment of urticaria. First- and second-generation antihistamines are considered safe to use in pregnancy.

Pregnancy Category B (Table 3)
- *Chlorpheniramine maleate*: First-generation antihistamine
  - *Mechanism of action*: H1 histamine receptor inverse agonist. It has anticholinergic and transient sedative effects.
  - *Pharmacokinetics*: Oral bioavailability is 34%. The onset of action is 0.5–1 hour; the duration of action is 2 days.
  - *Dosage*: 4 mg every 6 hours; maximum 24 mg/day
  - *Side effects*: Frequent drowsiness, dry mouth, dizziness, and irritability with intermittent therapy
- *Cetirizine*: Second-generation antihistamines
  - *Mechanism of action*: Acts by inhibiting adhesions of eosinophils, chemotaxis of eosinophils and neutrophils
  - *Pharmacokinetics*: The onset of action takes 1 hour and the duration of action is 24 hours. 70% excreted unchanged in urine within 72 hours and 10% excreted in feces.
  - *Dosage*: 10 mg once daily
  - *Side effects*: Sedation, headache, dry mouth, fatigue, and nausea
- *Levocetirizine*: Second-generation antihistamines
  - *Mechanism of action*: Acts by inhibiting adhesions of eosinophils, chemotaxis of eosinophils and neutrophils
  - *Pharmacokinetics*: The onset of action takes 1 hour and the duration of action is 24 hours.
  - *Dose*: 5 mg once daily
  - *Side effects*: Asthenia, drowsiness, dry mouth
- *Loratadine*: Second-generation antihistamines
  - *Mechanism of action*: Acts by inhibiting adhesions of eosinophils, chemotaxis of eosinophils and neutrophils
  - *Pharmacokinetics*: Extensively metabolized to an active metabolite descarboethoxyloratadine. Excreted in urine and feces
  - *Dose*: 10 mg once daily
  - *Side effects*: Drowsiness, somnolence, insomnia, headache, fatigue, dry mouth, pharyngitis, dizziness, gastrointestinal disturbances
- *Fexofenadine*: Second-generation antihistamines
  - *Mechanism of action*: H1 receptor antagonist
  - *Pharmacokinetics*: Rapid onset of action. Food decreases oral absorption. Excreted unchanged in urine and feces
  - *Dose*: 180 mg once daily
  - *Side effects*: Headache, drowsiness, nausea

TABLE 3: Pregnancy category B drugs used in the management of urticaria.

Drug	Generation	Mechanism of action	Pharmacokinetics	Dosage	Side effects
Chlorphenira-mine maleate	First-generation antihistamine	H1 histamine receptor inverse agonist. Anticholinergic and transient sedative effects	Oral bioavailability is 34%. Onset of action is 0.5–1 hour; duration of action is 2 days	4 mg every 6 hours; maximum 24 mg/day	Frequent drowsiness, dry mouth, dizziness, irritability with intermittent therapy
Cetirizine	Second-generation antihistamine	Inhibits adhesions of eosinophils, chemotaxis of eosinophils and neutrophils	Onset of action takes 1 hour; duration of action is 24 hours. 70% excreted unchanged in urine within 72 hours; 10% excreted in feces	10 mg once daily	Sedation, headache, dry mouth, fatigue, nausea
Levocetirizine	Second-generation antihistamine	Inhibits adhesions of eosinophils, chemotaxis of eosinophils and neutrophils	Onset of action takes 1 hour; duration of action is 24 hours	5 mg once daily	Asthenia, drowsiness, dry mouth
Loratadine	Second-generation antihistamine	Inhibits adhesions of eosinophils, chemotaxis of eosinophils and neutrophils	Extensively metabolized to an active metabolite descarboethoxy-loratadine. Excreted in urine and feces	10 mg once daily	Drowsiness, somnolence, insomnia, headache, fatigue, dry mouth, pharyngitis, dizziness, gastrointestinal disturbances
Fexofenadine	Second-generation antihistamine	H1 receptor antagonist	Rapid onset of action. Food decreases oral absorption. Excreted unchanged in urine and feces	180 mg once daily	Headache, drowsiness, nausea
Omalizumab	Monoclonal antibody that targets immunoglobulin E (IgE)	Recently assigned a pregnancy category B by the FDA. Considered safe and successful after risk-benefit evaluation in pregnant women with uncontrolled chronic urticaria	Omalizumab works by binding to IgE. By targeting and neutralizing IgE, omalizumab prevents IgE from attaching to mast cells and basophils	5–600 mg by subcutaneous injection every 2 or 4 weeks	Headache, upper respiratory tract infections, sinusitis, sore throat, viral infections, fatigue

- *Omalizumab*: It has been recently assigned a pregnancy category B by the Food and Drug Administration (FDA). Thus, it can be considered as a safe and successful therapeutic alternative, after careful consideration of the risk–benefit profile in pregnant women with uncontrolled chronic urticaria.
  - *Mechanism of action*: Monoclonal antibody that targets immunoglobulin E (IgE)
  - *Dose*: 5–600 mg by subcutaneous injection every 2 or 4 weeks
  - *Side effects*: Headache, upper respiratory tract infections, sinusitis, sore throat, viral infections, fatigue

Pregnancy Category C

- *Hydroxyzine*: First-generation antihistamines
  - *Mechanism of action*: Inverse agonist of H1 receptors
  - *Pharmacokinetics*: Onset 15–30 minutes after oral intake
  - *Dose*: 25 mg at night, can be increased to twice or thrice a day
  - *Side effects*: Transient drowsiness and dry mouth
- *Desloratadine*: Second-generation antihistamines
  - *Mechanism of action*: Reduces adhesions and chemotaxis of eosinophils
  - *Pharmacokinetics*: Major active metabolite of loratadine and about 5 times more potent than loratadine in suppressing wheal
  - *Dose*: 5 mg once daily
  - *Advantages*: Nonsedating antihistamines, no anticholinergic activity
- *Corticosteroids*: These are used in severe cases of urticaria that do not respond to antihistamines, but their use during pregnancy is controversial due to potential risks to fetal development.

CONCLUSION

Estrogen and progesterone levels, which rise dramatically in pregnancy, probably play a role in at least some urticarial rashes and angioedema states. The influence of estrogens on bradykininergic angioedema of HAE type I/II is the most prominent, and they might aggravate the disease, especially in the first and last trimesters of pregnancy. HAE attacks during pregnancy are more common in the abdomen, probably because of the enormous changes in the uterus and microtrauma during fetal development. Factors associated with a more aggressive course in pregnancy include a disease onset early in life, bearing a fetus with C1EI deficiency, and disease exacerbation during menses. Delivery in patients with HAE type I/II usually is uneventful, and C1EI concentrate is not indicated routinely. Pregnancy has a variable impact on the course of HAE type III. Progesterone and estrogen dermatitis, which tends to fluctuate during the menstrual cycle, usually remits during pregnancy, although exacerbation is described in some case reports. Chronic urticaria is unlikely to flare in pregnancy. Special dermatoses of pregnancy include PUPPP and pemphigoid gestationis, with urticarial-like lesions that occur during the second or third trimester of pregnancy and resolve after delivery. Sex hormones might play some role in the pathogenesis of disease.

SUGGESTED READINGS

1. Kaplan AP. In: Adkinson Jr NF, Busse WW, Bochner BS, Holgate ST, Simons FER, Lemanske RF (Eds). Middleton's Allergy: Principles and Practice. 7th edition. Philadelphia: Elsevier; 2009. pp. 1064-7.
2. Greaves M. Chronic urticaria. J Allergy Clin Immunol. 2000;105(4):664.
3. Zaitsu M, Narita S, Lambert KC, Grady JJ, Estes DM, Curran EM, et al. Estradiol activates mast cells via an ongenomic estrogen receptor-alpha and calcium influx. Mol Immunol. 2007;44:1977-85.
4. Narita S, Goldblum RM, Watson CS, Brooks EG, Estes DM, Curran EM, et al. Environmental estrogens induce mast cell degranulation and enhance IgE-mediated release of allergic mediators. Environ Health Perspect. 2007;115:48-52.
5. Vasconcelos C, Xavier P, Vieira AP, Martinho M, Rodrigues J, Bodas A, et al. Autoimmune progesterone urticaria. Gynecol Endocrinol. 2000;14(4):245-7.
6. Roth MM. Pregnancy dermatoses: diagnosis, management, and controversies. Am J Clin Dermatol. 2011;12(1):25-41.
7. Toms-Whittle LM, John LH, Griffiths DJ, Buckley DA. Autoimmune progesterone dermatitis: a diagnosis easily missed. Clin Exp Dermatol. 2011;36(4):378-80.
8. Hide M, Francis DM, Grattan CEH, Hakimi J, Kochan JP, Greaves MW. Autoantibodies against the high affinity IgE receptor as a cause of histamine release in chronic urticaria. N Engl J Med. 1993;328:1599-604.
9. Agostoni A, Cicardi M. Hereditary and acquired C1-inhibitor deficiency: biological and clinical characteristics in 235 patients. Medicine (Baltimore). 1992;71:206-15.
10. Georgy MS, Pongracic JA. Chapter 22: hereditary and acquired angioedema. Allergy Asthma Proc. 2012;33(Suppl 1):S73-6.
11. Bork K, Hardt J, Schicketanz KH, Ressel N. Clinical studies of sudden upper airway obstruction in patients with hereditary angioedema due to C1 esterase inhibitor deficiency. Arch Intern Med. 2003;163:1229-35.
12. Cunningham DS, Jensen JT. Hereditary angioneurotic edema in the puerperium. A case report. J Reprod Med. 1991;36(4):312-3.
13. Cox M, Holdcroft A. Hereditary angioneurotic oedema: current management in pregnancy. Anaesthesia. 1995;50:534-49.
14. Zuraw BL, Bork K, Binkley KE, Banerj Ai, Christiansen SC, Castaldo A, et al. Hereditary angioedema with normal C1 inhibitor function: consensus of an international expert panel. Allergy Asthma Proc. 2012;33 Suppl 1:S145-56.
15. Matz H, Orion E, Wolf R. Pruritic urticarial papules and plaques of pregnancy: polymorphic eruption of pregnancy (PUPPP). Clin Dermatol. 2006;24(2):105-8.
16. Jenkins RE, Shornick J. Pemphigoid gestationis. In: Black MM, Ambros-Rudolph C, Edwards L, Lynch PJ (Eds). Obstetric and Gynecologic Dermatology, 3rd edition. London: Mosby; 2008. pp. 37-4.

CHAPTER 16

Urticaria in Elderly: Causes, Management and Consideration

Kalpana Pathak

INTRODUCTION

Population demography is changing worldwide. Global life expectancy has doubled over the past century due to improved healthcare and medical advancements. This has led to increased geriatric population around the world. According to the World Health Organization (WHO), people aged 65 years and above are considered to be elderly people. Chronic urticaria is considered to be the most common pruritic condition in older age groups. As such, precise data on the prevalence of chronic urticaria in elderly patients is lacking; however, among all patients with chronic urticaria, 4.1–5.5% belong to the elderly age group.

Chronic urticaria in older population is equally distributed in both genders. In old age, structural and physiological skin changes happen. The dermal thickness reduces by 20%, the dermal layer loses 50% of mast cells, and there is 60% reduction in basal and cutaneous blood flow. Immune function remodeling happens in old age (immunosenescence) leading to reduction in total and naive B cells and decreased antibody response. This leads to fewer wheals and angioedema, reduced frequency of associated physical urticaria, and lower autologous serum skin test (ASST) positivity. All this can contribute to the underdiagnosis of chronic urticaria as pruritus is a common occurrence in the elderly age group.

Various comorbidities are found to be in association with urticaria in elderly **(Box 1)**. Gastrointestinal disorders, coronary and cerebrovascular diseases are common. Other common associations are dyslipidemias, chronic kidney disease, obesity, hypertension, diabetes mellitus, thyroid disorders, malignancy, and autoimmune disorders.

DIAGNOSTIC APPROACH

The diagnostic approach of chronic urticaria in elderly remains the same standard approach as in the adult age group. It aims to exclude differential diagnoses and identify exacerbating or stimulating factors and any underlying causes. As comorbidities and polypharmacotherapy are quite common in this age group, the

---

Box 1: Associated comorbidities.

- *Gastrointestinal diseases (most common)*: Helicobacter pylori infection, intestinal parasites, reflux esophagitis, inflammation of bile duct or gallbladder
- Coronary artery disease
- Cerebrovascular disease
- *Thyroid disorders*: Hyperthyroidism, hypothyroidism, Graves' disease, Hashimoto's disease
- *Metabolic disorders*: Dyslipidemia, diabetes mellitus, obesity, hypertension
- *Autoimmune disorders*: Systemic lupus erythematosus (SLE), Raynaud's disease, rheumatoid arthritis
- *Malignancy*: Gastrointestinal, hematological

Box 2: Basic clinical investigations.

- Complete blood count and differential blood count (absolute eosinophil count and absolute basophil count)
- C-reactive protein
- Erythrocyte sedimentation rate
- Serum total IgE
- Thyroid function test, antithyroid peroxidise antibodies

---

possibilities of underlying internal pathologies such as infections, autoimmune diseases, malignancy, and drug-induced allergies [aspirin and angiotensin-converting enzyme (ACE) inhibitors] should be ruled out through detailed clinical history and physical examination. Basic diagnostic workup **(Box 2)** includes complete blood count, erythrocyte sedimentation rate (ESR), C-reactive protein, serum total immunoglobulin E (IgE), thyroid function tests, and antithyroid peroxidase antibodies. Apart from these, other laboratory investigations can be done to rule out comorbidities and ascertain functioning of organs that may interfere with treatment protocol by means of kidney function tests (KFT) and liver function tests (LFT).

CONDITIONS MIMICKING URTICARIA

Wheals and angioedema are not specific for chronic urticaria. The physician should be well aware about differential diagnoses, especially in cases which are refractory to standard treatment. Wheals usually without angioedema are common in urticarial vasculitis, maculopapular cutaneous mastocytosis, bullous pemphigoid, and autoinflammatory disorders like Schnitzler syndrome or cryopyrin-associated periodic syndromes. Patients who exclusively develop angioedema but not wheals may have bradykinin-mediated angioedema such as acquired idiopathic angioedema or hereditary angioedema. It is quite commonly seen with the use of an ACE inhibitor in the treatment of arterial hypertension in older individuals.

Urticarial vasculitis (UV) is characterized by painful urticarial rashes and histopathological features of leukocytoclastic vasculitis. It is a complement-mediated disease and is considered a type 3 hypersensitivity reaction. Patients with UV may have normal (normocomplementemic) or reduced complement levels (hypocomplementemic). Also, UV may occur as a primary disorder or secondary to an underlying autoimmune disorder. The disease is mainly seen in the middle age group; however, there are reports of UV in elderly up to 90 years of age. The hallmark symptoms of urticarial vasculitis are pain and burning sensation in lesions, in contrast to pruritus in urticaria. The lesions of urticaria resolve in hours but in UV, lesions can persist for days and may heal with bruising or hyperpigmentation.

Autoinflammatory urticarial syndromes are rare and debilitating chronic skin disorders. These present with urticarial lesions usually sparing face and do not respond to antihistamines. Cutaneous histopathology shows neutrophil-rich infiltrates. Blood investigations may reveal neutrophilic leukocytosis, raised CRP, ESR, and serum amyloid A. Cryopyrin-associated periodic syndrome is a hereditary autoinflammatory disorder presenting commonly in early childhood and is characterized by fever, urticarial rash, systemic features like fatigue, headache, arthralgia, myalgia, hearing loss, ocular inflammation, and/or bone lesions. Schnitzler syndrome is an acquired autoinflammatory disease that usually presents later in life with clinical features of recurrent fever, urticarial lesions, arthralgia, arthritis, myalgia, lymphadenopathy, hepatosplenomegaly, and monoclonal gammopathy (mostly IgM class).

Adult-onset Still disease is a rare systemic inflammatory disease and usually manifests with high fever, arthralgia, hepatosplenomegaly, lymphadenopathy, and an erythematous evanescent rash that accompanies the fever spike. Urticarial eruptions have also been reported in a number of patients. The inflammatory markers like ferritin, ESR, and C-reactive protein are raised while antinuclear antibody (ANA) and rheumatoid factor are negative.

Bullous pemphigoid is an autoimmune bullous disorder quite frequent in the older age group of 65–75 years. It has a male preponderance. The onset is characterized by a nonbullous phase which may last for weeks to months and is marked by pruritic urticarial plaques or eczematous patches. Later, tense hemorrhagic bullae may form over urticarial or eczematous lesions. Therefore, in elderly patients with a long-lasting pruritic urticarial or eczematous rash, a possibility of bullous pemphigoid should be kept.

TREATMENT

There are no specific guidelines or recommendations for the management of urticaria in elderly patients. Hence, the treatment protocol for general population is followed. The treatment involves a multipronged approach:
- Avoiding the known triggers
- Nonpharmacological measures to reduce skin hyper-responsiveness, like keeping the skin well hydrated by using emollients and avoiding the precipitating factors like scratching, wearing occlusive clothes, exposure to extreme variations of temperature like too hot or cold temperatures, etc.
- Pharmacotherapy

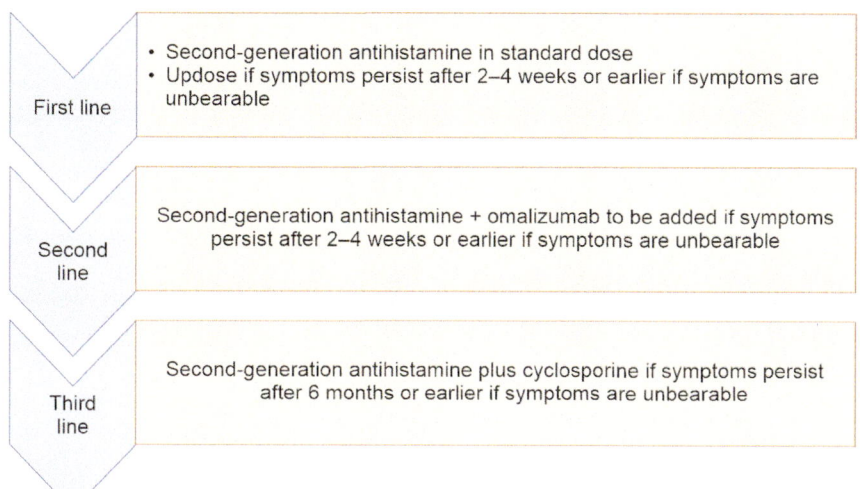

FLOWCHART 1: Algorithm for treatment.

According to the current GA²LEN and Indian consensus statement, all patient population should be treated with a stepwise approach **(Flowchart 1)** of starting with the standard dosing of second-generation antihistamine and updosing up to four-fold in the absence of a satisfactory clinical response. Addition of omalizumab and cyclosporine constitutes second line and third line of treatment, respectively. Pharmacological treatment in elderly patients can be challenging due to age-related changes in physiology, pharmacokinetics, and pharmacodynamics. Chances of drug interactions and side effects are high due to comorbidities and polypharmacy.

Second-generation Antihistamines

First-generation antihistamines cross the blood–brain barrier; hence, they may cause cognitive impairment, memory, disturbance, and sedation. These medicines also affect circadian rhythm. In addition, as these medications have anticholinergic, antiestrogenic, and antidopaminergic functions, these may cause or worsen urinary retention, arrhythmia, postural, hypotension, etc. The GA²LEN position paper recommends avoiding these in general population as side effects are more pronounced. The American Geriatric BEERS Criteria 2023 also recommend to avoid first-generation antihistamines owing to their side-effect potential. Considering the above factors, second-generation, nonsedating antihistamines are first-line treatment. No recommendation can be made on the most preferred antihistamine. Among the second-generation agents, levocetirizine, desloratadine, bilastine, ebastine, and fexofenadine are commonly used. If symptoms persist with standard dose, a dose escalation of up to four times is advised. However, updosing in the elderly may have a lower safety profile and an increased risk of drug interactions and adverse effects due to comorbidities, polypharmacotherapy, and renal or hepatic impairment **(Table 1)**.

TABLE 1: Dose adjustment of drugs in elderly patients.		
Drug	**Elderly**	**Dose adjustment**
Bilastine	No dose adjustment	No dose adjustment in renal or hepatic insufficiency
Cetirizine	No dose adjustment if renal function normal	Dose adjustment required in renal or hepatic insufficiency
Levocetirizine	No dose adjustment if renal function normal	No dose adjustment in hepatic impairment but required in renal impairment
Desloratadine	No dose adjustment	Caution suggested in severe renal impairment
Loratadine	No dose adjustment	No dose adjustment in renal impairment but required in hepatic insufficiency
Ebastine	No dose adjustment	No dose adjustment in renal impairment. Contraindicated in severe liver impairment. Caution for patients with mild-to-moderate liver impairment
Fexofenadine	No dose adjustment	Dose adjustment in renal impairment

Omalizumab

Various studies have found omalizumab to be safe and effective in patients with refractory chronic urticaria in ages 65 years and above. Dose adjustment based on age, gender, weight, concomitant therapies like second-generation antihistamine, leukotriene receptor antagonist, or baseline IgE investigation is not required in the treatment of patients with chronic urticaria. This aspect holds importance as a percentage of elderly population is increasing globally and urticaria has a huge impact on the quality of life. At clinical dosage, omalizumab clearance is predominantly by the reticuloendothelial system, so it can be given to older patients with renal or hepatic impairment as well.

Cyclosporine

Cyclosporine has well-known dose-dependent adverse effects like arterial hypertension and nephrotoxicity which require careful monitoring. The clearance of cyclosporine decreases with age, and hence older patients may have a large proportion of drug in blood. Cyclosporine is a substrate of CYP 3A and P glycoprotein, both of which are important for elimination of many drugs. Hence, it has a high propensity to cause drug interactions, especially in elderly patients on multiple medications. Therefore, its use in geriatric patients should be reserved to severe refractory cases and therapy should be started with the lowest possible dose of cyclosporine.

CONCLUSION

Elderly patients are growing worldwide and constitute a distinctive subset of patients owing to associated comorbidities, multiple medications, and physiological limitations. Chronic urticaria in the elderly is not an uncommon condition. If not managed properly, it may severely affect the patient's quality of life. Hence, appropriate diagnostic tools should be used to diagnose the disease as urticaria could be an underdiagnosed condition in the elderly. When prescribing treatment, comorbidities, organ insufficiency (renal and/or hepatic impairment), drug interactions, and adverse effects of prescribed drugs should be carefully monitored. There is a vast scope of further research to understand urticaria in elderly as the available data regarding its epidemiology, clinical features, and safety of treatment options being offered is too limited.

SUGGESTED READINGS

1. Buxbaum JD, Chernew ME, Fendrick AM, Cutler DM. Contributions of public health, pharmaceuticals, and other medical care to US life expectancy changes, 1990-2015. Health Aff. 2020;39(9):1546-56.
2. World Health Organization (WHO). (2021). Decade of healthy ageing: baseline report: summary. Geneva: World Health Organization. [online] Available from https://www.who.int/publications/i/item/9789240017900. [Last accessed October, 2024].
3. Ward JR, Bernhard JD. Willan's itch and other causes of pruritus in the elderly. Int J Dermatol. 2005;44(4):267-73.
4. Thaipisuttikul Y. Pruritic skin diseases in the elderly. J Dermatol. 1998;25(3):153-7.
5. Chuamanochan M, Kulthanan K, Tuchinda P, Chularojanamontri L, Nuchkull P. Clinical features of chronic urticaria in aging population. Asian Pac J Allergy Immunol. 2016;34(3):201-5.
6. Ban G-Y, Kim M-Y, Yoo H-S, Nahm D-H, Ye Y-M, Shin Y-S, et al. Clinical features of elderly chronic urticaria. Korean J Intern Med. 2014;29(6):800-6.
7. Juhlin L. Recurrent urticaria: clinical investigation of 330 patients. Br J Dermatol. 1981;104(4): 369-81.
8. Magen E, Mishal J, Schlesinger M. Clinical and laboratory features of chronic idiopathic urticaria in the elderly. Int J Dermatol. 2013;52:1387-91.
9. Farage MA, Miller KW, Elsner P, Maibach HI. Functional and physiological characteristics of the aging skin. Aging Clin Exp Res. 2008;20:195-200.
10. Xu W, Wong G, Hwang YY, Larbi A. The untwining of immunosenescence and aging. Semin. Immunopathol. 2020;42:559-72.
11. Kulthanan K, Rujitharanawong C, Munprom K, Trakanwittayarak S, Phumariyapong P, Prasertsook S, et al. Prevalence, Clinical Manifestations, Treatment, and Clinical Course of Chronic Urticaria in Elderly: A Systematic Review. J Asthma Allergy. 2022;15:1455-90.
12. Maurer M, Magerl M, Metz M, Siebenhaar F, Weller K, Krause K. Practical algorithm for diagnosing patients with recurrent wheals or angioedema. Allergy. 2013;68(6):816-9.
13. Davis MDP, van der Hilst JCH. Mimickers of Urticaria: Urticarial Vasculitis and Autoinflammatory Diseases. J Allergy Clin Immunol Pract. 2018;6(4):1162-70.
14. Matos AL, Figueiredo C, Gonçalo M. Differential Diagnosis of Urticarial Lesions. Front Allergy. 2022;3:808543.
15. Criado RF, Criado PR, Vasconcellos C, Carlos M Szajubok J, Michalany NS, Kadunc BV, et al. Urticaria as a cutaneous sign of adult-onset Still's disease. J Cutan Med Surg. 2006;10(2): 99-103.
16. Lamberts A, Meijer JM, Pas HH, Diercks GFH, Horváth B, Jonkman MF. Nonbullous pemphigoid: Insights in clinical and diagnostic findings, treatment responses, and prognosis. J Am Acad Dermatol. 2019;81(2):355-63.
17. Zuberbier T, Abdul Latiff AH, Abuzakouk M, Aquilina S, Asero R, Baker D, et al. The international EAACI/GA^{2}LEN/EuroGuiDerm/APAAACI guideline for the definition, classification, diagnosis, and management of urticaria. Allergy. 2022;77(3):734-66.

18. Godse K, Patil A, De A, Sharma N, Rajagopalan M, Shah B, et al. Diagnosis and Management of Urticaria in Indian Settings: Skin Allergy Research Society's Guideline-2022. Indian J Dermatol. 2022;67(6):732-43.
19. Antia C, Baquerizo K, Korman A, Alikhan A, Bernstein JA. Urticaria: a comprehensive review: treatment of chronic urticaria, special populations, and disease outcomes. J Am Acad Dermatol. 2018;79:617-33.
20. Church MK, Maurer M, Simons FER, Bindslev-Jensen C, Van Cauwenberge P, Bousquet J, et al. Risk of first-generation H1-antihistamines: a GA2LEN position paper. Allergy. 2010;65:459-66.
21. By the 2023 American Geriatrics Society Beers Criteria® Update Expert Panel. American Geriatrics Society 2023 updated AGS Beers Criteria® for potentially inappropriate medication use in older adults. J Am Geriatr Soc. 2023;71(7):2052-81.
22. Guillen-Aguinaga S, Jauregui Presa I, Aguinaga-Ontoso E, Guillen-Grima F, Ferrer M. Updosing nonsedating antihistamines in patients with chronic spontaneous urticaria: a systematic review and meta-analysis. Br J Dermatol. 2016;175(6):1153-65.
23. Hansen J, Klimek L, Hörmann K. Pharmacological management of allergic rhinitis in the elderly: safety issues with oral antihistamines. Drugs Aging. 2005;22(4):289-96.
24. Martina E, Damiani G, Grieco T, Foti C, Pigatto PDM, Offidani A. It is never too late to treat chronic spontaneous urticaria with omalizumab: real-life data from a multicenter observational study focusing on elderly patients. Dermatol Ther. 2021;34: e14841.
25. Nettis E, Cegolon L, Di Leo E, Canonica WG, Detoraki A, Italian OCUReL Study Group. Omalizumab in elderly patients with chronic spontaneous urticaria: an Italian real-life experience. Ann Allergy Asthma Immunol. 2018;120(3):318-23.
26. Labrador-Horrillo M, Ferrer M. Profile of omalizumab in the treatment of chronic spontaneous urticaria. Drug Des Devel Ther. 2015;9:4909-15.
27. Patruno C, Fabbrocini G, Cillo F, Torta G, Stingeni L, Napolitano M. Chronic Urticaria in Older Adults: Treatment Considerations. Drugs Aging. 2023;40(3):165-77.

CHAPTER
17

Urticarial Vasculitis

Neha Rani, Sanjeev Gupta, Aneet Mahendra

INTRODUCTION

Urticarial vasculitis (UV), earlier referred to as hemorrhagic urticaria, was initially described in 1890 by Wills and Lond. The histopathological identification of vasculitis in association with urticaria was reported in 1956. UV is characterized by chronic or recurrent urticarial wheals associated with histopathological evidence of leukocytoclastic vasculitis. It arises from the inflammation affecting the small blood vessels in the skin. It can be localized to the skin or may extend systemically to involve various organs such as musculoskeletal, renal, pulmonary, ocular, or gastrointestinal systems. UV is categorized into two types: Hypocomplementemic UV (HCUV) and normocomplementemic UV (NCUV). This characterization of UV is necessary as the hypocomplementemic type may have systemic involvement and is sometimes called HCUV syndrome, whereas the NCUV usually is a benign, self-limiting disease. The pathophysiology of UV is incompletely understood. The diagnosis is made histopathologically from a lesional skin biopsy. A thorough clinical and laboratory workup is essential as there is potential multisystem involvement. Management of UV is difficult and includes various drugs such as antihistamines, nonsteroidal anti-inflammatory drugs (NSAIDs), oral corticosteroids, antimalarials, immunosuppressive agents, and biologics.

Synonyms:
- Urticarial vasculitis
- Urticarial venulitis
- McDuffie syndrome

EPIDEMIOLOGY

- UV is a rare skin disease and its exact prevalence worldwide remains unknown. The lifetime prevalence may be in the region of 0.025%. It is a rare disease occurring in 1–20% of patients presenting with a chronic urticarial disease.
- *Age*: Peak incidence is in the fourth decade. The median age at the diagnosis ranges from 35 to 51 years.

- HCUV peaks in the fifth decade.
- Both types of UV are rare in children and even rarer in infants.
- Women are affected more often than men and HCUV tends to be more frequent during the fourth to sixth decade.
- Ethnic predisposition is unknown in UV.

Genetics: UV is not known to be familial, but the concordance of HCUV was described in identical twins. Recently, homozygous mutations in *DNASE1L3* which encodes an endonuclease have been identified in two families with autosomal recessive HCUV.

Environmental factors: Various factors are implicated as potential causes including drugs, infections, and physical factors. Drugs that are implicated in UV include cimetidine, procarbazine, diltiazem, potassium iodide, fluoxetine, infliximab procainamide, enalapril, NSAIDs, antidepressants, sulfamethoxazole–trimethoprim, and etanercept. Infections include hepatitis B, hepatitis C, tuberculosis, infectious mononucleosis, streptococcus, mycoplasma, COVID-19, influenza A/H1N1, trichomoniasis, Epstein–Barr virus, and Lyme disease. Occasionally, it can be precipitated by exercise and exposure to sunlight or cold environment.

Associated diseases: Many diseases are associated with UV although it is not known whether these represent a causal relationship or a coincidence.
- *Connective tissue disorders*: Systemic lupus erythematosus (SLE), Sjögren disease, systemic sclerosis
- *Infections*: Chronic hepatitis B and C infections, infectious mononucleosis, Lyme borreliosis
- *Hematological disorders*: Essential cryoglobulinemia, idiopathic thrombocytopenia, monoclonal gammopathy, serum sickness, serum sickness-like reaction
- *Hematological malignancies*: Hodgkin lymphoma, IgA myeloma, acute myelogenous leukemia
- *Thyroid dysfunction*
- *Malignancy*: Adenocarcinoma of colon
- *Syndromes*: Schnitzler syndrome, Muckle–Wells syndrome, Cogan syndrome

PATHOPHYSIOLOGY

Urticarial vasculitis is a form of small-vessel vasculitis and is categorized as immune-complex-mediated disease. It predominantly affects postcapillary venules in superficial dermis. UV is an example of type 3 immune reaction, involving the formation of immune complexes in bloodstream which later accumulate in the blood vessel wall. These immune complexes then lead to vascular endothelial damage. This process activates the complement system through the classical pathway. Complements C3 and C5a are anaphylatoxins and play a role in mast cell degranulation and cytokine production. This leads to the release of mast cell mediators including tumor necrosis factor α (TNF-α), histamine, prostaglandins, heparin, platelet-activating factors, leukotrienes, etc., contributing to edema and tissue reactions. The primary antibodies involved are IgG or IgM, occasionally IgA although the specific antigens often remain unidentified. Another common feature of UV is the deposition of IgG, IgM, and C3 within and around the blood vessel wall.

Various factors thought to be pathogenic in UV include:
- Circulating immune complexes
- Activation of complement via classical pathway
- Activation of mast cell
- Proinflammatory cytokines production
- Activation and damage of endothelial cell
- Inflammatory cell infiltration
- Neutrophil karyorrhexis
- Fibrin deposition

Mast cell activation: Activation of mast cell occurs early in the vasculitic lesions. Mast cell activation results in the release of proinflammatory cytokines like TNF-α, histamine, prostaglandins, heparin, platelet-activating factor, and leukotrienes. Patients with UV also have elevated serum levels of interleukin 6 (IL-6) and IL-1 receptor antagonists. Patients with UV also have elevated serum levels of IL-6 and IL-1 receptor antagonists.

Endothelial cell damage: The mechanism of action of endothelial cell activation and damage is not known clearly. On microscopic examination, endothelial cell involvement is characterized by swelling and necrosis. Endothelial cell activation is reflected by upregulation of cell adhesion molecules. In vasculitis, activation of endothelial cells results in loss of anticoagulant and fibrinolytic properties which leads to fibrin deposition and fibrinoid degeneration of affected blood vessels. This also leads to the recruitment of inflammatory cells into perivascular infiltrates. This is not understood whether this activation of endothelial cells is caused by antiendothelial antibodies or complement activation or transmigration of inflammatory cells.

Autoantibodies: A spectrum of autoantibodies has been observed such as antinuclear antibody (ANA), extractable nuclear antigen antibody (ENA), antiphospholipid antibody, and antiendothelial antibody. The pathogenic importance of these autoantibodies is not known, and further research is required to unravel their clinical relevance.

Inflammatory cells: The dynamic nature of inflammatory infiltrates has been observed in UV. In serial biopsies taken from a patient of UV, the first cells recruited at 3 hours were eosinophils, followed by predominance of neutrophils at 24 hours. Histological studies have also shown extracellular deposition of neutrophil elastase and eosinophil peroxidase. Neutrophil-rich infiltration with leukocytoclasis is another common feature. In lesions older than 48 hours, lymphocytes constitute the predominant cells in perivascular infiltrate.

CLINICAL FEATURES

When to suspect urticarial vasculitis?
- Urticarial wheals lasting for more than 24 hours
- Lesions heals with hyperpigmentation/purpura
- Features of systemic involvement, especially pulmonary, gastrointestinal, and renal systems

Patients present with recurrent, indurated wheals that heal with residual hyperpigmentation, and wheals are usually painful rather than itchy and last longer than 24 hours. These features distinguish UV from chronic urticaria in which the wheals resolve within 24 hours, itching is intense rather than pain, and no residual pigmentation is observed. UV wheals tend to be nonblanchable or partially blanchable with central dark-red or brown macules. The size of the lesions may range from 0.5 to 5 cm in diameter whereas in urticaria, the wheals can coalesce and become much larger. UV may be associated with fatigue, malaise, or fever.

In a number of patients, wheals in UV are indistinguishable from urticaria. UV may be an underlying disease in 20% of patients with chronic urticaria not responding to treatment with antihistamines. In addition to wheals, other cutaneous manifestations in UV may occur such as livedo reticularis, Raynaud's phenomenon, bullous lesions, and angioedema.

Normocomplementemic UV usually has only cutaneous manifestations with limited systemic involvement, whereas HCUV with low C3 and C4 may develop systemic disease involving the lungs, kidneys, and eyes. Extracutaneous manifestations of HCUV include fever, myalgia, fatigue, malaise, conjunctivitis, arthralgia, nephritis, episcleritis, and cardiac valve involvement. A subset of HCUV patients exhibit anti-C1q antibodies and represent a distinct entity. Anti-C1q antibodies target the collagen-like region of C1q and these have been identified in patients of SLE, often linked to glomerulonephritis. However, not all SLE patients with anti-C1q antibodies develop UV. Approximately 5–10% of SLE patients experience UV and 28–47% of SLE patients display anti-C1q antibodies.

Joint involvement is seen very commonly and usually presents as arthralgia and joint stiffness and occasionally with arthritis or synovitis. Patients with HCUV may have gastrointestinal involvement and present with symptoms such as nausea, vomiting, abdominal pain, diarrhea, or intestinal bleeding. In some, there may be persistent microscopic hematuria or proteinuria.

There may be ***pulmonary involvement*** in 20–30% of patients which may increase up to 50% in patients with HCUV. Patients present with cough, dyspnea or hemoptysis, and occasionally chronic obstructive pulmonary disease (COPD). The precise cause of obstructive lung disease remains unclear; factors such as pulmonary capillary vasculitis, dysfunction of alpha-1 antitrypsin, and binding of anti-C1q antibody to surfactant protein in alveoli are potential contributors. Lung biopsy on these patients shows features of leukocytoclastic vasculitis. Pulmonary involvement happens to be more severe in smokers and in patients with HCUV. Therefore, screening of chronic obstructive pulmonary disease (COPD) is crucial and smoking cessation is strongly recommended in all patients.

Pleuritis can be seen, often manifesting as chest pain or shortness of breath. These complications are recalcitrant to treatments, with many patients requiring lung transplantation. Overall, pulmonary involvement is associated with poor prognosis and is the most common cause of mortality in UV patients. Upper respiratory tract infections may occur as well.

Renal involvement can be seen in 9-60% patients of HCUV. Most frequently, patients show evidence of glomerular impairment resulting from membranoproliferative glomerulonephritis. Other findings on renal histology include extracapillary, extramembranous, mesangial, crescentic, focal proliferative, and segmental hyalinosis glomerulonephritis. Some patients may have associated diffuse interstitial involvement. The most common symptoms are hematuria and proteinuria. A small minority of patients may develop renal failure requiring dialysis. However, even patients with extensive kidney involvement carry a fairly good prognosis.

Gastrointestinal involvement may occur in up to 30% of patients of UV, manifesting as abdominal pain, diarrhea, nausea, and vomiting. Cases of intestinal ischemia secondary to UV have also been reported.

Other clinical features can be seen including adenopathy, splenomegaly, or hepatomegaly. Rare presentations include pseudotumor cerebri, optic nerve atrophy, episcleritis, uveitis, scleritis, and conjunctivitis. In HCUV cardiac valvulopathy, pericarditis, pericardial effusion, cranial nerve palsies, transverse myelitis, and Jaccoud arthropathy can be seen sometimes.

To distinguish between NCUV and HCUV, serial testing of serum complement levels is required over time.

Hypocomplementemic UV with systemic symptoms is called HCUV syndrome (HCUVS) and is recognized only in about 5% of patients with UV.

Diagnostic criteria for HCUVS:
- Biopsy-proven vasculitis
- Arthralgia or arthritis
- Uveitis or episcleritis
- Recurrent abdominal pain
- Glomerulonephritis
- Decreased C1q or presence of anti-C1q autoantibodies

All systemic features in a patient are not required to make a diagnosis of UV.

HISTOPATHOLOGY

Classical histopathological changes in a fully developed UV lesion are as follows:
- Endothelial cell damage
- Swelling and loss of integrity of vessel wall
- Fibrin deposits in affected postcapillary venules
- Neutrophil-predominant perivascular infiltrates
- Leukocytoclasis
- Erythrocyte extravasation

However, all of these changes may not be seen on histopathology, thus causing diagnostic uncertainty in the patients of UV.

Direct immunofluorescence (DIF): IgG, IgM, and/or C3 are seen within or around the blood vessels of lesions more frequent in patients of HCUV. These immunoglobulin deposits can also be seen at the dermoepidermal junction (DEJ). Some studies suggest that 70% of UV patients with immunoglobulin deposition at the DEJ eventually develop glomerulonephritis.

In NCUV, there may be a predominance of eosinophils as compared to HCUV which shows neutrophil-predominant perivascular infiltrates and dermal neutrophilia.

Lesions older than 48 hours show lymphocytic predominance perivascular infiltration. Lymphocytic vasculitis is not a common feature of UV; therefore, histological diagnosis in these cases is made on evidence of vessel damage with fibrinoid degeneration.

DIFFERENTIAL DIAGNOSIS

It may be difficult sometimes to differentiate lesions of UV from urticaria clinically as well as on histopathology, where some of the characteristic histopathological findings of UV are not seen on skin biopsy. Numerous patients with intermediate histological findings have confirmed that there is a continuum of histological changes between UV and urticaria; therefore, there may not be a clear-cut distinction between urticaria and UV. Thus, the concept of minimal diagnostic histological criteria for UV has been proposed. Therefore, in difficult-to-diagnose cases, leukocytoclasia or/and fibrin deposition with or without erythrocyte extravasation may be sufficient for diagnosis **(Table 1)**.

Further research is warranted to increase the accuracy of diagnosis of UV in difficult cases.

CLASSIFICATION OF SEVERITY

Severity ranges from a mild disease to a life-threatening disease. Patients with only cutaneous involvement generally have a milder disease. In patients with HCUVS, systemic involvement can be associated and it may be very severe and refractory to the treatment.

COMPLICATIONS AND COMORBIDITIES

Urticarial vasculitis may be associated with renal involvement. In early stages, there can be microscopic hematuria or proteinuria but later in the disease, it may progress to renal failure. Kidney biopsy may show features of glomerulonephritis. UV patients, who display immunoglobulin and complement deposition at DEJ on DIF are more likely to develop glomerulonephritis.

TABLE 1: Differentiating features of urticaria and urticarial vasculitis.

Features	Urticaria	Urticarial vasculitis
Wheal duration	<24 hours	>24 hours
Pain	No	Yes
Purpura/residual hyperpigmentation	No	Yes
Systemic involvement	Uncommon	Common
Leukocytoclasia	No	Yes
Complement levels	Normal	Normal or low (HCUV)
Response to antihistamines	Good	Poor

(HCUV: hypocomplementemic urticarial vasculitis)

Chronic obstructive pulmonary disease is thought to be a life-threatening complication of UV which occurs later in the disease course.

Other common comorbidities associated with UV include connective tissue diseases and hematological malignancies. UV may be the first presentation of these diseases. Other comorbidities in UV patients can be chronic viral infections such as hepatitis B and C.

DISEASE COURSE AND PROGNOSIS

Urticarial vasculitis is a self-limiting condition in most of patients but may last for several years in some patients. NCUV which tends to have only cutaneous involvement is considered a benign disease with a good prognosis. Conversely, HCUV/HCUVS is associated with frequent systemic involvement and carries a more severe course. These patients are at a higher risk of developing SLE, COPD, or laryngeal angioedema which can be fatal. The prognosis of UV depends upon the systemic involvement. In some patients, it may precede the onset of hematological or other connective tissue disorders. More than 50% of patients with HUVS may develop SLE.

INVESTIGATIONS

- All patients of UV should undergo a routine laboratory workup including complete blood count (CBC), erythrocyte sedimentation rate (ESR), biochemistry, liver function test (LFT), renal function tests, urine routine examination, and microscopy.
- Testing for hepatitis B and C.
- In cases of abnormal urine routine examination, 24-hour urine and creatine clearance should be done.
- Complement levels (CH50, C3, C4, and anti-C1q) should be done to differentiate NCUV and HCUV.

- Antibody screening includes ANA, ENA, Rheumatoid Arthritis Factor, and circulating immune complexes.
- Chest X-ray and pulmonary function testing should be done in cases where there is suspicion of pulmonary involvement.
- Ophthalmic examination should be done if eye involvement is suspected.
- A confirmatory diagnosis is made on histopathology from a lesional skin biopsy. Multiple skin biopsies may be needed for confirmatory diagnosis. Routine DIF is not recommended unless there is suspicion of HCUVS **(Box 1)**.

Renal function tests are very important in cases of UV. It may be symptomatic or many cases may have silent renal involvement. Strict monitoring of microscopic hematuria and proteinuria is to be done along with blood pressure monitoring. Renal biopsy with immunofluorescence may be diagnostic in many silent suspected cases but may not be sensitive. Membranoproliferative glomerulonephritis is the most common pattern in renal biopsy.

MANAGEMENT (BOX 2)

Urticarial vasculitis poses a treatment challenge as there are no drugs approved by the US Food and Drug Administration (FDA) for this condition. Treatment strategies are based on limited information from the case studies. Before initiating the treatment, it is crucial to address any underlying condition that might be responsible for the UV.

First-line treatment: H1 antihistamines, oral antibiotics (doxycycline), and NSAIDs.

Antihistamines provide symptomatic relief in some patients. Preferably, sedative antihistamines are preferred. Some studies state that there is not much role of H1 blocker antihistamines in UV. Among the NSAIDs, indomethacin is the preferred one. Many studies advocate the benefit of indomethacin in UV cases.

Second-line treatment: If the patient does not respond to first-line treatment,
- Dapsone 75–100 mg/day
- Colchicine 1–1.5 mg/day

Box 1: Investigations to be done in case of urticarial vasculitis (UV).

Initial workup:	Extended workup:
• Lesional skin biopsy (diagnostic)	• DIF
• CBC	• CH50, anti-C1q antibodies
• ESR	• Renal function tests
• C3, C4	• 24-Hour urine protein and creatinine clearance
• ANA	• Cryoglobulins
• ENA	• Serum protein electrophoresis
• Hepatitis B and C serology	• Chest X-ray, pulmonary function test
• Circulating immune complexes	• Assessment of visual acuity and slit-lamp examination
• Urine complete examination	
• Renal function tests	• Serum D-dimer levels

(ANA: antinuclear antibody; CBC: complete blood count; DIF: direct immunofluorescence; ENA: extractable nuclear antigen antibody; ESR: erythrocyte sedimentation rate)

> **Box 2: Different drugs which can be used in UV treatment.**
>
> *First-line treatment*:
> - Nonsedating antihistamines
> - Non-steroidal anti-inflammatory drugs (NSAIDs)
>
> *Second-line treatment*:
> - Dapsone
> - Colchicine
> - Hydroxychloroquine (HCQ)
> - Short-course oral corticosteroids
>
> *Third-line treatment*:
> - Azathioprine
> - Cyclosporine
> - Mycophenolate mofetil
> - Methotrexate
> - Intravenous immunoglobulins
> - Cyclophosphamide
> - Biological agents

- HCQ 400 mg/day
- Azathioprine 50–100 mg/day

In case the patient does not respond with first-line therapy, the second-line drugs are preferred. The duration of therapy of these drugs is not documented. That can be titrated as per response and strict regular follow-up.

Third-line treatment:
- Oral corticosteroids can be used for short-term treatment.
- For severe refractory cases, immunosuppressive agents may be beneficial, e.g., methotrexate, cyclophosphamide, azathioprine, cyclosporine, and mycophenolate mofetil.
- Other modalities include intravenous immunoglobulin (IVIg), intramuscular gold, and plasmapheresis.

Recent studies show the effectiveness of biological therapies. Biologicals that have shown efficacy in UV in different small studies include:
- Anakinra (IL-1 receptor antagonist)
- Canakinumab (humanized anti-IL-1b)
- Tocilizumab (anti-IL-6) in patients with UV-associated SLE
- Omalizumab (anti-IgE) in NCUV
- Rituximab (anti-CD20)

By including biological medicines in the regimen for treating UV, the toxicity problem related to conventional treatment, particularly long-term oral corticosteroids, may be mitigated.

The choice of treatment for UV should take comorbidities into account; for example, patients of UV associated with SLE may respond to dapsone.

Treatment for hepatitis C may cause UV suppression in patients with concurrent hepatitis C infection.

CONCLUSION

- Urticarial vasculitis (UV) is a rare clinicopathological disorder.
- It is characterized by urticarial wheals and features of leukocytoclastic vasculitis on histopathology.
- A lesional skin biopsy is considered as gold standard for diagnosis of UV.
- Systemic involvement can be seen along with cutaneous features.

SUGGESTED READINGS

1. Gu SL, Jorizzo JL. Urticarial vasculitis. Int J Womens Dermatol. 2021;7(3):290-7.
2. Kolkhir P, Bonnekoh H, Kocatürk E, Hide M, Metz M, Sánchez-Borges M, Krause K, Maurer M. Management of urticarial vasculitis: A worldwide physician perspective. World Allergy Organ J. 2020;13(3):100107.
3. Kolkhir P, Grakhova M, Bonnekoh H, Krause K, Maurer M. Treatment of urticarial vasculitis: a systematic review. J Allergy Clin Immunol. 2019;143:458-66.
4. Chang S, Carr W. Urticarial vasculitis. Allergy Asthma Proc. 2007;28(1):97-100.

CHAPTER 18

Urticaria Mimickers: A Comprehensive Guide to Differential Diagnosis

Rohit Batra, Anushruti Aggarwal, Sanjeev Gupta

INTRODUCTION

Urticaria is a common dermatological condition characterized by transient, pruritic wheals that can appear anywhere on the skin. It is often a benign condition, typically self-limiting, but it can also present in chronic forms that significantly impact a patient's quality of life. Urticaria is typically classified into acute (lasting less than 6 weeks) and chronic (lasting 6 weeks or more) based on duration. It can also be categorized into spontaneous and inducible types, based on its etiology.

While urticaria is generally easy to diagnose based on its clinical presentation, there are numerous conditions that can mimic its appearance, leading to potential misdiagnosis. Mismanagement stemming from incorrect diagnosis can have serious consequences, especially in conditions that require specific treatments or that are associated with systemic involvement. This chapter aims to provide a detailed overview of the various conditions that can mimic urticaria, offering clinicians a comprehensive guide to differential diagnosis, supported by clinical and laboratory clues.

Understanding the differential diagnoses of urticaria is particularly important when dealing with chronic urticaria or when urticaria is associated with systemic symptoms. The diagnostic process should involve a thorough patient history, detailed physical examination, and appropriate laboratory investigations to avoid misdiagnosis and ensure optimal patient care.

OVERVIEW OF URTICARIA

Urticaria is a condition characterized by the sudden onset of wheals, which are raised, erythematous, and pruritic lesions. These lesions are transient, lasting less than 24 hours, and do not leave any residual marks upon resolution. Urticaria may also be accompanied by angioedema, which involves deeper swelling of the skin and subcutaneous tissues, often affecting the face, lips, and extremities.

Chronic urticaria is a more challenging condition, with symptoms persisting for 6 weeks or longer. In many cases, chronic urticaria is idiopathic, meaning no specific cause can be identified. However, autoimmune mechanisms are believed to play a role in a significant proportion of cases.

DIFFERENTIAL DIAGNOSIS OF ACUTE URTICARIA

Acute urticaria typically appears suddenly and resolves within 6 weeks. It can be caused by various factors, including allergic reactions, infections, and physical stimuli. The key dermatological and systemic disorders that can mimic acute urticaria are given in the following text.

Dermatological Disorders

- *Viral exanthems*:
    - *Clinical features*: Viral infections often cause rashes that may resemble urticaria, particularly in children. Common culprits include enteroviruses, Epstein–Barr virus, and parvovirus B19.
    - *Distinguishing features*: Viral exanthems typically present with a more diffuse and symmetric rash, accompanied by systemic symptoms like fever, malaise, and lymphadenopathy.
- *Erythema multiforme (EM)*:
    - *Clinical features*: EM presents with target lesions, which are erythematous macules with a central clearing and an outer ring of erythema. These lesions often appear on the acral surfaces, such as the hands and feet, and may be accompanied by mucosal involvement in more severe cases. EM is often triggered by infections, particularly herpes simplex virus (HSV), or by certain medications.
    - *Pathophysiology*: EM is considered a hypersensitivity reaction, most commonly following infections or drug exposure. The characteristic rash is due to a cytotoxic immune response targeting keratinocytes.
    - *Diagnostic clues*: Fixed lesions lasting longer than 24 hours, negative Darier's sign, and mucosal involvement in severe cases are key distinguishing features from urticaria.
- *Drug reactions*:
    - *Clinical features*: Drug-induced urticaria and angioedema are common, but other drug reactions can mimic urticaria. Fixed drug eruptions present as erythematous plaques that recur at the same site with re-exposure to the offending drug. Stevens–Johnson syndrome/toxic epidermal necrolysis (SJS/TEN) presents with widespread erythema, necrosis, and detachment of the epidermis, often starting with a prodrome of fever and malaise.
    - *Pathophysiology*: Drug reactions can involve various immune-mediated mechanisms, including type I hypersensitivity (e.g., IgE-mediated), type III hypersensitivity (immune complex-mediated), and type IV hypersensitivity (T-cell-mediated).
    - *Diagnostic clues*: A detailed drug history, the timing of symptom onset relative to drug exposure, and the presence of systemic symptoms (e.g., fever,

mucosal involvement) are critical in identifying drug-induced conditions. Skin biopsy and patch testing may also aid in diagnosis.
- *Papular urticaria*:
  - *Clinical features*: Papular urticaria is a hypersensitivity reaction to insect bites, commonly seen in children. It presents with recurrent pruritic papules, often on the lower extremities. The lesions can persist for several days, unlike the transient wheals of urticaria.
  - *Pathophysiology*: The condition is caused by an exaggerated immune response to insect bites, leading to persistent pruritic papules.
  - *Diagnostic clues*: A history of insect exposure, the localized distribution of the lesions, and their persistence distinguish papular urticaria from classic urticaria.

Systemic Disorders
- *Anaphylaxis*:
  - *Clinical features*: Anaphylaxis is a severe, systemic allergic reaction that can present with acute urticaria, angioedema, and potentially life-threatening symptoms such as bronchospasm and hypotension.
  - *Distinguishing features*: The rapid onset of symptoms following exposure to a known allergen, along with systemic involvement, is characteristic of anaphylaxis.
- *Serum sickness*:
  - *Clinical features*: Serum sickness is an immune-complex-mediated hypersensitivity reaction that occurs after exposure to foreign proteins or certain medications. It presents with urticarial rash, fever, arthralgia, and lymphadenopathy.
  - *Distinguishing features*: The delayed onset of symptoms (typically 1–3 weeks after exposure), along with the presence of systemic symptoms like fever and joint pain, distinguishes serum sickness from acute urticaria.
- *Autoimmune disorders*:
  - *Clinical features*: Autoimmune conditions, such as systemic lupus erythematosus (SLE), can occasionally present with an acute urticarial rash. SLE is an autoimmune disease with a wide range of clinical manifestations. Cutaneous features include a malar rash, photosensitivity, and nonscarring alopecia. Systemic involvement may include nephritis, arthritis, serositis, and central nervous system (CNS) disease. Other autoimmune diseases such as dermatomyositis and systemic sclerosis can also present with skin findings that mimic urticaria. Dermatomyositis presents with a heliotrope rash and Gottron's papules, while systemic sclerosis may present with sclerodactyly and digital ulcers.
  - *Pathophysiology*: Autoimmune diseases involve the immune system attacking the body's own tissues, leading to inflammation and tissue damage. The skin manifestations of these diseases are often part of a broader systemic involvement.
  - *Diagnostic clues*: A positive antinuclear antibody (ANA) test, anti-double-stranded DNA (anti-dsDNA) antibodies, and systemic symptoms such as

arthritis, nephritis, and serositis are crucial in differentiating SLE from urticaria. The presence of systemic symptoms (e.g., muscle weakness, Raynaud's phenomenon), specific autoantibodies (e.g., anti-Jo-1 in dermatomyositis, anti-Scl-70 in systemic sclerosis), and a detailed history and physical examination are essential for differentiating from urticaria.

DIFFERENTIAL DIAGNOSIS OF CHRONIC URTICARIA

Chronic urticaria lasts for 6 weeks or longer and can be more challenging to diagnose due to its chronic nature and the wide range of potential mimickers. The primary dermatological and systemic disorders that can mimic chronic urticaria are given in the following text.

Dermatological Disorders

- *Urticarial vasculitis*:
  - *Clinical features*: Urticarial vasculitis is characterized by urticarial lesions that persist for more than 24 hours, often with associated purpura and systemic symptoms such as fever, arthralgia, or abdominal pain. Unlike typical urticaria, these lesions often resolve with hyperpigmentation.
  - *Pathophysiology*: Urticarial vasculitis involves immune complex deposition in small blood vessels, leading to complement activation and inflammation. This distinguishes it from classic urticaria, where immune complex deposition is not a feature.
  - *Diagnostic clues*: The diagnosis of urticarial vasculitis can be confirmed by skin biopsy, which shows leukocytoclastic vasculitis. Complement levels (C3, C4) may be low, and this is particularly suggestive in cases of hypocomplementemic urticarial vasculitis.
  - *Management*: Treatment may involve antihistamines, nonsteroidal anti-inflammatory drugs (NSAIDs), or immunosuppressants like corticosteroids or hydroxychloroquine.
- *Bullous pemphigoid*:
  - *Clinical features*: Bullous pemphigoid typically presents in elderly patients with pruritic urticarial plaques that may develop into tense blisters. The lesions are often found on the flexural areas of the skin, such as the inner thighs and the abdomen.
  - *Pathophysiology*: Bullous pemphigoid is an autoimmune blistering disease caused by IgG antibodies targeting hemidesmosomes, which are structures that anchor the epidermis to the dermis.
  - *Diagnostic clues*: A biopsy with direct immunofluorescence will show linear IgG and C3 deposition at the dermoepidermal junction, which is diagnostic of bullous pemphigoid. The presence of blisters and the chronicity of lesions distinguish this condition from urticaria.
- *Eosinophilic dermatoses*:
  - *Clinical features*: Conditions like Wells syndrome (eosinophilic cellulitis) can present with urticarial plaques. These plaques are typically indurated and may evolve into blistered or necrotic lesions.

- *Distinguishing features*: The presence of tissue eosinophilia on biopsy and the indurated nature of the plaques help distinguish eosinophilic dermatoses from chronic urticaria.
- *Annular erythemas*, such as erythema annulare centrifugum (EAC) and other reactive erythemas, can mimic urticarial lesions due to their annular or ring-like appearance, which might be mistaken for resolving urticarial wheals.
  a. EAC:
     - *Clinical features*: Annular, erythematous plaques with trailing scale, expanding centrifugally
     - *Distinguishing features*: The annular shape with a trailing scale, centrifugal expansion, and histopathology showing perivascular lymphocytic infiltrate ("coat-sleeve" cuffing).
     - *Management*: Identifying and addressing underlying causes, with lesions often resolving spontaneously
  b. *Erythema marginatum:*
     - *Clinical features*: Nonpruritic, erythematous rings, often linked to rheumatic fever
     - *Distinguishing features*: Association with streptococcal infection and rheumatic fever, nonpruritic nature
     - *Management*: Focuses on managing rheumatic fever with antibiotics and anti-inflammatory medications.
  c. Erythema gyratum repens
     - *Clinical features*: Rapidly progressing concentric rings, often associated with malignancies
     - *Distinguishing features*: The wood-grain appearance, rapid progression, and strong link to internal malignancies
     - *Management*: Involves identifying and treating the underlying malignancy
- *Annular discoid lupus erythematosus (DLE)*:
  - *Clinical features*:
    – *Appearance*: Annular DLE presents with erythematous, scaly plaques that may have central atrophy and hyperpigmentation. The lesions are often found on sun-exposed areas like the face, neck, and scalp.
    – *Symptoms*: These lesions are typically asymptomatic or mildly pruritic, unlike the intensely pruritic wheals of urticaria.
    – *Chronicity*: DLE is a chronic condition, with lesions persisting for months to years, which is different from the transient nature of urticarial lesions.
  - *Distinguishing features*:
    – *Distribution*: Predominantly affects sun-exposed areas, whereas urticaria can occur anywhere on the body
    – *Histopathology*: DLE shows hyperkeratosis, follicular plugging, and a lymphocytic infiltrate at the dermoepidermal junction, features that are not seen in urticaria.
    – *Association*: DLE can be associated with SLE, so systemic symptoms or serology (e.g., positive ANA) may aid in distinguishing it from urticaria.

- *Management*:
  - Treatment: DLE requires immunosuppressive therapy, sun protection, and topical corticosteroids, contrasting with the antihistamines typically used for urticaria.
- *Annular sarcoidosis*:
  - *Clinical features*:
    - Appearance: Annular sarcoidosis presents as nonpruritic, reddish-brown plaques that often have a raised, annular border with central clearing. These lesions are typically found on the face, neck, and trunk.
    - Symptoms: The lesions are generally nonpruritic and asymptomatic, which contrasts with the pruritic nature of urticarial wheals.
  - *Distinguishing features*:
    - Systemic involvement: Sarcoidosis often involves multiple organs (lungs, eyes, lymph nodes), and systemic symptoms such as cough, dyspnea, or uveitis may be present, aiding differentiation.
    - Histopathology: Biopsy reveals noncaseating granulomas, a hallmark of sarcoidosis, absent in urticaria.
    - Chronicity: Lesions persist and may evolve slowly over months, unlike the transient nature of urticaria.
  - *Management*:
    - Treatment: Management includes systemic corticosteroids or immunosuppressive agents, depending on organ involvement, unlike the antihistamines used for urticaria.
- *Leprosy (Hansen's disease)*:
  - *Clinical features*:
    - Appearance: Leprosy can present with annular or hypopigmented patches, which may be anesthetic. These lesions are usually found on cooler parts of the body, such as the face, ears, and extremities.
    - Symptoms: Anesthesia or hypoesthesia within the lesions is a key distinguishing feature, whereas urticarial lesions are typically pruritic and have normal sensation.
  - *Distinguishing features*:
    - Nerve involvement: The presence of peripheral nerve thickening and sensory loss is characteristic of leprosy and not seen in urticaria.
    - Histopathology: Skin biopsy may reveal acid-fast bacilli and granulomatous inflammation, distinguishing it from urticaria.
    - Systemic signs: Advanced leprosy can involve deformities and systemic signs, absent in urticaria.
  - *Management*:
    - Treatment: Multidrug therapy (MDT) is used for leprosy, a specialized treatment approach not relevant for urticaria.

Systemic Disorders

- *Connective tissue diseases*:
  - Clinical features: Diseases such as SLE and dermatomyositis can present with chronic urticarial lesions as part of their cutaneous manifestations.

- *Distinguishing features*: The presence of systemic symptoms, such as arthritis, fatigue, and specific cutaneous features (e.g., heliotrope rash in dermatomyositis), alongside positive autoimmune serologies, are key distinguishing factors.
- *Chronic infections*:
  - *Clinical features*: Chronic infections like *Helicobacter pylori*, hepatitis B and C, and parasitic infestations can manifest as chronic urticaria. Patients may also present with gastrointestinal complaints, fatigue, and intermittent fever.
  - *Distinguishing features*: A thorough history, positive serological tests for chronic infections, and improvement of urticaria with treatment of the underlying infection help distinguish these from other causes.
- *Malignancies*:
  - *Clinical features*: Certain malignancies, particularly lymphomas, can present with chronic urticaria. The urticaria is often resistant to treatment and may be associated with systemic symptoms like weight loss, night sweats, and lymphadenopathy.
  - *Distinguishing features*: Persistent urticaria, especially when resistant to treatment, coupled with "B symptoms" and abnormal findings on imaging or biopsy, strongly suggest an underlying malignancy.
- *Cryoglobulinemia*:
  - *Clinical features*: Cryoglobulinemia presents with palpable purpura, arthralgia, Raynaud's phenomenon, and systemic involvement such as glomerulonephritis. The skin lesions may resemble urticaria but are usually more persistent and may ulcerate.
  - *Pathophysiology*: Cryoglobulins are immunoglobulins that precipitate at low temperatures and cause immune complex-mediated vasculitis. This leads to inflammation and damage in small blood vessels, particularly in the skin and kidneys.
  - *Diagnostic clues*: The presence of serum cryoglobulins, cold-induced symptoms, and low complement levels, particularly C4, are key diagnostic features. A history of associated conditions, such as hepatitis C, should also raise suspicion.

DISTINGUISHING ACUTE FROM CHRONIC URTICARIA MIMICKERS

While acute and chronic urticaria share some common features, the conditions that mimic them can differ significantly. The key points in distinguishing these mimickers include the following:
- *Duration*: Acute urticaria mimickers often have a rapid onset and resolution, whereas chronic mimickers are associated with long-standing conditions.
- *Systemic symptoms*: Acute mimickers may involve systemic allergic responses or infections, while chronic mimickers often involve autoimmune or systemic disorders with more insidious onset and progression.

- *Histopathological findings*: Acute mimickers typically show nonspecific inflammation, while chronic mimickers like urticarial vasculitis or bullous pemphigoid reveal specific histopathological features.
- *Response to treatment*: Acute mimickers usually respond well to antihistamines and avoidance of triggers, while chronic mimickers may require more complex management, including immunosuppressive therapies or treatment of underlying systemic conditions.

DIAGNOSTIC APPROACH

Given the broad differential diagnosis for urticaria-like conditions, a systematic approach is essential to avoid misdiagnosis. The following steps outline the recommended approach:

1. *Patient history*:
   - Obtain a detailed history, including the duration and frequency of the rash, associated symptoms (e.g., fever, arthralgia), triggers (e.g., medications, foods, infections), and family history.
   - Inquire about any recent changes in medications, including over-the-counter drugs and supplements.
   - Review the patient's medical history for any underlying autoimmune or systemic conditions.
2. *Physical examination*:
   - Conduct a thorough cutaneous examination, noting the distribution, morphology, and duration of the lesions.
   - Examine for any systemic signs, such as lymphadenopathy, hepatosplenomegaly, or signs of systemic autoimmune disease.
   - Assess for any signs of angioedema, especially in cases where hereditary angioedema is suspected.
3. *Laboratory investigations*:
   - Basic blood work, including complete blood count (CBC), erythrocyte sedimentation rate (ESR), and C-reactive protein (CRP), can help identify underlying infections or inflammatory processes.
   - Specific tests such as ANA, C3, C4, and cryoglobulins should be considered in cases where autoimmune or vasculitic causes are suspected.
   - Skin biopsy with histopathological examination and direct immunofluorescence may be necessary for conditions like urticarial vasculitis, bullous pemphigoid, or other vesiculobullous disorders.
4. *Specialized tests*:
   - Patch testing for contact dermatitis
   - Genetic testing for hereditary angioedema if clinically indicated.
   - Imaging studies (e.g., CT scan, MRI) may be necessary if systemic involvement is suspected (e.g., lymphadenopathy, organomegaly).

CONCLUSION

Urticaria mimickers encompass a broad range of dermatological and systemic conditions that require careful differentiation from true urticaria. A thorough understanding of these conditions, coupled with a systematic diagnostic approach, is essential for accurate diagnosis and optimal patient management. By identifying the underlying cause, clinicians can tailor treatment to address the specific condition, improving patient outcomes and preventing potential complications.

SUGGESTED READINGS

1. Zuberbier T, Aberer W, Asero R, Abdul Latiff AH, Baker D, Ballmer-Weber B, et al. The EAACI/GA²LEN/EDF/WAO guideline for the definition, classification, diagnosis, and management of urticaria. Allergy. 2018;73(7):1393-414.
2. Kaplan AP. Urticaria and angioedema. In: Franklin Adkinson N, Bochner BS, Wesley Burks A, Busse WW, Holgate ST, Lemanske RF, et al. Middleton's Allergy: Principles and Practice. 8th ed. Philadelphia: Elsevier; 2013.
3. Greaves MW. Chronic urticaria. J Allergy Clin Immunol. 2000;105(4):664-72.
4. Grattan CEH, Black AK. Urticarial vasculitis and other urticarial syndromes. In: Bolognia JL, Schaffer JV, Cerroni L (Eds). Dermatology, 4th edition. Philadelphia: Elsevier; 2018.
5. Schaefer P. Acute and chronic urticaria: evaluation and treatment. Am Fam Physician. 2017;95(11):717-24.
6. Magerl M, Borzova E, Giménez-Arnau A, Grattan CEH, Lawlor FJ, Matos Benavides L, et al. Physical urticarias: classification and diagnostic guidelines. Allergy. 2016;71(4):563-74.
7. Maurer M, Weller K, Bindslev-Jensen C, Giménez-Arnau A, Bousquet PJ, Bousquet J, et al. Unmet clinical needs in chronic spontaneous urticaria. Allergy. 2011;66(3):317-30.

CHAPTER 19

Mast Cell Disorders

Rohit Batra, Anushruti Aggarwal, Sanjeev Gupta

INTRODUCTION

Mastocytosis encompasses a spectrum of rare, often complex disorders marked by the pathological accumulation and activation of mast cells within the skin, bone marrow, gastrointestinal tract, liver, spleen, and other organs. This multifaceted condition includes both cutaneous and systemic forms, ranging from mild, skin-limited cases to aggressive subtypes with significant organ involvement and life-altering symptoms.

Advances in understanding mast cell biology, particularly the role of genetic mutations such as the KIT D816V mutation, have provided crucial insights into the disease's pathogenesis, classification, and management. This chapter aims to comprehensively address the epidemiology, classification, pathophysiology, diagnosis, and therapeutic approaches to mastocytosis, with an emphasis on recent developments that are reshaping patient care.

DEFINITION AND CLASSIFICATION

Mastocytosis is a heterogeneous group of disorders, characterized by the accumulation of neoplastic mast cells in the skin and various other organs. It can present with either cutaneous or systemic involvement. Various internal organs, such as the bone marrow, spleen, lymph nodes, and the gastrointestinal (GI) tract can be involved.

Classification of Mast Cell Disorders

There are two classifications—by (i) the World Health Organization (WHO) and another by (ii) the International Consensus Classification (ICC). As such there is no major difference between these two classifications.

WHO Classification
- *Cutaneous mastocytosis*: Urticaria pigmentosa or maculopapular cutaneous mastocytosis, diffuse cut mastocytosis, and mastocytoma

- *Systemic mastocytosis*: Indolent type, associated with nonmast cell blood disorders, aggressive type, mast cell leukemia (MCL)/sarcoma, and extracutaneous mastocytoma

EPIDEMIOLOGY

It is an uncommon disease with low prevalence. Childhood type usually manifests in first 2 years of age, while adult type in third to 6th decade. As such, there is no gender preference.

MAST CELL BIOLOGY

Mast cells are part of the innate and adaptive immune system. They are derived from bone marrow progenitors. Mast cells accumulate at inflammatory sites associated with atopy, wound healing, and malignancies. They interact with the external environment and are predominantly located in close proximity of blood vessels and sensory nerves.

Origin and Development

- Mast cells are derived from hematopoietic stem cells in the bone marrow. They undergo differentiation into mature mast cells in peripheral tissues, where they reside long term.
- Mast cells are found in loose (areolar) connective tissue throughout the body, in virtually every organ. They are responsible for the inflammatory cascade. Mast cells can degranulate, releasing inflammatory mediators into the extracellular space when induced by the immune system. Mast cells are associated with many pathologies, including type I hypersensitivity reactions, mastocytosis, mast cell activation syndrome, and urticarial syndromes.

Functions of Mast Cells

Mast cells are mononuclear cells. They contain small secretory granules, ranging in size from 0.2 to 0.8 μm. IgE receptors are found in the plasma membrane, which bind the Fc region of circulating IgE, and the two crosslink to induce cell degranulation.

Two major types of mast cell have been identified and are distinguished by the content of their secretory granules. MC(T) cells contain granules with mostly tryptase. MC(T) cells are found near mucosal tissue that is exposed to the outside world, i.e., gastrointestinal or respiratory mucosa. These cells act predominantly in the immune response. MC(TC) cells contain tryptase as well as chymase and carboxypeptidase in the secretory granules. The majority of MC(TC) cells are found in the submucosa and connective tissue adjacent to the conjunctiva and skin, often near blood and lymphatic vessels. These cells play a pivotal role in tissue repair.

The mast cell functions as part of the body's innate immune system. When membrane-bound IgE binds a foreign substance and two Fc receptors crosslink, the mast cell immediately releases a large number of mediators into the nearby extracellular space via degranulation. Granules are contained within a lipid membrane which fuses with the plasma membrane. The most important cytokines released is histamine. Histamine induces white blood cell chemotaxis, airway smooth muscle constriction, and increased vascular permeability. Other mediators released from the granules include tryptase, chymase, and tumor necrosis factor alpha (TNF-α).

Mast cells synthesize and release prostaglandins and leukotrienes, which have proinflammatory effects. Finally, cytokine production is increased due to an increase in gene transcription.

The inflammatory effect of the mast cell is used by the innate immune system as first line of defense. MC(T) cells are the predominant cell type in the immune response. When a foreign protein is encountered, the proinflammatory effects exerted by the mast cells result in recruitment of circulating immune cells. Cytokines released also have direct effects on local tissue, such as increased mucus production or increased gut peristalsis to reduce pathogen invasion.

Mast cells also play a role in tissue repair and angiogenesis. Upon injury, MC(TC) release procoagulant cytokines, leukotrienes, and platelet-activating factor. Later, heparin, tryptase, and tissue plasminogen activator (tPA) from the cell modulate blood flow to increase nutrient and immune cell delivery. Inflammatory mediators promote the differentiation and growth of fibroblasts and endothelial cells. Mast cells also possess many angiogenic cytokines such as vascular endothelial growth factor (VEGF) and basic fibroblast growth factor (FGF-2). Finally, mast cells have been implicated in the wound contraction and the regeneration of nerve fibers.

- *Mast cell mediators*: These are of two types—(i) Preformed mediators, and (ii) newly synthesized mediators. Preformed mediators are the ones stored in granules and released rapidly during degranulation. These include:
  - *Histamine*: Causes vasodilation, increases vascular permeability, and induces smooth muscle contraction
  - *Tryptase and other proteases*: Serves as a marker for mast cell activation and plays a role in tissue remodeling and inflammation
  - *Heparin*: An anticoagulant that also aids in tissue repair
- *Newly synthesized mediators are formed upon activation*:
  - *Leukotrienes and prostaglandins*: Potent bronchoconstrictors, promoting inflammation and allergic symptoms.
  - *Cytokines*: TNF-α, interleukin 4 (IL-4), IL-13—promoting inflammation and contributing to chronic allergic responses.

PATHOPHYSIOLOGY OF MASTOCYTOSIS

The pathophysiology involves both genetic and molecular alterations, as well as complex interactions with the surrounding tissue environment.

Genetic Basis
- *KIT gene mutation*:
  - The most common and critical genetic mutation in mastocytosis involves the *KIT proto-oncogene*, which encodes the transmembrane receptor tyrosine kinase known as CD117.
  - The *D816V point mutation* in the *KIT* gene is found in over 90% of cases of systemic mastocytosis. This mutation results in the substitution of aspartic acid (D) with valine (V) at position 816, leading to constitutive activation of the KIT receptor.
  - *Constitutive activation of KIT*: The D816V mutation causes the KIT receptor to be constantly "on" independent of ligand binding [stem cell factor (SCF)]. This promotes uncontrolled mast cell growth, survival, and accumulation.
- *Additional mutations*:
  - Other less common mutations in *KIT* and other genes involved in signal transduction pathways (e.g., RAS, JAK2) can contribute to the disease's severity, especially in advanced forms such as aggressive systemic mastocytosis (ASM) or MCL.

Mast Cell Accumulation and Tissue Infiltration
- The aberrantly activated KIT receptor leads to uncontrolled proliferation of mast cells, resulting in their accumulation in various tissues, including the skin, bone marrow, liver, spleen, and gastrointestinal tract.
- The infiltrating mast cells typically have abnormal morphology, including spindle shapes or atypical forms. They form dense clusters, particularly in the bone marrow and other extracutaneous organs, leading to tissue damage and dysfunction.

Mast Cell Mediator Release
- Mast cells contain granules rich in bioactive substances, including histamine, tryptase, heparin, prostaglandins, leukotrienes, and cytokines.
- In mastocytosis, these mediators are released either spontaneously or in response to triggers such as physical stimuli (heat, pressure), certain foods, medications, or stress.
- The excessive release of these mediators leads to symptoms such as flushing, pruritus, abdominal pain, diarrhea, hypotension, and anaphylaxis.
- *Role of KIT activation in mediator release:*
  - The KIT receptor not only drives mast cell proliferation but also contributes to the activation of downstream signaling pathways involved in degranulation and mediator release.
  - The key pathways include the PI3K-AKT, MAPK, and JAK-STAT pathways, which modulate survival, cytokine production, and mast cell activation.

Tissue Damage and Organ Dysfunction
- In advanced forms of systemic mastocytosis [e.g., ASM, systemic mastocytosis with associated hematologic neoplasm (SM-AHN)], the infiltrating mast cells cause significant tissue damage and organ dysfunction.
- *Bone marrow*: Extensive mast cell infiltration leads to fibrosis, impaired hematopoiesis, and cytopenias.
- *Liver and spleen*: Mast cell infiltration results in hepatosplenomegaly, portal hypertension, and hepatic dysfunction.
- *Gastrointestinal tract*: Involvement can cause malabsorption, diarrhea, and weight loss due to villous atrophy and inflammation.

Interaction with the Microenvironment
- The bone marrow and tissue microenvironment play a significant role in supporting mast cell growth and survival.
- *Stem cell factor (SCF)*: SCF, the ligand for KIT, is produced by stromal cells and is crucial for normal mast cell development. In mastocytosis, excess SCF can enhance mast cell proliferation and survival.
- *Cytokine networks*: Cytokines such as IL-6 and TNF-α, produced by both mast cells and surrounding cells, contribute to the inflammatory milieu, further promoting mast cell accumulation and tissue damage.

Progression to Advanced Disease
- While indolent forms of systemic mastocytosis are relatively stable, genetic and epigenetic changes can drive progression to more aggressive forms.
- *Clonal evolution*: Additional mutations in signaling or epigenetic regulators (e.g., *TET2, SRSF2, ASXL1*) can lead to more aggressive mast cell behavior, organ dysfunction, and the development of associated hematologic neoplasms (SM-AHN).
- *Impaired apoptosis*: Resistance to apoptosis is another hallmark of advanced mastocytosis, contributing to the accumulation of long-lived mast cells.

CLASSIFICATION OF MAST CELL DISORDERS

Cutaneous Mastocytosis
Urticaria Pigmentosa (Maculopapular Cutaneous Mastocytosis)
Urticaria pigmentosa (UP) is the most common form of cutaneous mastocytosis, primarily affecting the skin. It is characterized by the abnormal accumulation of mast cells in the skin, leading to various skin lesions. UP can occur in both children and adults, with the clinical course and prognosis varying between these age groups. It the most common variant of cutaneous mastocytosis, especially in children.
- *Pediatric UP*: In children, it mostly presents in the first year. It is characterized by brownish macules, papules or nodules, which can appear anywhere

on the body excluding palms and soles. These lesions are associated with itching. They may become urticarial (raised, red, and itchy) when rubbed or scratched, a reaction known as *Darier's sign*. Other symptoms may be recurrent diarrhea, acid reflux, urinary frequency, and headache. Many cases resolve spontaneously by adolescence, especially if the disease is limited to the skin. Prognosis is generally good, with few progressing to systemic mastocytosis.
- *Adult UP*: It can occur at any age but mostly occurs in the second or third decade. Adults often have more pigmented and stable lesions compared to children. The lesions are usually brownish macules or plaques that do not blister. Adults are at higher risk of developing systemic mastocytosis, where mast cells accumulate in internal organs such as the bone marrow, liver, spleen, and gastrointestinal tract. UP in adults tends to persist and is more likely to progress to systemic mastocytosis. The prognosis depends on whether there is systemic involvement. Indolent systemic mastocytosis (ISM) has a relatively good prognosis, whereas aggressive forms are associated with a worse outcome. Regular follow-up is important to monitor the progression of the disease, especially in adults, to detect any signs of systemic involvement.

Diffuse Cutaneous Mastocytosis

It is a rare but severe form in which mast cells infiltrate the skin diffusely. It presents as widespread skin thickening, bullae, and a higher risk of systemic symptoms.

Mastocytoma of the skin: Solitary, nodular lesions often seen in infants, usually resolving with age.

Systemic Mastocytosis

Types and Classification of Systemic Mastocytosis

The WHO classifies systemic mastocytosis into several subtypes based on clinical severity, prognosis, and the extent of organ involvement:
- *ISM:*
  - *Clinical features*: ISM is the most common and least severe form. Patients typically have stable disease with a good prognosis. Mast cells infiltrate one or more extracutaneous organs (e.g., bone marrow, gastrointestinal tract) but without significant organ dysfunction
  - *Symptoms*: The disease is usually mild and chronic, with symptoms caused by the release of mast cell mediators (e.g., flushing, pruritus, gastrointestinal discomfort). Skin involvement is common (e.g., UP)
  - *Prognosis*: Excellent, with near-normal life expectancy
- *Smoldering systemic mastocytosis (SSM)*:
  - *Clinical features*: SSM is more severe than ISM and is associated with a higher mast cell burden and more significant organ involvement. However, it is still not aggressive.

- *Symptoms*: Patients may show signs of organomegaly (e.g., splenomegaly, hepatomegaly), anemia, or mild cytopenias. The disease remains stable for years but may progress to more severe forms.
  - *Prognosis*: Intermediate, with a risk of progression to more aggressive forms
- ASM:
  - *Clinical features:* ASM is characterized by extensive infiltration of organs by mast cells, leading to organ dysfunction without the development of overt MCL. It involves severe systemic symptoms and may result in organ damage (e.g., liver failure, malabsorption due to gastrointestinal involvement).
  - *Symptoms*: Includes severe cytopenias, ascites, malabsorption, and weight loss. Mediator-related symptoms are still present but are overshadowed by the organ dysfunction.
  - *Prognosis*: Poor, with significantly reduced survival, often due to organ failure
- SM-AHN:
  - *Clinical features*: SM-AHN involves the coexistence of SM with another clonal hematologic disorder (e.g., myelodysplastic syndrome, chronic myelomonocytic leukemia, or myeloproliferative neoplasms).
  - *Symptoms*: Patients present with symptoms of both systemic mastocytosis and the associated hematologic malignancy, which complicates management and worsens the prognosis.
  - *Prognosis*: The prognosis depends on the nature and aggressiveness of the associated hematologic neoplasm, which usually dominates the clinical picture.
- MCL:
  - *Clinical features*: MCL is the rarest and most aggressive form of SM. It is defined by the presence of a large number of circulating mast cells and extensive infiltration of the bone marrow and other organs.
  - *Symptoms*: Patients present with severe cytopenias, extensive organ involvement, hepatosplenomegaly, and a rapid clinical course. Mediator-related symptoms may be overshadowed by the severe systemic involvement.
  - *Prognosis*: Extremely poor, with median survival typically <6 months.
- *Mast cell sarcoma*:
  - *Clinical features*: This is a rare, highly malignant form characterized by a tumor of poorly differentiated mast cells. It is typically aggressive and progresses rapidly.
  - *Symptoms*: Presents with a mass lesion, and rapid dissemination is common
  - *Prognosis*: Very poor, with rapid progression and resistance to treatment

Mast Cell Activation Syndrome

In mast cell activation syndrome (MCAS), mast cells are abnormally activated, leading to the release of mediators such as histamine, tryptase, prostaglandins, leukotrienes, and other inflammatory molecules.

This release occurs spontaneously or in response to triggers such as foods, stress, temperature changes, medications, or environmental factors.

Unlike systemic mastocytosis, which involves an increased number of mast cells, MCAS typically involves normal mast cell counts but with excessive activation and mediator release. It can be:
- *Primary MCAS (monoclonal/clonal)*: Typically involves clonal mast cell populations, often associated with the KIT D816V mutation
- *Secondary MCAS*: Occurs due to other conditions such as allergies, infections, or autoimmune diseases, where mast cells are inappropriately activated
- *Idiopathic MCAS*: No identifiable cause; patients present with episodes of mast cell activation symptoms without obvious triggers or clonal populations

DIAGNOSTIC CRITERIA

The WHO Criteria for Systemic Mastocytosis
- *Major criterion*: Multifocal, dense infiltrates of mast cells in bone marrow or other extracutaneous organs
- *Minor criteria*: Include KIT mutation (especially D816V), aberrant CD2/CD25 expression, atypical mast cell morphology, and elevated serum tryptase levels (>20 ng/mL)
- Diagnosis of systemic mastocytosis requires either one major and one minor criterion or three minor criteria.

Diagnostic Challenges
Emphasize the difficulty in distinguishing mast cell disorders from conditions with overlapping symptoms such as chronic urticaria, idiopathic anaphylaxis, and gastrointestinal disorders. The episodic nature of symptoms can delay diagnosis.

Laboratory Investigations
- *Serum tryptase levels*: Elevated tryptase (>20 ng/mL) is a key marker of systemic mast cell activation. Tryptase levels peak during acute episodes of mast cell degranulation (e.g., anaphylaxis).
- *Bone marrow biopsy*: Essential for diagnosing systemic mastocytosis. Look for dense infiltrates of spindle-shaped mast cells (>15 mast cells in aggregates) and aberrant expression of markers such as CD25 and CD2.
- *Molecular testing*: KIT mutation testing (especially for D816V) is critical for confirming clonal mast cell disease. Polymerase chain reaction (PCR)-based assays are typically used.

MANAGEMENT AND TREATMENT

General Management Principles
- The management of mastocytosis varies depending on the type (cutaneous or systemic) and the severity of symptoms.

- Treatment is mainly symptomatic and aimed at controlling the release and effects of mast cell mediators.

Educating patients about potential trigger is crucial. These include physical triggers such as heat, exertion, nonsteroidal anti-inflammatory drugs (e.g., aspirin, ibuprofen, diclofenac), insects, and radiocontrast media.

Pharmacological Management

- *Antihistamines:*
  - *H1-antihistamines*: Used to control pruritus, flushing, urticaria, and other allergic symptoms, e.g., cetirizine, loratadine, fexofenadine, diphenhydramine
  - *H2-antihistamines*: Used to reduce gastric hypersecretion, abdominal pain, and peptic ulcer disease, e.g., ranitidine, famotidine, cimetidine
- *Mast cell stabilizers*: These help in reducing the release of mediators from mast cells, *e.g.,* cromolyn sodium, particularly effective in gastrointestinal symptoms and cutaneous mastocytosis
- *Leukotriene inhibitors*: Leukotriene receptor antagonists may be used to reduce mediator-related symptoms such as bronchospasm and gastrointestinal discomfort, e.g., montelukast and zafirlukast
- *Corticosteroids*:
  - *Topical steroids*: Used in cutaneous mastocytosis to reduce pruritus and lesions. Topical corticosteroids (e.g., 0.05% clobetasol propionate twice daily for up to 6 weeks for UP on the body in adults but not the face)
  - *Systemic steroids*: May be used in severe cases of systemic mastocytosis, particularly when there is organ involvement or anaphylaxis
- *Epinephrine*: Essential for managing anaphylaxis in patients with systemic mastocytosis. Patients are often prescribed self-injectable epinephrine (e.g., epipen) and trained on its use.
- *Tyrosine kinase inhibitors (TKIs)*: In advanced systemic mastocytosis, particularly with D816V KIT mutation, TKIs such as midostaurin can be effective. Other TKIs such as imatinib may be useful in KIT mutation-negative cases.
- *Immunotherapy*: *Omalizumab (anti-IgE therapy)* has been used off-label to control symptoms related to mast cell activation, especially in patients with recurrent anaphylaxis or severe systemic symptoms.
- *Cytoreductive therapy*: Indicated in ASM and MCL where there is significant organ damage. *Medications such as* cladribine (2-CDA), interferon-alpha are administered or more intensive chemotherapy is given depending on the case.
- *Bone marrow transplantation*: Considered in selected cases of advanced mastocytosis with poor prognosis, especially in young patients or those with mast cell leukemia.

Supportive Care

- *Pain management*: Nonsteroidal anti-inflammatory drugs (NSAIDs) are generally avoided due to the risk of exacerbating symptoms. Acetaminophen is preferred.

- *Psychological support*: Anxiety and depression may occur due to chronic symptoms and the unpredictable nature of the disease.

PROGNOSIS OF MASTOCYTOSIS

- *Cutaneous mastocytosis*:
  - Generally, it has a good prognosis, especially in children where it often regresses spontaneously by adolescence.
  - In adults, it tends to persist but is less likely to progress to systemic disease.
- *ISM*:
  - ISM has a favorable prognosis with a normal life expectancy, though symptoms may persist lifelong.
- *SSM*:
  - Intermediate prognosis; patients have a higher risk of progression to aggressive disease.
- *ASM*:
  - Poor prognosis due to significant organ damage.
  - Median survival is reduced, with a range from 2 to 4 years depending on the severity of organ involvement.
- *MCL*:
  - The prognosis is very poor, with a median survival of <1 year.
- *Mastocytosis-associated with hematologic neoplasms (AHN)*:
  - Prognosis depends on the type of associated hematologic neoplasm, which often drives the overall survival outcome.

REGULAR MONITORING AND FOLLOW-UP

- Patients with systemic involvement require regular monitoring for disease progression and organ dysfunction.
- Periodic bone marrow biopsies and serum tryptase levels are often used to assess disease status.
- Follow-up care also includes managing secondary complications such as osteoporosis, particularly in systemic cases.

CONCLUSION

Effective management of mastocytosis requires a tailored, multidisciplinary approach that considers disease subtype, symptom severity, and potential complications. Treatments primarily target the control of mast cell mediator release, symptomatic relief, and reduction of mast cell burden in advanced cases. Although cutaneous mastocytosis generally has a favorable prognosis, systemic forms may progress, underscoring the need for vigilant monitoring. Emerging targeted therapies, particularly tyrosine kinase inhibitors for cases involving KIT mutations, offer promising avenues for improved outcomes. Continued research into the genetic and molecular underpinnings of mastocytosis will be vital to refining therapeutic strategies and enhancing patient quality of life.

SUGGESTED READINGS

1. Valent P, Akin C, Arock M, Brockow K, Butterfield JH, Carter MC, et al. Definitions, criteria and global classification of mast cell disorders with special reference to mastocytosis: a consensus proposal. Leukemia Res. 2001;25(7):603-25.
2. Metcalfe DD. Mast cells and mastocytosis. Blood. 2008;112(4):946-56.
3. Valent P, Akin C, Metcalfe DD. Mastocytosis: 2016 updated WHO classification and novel emerging treatment concepts. Blood. 2017;129(11):1420-7.
4. Horny HP, Metcalfe DD, Bennett JM, et al. Mastocytosis. In: Swerdlow SH, Campo E, Harris NL Jaffe ES, Pileri SA, Stein H, Thiele J (Eds). WHO Classification of Tumours of Haematopoietic and Lymphoid Tissues, 4th edition. Lyon: IARC Press; 2017. pp. 62-9.
5. Escribano L, Akin C. Urticaria pigmentosa and cutaneous mastocytosis. In: Bolognia JL, Jorizzo JL, Schaffer JV (Eds). Dermatology, 4th edition. Philadelphia: Elsevier; 2017. 1285-95.
6. Castells M, Austen KF. Mastocytosis: Mediator-related symptoms and treatment. Best Pract Res Clin Haematol. 2006;19(3):495-516.
7. Valent P, Escribano L, Broesby-Olsen S, Hartmann K, Grattan C, Brockow K, et al. Proposed diagnostic algorithm for patients with suspected mastocytosis: A proposal of the European Competence Network on Mastocytosis. Leukemia. 2014;28(7):1223-32.
8. Pardanani A. Systemic mastocytosis in adults: 2021 update on diagnosis, risk stratification and management. Am J Hematol. 2021;96(4):508-25.
9. Arock M, Sotlar K, Akin C, Broesby-Olsen S, Hoermann G, Escribano L, et al. KIT mutation analysis in mast cell neoplasms: Recommendations of the European Competence Network on Mastocytosis. Leukemia. 2015;29(6):1223-32.
10. Alvarez-Twose I, Gonzalez-de-Olano D, Sanchez-Munoz L, Jara-Acevedo M, Teodosio C, García-Montero A, et al. Validation and prognostic value of the REMA score for systemic mastocytosis. Blood. 2012;120(13):2629-39.
11. Gotlib J. Clinical practice. Mastocytosis. N Engl J Med. 2017;376(8):742-52.
12. Horny HP, Sotlar K, Valent P. Mastocytosis: state of the art. Pathobiology. 2021;88(2):66-82.
13. Carter MC, Robyn JA, Bressler PB, Metcalfe DD, Quezado Z. Pediatric mastocytosis: routine anesthetic management for a complex disease. Anesth Analg. 2008;107(2):422-7.
14. Akin C, Metcalfe DD. Systemic mastocytosis. Annu Rev Med. 2004;55:419-32.
15. Theoharides TC, Valent P, Akin C. Mast cells, mastocytosis, and related disorders. N Engl J Med. 2015;373(2):1885-6.
16. Valent P, Sperr WR, Sotlar K, Sabbagh AA, Nawaz Z, Akiki SJ, et al. Chronic myelomonocytic leukemia and mastocytosis: a clinicopathological study of a rare association. J Clin Pathol. 2005;58(10):1186-91.
17. Broesby-Olsen S, Fenger RV, Kristensen TK. Mastocytosis in children and adults: a review of current guidelines. Br J Haematol. 2015;169(4): 515-24.
18. Valent P, Sperr WR, Akin C, Horny H-P, Arock M, Lechner K, et al. Diagnosis and treatment of systemic mastocytosis: state of the art. Br J Haematol. 2003;122(5):695-717.
19. Horny HP, Sotlar K, Valent P. Mastocytosis: an update on classification and management. Acta Haematologica. 2021;144(4):324-9.
20. Arock M, Vaes M, Rhodes A, Valent P. Current treatment options in patients with mastocytosis: status in 2021 and future perspectives. Eur J Haematol. 2021;107(6):517-37.

CHAPTER 20

Skin Prick Test in Urticaria

Neeraj Gupta

INTRODUCTION

Urticaria, commonly known as hives, is a skin condition characterized by the sudden appearance of raised, red, and itchy welts on the skin. It can be triggered by various factors, including allergens, medications, infections, and stress. Diagnosing the underlying cause of urticaria is crucial for its effective management and treatment. A detailed history about symptomatology, antecedent events, atopy, and triggering and relieving factors is often sufficient to identify the cause. Acute urticaria is often precipitated by concurrent viral illnesses and is usually self-limiting which seldom demands any diagnostic workup. Long-term symptoms (lasting over 6 weeks) might be mediated by immediate hypersensitivity to some allergens like food, house dust mites, cockroaches, pollens, or molds. One of the diagnostic tools employed in identifying culprit allergens associated with urticaria is the skin prick test (SPT).

WHAT IS A SKIN PRICK TEST?

The SPT is a simple and reliable in vivo diagnostic procedure used to identify allergen sensitivities in individuals suspected of having allergic conditions, including urticaria. During the test, small amounts of suspected allergens are introduced into the skin through a prick or scratch. The skin's reaction to these allergens is then observed after a specific period, usually around 15 minutes.

PRINCIPLE

The SPT is based on immediate (type I) hypersensitivity reaction. The offending allergen, after coming in contact with atopic individuals, is recognized by T-helper 2 (Th2) cells, which in turn stimulate B cells followed by plasma cells to produce abundant amounts of immunoglobulin E (IgE) with subsequent release in systemic circulation. These free IgE molecules can be detected during different in vitro tests (total and specific IgE). Due to their high affinity, released

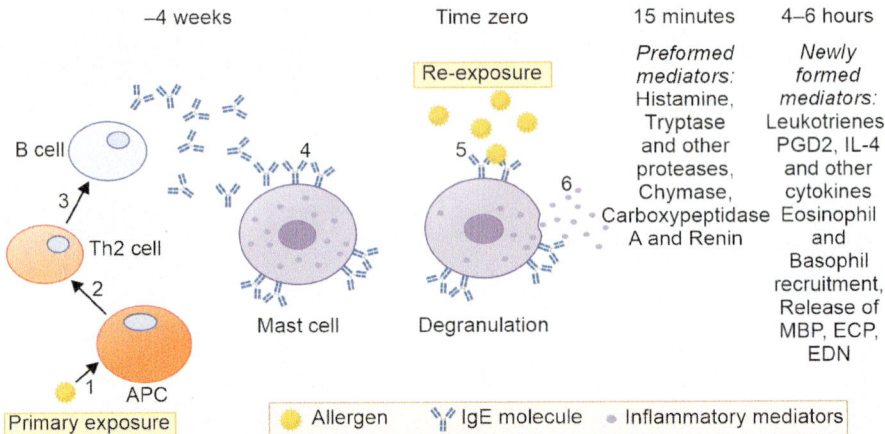

FIG. 1: Immediate hypersensitivity (type 1) reaction. **1**: Primary exposure of allergen; **2**: Allergen presentation to Th2 cells; **3**: Stimulation of B cells and production of IgE antibodies by plasma cells; **4**: Binding of IgE molecules to mast cells; **5**: Allergen binding to mast cell-bound IgE on re-exposure; **6**: Mast cell degranulation followed by mediator release.

[APC: antigen (allergen) presenting cell; ECP: eosinophil cationic protein; EDN: eosinophil-derived neurotoxin; PGD2: prostaglandin D2; IL: interleukin; MBP: eosinophil-derived granule major basic protein; Th2: T-helper].

IgE molecules immediately bind to the surface of mast cells and basophils with their Fc component. During the re-exposure (either during SPT or challenge/provocation tests), the same allergen gets attached to the Fab portion of two consecutive similar IgE molecules bound to mast cells. This triggers the bursting of mast cells with release of preformed mediators (like histamine and others) followed by appearance of wheal and flare reaction within 15 minutes post prick procedure. **Figure 1** demonstrates type 1 hypersensitivity reaction. The quantitative assessment of wheal is indicative of immediate hypersensitive reaction to the tested allergen.

PROCEDURE

1. *Preparation*:
   - *Patient*: Before conducting the SPT, the healthcare provider should gather detailed information about the patient's medical history, including their symptoms, potential triggers with possible temporal associations, and previous allergic reactions. It is essential to inform the patient and/or caregivers about the procedure and any associated risks beforehand. **Table 1** enumerates the drugs to be withheld before performing SPT.
   - *Personnel*: SPT should be performed by a qualified and experienced technician or physician in the allergist's office.
   - *Equipment and infrastructure*: Though SPT is a safe procedure and usually done as an outpatient or office procedure, it still carries a theoretical risk of a mild allergic reaction which is rarely severe enough to cause anaphylaxis. One has to be prepared and vigilant enough to deal with any unexpected

TABLE 1: Medications to be stopped before performing SPT.

Name (group) of medication	Duration of withholding
First-generation antihistamines (e.g., chlorpheniramine, diphenhydramine, hydroxyzine, and promethazine)	5 days
Second-generation antihistamines (e.g., cetirizine, desloratadine, bilastine, and fexofenadine)	7 days
H_2 blockers (e.g., ranitidine, cimetidine, and famotidine)	2 days
Short-term topical or systemic steroids (<1 week)	No need to stop
Long-term topical or systemic steroids (≥1 week)	21 days
Tricyclic (e.g., amitriptyline, imipramine, and nortriptyline) and atypical (e.g., bupropion, mirtazapine, and trazodone) antidepressants	14 days
Benzodiazepines (e.g., alprazolam, clonazepam, diazepam, lorazepam, and midazolam)	7 days
Beta-blockers (tablets and eye drop)	5 days
Antihistamine nasal spray (e.g., azelastine)	1 day
Antihistamine eye drops (e.g., azelastine and olopatadine)	1 day
Immunomodulators (e.g., omalizumab)	6 months

untoward reaction during the immediate postprocedure observation time. A written informed consent from the patient and/or caregivers is essential before performing the procedure. An emergency tray with all resuscitation supplies, oxygen, and prefilled adrenaline syringe should be ready beforehand. The room should be well illuminated with comfortable temperature. An arm chair with backrest is preferable in the testing room. An adjacent waiting room with adequate facilities for comfortable resting and allergy testing information material should be available. Regionally relevant standardized allergen extracts, prick lancets, cleaning solution, gauze pieces, skin markers, and measuring scales are essential for performing the procedure.

2. *Selection of allergens*: Based on the patient's history and suspected triggers, a panel of allergens is selected for testing. Common allergens tested for urticaria may include pollen, dust mites, pet danders, foods, mold, and latex. It is advisable to reduce the number of test allergens to a maximum of 6–8 to obtain meaningful results.

3. *Selection and preparation of test area*: The patient's forearm is preferred for testing; however, the test can be performed in the upper back area, especially in young uncooperative children. The selected area is cleaned with alcohol-based solution (70% Ethanol plus 2.5% Chlorhexidine) followed by saline in order to remove any residual effect and dried adequately. Any residual alcohol might denature the test allergen protein, thus resulting in a false-negative reaction. The test area is marked with a skin marker pen for respective allergen identification. The marks should be at least 5 cm away from wrist or elbow joints with a minimum distance of 2 cm in between.

4. *Application of allergens and SPT procedure*: A small drop of each allergen solution is placed on the designated mark. Using a sterile lancet, the skin is then pricked through the drop, ensuring that a small amount of the allergen enters the skin's surface. The aim should be to introduce 0.3 µL of allergen at a depth of 1 mm. Ideally, separate lancets should be used for each allergen prick. The SPT is an epicutaneous procedure as the allergen is deposited in the epidermis only. Later, the test solution gradually diffuses down to dermis as per its concentration gradient where it finds the mast cells (with bound IgE in case of a previously sensitized individual) in order to initiate type-1 hypersensitivity reaction. The SPT is a bloodless and painless technique if performed appropriately as the epidermis lacks any blood vessels or pain fibers. Histamine (positive control) and normal saline (negative control) are also instilled along with test allergens during the procedure. **Figure 2** depicts the SPT procedure.
5. *Observation*: The patient is instructed not to scratch the tested area during the observation period. After 10–15 minutes, the test sites are examined for any signs of allergic reactions, such as redness, swelling, or itching. Appearance of wheal within a predefined time period is considered as the end point of test (10 minutes for histamine and 15 minutes for other allergens and negative control). The size of the wheal diameter (raised area) is measured and recorded **(Fig. 3)**.

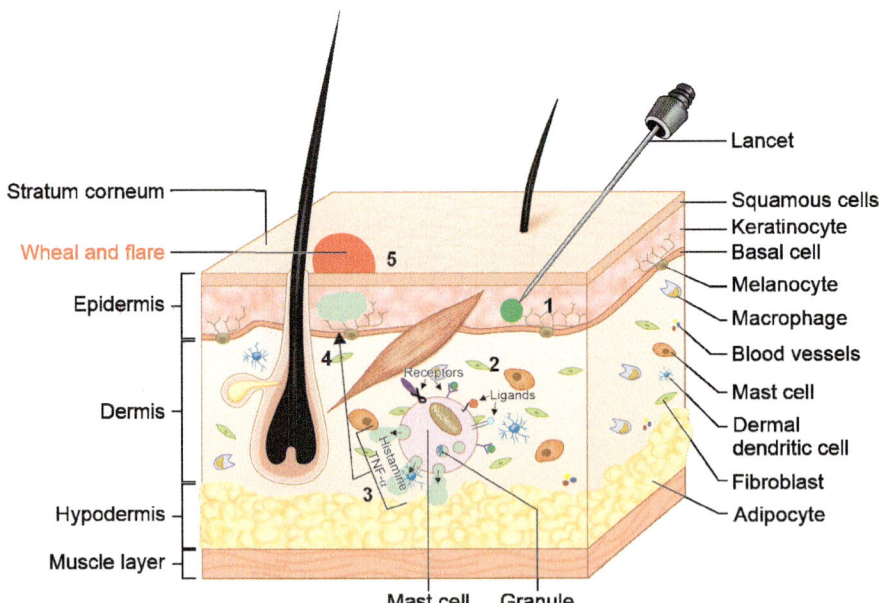

FIG. 2: Skin prick test (SPT) procedure. **1**: Epicutaneous delivery of allergen with lancet; **2**: Diffusion of allergen to dermis and binding to bound IgE on mast cells; **3**: Release of preformed mast cell mediators; **4**: Passive transfer of mediators to skin surface; **5**: Wheal and flare reaction within a specified time period.

CHAPTER 20: Skin Prick Test in Urticaria

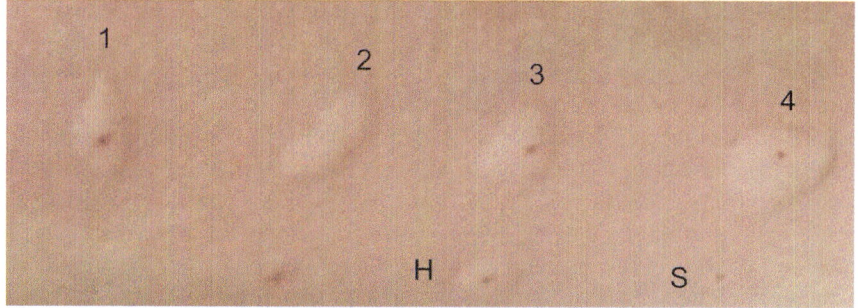

FIG. 3: Wheal and flare reaction during the skin prick test (SPT) procedure. H: Histamine (positive control); S: Normal saline (Negative control); **1, 2, 3,** and **4**: Test allergens.

TABLE 2: Interpretation of SPT.		
Controls	Test allergen	Interpretation
Negative—normal saline Positive—histamine		
Normal saline from 0 to 3 mm and histamine at least 3 mm or more than negative control	Irrespective	Test is valid
Normal saline > 3 mm or histamine < 3 mm than negative control	Irrespective	Test is invalid
Valid controls	Test allergen at least 3 mm or more than negative control (irrespective of histamine wheal size)	Tested allergen is positive
(mm: millimeter)		

6. *Interpretation*: The results are interpreted based on the size and appearance of the wheals. A positive reaction indicates that the patient is sensitized to the specific allergen tested **(Table 2)**. Allergy testing is only a marker of hypersensitivity and needs to be clinically correlated before labeling it as true allergy.

ROLE OF SKIN PRICK TEST IN URTICARIA

While urticaria is often nonallergic in nature, allergic triggers can still play a significant role in some cases. Skin prick testing plays a valuable role in the diagnosis and management of urticaria by identifying potential allergens that may trigger or exacerbate the condition in select cohort. The benefits of performing SPT in urticaria patients are as follows:
- *Targeted avoidance measures*: By pinpointing specific allergens that elicit a positive reaction, SPT helps healthcare providers in identifying potential triggers for urticaria episodes. This information enables patients to implement targeted avoidance strategies to minimize exposure to allergens.

- *Differentiation from nonallergic causes*: In cases where urticaria is suspected to be allergic in origin, SPT can help differentiate allergic urticaria from nonallergic forms. This information is crucial to stop any unnecessary avoidance of food by the patients.
- *Guiding treatment decisions*: Knowledge of allergens identified through SPT can guide treatment decisions, such as allergen immunotherapy (AIT) or targeted pharmacotherapy. For example, if a specific food allergen, insect, or mold is identified as a trigger, dietary modifications can be recommended. AIT is a process of immunological desensitization to the offending agent. This can be achieved by administration of gradually escalating doses of responsible allergen. AIT is commonly recommended using either subcutaneous injectable or sublingual liquid drops or tablets. The sublingual route has a better safety profile than the subcutaneous one at the cost of slightly compromised efficacy. Newer routes like oral or intralymphatic immunotherapy are under investigation and need more data before recommendation. AIT usually works best in conditions of rhinitis followed asthma. AIT can be offered in patients with urticaria due to pollen or dust mite with equivocal results.
- *Monitoring response to treatment*: SPT can also be used to monitor the effectiveness of allergen avoidance measures or immunotherapy over time. Changes in skin reactivity to allergens may indicate a response to treatment or the need for adjustments in management strategies.

FEASIBILITY OF SKIN PRICK TEST IN URTICARIA

Despite the potential benefits of this diagnostic modality in selected patients with urticaria, there can be feasibility limitations for the procedure.
- Unable to stop antihistamines due to chronic unremitting symptoms
- *Soon after anaphylaxis*: Need to wait for at least 4 weeks after a severe type-I hypersensitivity reaction in order to provide enough time for mast cell mediator regeneration
- *Extremes of age*: Though there are no age-specific absolute contraindications for performing SPT, it is still usually avoided in infants < 6 months or adults >65 years of age
- Patients with other comorbid conditions and unable to stop immunomodulators, steroids, or other medications (e.g., beta blockers)
- Uncooperative patients
- Unhealthy skin conditions
- Nonavailability of experts to perform and interpret the procedure correctly

COMPARISON OF SKIN PRICK TEST WITH SPECIFIC IgE TESTS IN URTICARIA

The SPT is considered as the gold standard test for demonstrating immediate hypersensitivity to a suspected allergen. It detects bound IgE and has high specificity when compared to specific IgE (in vitro) estimation. In vitro allergy diagnostic tests are based on detection of free IgE and have good sensitivity while compared to SPT. Though SPT should be preferred for allergy testing in a given patient, specific IgE can provide useful information in clinical conditions where SPT is not feasible.

CONCLUSION

The SPT is a valuable tool in the diagnostic workup of urticaria, helping to identify allergic triggers and guide treatment decisions. By accurately identifying allergens associated with urticaria, healthcare providers can tailor management strategies to effectively control symptoms and improve the quality of life for patients with this challenging condition. However, it is essential to interpret SPT results in the context of the patient's clinical history and other diagnostic findings to ensure accurate diagnosis and management.

KEY POINTS

- Diagnosis of urticaria is often historical and seldom requires a detailed investigational workup.
- Once performed and interpreted by qualified personnel, the SPT is a reliable test for demonstration of immediate hypersensitivity in a selected cohort of patients with urticaria.
- SPT results need clinical correlation before labeling it as evidence of allergy.
- SPT can guide the preventive and therapeutic pathways in order to provide precision medicine to the indigent.

SUGGESTED READINGS

1. Gupta N, Agarwal P, Sachdev A, Gupta D. Allergy Testing: An Overview. Indian Pediatr. 2019;56(11):951-7.
2. Koirala S, Paudel U, Pokhrel DB, Parajuli S. Skin Prick Test Positivity in Chronic Urticaria. J Nepal Health Res Counc. 2021;18(4):615-8.
3. Lote S, Gupta SB, Poulose D, Deora MS, Mahajan A, Gogineni JM, et al. Role of the Skin Prick Test in Urticaria Patients. Cureus. 2022;14(2):e21818.
4. Heinzerling L, Mari A, Bergmann KC, Bresciani M, Burbach G, Darsow U, et al. The skin prick test: European standards. Clin Transl Allergy. 2013;3(1):3.
5. Bains P, Dogra A. Skin prick test in patients with chronic allergic skin disorders. Indian J Dermatol. 2015;60(2):159-64.

CHAPTER 21

Patch Test in Urticaria

Sanjeev Gupta, Aditi Dabhra, Saurabh Swaroop Gupta

INTRODUCTION

Urticaria is a chronic skin condition characterized by pruritic raised areas known as wheals. While the cause in most cases remains unknown, certain substances like food, drugs, mechanical stimuli, temperature, latex, UV light, or even water might act as triggers. When the condition of urticaria continues for a duration of >6 weeks, it is classified as "chronic." Furthermore, in the absence of a discernible etiology, it is classified as "idiopathic." Chronic spontaneous urticaria (CSU), often referred to as chronic idiopathic urticaria, accounts for 66–93% of all instances of chronic urticaria (CU). CSU can significantly diminish a patient's quality of life and have a detrimental impact on the burden of healthcare costs.

The underlying cause of CSU is mostly associated with the degranulation of mast cell, which can be initiated by either immunological or nonimmune reactions. Immunological reactions, such as the production of IgE antibodies (known as an "allergic response"), the formation of immunological complexes, and the presence of autoimmune antibodies, bind to the mast cell receptors. Mast cell in response releases granules that contain histamine, leukotrienes, and other substances that lead to the development of wheals and the accompanying itching sensation.

> Unlike CSU, the pathomechanism of the allergic contact dermatitis (ACD) primarily involves T-cell responses mediated by antigen presentation cells (APCs). In addition to a distinct mechanism, the clinical presentation also varies, typically appearing as an erythematous plaque with well-defined boundaries that correspond to the area of contact. Occasionally, there may be scales, crusts, or fluid-filled vesicles. The patch test is widely regarded as the most reliable method for diagnosing delayed-type and cell-mediated reactions to exogenous substances and can also be employed to assess both immediate and delayed drug reactions.

Recent research has demonstrated the interconnection between mast cells and IgE in the formation of contact dermatitis (CD), and the involvement of APCs and CD4 T helper cells in the pathogenesis of CSU.

HISTORY OF PATCH TEST (TABLE 1)

- In 1847, Stadeler for the first time described Stadeler's blotting paper strip technique by which he reproduced onto the human skin the lesion caused by *Anacardium occidentale*. In this technique, balsam was applied over a 1 cm^2 area on the lower thorax and then this area was covered by blotting paper dipped in balsam and kept in place for 3 hours. The person experienced burning sensation with a red halo on the skin.
- A major advance in this field was made in the year 1895 by Jadassohn, known as the father of patch test, who established its role in dermatitis' medicamentosa. He applied certain chemicals onto the skin using blotting paper. He was able to reproduce CD-like picture in patients who were intolerant to substances like iodoform mercury salts. This is regarded as the first patch test.
- Bloch in Basel, in 1911, gave a detailed description of the procedure of patch testing in which the allergen is applied to the patient's back using a linen strip, covered with a large-sized piece of gutta percha and zine oxide adhesive plaster for its fixation and the strip left in place for 24 hours. Subsequently, the technique of patch testing has been used and modified extensively.

HISTORY OF PATCH TEST IN URTICARIA (TABLE 1)

- Initial research was carried out in the 1980s to determine the potential involvement of patch testing in the assessment of CU.
- In 2007, Guerra et al. also discussed the involvement of contact sensitization in CU, suggesting that it may contribute to the onset of urticaria. A study revealed that 41% of patients diagnosed with CSU exhibited positive results for contact allergens. Furthermore, complete healing was achieved by the use of contact avoidance strategies. Previous research has documented similar investigations with conflicting findings. Furthermore, certain investigations utilized the patch test approach using prevalent aeroallergen and food allergens rather than the typical contact allergens. For instance, it has been hypothesized that allergens from home dust mites might enter the outermost

Year	Event description
1847	Stadeler described the blotting paper strip technique for reproducing skin lesions caused by anacardium occidentale
1895	Jadassohn conducted the first patch test, establishing its role in diagnosing dermatitis medicamentosa
1911	Bloch provided a detailed description of patch testing, including allergen application and fixation methods
1980	Initial research on the involvement of patch testing in chronic urticaria assessment was carried out
2007	Guerra et al. discussed contact sensitization's role in chronic urticaria, suggesting that it contributes to onset

TABLE 1: Timeline of events in the history of patch test and its role in urticaria.

layer of the skin, known as the stratum corneum, and trigger the activation of Langerhans cells and mast cells.

PRINCIPLE OF PATCH TEST

- The rationale behind patch testing is that activated and antigen-specific T lymphocytes are present throughout the body, allowing for the application of patch test allergens onto unaffected skin, the most common site being the upper area of back, as the patch test strips are unlikely to be disturbed at this site. When the allergen is administered to an unaffected part of the skin, it elicits a distinct dermatitis reaction.
- The test serves as a miniature version of the disease being studied.
- The patch test is based on the absorption of a sufficient quantity of the allergen to induce a consistent inflammatory response.
- A positive patch test confirms the presence of allergic contact sensitivity in an individual, as long as it is performed correctly.
- Patch test reactions, when accurately interpreted, can provide as valid scientific evidence for identifying the source of dermatitis.
- Although these tests are not flawless bioassays, they are quite important for accurate diagnosis. The primary benefits of this method include the capacity to choose the specific location for application, the ability to limit it to a small area, and the use of a very low concentration of the test chemical.

PATCH TEST UNITS

- The initial patches were made of pieces of cotton soaked in allergen solutions.
- In 1972, Fregert introduced the Al test which consists of an elongated sheet of aluminum foil covered with a thin layer of polythene and having a central disc of filter paper of 10 mm diameter fixed to it. The antigens were required to be soaked into the paper discs and these strips were then to be strapped onto the patient's back with adhesive tape.
- Currently, the most prevalent method for applying allergens is the Finn chamber system, which was invented by Pirila in 1975. The object is composed of aluminum and possesses a diameter of 8 mm and a depth of 0.5 mm. Multiple patches can be applied simultaneously, and the response sites are smaller compared to the Al test method.
- In 1986, Kaur and Sharma utilized an indigenous version of the Finn chamber in India. The core sections of the metallic caps on the penicillin injectable vials were utilized.

TAPES

The contemporary adhesive tapes possess sufficient adhesion and maintain the patches in close proximity to the skin's surface. The tape utilized for fixing should ideally be nonallergenic, nonocclusive, and nonirritant. While using occlusive chambers like the Finn chamber, porous tapes, e.g., Micropore, Scanpor, and Norges plaster, may be used.

VEHICLES

The often-utilized vehicle is white petrolatum because of its replenishing properties and a minimal possibility for causing sensitization. Softisan, a hydrophilic substitute for lanolin, and plastibase have been proposed as alternate options.

ALLERGENS

- Currently, there are over 300 chemicals that may be purchased and used as allergens for patch testing. Additional series can be added to the conventional series of common allergens to specifically target individuals in certain groups, such as hairdressers, housewives, gardeners, dental technicians, and printers.
- While any chemical present in the environment has the potential to trigger CD as an allergen, it is advisable to utilize the standard series for conducting patch testing.
- By utilizing standardized series, it is feasible to identify around 70–80% of contact sensitivities.
- The concentration of the allergen, the solvent used for dilution, and the quantity applied have an impact on the outcomes of the patch testing. An optimal concentration of an allergen will elicit a mild response in an individual who has developed sensitivity to it while producing no response in an individual who has not developed sensitivity. The appropriate concentrations for patch testing have been determined for all common allergies.
- It is essential to utilize the precise quantity of the test material for each patch test. Excessive quantities should be avoided since they can contaminate the adjacent area and potentially extend beyond it.

TEST PROCEDURE

- During the test technique, small amounts of suspected antigens are placed to a specific area of healthy skin, typically the upper back, and covered with a fixing tape.
- The samples are left undisturbed for a period of 48 hours. After this time, they are removed and it is recommended to take the reading 1 hour after their removal.
- Antibiotics such as neomycin and corticosteroids might cause delayed reactions. Therefore, a second reading may be necessary at 72 or 96 hours to check for such reactions.

READING AND EVALUATION OF PATCH TEST RESULTS

- The patch test should be left on for a minimum of 1 day, with the majority of the work involving allergens already completed in the area for 2 days. This is now regarded the usual technique.

	TABLE 2: ICDRG grading for patch test result.
–	Negative
?/+	Doubtful reaction, faint erythema only
+	Weakly (nonvesicular) positive reaction. Erythema, infiltration, and possibly papules
++	Strong (vesicular) positive reactions. Erythema, infiltration, papules, and vesicles
+++	Extreme positive reactions. Intense erythema, infiltration, and coalescing vesicles. Bullous reaction
IR	Irritant reaction
NT	Not tested

- Well-known allergens are often evaluated at concentrations that, when exposed to a sensitized individual for 48 hours beneath a sealed patch, allow enough of the allergen to penetrate and trigger a reaction.
- The optimal schedule involves applying the regimen for a duration of 48 hours and then measuring the results 1 hour following its removal. This interval is implemented to allow the erythema, which is generated by the stripping action of tape after its removal, to subside.
- Certain allergens, such as neomycin and corticosteroids, may exhibit delayed positive reactions. Therefore, it is recommended to do a second reading on day 4 and day 7 to ensure accurate results. This also enables the distinction between genuine allergic and irritating reactions, as a positive allergic reaction will last for a few days, while the irritant reaction tends to subside.

The readings should be taken and graded according to the International Contact Dermatitis Research Group (ICDRG) scoring system **(Table 2)** which is as follows:

SOURCES OF ERROR

False-positive reactions can be seen due to:
- Excessive concentration/amount of allergen
- Uneven dispersion
- Contaminants
- Irritant vehicle
- Adhesive tape reactions
- Pressure effect of hard materials
- Current dermatitis at the patch-test site or distant site
- "Angry back" reaction
- Artifact

Angry back reaction: This phenomenon is a significant factor that leads to inaccurate positive responses. It is alternatively referred to as the "excited skin syndrome" or "status eczematicus." This phenomenon is known as hyper-reactivity of the skin at the site of the patch test due to the presence of active eczema. This condition makes the skin more sensitive and leads to false-positive reactions to allergens and greater sensitivity to irritants.

PROTOCOL TO EVALUATE CONTACT URTICARIA

According to the Von Krogh and Maibach study, it is important to observe both immediate and delayed responses when assessing a suspected case of contact urticaria. The recommendation is to remove a closed patch on the ventral forearm after 15–20 minutes to test for an immediate reaction. Simultaneously, delayed-type hypersensitivity testing should be performed on the back, and the results should be read after 48–96 hours. The suggestion of using this dual-testing procedure stems from the fact that delayed-type hypersensitivity might occur simultaneously in people with contact urticaria. The suggestion was made to adopt the term "contact dermatitis of immediate and delayed type" to describe patients who display these mixed reactions during patch test circumstances **(Flowchart 1)**.

If a positive response is detected at any stage, further assessment of the positive individual should be discontinued. Epinephrine and resuscitation tools should be easily accessible when doing tests for contact urticaria.

OTHER TYPES OF PATCH TEST

- *Open test*: During these tests, a liquid test substance is placed to a skin region with a diameter of approximately 1 cm and left to dry. These reactions may occur earlier and are less intense compared to a closed patch test reaction.

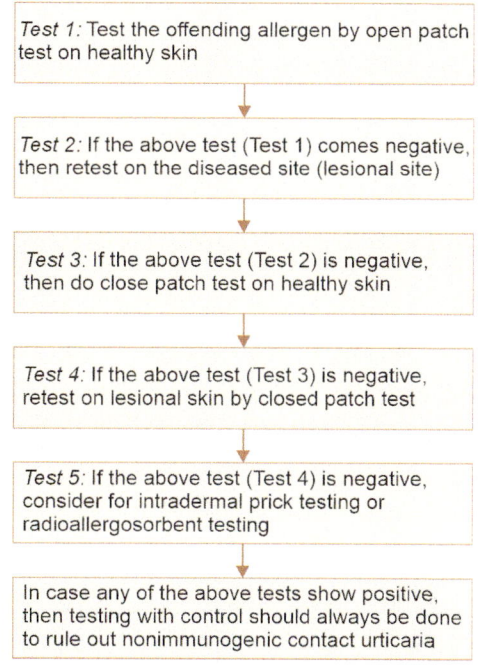

FLOWCHART 1: Protocol to detect contact urticaria.

Therefore, an open test is more appropriate as a fundamental screening test for less familiar allergens.

If there is uncertainty, and the historical evidence points toward CD but both open and closed tests yield negative results, it is advisable to repeat the test. This is especially beneficial in the treatment of dermatitis related to cosmetics and clothing.

- *Photopatch test*: This particular patch test is most appropriate for patients who have a history of eczema on areas of the skin that are exposed to light and where the condition tends to aggravate upon exposure to sunlight. This testing method primarily involves patch testing, followed by irradiation of the test area to induce the production of a photoantigen. The antigens are administered simultaneously. After a duration of 24 hours, the patches are taken off and the test location is exposed to UVA light with an intensity of 10–15 J/cm^2. Subsequently, the patches are substituted, and the ultimate measurement is obtained 48 hours following exposure to radiation. Substances that can cause photocontact dermatitis include scents, sunscreens, antibacterial agents, colors, medications such as sulfonamides, phenothiazines, psoralens, and thiazides, as well as coal tar derivatives.
- *Semiopen test*: It can be used when testing certain emulsifiers, solvents, or other irritant substances.
- *Repeat open application test (ROAT)*: This test is beneficial for cases where there is uncertainty over a positive patch test result caused by preparations containing a low concentration of the allergen in question. During this experiment, chemicals are administered twice daily for a duration of 7 days. The upper arm or the flexor surface of the forearm is the most frequently encountered location for the test. A minimum surface area of 5 cm^2 should be used.

STUDIES (TABLE 3)

- A study was done by Boonk et al. in 1981 on 164 patients with chronic recurrent urticaria to examine the effectiveness of skin tests. Patch tests were performed using the standard series of the International Contact Dermatitis Research Group and a series of penicillins. The results showed positive reactions in 22% patients (35 out of 162) for the standard series and in 6.9% patients (11 out of 158) for the penicillin series. A total of 21.5% (33 out of 152) positive intracutaneous tests were found for cilligen (a penicilloyl polylysine product from Sigma Chemical Company that is used to screen for penicillin allergies) and/or penicillin G. 35% (51 out of 147) of the patients exhibited positive intracutaneous testing with inhalants. The scratch tests conducted with food allergens yielded positive reactions in 12.5% of the participants (12 out of 95). There was no discernible disparity in outcomes between individuals diagnosed with idiopathic urticaria or angioedema and those diagnosed with physical urticaria. The significance of these observations is being analyzed. The majority of individuals with a penicillin allergy were

TABLE 3: Key studies and findings related to patch testing in chronic urticaria.

Year	Author	Result
1981	WJ Boonk et al.	Studied 164 chronic recurrent urticaria patients with patch tests; found positive reactions in 22 patients (13.4%) for standard allergens and in 11 patients (6.9%) for penicillin series. Dietary exclusion of milk and products had a 50% success rate
1982	RP Warin et al.	Conducted patch and challenge tests on 56 chronic urticaria patients; positive reactions observed for balsam of Peru, cinnamon, cloves, and nickel
2007	Laura Guerra et al.	Investigated contact allergy in chronic urticaria; 41% (50/121) had positive patch tests for contact allergens; all showed remission within 1 month after avoidance
2008	Ashima Deb Sharma	Evaluated patch testing for diagnosing CU using Indian standard battery; 11 out of 57 patients had positive reactions; allergen avoidance led to complete resolution in 9 patients within 2–3 weeks
2011	Eli Magen et al.	Retrospective study on severe CIU patients; patch tests revealed sensitization to nickel sulfate (9.3%), potassium dichromate (4.7%), and others; significant improvement in CUSS after allergen avoidance
2016	Hao Chen et al.	Studied allergic contact sensitization in central Chinese CU patients; 42.9% sensitization rate; allergen avoidance significantly improved CU severity over 4 weeks
2020	Deniz Ozceker et al.	Investigated food additive sensitization in children with CSU using APT; 14.1% showed sensitization, none in controls; suggested APT tests could help identify dietary triggers

(APT: atopy patch test; CSU: chronic spontaneous urticaria; CU: chronic urticaria)

advised to follow a diet that excludes milk and milk products. This endeavor achieved a success rate of 50%.
- In a study done by Warin et al. in 1982, a total of 56 patients diagnosed with CU underwent patch testing, specifically focusing on the initial wheal reaction to several materials. Subsequently, challenge tests were conducted using most of the same chemicals. Positive initial patch tests were frequently observed in those exposed to balsam of Peru and cinnamon, indicating a reaction that is commonly experienced in a large number of normal patients. Two patients who had positive instant patch tests to cinnamon and two patients who had positive quick patch tests to cloves also had positive challenge tests to the same substances. If other substances with a comparable effect are discovered, the use of immediate patch tests in evaluating CU is more likely to be beneficial. Out of the four patients, all of them exhibited positive results in immediate patch testing for nickel. Additionally, one of these patients also tested positive for nickel in a patch test conducted after 48 hours. Two further patients exhibited exclusively positive 48-hour patch testing for nickel. Nevertheless, none of these patients exhibited a favorable response during the nickel challenge test.

- In 2007, Guerra et al. conducted an experiment to investigate the notion that contact allergy contributes to CU. As part of the diagnostic process, they used the Italian series of patch tests. Out of the 121 individuals diagnosed with CU, 50 of them, which accounts for 41% of the total, had positive results for contact allergens. All patients achieved complete remission within 1 month as a result of implementing avoidance measures. Testing for contact sensitization can be beneficial in managing CU.
- In 2016, Chen et al. investigated the incidence and distribution of allergic contact sensitization in CU patients in central China and assessed the effectiveness of allergen avoidance in managing CU. Patch tests with 20 allergens were conducted on subjects, revealing a 42.9% sensitization rate. Men commonly reacted to potassium dichromate, benzene mix, and carba mix, while women frequently reacted to nickel sulfate. Sensitization rates varied by age and occupation. The study found that allergen avoidance significantly improved CU severity over 4 weeks, with severity scores dropping from 20 to 12 in the avoidance group compared to 15 to 14 in the control group. These findings suggest that contact allergens contribute to CU's pathogenesis and that allergen avoidance is beneficial in its management.
- In 2011, Magen et al. retrospectively examined severe CIU patients to determine the frequency of sensitization to patch test allergens and the impact of allergen avoidance on CIU remission. Forty-three subjects were patch tested using TRUE (thin-layer rapid-use epicutaneous) test, revealing sensitization to nickel sulfate (9.3%), potassium dichromate (4.7%), and several other allergens in smaller percentages. Patients with positive patch test results showed significant improvement in Chronic Urticaria Severity Score (CUSS) after 1 month of allergen avoidance.
- In a study done in 2020 by Ozceker et al., they investigated the prevalence of sensitization to food additives in children with CSU using atopy patch tests (APT). APTs were conducted on 120 children with CSU and 61 healthy controls, testing for 23 different food additives. Results showed that 14.1% of children with CSU were sensitized to food additives, while none of the controls had positive APT results. Azorubine and Cochineal red were the most common allergens, with sensitization rates of 5.8% and 6.7%, respectively. The study concludes that there may be an association between food additives and CSU, suggesting that APT tests could be useful in identifying dietary triggers and managing CSU more effectively.
- In 2008, Deb Sharma conducted a study and aimed to evaluate the role of patch testing in diagnosing the etiology of CU using the Indian standard battery of allergens approved by the Contact and Occupational Dermatitis Forum of India (CODFI). Fifty-seven CU patients underwent patch testing, and those with positive reactions were advised to avoid the identified allergens and restrict related allergens in their diet for 6 weeks. Results showed that 11 patients had positive reactions; of these, 9 experienced complete resolution of CU symptoms within 2–3 weeks of avoidance, and this improvement persisted for 6 weeks. The remaining two patients showed partial recovery. The study concludes that patch testing is a safe, simple, and cost-effective method for diagnosing the causes of CU before considering more expensive investigations.

CONCLUSION

- Patch testing plays a crucial role in identifying triggers in urticaria, particularly when contact allergens contribute to symptoms specially in contact urticaria.
- By pinpointing specific allergens, such as metals, preservatives, or fragrances, patch tests enable antigen specific avoidance strategies that can significantly improve patient outcomes.
- This diagnostic tool is especially valuable in cases of contact urticaria or when urticaria is linked to delayed hypersensitivity reactions, providing personalized insights for effective management.

SUGGESTED READINGS

1. Von Krogh G, Maibach HI. The contact urticaria syndrome-an updated review. J Am Acad Dermatol. 1981;5:328-42.
2. Boonk WJ, van Ketel WG. Skin testing in chronic urticaria. Dermatologica. 1981;163(2):151-9.
3. Warin RP, Smith RJ. Chronic urticaria Investigations with patch and challenge tests. Contact Dermatitis. 1982;8(2):117-21.
4. Guerra L, Rogkakou A, Massacane P, Gamalero C, Compalati E, Zanella C, et al. Role of contact sensitization in chronic urticaria. J Am Acad Dermatol. 2007;56(1):88-90.
5. Chen H, Liu G, Huang N, Li W, Dong X, Zhu R. Incidence of allergic contact sensitization in central Chinese subjects with chronic urticaria. An Bras Dermatol. 2016;91(2):168-72.
6. Magen E, Mishal J, Menachem S. Impact of contact sensitization in chronic spontaneous urticaria. Am J Med Sci. 2011;341(3):202-6.
7. Ozceker D, Dilek F, Yucel E, et al. Can allergy patch tests with food additives help to diagnose the cause in childhood chronic spontaneous urticaria? Postepy Dermatol Alergol. 2020;37(3):384-9.
8. Sharma AD. Use of patch testing for identifying allergen causing chronic urticaria. Indian J Dermatol Venereol Leprol. 2008;74:114-7.

CHAPTER 22

Oral Challenge Test

Payal Chauhan, Ria Sharma

INTRODUCTION

The term "urticaria" is more commonly used to describe a condition characterized by transient itchy weals, angioedema, or both. Urticaria can be either spontaneous or inducible.

Urticaria is often a result of an allergic reaction, where histamine and other mediators are released into the skin. While antihistamines and other medications are the mainstay of treatment, desensitization and oral challenge tests are an emerging approach aimed at reducing the severity of reactions over time. This chapter delves into the fundamental principles and practical applications of desensitization, a therapeutic technique designed to increase a patient's tolerance to allergens through gradual and controlled exposure.

Here we discuss about the desensitization procedures that had been tried in the following inducible urticaria:
- *Drug-induced urticaria*: Primarily caused by aspirin or nonsteroidal anti-inflammatory drugs (NSAIDs), antineoplastic, antibiotics, and antitubercular drugs
- *Cholinergic urticaria*: With pronounced hypersensitivity to a patient's own sweat

In addition to desensitization, this chapter explores oral challenge tests, which play a pivotal role in the accurate diagnosis and confirmation of specific allergens responsible for triggering urticarial reactions. These tests involve the controlled administration of potential allergens to observe and assess the body's response, providing valuable insights into the precise causes of urticaria.

MECHANISM OF URTICARIA

Understanding a brief overview of mechanisms underlying urticaria is crucial for comprehending how desensitization might work. When cutaneous mast cells are activated, they release a variety of mediators, with histamine being the most prominent, which leads to increased permeability of blood vessels, leading to the development of urticaria. The clinical effectiveness of antihistamines in treating urticaria supports this theory. Mast cells can be triggered through both allergic and nonallergic pathways. The allergic pathway gets activated when two adjacent subunits of high-affinity immunoglobulin E (IgE) receptors are cross-linked. This process releases preformed histamine, interleukin-4 (IL-4), proteases, prostaglandin D2, IL-8, leukotriene 4, and tumor necrosis factor (TNF-alpha). Nonallergic activation can be triggered by various substances, including neuropeptides (like substance P), radiocontrast media, drugs (such as morphine, vancomycin, and codeine), and certain foods such as strawberries.

MECHANISM OF DESENSITIZATION

The aim of desensitization is to change the antibody response from being primarily IgE-mediated to being primarily IgG-mediated, which can bind to allergens and prevent the activation pathways mediated by IgE. This involves administering gradually increasing doses of the allergen, starting with very small amounts. Over time, this regimen redirects the immune response from being driven by TH2 cells, which promote IgE production, to being driven by TH1 cells, which suppress production of IgE. Recent findings also indicate that at the site of allergic reaction, desensitization is associated with a decrease in the number of inflammatory cells seen during the late phase, further alleviating symptoms.

TYPES OF URTICARIAS IN WHICH DESENSITIZATION HAS BEEN TRIED

Drug-induced Urticaria

Numerous drugs can trigger urticaria via allergic or nonallergic pathways. Allergic urticaria is a type I hypersensitivity reaction mediated by IgE antibodies, presenting as a skin condition. Conversely, certain drugs can cause urticarial lesions through nonimmunological mechanisms without prior sensitization, as they directly induce mast cell mediator release. These drugs include opiates, codeine, amphetamine, polymyxin B, atropine, muscle relaxants, hydralazine, pentamidine, quinine, and radiocontrast media. Whether the reaction is mediated by IgE or not, mast cells are crucial effector cells in the most immediate drug reactions; therefore, the desensitization process works by inhibiting mast cell degranulation and cytokine production.

Drug desensitization was developed to safely reintroduce essential medicines to individuals who have experienced hypersensitivity reactions (both IgE- and non-IgE-mediated). Since drug desensitization can induce brief tolerance to the offending medication and given that certain medications (such as biologic agents and chemotherapy) are administered at extended intervals, each subsequent dose must be preceded by a desensitization procedure to maintain tolerance.

Drug Desensitization Protocols

There are two primary desensitization protocols currently in use: "Rapid drug desensitization (RDD)" and "slow drug desensitization (SDD)." RDD is typically used for acute reactions, which generally involve doubling the dose every 15 minutes until reaching the therapeutic level. On the other hand, SDD is used for delayed type of hypersensitivity reactions involving T cells and can be administered either through oral administration or intravenously. However, there is no established consensus on the particular protocols for SDD, such as the starting dose, the increments between doses, or the intervals between dosing steps. More research and clinical experience are necessary to determine the efficacy and appropriate protocols for desensitization in delayed reactions.

Rapid Drug Desensitization

Rapid drug desensitization induces mast cell tolerance to an antigen by internalizing FcεRI. This can occur via gradual crosslinking at low antigen levels, the reduction of activating signal transduction elements like Syk kinase, and subthreshold mediator depletion. These mechanisms are believed to play a role in cellular insensitivity to particular activating doses of the allergen. Following desensitization, the expression of Syk protein—a tyrosine protein kinase crucial for transmitting activation signals in mast cells and basophils—is diminished. This decrease hinders FcεRI activation by preventing IgE binding to the sensitized drug. Furthermore, the involvement of T cells has become significant. It has been proposed that desensitization might reduce immunological memory, as evidenced by the decreased severity of "drug hypersensitivity reactions (DHR)" and the reduced incidence of "breakthrough reactions (BTRs)" throughout the desensitization procedure. Currently, desensitization is used for DHR to a variety of medications, including antibiotics, aspirin/NSAIDs, antineoplastic agents, and antitubercular drugs.

- *Aspirin- or NSAID-induced cutaneous reactions protocols*: Silberman and his associates successfully implemented the given protocol to quickly desensitize patients who were hypersensitive to aspirin. They began with a dose of 1 mg, doubling it every 30 minutes until reaching a final dose of 100 mg, with the entire procedure lasting 3.5 hours. Another approach used five sequential doses (5, 10, 20, 40, and 75 mg), completing the procedure in 2.5 hours. None of the patients received pretreatment with antihistamines or corticosteroids, and β-blockers were discontinued 24 hours before desensitization.

  Schaefer and Gore have successfully implemented a protocol which lasted for 3 days with at least 3 hours between each dose increase. On day 1, only a placebo was given; on day 2, aspirin doses were increased to 30, 60, and 120 mg; and on day 3, aspirin doses were increased to 150, 325, and 650 mg.

  Wong and his associates conducted challenge-desensitization trials on 11 patients, with 10 patients receiving pretreatment with antihistamines. One patient, due to a fragile clinical condition, received 60 mg of prednisolone the evening prior and the morning of desensitization. Dosing was individualized and administered at 10–30-minute intervals with the following increasing doses: "0.1, 0.3, 1, 3, 10, 30, 40, 81, 162, and 325 mg" though the necessity of the last two doses could be determined based on the required therapeutic dosage. Water-based dilutions were prepared using dispersible aspirin tablets for oral administration.

Antineoplastic Drug-induced Cutaneous Reaction Protocols

Antineoplastic agents are frequently administered at consistent intervals, raising the likelihood of sensitization to these medications. Common culprits include taxanes (such as docetaxel and paclitaxel), monoclonal antibodies (such as infliximab, rituximab, bevacizumab, and trastuzumab), and platinum compounds (such as oxaliplatin, cisplatin, and carboplatin).

A protocol developed by the "Adverse Drug Reaction and Desensitization Program at Brigham and Women's Hospital" has gained global recognition. In this protocol, "the solution of the offending drug (1:1) is diluted to 1:10, 1:100, and occasionally 1:1000, with the concentration and infusion rate gradually increased over 15 minutes." This multibag approach is successfully completed by the majority of patients without encountering serious BTRs. Protocols involving multiple bags necessitate extensive effort and time for bag changes and dilution, thereby increasing the risk of medical staff's exposure to antineoplastic agents. Furthermore, prolonged dilution and administration may compromise the stability of the drug. To address these challenges, a protocol involving one bag was introduced, employing a uniform concentration while adjusting the administration rate. The one-bag protocol commenced at a rate of 0.1 mL/h utilizing a syringe pump with high precision without any dilution, with the dosage doubling every 15 minutes. To ensure the precise delivery of minute solution volumes in this protocol, 5% dextrose water was infused at a constant rate of 10 mL/h through a side stream throughout the entire desensitization procedure. Both protocols included the administration of premedications, comprising H2-receptor antagonist (famotidine 20 mg), montelukast (10 mg), and H1-receptor antagonist (fexofenadine 180 mg).

Antibiotics: Beta-lactam antibiotics encompass penicillins (PCNs), cephalosporins, carbapenems, and monobactams. Avoiding this extensive group of antibiotics is challenging when patients need these medications for infections. Desensitizing patients to antimicrobials is considered a last-ditch effort when no other treatments are available, requiring the anticipated benefits to outweigh the associated risks of drug exposure. Despite its potential adverse effects, PCN remains the preferred treatment for all stages of syphilis, especially in pregnant women with the infection.

In a research conducted by Wendel et al., 15 pregnant women with syphilis underwent oral PCN desensitization **(Table 1)**. While some experienced mild allergic reactions, these did not interfere with the treatment. According to clinical and serological criteria, all maternal infections were successfully treated, and all infants born to date have shown no clinical or serological signs of infection.

Intravenous desensitization involving continuous infusion of doses at 15–30-minute intervals, followed by the intravenous delivery of the complete therapeutic dose, has been performed.

There are case reports on desensitization to antifungal medications such as micafungin, voriconazole, and fluconazole, as well as antiviral medications like acyclovir, ribavirin, and valganciclovir.

- *Antitubercular drugs*: Allergic reactions to various antitubercular drugs pose a major obstacle and are rarely documented in clinical research. Withdrawing

TABLE 1: Oral penicillin desensitization protocol.

Steps	Penicillin V (units/mL)	Amount (mL)	Dose (units)	Cumulative dose (mg)
1.	1,000	0.1	100	100
2.	1,000	0.2	200	300
3.	1,000	0.4	400	700
4.	1,000	0.8	800	1,500
5.	1,000	1.6	1,600	3,100
6.	1,000	3.2	3,200	6,300
7.	1,000	6.4	6,400	12,700
8.	10,000	1.2	12,000	24,700
9.	10,000	2.4	24,000	48,700
10.	10,000	4.8	48,000	96,700
11.	80,000	1.0	80,000	176,700
12.	80,000	2.0	160,000	336,700
13.	80,000	4.0	320,000	656,700
14.	80,000	8.0	640,000	1,296,700

Notes: Observation period: 30 minutes before parenteral administration of penicillin. Interval between doses: 15 minutes; elapsed time: 3 hours 45 minutes; cumulative dose: 1.3 million units. Specific amount of drug was diluted in 30 mL of water and then given orally.

Source: Wendel GD, Stark BJ, Jamison RB, Molina RD, Sullivan TJ. Penicillin Allergy and Desensitization in Serious Infections during Pregnancy. N Engl J Med. 1985;312:1229-32.

the first-line drugs due to hypersensitivity can drastically reduce the effectiveness of tuberculosis treatment.

Three different reintroduction methods have been utilized for patients experiencing severe cutaneous adverse reactions (SCARs) related to anti-TB drugs. The first method involved replacing all drugs in the anti-TB regimen that caused SCARs with alternative drugs at full therapeutic doses. The second method was a graded challenge, where the stopped drugs were reintroduced one by one, with a 2–3-day interval between each dose, as outlined in **Table 2**. The third method involved gradually initiating tolerance through a desensitization procedure, starting with doses less than 1/10,000 of the prescribed amount and progressively increasing every 2 hours, as detailed in **Table 3**. For drugs that caused BTRs upon reintroduction, the interval was sometimes extended to 3 hours.

Cholinergic Urticaria

Cholinergic urticaria is characterized by the presence of small and itchy wheals which emerge in response to any stimulus that triggers sweating, such as intense physical exercise, consumption of spicy food, emotional stress, and increased body temperature. Research has shown that approximately 30% of cases of inducible urticaria and 5–7% of cases of all urticaria constitute cholinergic urticaria.

TABLE 2: A graded challenge protocol for first-line antitubercular drugs.

Drug	Day 1	Day 2	Day 3	Day 4	Day 4	Day 5	Day 6	Day 7	Day 8	Day 9	Day 10	Day 11	Day 12
Rifampin (mg)	150	300	450	600	600	600	600	600	600	600	600	600	600
Isoniazid (mg)					100	200	300	300	300	300	300	300	300
Pyrazinamide (mg)								500	1,000	1,500	1,500	1,500	1,500
Ethambutol (mg)											400	800	1,200

Source: Oh JH, Yun J, Yang MS, Kim JH, Kim SH, Kim S, et al. Reintroduction of Antitubercular Drugs in Patients with Antitubercular Drug-related Drug Reaction with Eosinophilia and Systemic Symptoms. J Allergy Clin Immunol Pract. 2021;9(9):3442-9.e3. [Erratum in: J Allergy Clin Immunol Pract. 2021;9(12):4509].

TABLE 3: Isoniazid desensitization protocol (target dose: 300 mg).							
Days	Steps	Concentration (mg/mL)	Amount (mL)	Time (h)	Administered dose (mg)	Cumulative dose (mg)
D1	1.	0.2	0.1		0.02	0.02
	2.	0.2	0.2	2	0.04	0.06
	3.	0.2	0.5	2	0.1	0.16
	4.	0.2	1	2	0.2	0.36
	5.	0.2	2	2	0.4	0.76
	6.	0.2	4	2	0.8	1.56
	7.	0.2	8	2	1.6	3.16
	8.	0.2	16	2	3.2	6.36
D2	9.	2	3		6	12.36
	10.	2	6	2	12	24.36
	11.	2	12	2	24	48.36
	12.	100 mg tab	0.5 tab	2	50	98.36
	13.	100 mg tab	1 tab	2	100	198.36
	14.	100 mg tab	2 tab	2	200	398.36
D3	15.	100 mg tab	3 tab		300	300

Source: Oh JH, Yun J, Yang MS, Kim JH, Kim SH, Kim S, et al. Reintroduction of Antituberculous Drugs in Patients with Antituberculous Drug-related Drug Reaction with Eosinophilia and Systemic Symptoms. J Allergy Clin Immunol Pract. 2021;9(9):3442-9.e3. [Erratum in: J Allergy Clin Immunol Pract. 2021;9(12):4509].

In a study done by Kozaru et al., patients with severe cholinergic urticaria and pronounced hypersensitivity to their own sweat underwent rapid desensitization using intradermal tests using autologous sweat. The effectiveness was determined by evaluating clinical symptoms, conducting intradermal tests with the patients' own sweat, and measuring histamine release from basophils when exposed to autologous sweat. After rapid desensitization, all patients showed decreased skin reactivity to their own sweat. Furthermore, two of the three patients with cholinergic urticaria exhibited reduced histamine release from basophils in response to autologous sweat post-desensitization **(Tables 4 and 5)**.

ORAL CHALLENGE TESTS

Oral challenge tests are a diagnostic tool used to assess a patient's sensitivity or allergic response to a specific substance by administering it orally under controlled conditions. These tests are particularly valuable in the diagnosis of food allergies, drug hypersensitivity, and other allergic reactions where ingestion is the primary route of exposure.

Oral food challenges (OFCs) are valuable for confirming or ruling out the possibility of a food allergy, regardless of whether it is IgE-mediated or not. They are also used to evaluate the tolerability of a food in children with a history of food allergy and to determine the threshold dose that triggers a reaction.

TABLE 4: Patients who showed positive reaction for 1/1000 diluted sweat.

Steps	Solution dilution	Volume
1.	1/1,000	0.02
2.	1/1,000	0.03
3.	1/1,000	0.05
4.	1/1,000	0.07
5.	1/1,000	0.1
6.	1/1,000	0.15
7.	1/100	0.02
8.	1/100	0.03
9.	1/100	0.05
10.	1/100	0.07
11.	1/100	0.1
12.	1/100	0.15
13.	1/100	0.2
14.	1/1000	0.02

Source: Kozaru T, Fukunaga A, Taguchi K, Ogura K, Nagano T, Oka M, et al. Rapid desensitization with autologous sweat in cholinergic urticaria. Allergol Int. 2011;60(3):277-81.

TABLE 5: Patients who showed positive reaction for 1/100 diluted sweat.

Steps	Solution dilution	Volume
1.	1/100	0.02
2.	1/100	0.03
3.	1/100	0.05
4.	1/100	0.07
5.	1/100	0.1
6.	1/100	0.15
7.	1/100	0.2
8.	1/100	0.02

Source: Kozaru T, Fukunaga A, Taguchi K, Ogura K, Nagano T, Oka M, et al. Rapid desensitization with autologous sweat in cholinergic urticaria. Allergol Int. 2011;60(3):277-81.

Additionally, OFCs are indicated for testing specific foods in patients sensitized to foods they have never consumed or for assessing cross-reactive foods that have not been previously introduced into the diet. The OFC can be administered in an "open, single-blind or double-blind challenge."

In an open OFC, the patient as well as their family members and the doctor are informed about the specific food being tested. This method is straightforward and cost-effective. In a single-blind OFC, only the doctor knows which food is being administered, reducing the potential for the patient's psychological factors to influence the results. In a double-blind placebo-controlled food challenge (DBPCFC), both the doctor and the patient are kept unaware of whether the administered substance is the actual food or a placebo, which helps to eliminate both the doctor's potential bias and the patient's psychological influence on the outcome. One commonly utilized protocol, as suggested by PRACTALL, involves seven progressively increasing doses of food with a semilogarithmic rise in protein levels: 3, 10, 30, 100, 300, 1000, and 3000. The initial amount being administered must always be less than the dose that previously triggered an allergic reaction.

Currently, there is no universally accepted standard for determining a positive result in a challenge for food allergies mediated by IgE. The choice to stop dosing depends on several factors, including the individual's clinical history, the protocols of the study, and the objective of the challenge (whether for diagnosing a food allergy, assessing tolerance, or identifying the threshold dose that triggers a reaction).

The outcomes of an OFC can be categorized as follows:
- *Positive*: When clear objective signs of an allergic reaction are observed or when there are repeated (at least three times) or multiple subjective symptoms affecting several organ systems
- *Negative*: When no symptoms are observed
- *Inconclusive*: If the test is halted before the full dose of food is consumed, indicating partial tolerance at best.

CONCLUSION

- Desensitization and oral challenge tests are indispensable tools in the comprehensive management of urticaria. These methodologies not only enhance our understanding of individual allergen sensitivities but also provide a pathway to more effective and personalized treatment strategies. As research and clinical practices continue to evolve, the integration of these tests will remain a cornerstone in the fight against this complex and often challenging condition.
- The goal of creating desensitization protocols for drug hypersensitivities is to enable the safe administration of critical medications while safeguarding patients from both IgE and non-IgE allergic reactions including anaphylaxis to aspirin/NSAIDs, antibiotics, antineoplastic, and other drugs.
- Desensitization procedures should be performed exclusively in environments that offer dedicated nurse–patient care and have immediate access to resuscitation staff and equipment. Once a desensitization is successfully completed, subsequent desensitizations can be carried out in either outpatient or inpatient settings, provided they maintain similar conditions, particularly for patients undergoing chemotherapy or monoclonal antibody treatments.
- Training specialists in oncology and allergy, pharmacists and nurses will promote the careful application of desensitization protocols for patients with hypersensitivity reactions who require first-line treatments.

- Oral challenge tests offer a precise diagnostic approach, confirming specific triggers and aiding in the development of targeted therapies. Together, these approaches empower healthcare providers to offer more nuanced and effective care, ultimately improving patient outcomes and quality of life for those suffering from urticaria.

SUGGESTED READINGS

1. Zuberbier T, Aberer W, Asero R, Bindslev-Jensen C, Brzoza Z, Canonica GW. The EAACI/GA(2) LEN/EDF/WAO guideline for the definition, classification, diagnosis, and management of urticaria: the 2013 revision and update. Allergy. 2014;69:868-87.
2. Warin RP, Champion RH. Urticaria. London: WB Saunders; 1974.
3. Kobza Black A, Champion RH. Urticaria. In: Champion RH, Burton JL, Burns DA, Breathnac SM (Eds). Textbook of Dermatology, 6th edition. New Jersey: Blackwell Science; 1998. pp. 2113-39.
4. Janeway CA Jr, Travers P, Walport M, Shlomchik MJ. Effector mechanisms in allergic reactions. In: Immunobiology: The Immune System in Health and Disease. 5th edition. New York: Garland Science; 2001.
5. Mathelier-Fusade P. Drug-induced urticarias. Clin Rev Allergy Immunol. 2006;30(1):19-23.
6. Vultaggio A, Matucci A, Nencini F, Bormioli S, Vivarelli E, Maggi E. Mechanisms of Drug Desensitization: Not Only Mast Cells. Front Pharmacol. 2020;11:590991.
7. Siripassorn K, Ruxrungtham K, Manosuthi W. Successful drug desensitization in patients with delayed-type allergic reactions to anti-tuberculosis drugs. Int J Infect Dis. 2018;68:61-8.
8. Ban GY, Jeong YJ, Lee SH, Shin SS, Shin YS, Park HS, et al. Efficacy and tolerability of desensitization in the treatment of delayed drug hypersensitivities to anti-tuberculosis medications. Respir Med. 2019;147:44-50.
9. Oka T, Rios J, Tsai M, Kalesnikoff J, Galli SJ. Rapid desensitization induces internalization of antigen-specific IgE on mouse mast cells. J Allergy Clin Immunol. 2013;132)(4):922-32.e16
10. Odom S, Gomez G, Kovarova M, Furumoto Y, Ryan JJ, Wright HV, et al. Negative regulation of immunoglobulin E-dependent allergic responses by Lyn kinase. J Exp Med. 2004;199: 1491-502.
11. Silberman S, Neukirch-Stoop C, Steg PPG. Rapid desensitisation procedure for patients with ASA hypersensitivity undergoing coronary stenting. Am J Cardiol. 2005;95:509-10.
12. Schaefer OP, Gore JM. Aspirin sensitivity: the role for aspirin challenge and desensitization in postmyocardial infarction patients. Cardiology. 1999;91(1):8-13.
13. Wong JT, Nagy CS, Krinzman SJ, Maclean JA, Bloch KJ. Rapid oral challenge-desensitization for patients with aspirin-related urticaria-angioedema. J Allergy Clin Immunol. 2000;105(5): 997-1001.
14. Lee CW, Matulonis UA, Castells MC. Carboplatin hypersensitivity: a 6-h 12-step protocol effective in 35 desensitizations in patients with gynecological malignancies and mast cell/IgE-mediated reactions. Gynecol Oncol. 2004;95(2):370-6.
15. Lee JH, Moon M, Kim YC, Chung SJ, Oh J, Kang DY, et al. A One-bag Rapid Desensitization Protocol for Paclitaxel Hypersensitivity: A Noninferior Alternative to a Multi-bag Rapid Desensitization Protocol. J Allergy Clin Immunol Pract. 2020;8(2):696-703.
16. Wendel GD, Stark BJ, Jamison RB, Molina RD, Sullivan TJ. Penicillin allergy and desensitization in serious infections during pregnancy. N Engl J Med. 1985;312:1229-32.
17. de Groot H, Mulder WM, Terreehorst I. Utility of desensitisation for allergy to antibiotics. Neth J Med. 2012;70(2):58-62.
18. Ward SL, Maciag MC, Jones S, Lee J, Lee J, Broyles AD. Successful Rapid Desensitization to Micafungin in a Pediatric Patient. Pediatr Allergy Immunol Pulmonol. 2021;34(3):106-8.
19. Jean T, Kwong K. Successful desensitization of voriconazole in an immunosuppressed pediatric patient. J Allergy Clin Immunol Pract. 2015;3:637-8.

20. Randolph C, Kaplan C, Fraser B. Rapid desensitization to fluconazole (Diflucan). Ann Allergy Asthma Immunol. 2008;100:616-7.
21. Gülen TA, Özden G, Turanç T. Ciddi Asiklovir Alerjisinde İntravenöz Asiklovir Desensitizasyon Tedavisi: Herpes Ensefaliti Olgusu [Treatment with Intravenous Acyclovir Desensitization for Severe Acyclovir Allergy: A Case of Herpes Encephalitis]. Mikrobiyol Bul. 2022;56(2):371-6. [in Turkish].
22. Ladd AM, Martel-Laferriere V, Dieterich D. Successful desensitization to ribavirin in a patient with chronic hepatitis C. J Clin Gastroenterol. 2012;46:716-7.
23. Gonzalez-Estrada A, Fernandez J. Novel valganciclovir desensitization protocol. Transplantation. 2014;98:e50-1.
24. Oh JH, Yun J, Yang MS, Kim JH, Kim SH, Kim S, et al. Reintroduction of Antituberculous Drugs in Patients with Antituberculous Drug-related Drug Reaction with Eosinophilia and Systemic Symptoms. J Allergy Clin Immunol Pract. 2021;9(9):3442-9.e3. [Erratum in: J Allergy Clin Immunol Pract. 2021;9(12):4509].
25. Kontou-Fili K, Borici-Mazi R, Kapp A, Matjevic LJ, Mitchel FB. Physical urticaria: Classification and diagnostic guidelines. An EAACI position paper. Allergy. 1997;52:504-13.
26. Kozaru T, Fukunaga A, Taguchi K, Ogura K, Nagano T, Oka M, et al. Rapid desensitization with autologous sweat in cholinergic urticaria. Allergol Int. 2011;60(3):277-81.
27. Nowak-Wegrzyn A, Assa'ad AH, Bahna SL, Bock SA, Sicherer SH, Teuber SS. Adverse Reactions to Food Committee of American Academy of Allergy, Asthma and Immunology. Work Group report: Oral food challenge testing. J Allergy Clin Immunol. 2009;123:S365-83.
28. Calvani M, Bianchi A, Reginelli C, Peresso M, Testa A. Oral Food Challenge. Medicina (Kaunas). 2019;55(10):651.
29. Sampson HA, Gerth van Wijk R, Bindslev-Jensen C, Sicherer S, Teuber SS, Burks AW, et al. Standardizing double-blind, placebo-controlled oral food challenges: American Academy of Allergy, Asthma and Immunology–European Academy of Allergy and Clinical Immunology PRACTALL consensus report. J Allergy Clin Immunol. 2012;130:1260-74.
30. Grabenhenrich LB, Reich A, Bellach J, Trendelenburg V, Sprikkelman AB, Roberts G, et al. A new framework for the documentation and interpretation of oral food challenges in population-base and clinical research. Allergy. 2017;72:453-61.
31. Castells M. Rapid desensitization for hypersensitivity reactions to medications. Immunol Allergy Clin North Am. 2009;29(3):585-606.

Autologous Serum Skin Test

Neha Rani, Sanjeev Gupta, Aditi Dabhra

INTRODUCTION

Chronic urticaria is characterized by erythematous, pruritic wheals that persist daily or almost daily for a duration more than 6 weeks. The etiology of chronic urticaria can be multifactorial, including idiopathic causes, chronic infections, infestations, pseudoallergens, atopic conditions, and noninfectious inflammatory diseases.

Chronic idiopathic urticaria is subdivided into two types: Chronic autoimmune criteria (CAU) and chronic spontaneous urticaria (CSU).

Chronic autoimmune urticaria is thought to be due to autoantibodies against FcεR1α receptors of immunoglobulin E (IgE) over mast cells and basophils, or directly against IgE. The presence of these autoantibodies can be demonstrated by autologous serum skin test (ASST).

ROLE OF AUTOLOGOUS SERUM SKIN TEST IN URTICARIA

- ASST is used for the diagnosis of autoimmune urticaria (AIU) since 1940.
- This in vivo test helps to identify the presence of circulating functional autoantibodies by injecting a patient's autologous serum into their skin and observing the reaction.
- A positive ASST test is associated with autoimmune cause and signifies a prolonged disease course and poor response to routine therapy.
- The ASST plays a crucial role in the diagnosis and management of chronic urticaria, particularly CAU.
- In clinical practice, the ASST helps to differentiate between autoimmune and nonautoimmune forms of chronic urticaria. This distinction is important as it can guide treatment decisions. Patients with a positive ASST may benefit from immunomodulatory therapies, such as corticosteroids, cyclosporine, or omalizumab, which target the underlying autoimmune process.
- Furthermore, the ASST can be used to monitor the effectiveness of these treatments. A decrease in the wheal response over time may indicate a reduction in the activity of the autoantibodies, reflecting a positive response to therapy.

INDICATIONS FOR AUTOLOGOUS SERUM SKIN TEST

Autologous serum skin test is indicated in suspected cases of AIU, especially when there is an inadequate response to antihistamines, even after updosing.

PRE-REQUIREMENTS

- Antihistamines should be discontinued at least 2–3 days before the test.
- Doxepin and Astemizole should be discontinued between 2 and 6 weeks.
- Before the test, it is advised that the patient abstains from taking immuno-suppressants for a period of 2 months.
- Before proceeding, it is necessary to obtain ethical approval or proper consent.
- The minimum age requirement is 18 years or older.
- The test area must be devoid of any lesions.

PROCEDURE

Approximately 2 cc of venous blood is collected in a sterile vacutainer and allowed to clot at room temperature for 30 minutes. The serum is then centrifuged at 2,000 RPM for 15 minutes. Following this, 0.05 mL of the autologous serum is injected intradermally into uninvolved skin using a 1 mL insulin syringe with a 30-gauge needle, at a site 2 cm below the cubital fossa on the left forearm. Similarly, 0.05 mL of 0.9% normal saline (negative control) is injected intradermally proximally, and 0.05 mL of histamine (positive control) is injected intradermally distally, at least 5 cm apart from each other. The results are read after 30 minutes **(Flowchart 1)**.

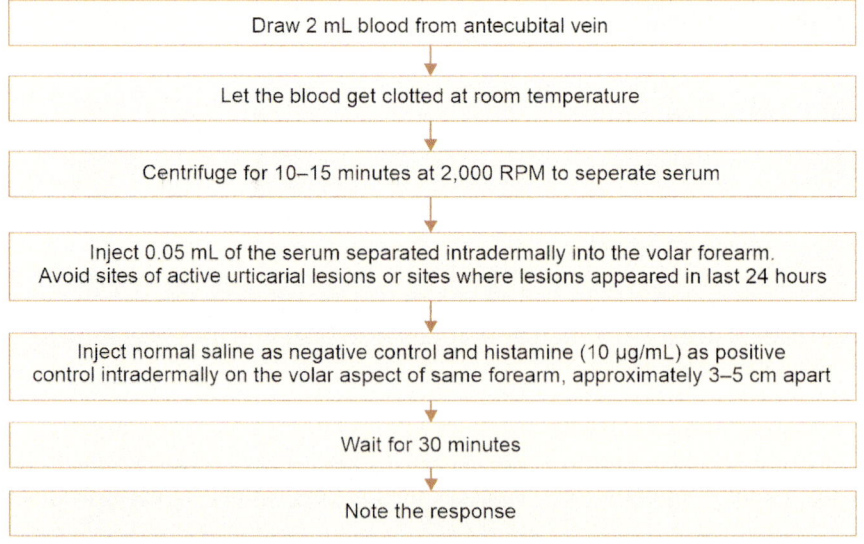

FLOWCHART 1: Procedure of autologous serum skin test (ASST).

INTERPRETATION OF AUTOLOGOUS SERUM SKIN TEST (TABLE 1)

- An indurated erythematous wheal at the site of autologous serum injection that is 1.5 mm larger than the wheal at the saline control site is considered positive.
- A positive result suggests the presence of functional antibodies, indicating an autoimmune component to the urticaria.
- When there is little or no reaction at the serum injection site or the wheal size is similar to or smaller than the control site, it is taken as negative.

CRITERIA FOR POSITIVITY

A positive test is a serum-induced wheal response with a diameter larger than 1.5 mm or greater than that of saline-induced response after 30 minutes. First, the maximum vertical ($d1$) and horizontal ($d2$) diameters of the wheals are measured and the average diameter (D) is calculated $[D = (d1 + d2)/2]$.

False-positive Autologous Serum Skin Test

A false-positive ASST occurs when the test shows the presence of functional autoantibodies in a patient who does not actually have CAU. False-positive results in the ASST can arise from various factors. Variation in injection techniques, such as differences in the volume and depth of injection, can lead to inconsistent skin responses. Additionally, individuals with dermographism are more likely to exhibit false-positive results. Patients with autoimmune thyroid disease may also have an increased propensity for false-positives due to underlying autoimmune mechanisms. Furthermore, children with allergic or nonallergic respiratory symptoms can display heightened skin reactivity, contributing to inaccurate ASST outcomes.

TABLE 1: Interpretation of autologous serum skin test.

Result	Wheal formation	Comparison with control	Implications
Positive result	A wheal (a raised, red, itchy bump) forms at the site of the serum injection	The wheal at the serum injection site is significantly larger (typically ≥1.5 mm larger) than the wheal at the saline control site	A positive result suggests the presence of functional autoantibodies, indicating an autoimmune component to the urticaria
Negative result	Little or no reaction at the serum injection site	The size of the wheal is similar to or smaller than the control injection site	A negative result suggests that the urticaria is less likely to be due to an autoimmune process and may be due to other triggers such as allergies, infections, or idiopathic causes

False-negative Autologous Serum Skin Test

False-negative results in the ASST can arise due to various factors, complicating the accurate diagnosis of CAU. Medications like antihistamines, corticosteroids, or other immunosuppressive drugs can suppress the skin reaction, leading to false-negatives. The timing of the test is crucial; performing it during periods of low disease activity or remission may result in insufficient circulating autoantibodies to trigger a detectable response. Technical errors, such as improper serum preparation, incorrect injection technique, or inadequate serum volume, can also contribute to false-negatives.

SIGNIFICANCE OF POSITIVE AUTOLOGOUS SERUM SKIN TEST RESULT

- A positive ASST denotes that a subset of population has an increased potential to develop urticaria due to endogenous causes as compared to the patients with a negative ASST.
- A positive ASST has also been found to correlate with severity and duration of disease.
- It has also been reported to correlate strongly with the patients with associated *Helicobacter pylori* IgG antibodies and who have intolerance to nonsteroidal anti-inflammatory drugs (NSAIDs).
- These patients with autoantibodies may need a higher dose of antihistamine or an additional immunomodulator.
- Recently, it has been found that a positive ASST may be an indicator of circulating vasoactive factors rather than specific autoantibodies. The significance of a negative ASST is still unclear.

AUTOLOGOUS PLASMA SKIN TEST

A similar test to the ASST is the autologous plasma skin test (APST). The primary difference between these tests lies in the preparation of the blood sample. For the APST, a venous blood sample is collected in a sterile tube containing 0.125 mol/L sodium citrate. The blood sample is then kept at room temperature for 30 minutes before being centrifuged at 2,500 RPM for around 10 minutes.

STUDIES ON AUTOLOGOUS SERUM SKIN TEST (TABLE 2)

In a prospective study conducted at Baghdad Teaching Hospital, 54 patients diagnosed with CIU were evaluated using the ASST to detect AIU. The study found that 40.7% of the patients tested positive for ASST, indicating autoimmune involvement. Statistical analysis showed no significant differences between patients with positive and negative ASST results in terms of age, sex, severity score, duration of disease, or frequency of attacks. However, there was a significant association ($p = 0.004$) between positive ASST results and the distribution of wheals on the face and extremities. This suggests that ASST is a valuable tool

for identifying AIU cases among CIU patients, particularly in those with wheals predominantly on the face and extremities. The study concludes that ASST is a simple and cost-effective test for distinguishing AIU from other forms of chronic urticaria, aiding in appropriate management strategies.
- In a study comparing the ASST and APST for diagnosing CAU in patients with chronic CSU, researchers found significant differences in test positivity between patients and healthy controls. ASST and APST were positive in 62% and 42% of CSU patients, respectively, compared to 10% and 6% in controls. The study highlighted that both tests can effectively detect autoimmunity associated with urticaria, although APST showed higher sensitivity.

TABLE 2: Overview of various studies on ASST.

Study	Location	Patients (n)	Positive ASST (%)	Key Findings
1	Baghdad Teaching Hospital	54	40.7	• ASST is valuable for detecting AIU, particularly in patients with wheals on face and extremities • No significant differences in demographic or disease characteristics between ASST-positive and -negative patients except for wheal distribution ($p = 0.004$).
2	Not specified	CSU patients versus controls	ASST: 62 APST: 42	ASST and APST effectively detect autoimmunity in CSU patients; APST shows higher sensitivity. Thyroid autoantibodies were present in CSU patients but not significantly different from controls
3	North India tertiary hospital	58	44.8	ASST-positive patients had longer disease duration, higher severity, and more generalized involvement. Positivity correlated with lower AEC and serum IgE levels, suggesting potential biomarkers for AIU
4	South India tertiary care hospital	48	41.6	ASST identifies CAU among CSU patients without significant differences in demographics, clinical characteristics, systemic symptoms, atopy, or other autoimmune conditions between positive and negative ASST groups
5	Review article	Not applicable	Not applicable	ASST is a useful tool for diagnosing AIU by detecting functional autoantibodies against IgE receptors, although its correlation with AIU remains complex. It aids in identifying patients who may benefit from targeted therapies despite limitations

Additionally, thyroid autoantibodies were found in a subset of CSU patients but did not significantly differ from controls. The findings underscore the utility of ASST and APST in diagnosing CAU and suggest the importance of assessing thyroid autoantibodies even in euthyroid CSU patients.

- In a descriptive study from a tertiary hospital in North India, the role of the ASST in CSU was investigated, focusing on its correlation with biochemical markers. Out of 58 enrolled patients, ASST was positive in 44.8% of cases, indicating its utility in identifying AIU, a subset known for its severity and resistance to conventional treatments. ASST-positive patients exhibited longer disease duration, higher disease severity, and more generalized involvement compared to ASST-negative patients. Biochemically, ASST positivity correlated with lower absolute eosinophil counts (AEC) and significantly lower serum IgE levels, suggesting that these markers could aid in diagnosing AIU. The study highlights ASST as a practical diagnostic tool and underscores the potential of AEC and IgE as additional markers in diagnosing AIU.
- In another study conducted in a tertiary care hospital in South India, ASST was used to assess CAU among patients with CSU. Among the 48 patients studied, 41.6% were ASST positive, indicating the presence of autoantibodies against the FcϵR1α receptor. There was no significant difference found between ASST-positive and -negative patients concerning demographics, clinical characteristics of urticaria (such as weal morphology, duration, severity), systemic symptoms, atopy, or association with other autoimmune conditions. This study underscores the utility of ASST as a diagnostic tool for identifying CAU in a clinical setting, although larger studies would be needed to confirm these findings more robustly.
- Another article on ASST provides a comprehensive overview of its methodology, interpretation, and clinical applications in diagnosing AIU. ASST, introduced by Grattan et al. in 1986, involves intradermal injection of autologous serum to detect functional autoantibodies against IgE or its receptors in chronic urticaria patients. The test's sensitivity and specificity are enhanced when patients discontinue antihistamines and immunosuppressants prior to testing. Positive ASST results are characterized by a wheal larger than saline control with associated erythema. Despite its utility, ASST's correlation with AIU remains complex, as evidenced by variations in positive rates and clinical implications across studies. It serves as a valuable tool in clinical practice for identifying patients likely to benefit from targeted therapeutic interventions, despite inherent limitations and ongoing research to refine its diagnostic accuracy and clinical relevance.

OTHER TESTS TO DETECT AUTOANTIBODIES

ELISA and Western Blot

- Autoantibodies in the patient's serum can be detected through serum-induced histamine release from the basophils of healthy donors, utilizing enzyme-linked immunosorbent assay (ELISA) or Western blot assays.

- In the context of ELISA, the patient's serum is added to a plate coated with the target antigen, and the binding of antibodies to this antigen is detected through a colorimetric reaction, indicating the presence of autoantibodies.
- Western blotting involves separating proteins by gel electrophoresis, transferring them to a membrane, and probing the membrane with the patient's serum. The presence of autoantibodies is visualized by detecting antibody–antigen interactions using labeled secondary antibodies.
- However, these methods cannot differentiate between functional histamine-releasing autoantibodies and nonfunctional autoantibodies.
- Functional autoantibodies can actively induce histamine release from basophils, leading to the clinical manifestations of chronic urticaria.
- Nonfunctional autoantibodies, although present, do not trigger this histamine release and thus do not contribute to the symptoms.
- Additionally, these tests are typically conducted only in specialized centers and are time-consuming.

Basophil Histamine Release Test

- The in vivo basophil histamine release test remains the gold standard for detecting functional antibodies in patients with CAU.
- This assay involves stimulating basophils from healthy donors with the patient's serum and subsequently measuring histamine release which indicates the presence of functional autoantibodies.
- The process is inherently time-consuming. Isolating basophils, preparing the serum, incubating the cells, and measuring histamine release involve several steps that can take several hours. This time-intensive nature makes the test less practical for routine clinical use.
- However, its application is limited due to the requirement for healthy donor basophils, its time-consuming nature, and its potential to overlook nonfunctional autoantibodies.

Measurement of CD63 and CD203 Expression

- Another novel method for diagnosing CAU is the measurement of CD63 and CD203 expression by donor basophils following incubation with the patient's serum.
- This approach leverages the specific markers expressed on the surface of basophils upon activation and degranulation, providing a functional assessment of autoantibodies present in the patient's serum.
- Upon activation, basophils express increased levels of certain surface markers, notably CD63 and CD203. CD63 is a marker of degranulation, appearing on the cell surface when intracellular granules fuse with the plasma membrane. CD203 is another activation marker expressed during the immune response.
- The expression of CD63 and CD203 is typically measured using flow cytometry, a technique that allows for the precise quantification of these markers on individual cells. Fluorescently labeled antibodies specific to CD63 and CD203

are used to stain the basophils, and the fluorescence intensity is measured, providing an indication of basophil activation.
- This method is highly specific and sensitive to basophil activation, providing a direct functional assessment of autoantibodies' ability to induce basophil degranulation, which correlates with clinical symptoms.
- However, it has limitations, including the requirement for specialized equipment and expertise for flow cytometry, which can be costly and not widely available.
- Additionally, the technique necessitates fresh basophils from healthy donors, requiring careful handling and immediate processing. Standardization of assay conditions is also critical to ensure consistent and reproducible results.

ADVANTAGES OF AUTOLOGOUS SERUM SKIN TEST

- ASST is a relatively reliable, easy in vivo technique with a sensitivity of 70% and a specificity of 80%.
- The ASST offers several advantages over tests like ELISA, Western blot assays, basophile histamine release test, and the measurement of CD63 and CD203 expression on donor basophils.
- It is simpler to perform and is more accessible for routine clinical use, requiring only the intradermal injection of the patient's serum and observation of the reaction, without the need for specialized equipment or expertise.
- The ASST provides a direct in vivo functional assessment of autoantibodies, demonstrating the presence of functional autoantibodies through a wheal-and-flare response, unlike ELISA and Western blot assays, which cannot differentiate between functional and nonfunctional autoantibodies.
- It is a simple office based procedure/bedside test and results can be obtained in a short period, typically within 30 minutes, making it faster than the more time-consuming procedures required for other tests.
- Additionally, the ASST is cost-effective, requiring no expensive reagents or sophisticated instruments, and offers clinically relevant information that can guide treatment strategies effectively.
- Overall, the ASST is a practical, cost-effective, and clinically valuable alternative to more complex and resource-intensive tests for diagnosing CAU.

DISADVANTAGE OF AUTOLOGOUS SERUM SKIN TEST

Autologous serum skin test should be done by an experienced investigator as a poor technique can lead to either a false-positive or a false-negative result.

KEY POINTS

- Autologous serum skin test (ASST) is a simple office procedure that does not require any advanced equipment.
- ASST is usually performed in patients with inadequate response to antihistamines, even after updosing.

- Positive results can indicate autoimmunity.
- Individuals who test positive for ASST can be scheduled for autologous blood therapy and autologous serum therapy.

CONCLUSION

Autologous serum skin test is a rapid in vivo diagnostic test used for the diagnosis of AIU. CAU is thought to be due to autoantibodies against FcεRIα receptors of IgE over mast cells and basophils, or directly against IgE. The presence of these autoantibodies can be demonstrated by ASST. Thus, ASST is used to differentiate the patients with and those without circulating functional autoantibodies, and thus helpful in the diagnosis of CAU.

Despite being the most accessible and useful test for diagnosing CAU, a positive ASST is not synonymous to AIU. The significance of negative ASST also remains unclear. Its reactivity strongly correlates in patients who have intolerance to NSAIDs. ASST is time consuming, needs expertise, and requires stoppage of antihistamines prior to the test. Moreover, the test is not standardized, with various methods described in the literature and different criteria for positive result. Nevertheless, ASST offers a simple screening test for a subset of patients with chronic urticaria who are likely to have an endogenous cause. It has good sensitivity and even better sensitivity in detecting autoantibodies in children as well. Therefore, it can be reasonably used as a predictive clinical test to diagnose AIU, especially in situations where the basophil histamine-releasing test is not available.

SUGGESTED READINGS

1. Al-Hamamy HR, Hameed AF, Abdulhadi AS. Autologous Serum Skin Test as a Diagnostic Aid in Chronic Idiopathic Urticaria. ISRN Dermatol. 2013:2013:291524.
2. Kumaran MS, Mangal S, Narang T, Parsad D. Autologous Serum and Plasma Skin Tests in Chronic Spontaneous Urticaria: A Reappraisal. Indian Dermatol Online J. 2017;8(2):94-9.
3. Mir MM. Autologous serum skin test in chronic spontaneous urticaria and its correlation with biochemical markers- A descriptive study from a tertiary hospital of North India. IP Indian J Clin Exp Dermatol. 2022;8(3):147-51.
4. Vikramkumar AG, Kuruvila S, Ganguly S. Autologous serum skin test as an indicator of chronic autoimmune urticaria in a tertiary care hospital in South India. Indian Dermatol Online J. 2014;5(Suppl 2):S87-91.
5. Vohra S, Sharma NL, Mahajan VK. Autologous serum skin test: Methodology, interpretation and clinical applications. Indian J Dermatol Venereol Leprol. 2009;75:545-8.

CHAPTER 24

Autologous Blood/Serum Therapy in Urticaria

Neha Rani, Sanjeev Gupta

INTRODUCTION

Autologous blood therapy (ABT)/autologous serum therapy (AST)/autohemotherapy (AHT) can be administered via various methods—intravenous injection, intramuscular injection, and local injection of the patient's own blood/serum in tendons, ligaments, joints, conjunctiva, wounds, and ulcers. Since the patient's own blood/serum is used, autologous blood/serum therapy minimizes the risk of immune reactions and transmission of infectious diseases, making it a preferred option in elective surgeries, orthopedic procedures, and chronic disease management.

Chronic autoimmune urticaria is caused by circulating autoantibodies and is diagnosed by a positive autologous serum skin test (ASST). So, autologous whole-blood therapy can be considered a therapeutic option in this subgroup of urticaria. In AHT, repeated intramuscular injections of autologous whole blood are given, and sometimes may be treated with ozone or ultraviolet light.

HISTORY OF AUTOLOGOUS BLOOD THERAPY

The concept of using blood for healing purposes is not a new one. In ancient cultures, blood was used for various purposes including healing rituals. Autologous blood therapy has been used in European medicine since the end of the 19th century. The idea of transfusing the patient's own blood was mentioned for the first time by Eulenburg and Landios in 1866. They proposed to treat gas poisoning with exchange transfusion. They suggested that blood withdrawn from the patients of gas poisoning could be transfused after poisonous gas has been eliminated. Halle surgeon von Volkmann first demonstrably considered the possibility of ABT in operative medicine in 1868. However, the first originally sourced ABT was performed by the Keil surgeon von Esmarch in a case of exarticulation of the thigh at the hip joint. He collected the blood that had been shed during the operation, defibrinated it, and reinjected it into a severed femoral vein. It has been gradually discarded from general medical use. Still, it holds value in conditions such as enhancement of the immune system, treatment of many dermatological diseases, ease of tendon and joint pain, and wound healing.

The major ozonated autohemotherapy (O3-AHT) was first described by Wherli and Steinbart in 1954; since then, after Wolff's modification, it has been used worldwide in age-related macular degeneration (AMD) with therapeutic effects and without any side effects. It has also shown therapeutic effects in patients with late stage of lower limb ischemia.

In Japan, intramuscular autologous blood injections have been used for chronic urticaria (CU). For dermatological diseases, whole-blood therapy has been tried in patients of pemphigus, severe dry eye due to Sjogren syndrome and rheumatoid arthritis, viral diseases such as herpes zoster, malignancies, and atopic dermatitis **(Table 1)**.

Mechanism of Action

The mechanism of action of ABT is still unclear. It is considered to act as a stimulation or a regulation therapy, which implies that a body self-healing reaction is elicited by a counterregulation to irritation. It is postulated to modulate the immune response to autologous antigens which are supposed to be involved in histamine release from basophils and mast cells. With intramuscular ABT, route of circulating histamine-releasing stimulators into the immune system is changed, thus causing some immunomodulation, which results in tolerance induction to histamine-releasing factors. Therefore, mild reactions such as bruises and soreness at the injection site have been regarded as inherent to the therapy. Another possible mechanism of ABT in chronic autoimmune urticaria is the stimulation of anti-idiotype production against these autoantibodies, which blocks the binding of these antibodies to their receptors on mast cells and basophils. Another possible mechanism could be the induction of tolerance to autoantigens or IgE or FcεRI. With autoimmunotherapy, these autoantigens are processed and presented by muscular dendritic cells to the immune system and elicit a different immune response that may convert a previously disease-

TABLE 1: History of autologous blood therapy (ABT).	
Year	Event
Ancient times	Blood used for various purposes, including healing rituals in ancient cultures
1866	Eulenburg and Landios first mentioned the idea of retransfusing a patient's own blood to treat gas poisoning by eliminating poisonous gas from the blood and retransfusing it
1868	Halle surgeon von Volkmann first considered the possibility of ABT in operative medicine
1868	Kiel surgeon von Esmarch performed the first originally sourced ABT by collecting shed blood during an operation, defibrinating it, and reinjecting it into the severed femoral vein during a case of exarticulation of the thigh at the hip joint
19th–20th century	Gradual decline in the general medical use of ABT
1954	Wherli and Steinbart were first to describe major ozonated autohemotherapy (O3-AHT)

causing antigen into a regulatory antigen, which activates regulatory T cells and suppresses effector T cells.

Indications

In Japan, intramuscular autologous blood injections have been used for CU. For other dermatological diseases, whole-blood therapy had been tried in patients of pemphigus, severe dry eye due to Sjögren syndrome and rheumatoid arthritis, viral diseases such as herpes zoster, malignancies, and atopic dermatitis.

For musculoskeletal system, AHT has been indicated in cases of mild-to-moderate arthrosis, tendon damage, ligament injuries, muscle injuries, and bursitis.

Ozonated AHT has shown positive effects in patients of dry AMD.

Dermatological diseases in which ABT is a treatment option include urticaria, eczema and herpes zoster, to name a few **(Box 1)**.

ROUTE OF ADMINISTRATION

Autologous blood therapy can be given as intramuscular injection, intravenous injection, or local injection in various sites, e.g., in tendons, ligaments, joints, conjunctivas, wounds, and ulcers.

Side Effects

Any major side effects of ABT have not been recorded till date. If the blood has not been manipulated before reinjection and standard hygiene procedure is followed, the risk of infection is very low. Some minor side effects such as soreness or bruising at the injection site could be observed, but are short-lived.

Advantages:
- Promotes self-healing potential of the body
- No risk of allergic reaction as patient's own blood is used
- Rapid treatment, requires less time

Box 1: Common diseases where autologous blood therapy (ABT) is used as a treatment option.

Dermatological diseases:
- Chronic urticaria
- Pemphigus vulgaris
- Herpes zoster
- Atopic dermatitis
- Rheumatoid arthritis
- Mild-to-moderate arthrosis
- Tendon damage
- Ligament injuries
- Muscle injuries
- Bursitis

Ophthalmic diseases:
- Age-related macular degeneration (AMD)
- Severe dry eye due to Sjogren syndrome
- Chronic urticaria
- Pemphigus vulgaris
- Herpes zoster
- Atopic dermatitis

Procedure:
- A venous blood sample is taken.
- The collected blood is given intramuscularly in the gluteal region.

As such, the technique of ABT is not standardized. Most of the people have modified it in their own way. In this technique, some amount of blood is withdrawn from the antecubital vein and reinjected in the deep intramuscular region, for instance, in the gluteus muscle. The amount of blood withdrawn may vary from 1 mL to start with and is gradually increased in subsequent visits up to 5 mL. Preferably, larger volumes should be avoided because of the risk of gluteal abscess formation. Some people prefer to heparinize the syringe before collecting blood so that the blood clotting is avoided in case there is some delay between blood collection and the injection at the site. The procedure can be repeated at weekly or at 10–15-day intervals. Later on, as per the response, the interval can be increased up to 8 weeks, although there is no standardization till date.

Contraindications

Autologous blood therapy is not indicated in patients with blood coagulation disorder, acute or chronic skin infections (HIV), malignancy or infection at the injection site.

AUTOLOGOUS SERUM THERAPY

Autologous serum therapy is a modification of ABT, in which autologous serum is used instead of whole blood. It is considered as less painful by some patients and also has been proven beneficial in urticaria.

Procedure:
- Collect 5 mL of blood in a plain sterilized vacutainer.
- Centrifugation at 3,000 RPM for 10 minutes.
- Separate the serum with a 5-mL syringe.
- 2.5 mL of separated serum is injected deep intramuscular into the gluteus muscle with a 22-G needle. The amount of serum can be increased gradually in subsequent visits up to 5 mL. As in ABT, larger volumes should be avoided because of the risk of gluteal abscess.
- Repeat the procedure weekly for 8 weeks; later, fortnightly injections can be given, though there is no standardization.

Both ABT and AST have been reported to show similar efficacy in urticaria patients. However, AST requires more time, expertise, equipment, and expenses than ABT.

Serum is the major constituent of whole blood. Thus, the volume injected for AST is half the volume required for ABT. Therefore, the net amount of serum injected in both AST and ABT is likely similar. As a result, ABT has more advantages over AST but increases the risk of local site soreness and bruising due to the larger volume used.

STUDIES (TABLE 2)

- In a study done by AK Bajaj et al. titled "Autologous serum therapy in chronic spontaneous urticaria," the authors aimed to assess the effectiveness of repeated autologous serum injections (ASIs) in patients with CU, particularly focusing on those with positive ASST results indicating autoimmune involvement. A cohort of 62 CU patients with positive ASST (group 1) underwent nine weekly ASIs, while 13 patients with negative ASST (group 2) served as controls. The results showed that 35.5% of ASST (+) patients were completely asymptomatic after treatment, with an additional 24.2% showing marked improvement. In contrast, 23% of ASST (–) patients achieved complete resolution, and another 23% showed significant improvement. Reductions in pruritus and antihistamine use were notable in both groups. The study concludes that AST is particularly effective for ASST (+) CU patients, but also beneficial, albeit to a lesser extent, for ASST (–) patients, suggesting its potential as a treatment option in recalcitrant cases of CU.
- In a study done by Panchami Debbarman et al. titled "Autologous serum therapy in CU," which was a double-blind, randomized controlled study aimed to evaluate the efficacy of autologous serum therapy (AST) in CU, particularly focusing on its impact on autoreactive urticaria (AU). A total of 111 patients were treated with either AST or placebo (normal saline injections) weekly for 9 weeks, alongside cetirizine as needed. The results demonstrated significant improvements in urticaria severity scores (TSS and UAS) starting as early as the 4th week in the AST group compared to placebo. The Dermatologic Life Quality Index (DLQI) also showed superior improvement with AST by the end of the study period. Interestingly, both AU and non-AU patients benefited similarly from AST, suggesting its efficacy extends beyond autoreactive mechanisms. Safety assessments indicated no significant adverse events related to AST. The study concludes that AST represents a promising therapeutic option for CU, offering potential relief and reducing the need for antihistamine medication, particularly beneficial in cases of autoreactive urticaria.
- In a systemic review done by Katja Oomen Welke titled "Intramuscular autologous blood therapy—a systematic review of controlled trials," which aimed to evaluate the efficacy and effector mechanisms of intramuscular autologous whole-blood therapy through a comprehensive analysis of prospective controlled trials. A meticulous search strategy identified eight studies meeting inclusion criteria, spanning various indications including urticaria, atopic dermatitis, ankylosing spondylitis, common cold, and respiratory tract infections. Despite varying study designs and methodologies, including differences in sample sizes and blinding protocols, the review highlighted significant methodological heterogeneity among the trials. Quality assessment using the Jadad score revealed a range from poorly to well-controlled trials, with only a minority achieving high scores due to issues such as small sample sizes and lack of blinding. This systematic review highlights significant heterogeneity among the eight randomized controlled trials (RCTs) assessing intramuscular autologous whole-blood therapy. Studies varied widely in design, sample sizes, controls, and treatment parameters, limiting the

CHAPTER 24: Autologous Blood/Serum Therapy in Urticaria

TABLE 2: Various studies performed to understand the effect of autologous serum therapy (AST) for the treatment of urticaria.

Study	Authors	Aim	Participants	Treatment	Results
Autologous serum therapy in chronic spontaneous urticaria	AK Bajaj et al.	Assess effectiveness of repeated autologous serum injections (ASIs) in chronic urticaria (CU) patients	62 CU patients with positive autologous serum skin test (ASST) (Group 1), 13 patients with negative ASST (Group 2)	Nine weekly ASIs (Group 1), no treatment (Group 2)	35.5% of ASST (+) patients asymptomatic, 24.2% showed marked improvement, 23% of ASST (–) patients asymptomatic, 23% showed significant improvement
Autologous serum therapy in chronic urticaria (double-blind, RCT)	Panchami Debbarman et al.	Evaluate efficacy of AST in CU, focusing on autoreactive urticaria (AU)	111 patients (treated with either AST or placebo, alongside cetirizine as needed)	Weekly injections for 9 weeks	Significant improvements in TSS and UAS scores from 4th week in AST group, superior DLQI improvement, no significant adverse events
Intramuscular autologous blood therapy (systematic review)	Katja Oomen Welke	Evaluate efficacy and effector mechanisms of intramuscular autologous whole-blood therapy	Various indications including urticaria, atopic dermatitis, ankylosing spondylitis, common cold, respiratory tract infections		Significant methodological heterogeneity, varying study designs, quality assessment revealed a range of poorly to well-controlled trials
Auto-hemotherapy in chronic urticaria	Abdolkarim Sheikhi et al.	Discuss potential of auto-hemotherapy, specifically intramuscular injections of autologous whole blood (AWB), for CU	Chronic urticaria patients, particularly ASST (+)	Intra-muscular injections of AWB	Auto-hemotherapy believed to modulate immune responses, potential mechanisms include anti-idiotype production, tolerance induction to IgE or FcεRI, regulatory T-cell activation

(DLQI: dermatology life quality index; IgE: immunoglobulin E; FcεRI: Fc epsilon RI; TSS: total severity score; UAS: urticaria activity score)

ability to draw quantitative conclusions. While some trials suggested potential benefits of autologous whole-blood therapy for conditions such as atopic eczema and ASST-positive urticaria, methodological issues such as small sample sizes and inadequate controls persisted across many studies. Effector mechanisms of autologous whole blood remain unclear, with only one study exploring potential immune-modulating effects. The review underscores the need for further high-quality RCTs with larger sample sizes to definitively establish the efficacy of autologous whole-blood therapy and to elucidate its mechanisms of action, which remain poorly understood at present.
- In a review done by Abdolkarim Sheikhi et al. titled "Autohemotherapy in chronic urticaria", the potential of autohemotherapy, specifically intramuscular injections of autologous whole blood, as a therapeutic option for CU, particularly in patients who test positive for ASST+ was discussed. CU, characterized by recurrent wheals and pruritus, affects a significant portion of the population with no identifiable external cause (chronic idiopathic urticaria). The recent evidence suggests an autoimmune basis in some CU cases, indicated by ASST positivity, which correlates with circulating histamine-releasing factors and autoantibodies. Autohemotherapy, though historically used and now re-examined, is believed to modulate immune responses by introducing autologous antigens via muscular injections, potentially inducing tolerance to histamine-releasing factors or their stimulators. Mechanisms proposed include anti-idiotype production against autoantibodies, tolerance induction to IgE or FcεRI, and regulatory T-cell activation, aiming to convert disease-causing antigens into regulatory ones. Further research is needed to validate these mechanisms and clarify the therapeutic efficacy of autologous whole blood in CU treatment.

CONCLUSION

The ABT/AST therapy can be termed as "old wine in a new bottle." There are equivocal results with this modality in urticaria, but as such there are no major side effects. Even though some trials reported beneficial effects of ABT, the efficacy of the same could not be ascertained. Therefore, further RCTs are required with higher quality and adequate sample size to determine the efficacy of ABT. The mechanism of action of ABT has yet to be scientifically determined. ABT or AST has shown effectiveness in ASST-positive patients with CU but a substantial number of ASST-negative patients have also been benefited from this treatment.

SUGGESTED READINGS

1. Bajaj AK, Saraswat A, Upadhyay A, Damisetty R, Dhar S. Autologous serum therapy in chronic urticaria: Old wine in a new bottle. Indian J Dermatol Venereol Leprol. 2008;74:109-13.
2. Debbarman P, Sil A, Datta PK, Bandyopadhyay D, Das NK. Autologous serum therapy in chronic urticaria: a promising complement to antihistamines. Indian J Dermatol. 2014;59(4):375-82.
3. Oomen-Welke K, Huber R. Intramuscular autologous blood therapy—a systematic review of controlled trials. BMC Complement Altern Med. 2019;19(1):248.
4. Sheikhi A, Azarbeig M, Karimi H. Autohemotherapy in chronic urticaria: what could be the autoreactive factors and curative mechanisms? Ann Dermatol. 2014;26(4):526-7.

CHAPTER 25

Diet in Urticaria

Manju Keshari

INTRODUCTION

Urticaria is a condition characterized by recurring episodes that significantly affect quality of life. Clinically, about half of patients exhibit only skin wheals, 10% experience angioedema, and 40% suffer from both. Each lesion typically lasts for 24 hours or less. The current guidelines classify urticaria as acute and chronic, depending on whether episodes persist for less than or more than 6 weeks (about 1 and a half months). Acute urticaria generally does not require extensive investigation since the trigger is often identifiable from the patient's history.

In contrast, chronic urticaria often lacks a clear trigger. The guidelines further categorize chronic urticaria into chronic spontaneous urticaria (CSU) and chronic inducible urticaria (CIU). The causes of CSU are often unknown, can occur at any age but are more prevalent among young adults, particularly in females. CIU includes conditions such as symptomatic dermographism, solar and heat urticaria, cold urticaria, delayed pressure urticaria, vibratory angioedema, cholinergic urticaria, contact and aquagenic urticaria.

PATHOGENESIS OF URTICARIA

Acute Urticaria

- *Mechanism*: Predominantly driven by IgE-mediated allergic reactions
- *Triggers*: Frequently caused by food allergens such as eggs, milk, peanuts, shellfish, and certain fruits

Chronic Urticaria

- *Mechanism*:
  - *Mast cell activation*: Central to the pathogenesis of chronic urticaria (CU)
    - *Histamine release*: Results in symptoms including itching, redness, and swelling

- *Other mediators*: Platelet-activating factor, leukotrienes, and prostaglandins that further amplify the inflammatory response
  - *Outcome*: Dermal edema presenting as characteristic urticarial lesions
- *Pathways of mast cell activation*:
  - *Immunological*: Involves IgE, IgG, or complement pathways. For instance, allergic reactions to dust mites or animal dander
  - *Nonimmunological*: Involves triggers such as transmembrane receptors or intracellular signals. Examples include physical factors such as exercise, pressure, or sunlight exposure

Nonimmunological Mechanisms

- *Triggers*: Include medications such as NSAIDs, infections such as bacterial or viral infections, certain foods such as chocolate or strawberries, and alcohol consumption
- *Characteristics*:
  - Food allergies are a rare cause of CU
  - To definitively identify food-induced CU, there are no reliable laboratory indicators or skin provocation tests

INVESTIGATIONS FOR FOOD ALLERGIES

When food allergy is suspected as a cause of urticaria, investigations might include detailed patient history, elimination diets, food diary analysis, skin prick tests (SPTs), or specific IgE blood tests to pinpoint the allergen.

Food Allergy Testing Methods

- *Skin prick testing:*
  - Can identify specific food allergens
  - Positive results do not always correlate with clinically relevant food-induced urticaria.
  - More useful in acute cases
- *Mast and basophil cell activation tests*:
  - More precise than measuring IgE levels
  - Supports the diagnosis of IgE-mediated food allergy
  - Promises more accurate identification of food triggers
- *Food challenge test*:
  - Also known as the *oral food challenge* (OFC)
  - Considered to be the gold standard in the diagnosis of food allergies that are non-IgE-mediated or IgE-mediated
- *Specific IgE (SIgE) testing*:
  - Indicates an allergy to certain foods, pollen, latex, mold, some medicines, dust mites, or insect venom from bites or stings
  - More helpful in diagnosing acute urticaria

CHRONIC URTICARIA AND DIAGNOSIS

Diagnostic Tests for Food-triggered Chronic Urticaria

The use of diagnostic tests such as the basophil activation test, mast cell activation tests, SIgE and the SPT identifying CU triggered by food in CSU has shown conflicting results. Most studies indicate low sensitivity for these tests and suggest they do not replace the food challenge test.

DIETARY PRACTICES AND CHRONIC URTICARIA

Food allergies are rarely the cause of CU, and the relationship between diet and CU is not clearly established. Many people restrict their diet, and dermatologists play a crucial role in helping patients find any reproducible connections between their dietary exposures and symptoms.

Pseudoallergens and Histamine-releasing Food

Pseudoallergens are chemicals that elicit hypersensitivity or intolerance reactions that mimic true allergic responses. These responses can be triggered by various substances, including additives in food, vasoactive histamine and other vasoactive compounds, and certain organic constituents found in vegetables, fruits, and spices.

Pseudoallergens may cause or exacerbate CU (hives) in a small percentage of patients. Preservatives, dyes, salicylates, and aromatic compounds are a few examples of pseudoallergens that are present in natural foods such as garlic, artichokes, tomatoes, certain fruits, and rhubarb as well as processed foods such processed meats and artificial sweeteners.

The symptoms of urticaria may be lessened by diet devoid of foods that release histamine and pseudoallergens. Food intolerance in CU is not a true allergy but involves food-related symptoms that are reproducible without immediate type 1 allergic reactions. Thus, foods that release histamine and pseudoallergens that could exacerbate urticaria include:
- Alcohol
- Food additives
- Flavoring agents
- Aromatic substances
- Preservatives
- Artificial colors
- Seafood
- Certain vegetables and fruits
- Fermented foods

Reactions to these foods are dose-dependent, with symptoms usually delayed by 4–12 hours, making it difficult for patients to identify specific triggers.

Histamine

Many people who suffer with CU reported that eating foods high in histamine, such aged cheese or red wine makes their symptoms worse. Not all foods high in histamine are classified as pseudoallergens. Mackerel, preserved meats, fermented cabbage, citrus fruits, and peanuts are some more popular foods high in histamine. A disparity between the breakdown of stored histamine and its accumulation leads to histamine intolerance.

Gluten

Autoimmune diseases, including celiac disease, have been linked to CU. Various case reports document patients with celiac disease developing CU following gluten ingestion. Different hypotheses imply that there may be a connection between celiac disease and CU, and that certain occurrences of chronic urticaria may represent cutaneous symptoms of the condition. The inflammatory reactions caused by celiac disease may lead to the stimulation of anti-IgE receptor antibodies and the activation of mast cells. A further factor in this syndrome may be increased gastrointestinal permeability, which allows antigens to pass through.

Alcohol

Numerous hypersensitivity responses have been linked to alcohol; urticaria is an uncommon but documented reaction. Drinking alcohol is known to raise total serum IgE levels. Several case reports have implicated alcohol consumption as a cause of urticaria; however, it is still unclear what causes mast cell activation pathophysiology. While the acute and long-term toxicological consequences of alcohol abuse are widely recognized, new research has focused on the lesser-known negative effects of alcohol intake, such as urticaria. The adverse effects are categorized as immunologic or nonimmunologic based on these investigations. Regarding urticarial responses to alcohol, three specific mechanisms have been proposed: (1) Direct effect of ethanol on mast cells, which results in their degranulation, (2) allergenic potential of ethanol metabolites, and (3) activation of endogenous opioid and prostaglandin receptors.

Caffeine

A few cases have mentioned caffeine hypersensitivity. Although coffee consumption is prevalent, urticaria caused by caffeine seems to be uncommon.

Lipids

Studies reveal that after ingesting aspirin, people with aspirin-induced urticaria have higher blood levels of arachidonic acid than age-matched controls. Fatty acids like arachidonic acid produce proinflammatory leukotrienes such leukotriene-B4, which has been shown to be a mediator of pruritus in a variety of inflammatory dermatoses.

Vitamin D

Adult patients with chronic urticaria are more likely to be deficient in vitamin D, according to a recent research. Patients with persistent urticaria had considerably lower serum 25[OH]D levels; however, symptoms improved after vitamin D supplementation.

Iron

Several case reports suggest a relationship between CU and low blood iron levels. Approximately 30% of patients with CU had low iron levels, and some of these patients' showed improvement or resolution of symptoms following iron treatment. Low ferritin levels have been associated with CU, particularly in males. In healthy individuals, about 3–6% of dietary nickel is typically absorbed. It has been shown that iron deficiency enhances the absorption of nickel, leading individuals with iron deficiency anemia to retain more nickel from their diet. Studies have shown that a combination of a low-nickel diet and high oral iron intake can significantly reduce the severity of urticarial activity, especially in nickel-sensitive individuals with iron deficiency.

DIAGNOSTIC AND THERAPEUTIC APPROACHES

Food Diaries, Oral Provocation Tests, and Elimination Diets

- *Food diaries*: Keeping an "urticarial diary" documenting symptom intensity, frequency, food intake, and other activities such as medication and stress can be helpful.
- *Elimination diets*: Patients adhere to a strict low-pseudoallergen diet for 3 weeks. Improvement in clinical manifestations suggests a diagnosis of CU due to intolerance.
- *Oral provocation tests (OPT)*: Used to confirm the diagnosis by reintroducing suspected triggers.

Monitoring and Assessment

The Urticaria Activity Score (UAS), a 0–3 point rating system that gauges the frequency of wheals and the intensity of itching, should be used to evaluate responses to the diet. Maximum points per day are 6 and weekly totals of 42 are obtained by adding these scores each day (UAS7). The degree of improvement is measured by comparing the use of on-demand antihistamine treatment prior to and following the diet, as well as UAS measurements.

Overall, while food-triggered chronic urticaria is rare, careful dietary management and monitoring can help identify and mitigate symptoms.

Urticaria Activity Score

In the past day, how many wheals have you observed?

Rating:
- *None*: 0
- *Mild*: 1 (<20 wheals in a 24-hour period)

- *Moderate*: 2 (20–50 wheals per day)
- *Severe*: 3 (>50 wheals per day)

In the past day, how bad has the itching been?

Rating:
- *None*: 0
- *Mild*: 1 (existing but not bothersome or grating)
- *Moderate*: 2 (difficult but does not obstruct regular daily activities or sleep)
- *Intense*: 3 (severe itch that is bothersome enough to prevent regular daily activities or sleep)

A safe, healthful, and inexpensive way to identify people with CSU who will benefit from avoiding pseudoallergens is to implement a pseudoallergen-free diet. **Table 1** describes in detail the food items allowed and prohibited in the pseudoallergen-free diet.

TABLE 1: Pseudoallergen-free diet.

Category of food	Allowed	Avoid
Fat	White butter (fresh), plant-based oils, ghee	Mayonnaise, margarine, and all other fats
Dairy products	Quark, fresh milk, and fresh cream (free of carrageen) natural yoghurt, fresh unseasoned cheese	All fermented dairy products (aged cheese, yogurt, sour cream), all other milk products
Simple food	Preservative-free bread and buns, chapati, sorghum, all millets, potatoes, rice, legumes, and durum noodles (without eggs)	All fermented foods (Idli, dosa), other food items (such as cakes, egg noodles, pasta, and pommes frites)
Salt and spices	Onions, sugar, chives, and salt	Garlic, herbs, and all other spices
Desserts	Not any	Anything sweet, even gum and sweeteners
Vegetables	All vegetables, except the forbidden ones, salad (cleaned thoroughly), broccoli, asparagus, Chinese cabbage, brussels sprouts, carrots, and zucchini	Chickpeas, mushroom, lettuce, eggplant, avocados, olives, pie plant, and artichokes, tomatoes all processed tomatoes, olives, paprika, fermented vegetables (sauerkraut, kimchi), overripe vegetables
Spreads	Honey, yogurt, and other products mentioned with dairy	Every other spread
Drinks	Coffee, milk, mineral water, and flavorless black tea	Alcohol, herbal tea, and all other drinks
Sea food	Caught frozen fish cooked at time of eating	All other seafood
Meat	Fresh meat	Unseasoned mincemeat, fresh self-made cold meat, aged sausages, meat (processed), smoked meat
Other		Food additives (dyes, preservatives, artificial sweeteners), chocolate, chewing gum, candy, eggs, strawberry, cherries

Provocative testing, which includes food additives (foods high in pseudoallergens for 2–4 days) is seen to aggravate the symptoms. Under infusion treatment and emergency standby conditions, this test should be conducted. Monitoring should be done for next 24 hours as there is risk of delayed reaction after provocation test.

Supplements and Remedies for Chronic Urticaria

Vitamin C
In the past, urticaria has been shown to improve with vitamin C at dosages of 1,000 mg three times a day. Furthermore, vitamin B12 deficiency has been discovered in one third of patients with CU, suggesting still another subject for possible future investigation.

Phenols
Fruits and vegetables include a class of phytonutrients called flavonoids, which are plant compounds that may prevent histamine from being released into in vitro mast cells. In allergic instances, quercetin at a dose of 500 mg three times a day has been demonstrated to be helpful. Flavonoids have anti-inflammatory, antiallergic, and antioxidant qualities. Flavonoids balance Th1/Th2 helper cells and prevent mast and basophil cell activation and associated cytokines through a variety of mechanisms, as demonstrated by recent clinical investigations.

CONCLUSION

About 50% of those with persistent urticaria are open to using drugs to alleviate their symptoms. Patients often request physicians to name the causative factors so they can cut them from their diet. In CSU, patients often associate the onset of symptoms with various activities, medications, or foods.

While most guidelines discourage the identification of food as a cause of chronic urticaria, it is common for patients to believe that the consumption of certain foods worsens their condition or causes it. However, few studies have been conducted to confirm or disprove this association. The self-reported prevalence of food as a trigger of CSU ranges from 13 to 80%, depending on diet and social customs of different populations. The exact reason for the high self-report rate is unknown. Patients often lack information about the disease and may name the last action they performed as a trigger, particularly since urticaria can spontaneously appear around mealtimes. Some studies have shown that food restrictions are not relevant in CSU and that diet modifications are ineffective.

However, determined patients may find that making dietary changes, such as giving up foods high in histamines, avoiding pseudoallergens, switching to a gluten-free diet, or cutting back on alcohol, is a more affordable way to manage their symptoms.

Furthermore, certain food supplements, including iron, vitamin D, vitamin C, and flavonoids, have been found effective in the treatment of urticarial symptoms in some studies.

SUGGESTED READINGS

1. Powell RJ, Leech SC, Till S, Huber PAJ, Nasser SM, Clark AT. BSACI guideline for the management of chronic urticaria and angioedema. Clin Exp Allergy. 2015;45(3):547-65.
2. NIAID-Sponsored Expert Panel; Boyce JA, Assa'ad A, Burks AW, Jones SM, Sampson HA, Wood RA, et al. Guidelines for the diagnosis and management of food allergy in the United States: summary of the NIAID-Sponsored Expert Panel report. J Allergy Clin Immunol. 2010; 126(6 Suppl):S1-58.
3. Zuberbier T, Aberer W, Asero R, Abdul Latiff AH, Baker D, Ballmer-Weber B, et al. The EAACI/GA2LEN/EDF/WAO guideline for the definition, classification, diagnosis and management of urticaria. The 2017 revision and update. Allergy. 2018;73:1393-414.
4. Nicolas JF. Chronic spontaneous urticaria is not an allergic disease. Eur J Dermatol. 2011;21:349-53.
5. Theoharides TC, Valent P, Akin C. Mast cells, mastocytosis, and related disorders. N Engl J Med. 2015;373(2):163-72.
6. Bergmann MM, Santos AF. Basophil activation test in the food allergy clinic: its current use and future applications. Medicina (Kaunas). 2019;55(10):651.
7. Thaiwat S, Nakakes A, Sangasapaviliya A. The effect of food avoidance in adult patients with chronic idiopathic urticaria. J Med Assoc Thailand. 2015;98(12):1162-8.
8. Kang M, Song W, Park H, Lim K-H, Kim S-J, Lee S-Y, et al. Basophil activation test with food additives in chronic urticaria patients. Clin Nutr Res. 2014;3(1):9-16.
9. Ebo DG, Heremans K, Beyens M, van der Poorten MM, Van Gasse AL, Mertens C, et al. Flow-based allergen testing: Can mast cells beat basophils? Clin Chim Acta. 2022;532:64-71.
10. Hsu M-L, Li L-F. Prevalence of food avoidance and food allergy in Chinese patients with chronic urticaria. Br J Dermatol. 2012;166(4):747-52.
11. Trujillo MJ, Rodriguez A, Gracia Bara MT, Matheu V, Herrero T, Rubio M, et al. Dietary recommendations for patients allergic to Anisakis simplex. Allergol Immunopathol (Madr). 2002;30(6):311-4.
12. Zuberbier T, Maurer M, Grattan C. Urticaria and Angioedema. Berlin, Heidelberg: Springer-Verlag; 2010.
13. Magerl M 1, Pisarevskaja D, Scheufele R, Zuberbier T, Maurer M. Effects of a pseudoallergen-free diet on chronic spontaneous urticaria: a prospective trial. Allergy. 2010;65(1):78-83.
14. Zuberbier T. The role of allergens and pseudoallergens in urticaria. J Investig Dermatol Symp Proc. 2001;6(2):132-4.
15. Supramaniam G, Warner JO. Artificial food additive intolerance in patients with angio-oedema and urticaria. Lancet. 1986;2(8512):907-9.
16. Maurer M, Grabbe J. Urticaria: its history-based diagnosis and etiologically oriented treatment. Dtsch Arztebl Int. 2008;105:458-65.
17. Reese I, Zuberbier T, Bunselmeyer B, Erdmann S, Henzgen M, Fuchs T, et al. Diagnostic approach for suspected pseudoallergic reaction to food ingredients. Dtsch Dermatol Ges. 2009;7:70-7.
18. Kaplan AP. Dietary therapy for chronic urticaria. Curr Allergy Asthma Rep. 2010;10(4):225-6.
19. Moneret-Vautrin DA. Allergic and pseudo-allergic reactions to foods in chronic urticaria. Ann Dermatol Venereol. 2003;130 Spec No 1:1S35-42.
20. Maurer M, Metz M, Magerl M, Siebenhaar F, Staubach P. Relevance of food allergies and intolerance reactions as causes of urticaria. Hautarzt. 2003;54:138-43.
21. Maurer M, Magerl M, Pisarevskaja D, Scheufele R, Zuberbier T. Effects of a pseudoallergen-free diet on chronic spontaneous urticaria: a prospective trial. Allergy. 2010;65(1):78-83.
22. Peroni DG, Paiola G, Tenero L, Fornaro M, Bodini A, Pollini F, et al. Chronic urticaria and celiac disease: A case report. Pediatr Dermatol. 2010;27(1):108-9.
23. Candelli M, Nista EC, Gabrielli M, Santarelli L, Pignataro G, Cammarota G, et al. Celiac disease and chronic urticaria resolution: A case report. Dig Dis Sci. 2004;49(9):1489-90.

24. Hautekeete ML, DeClerck LS, Stevens WJ. Chronic urticaria associated with coeliac disease. Lancet. 1987.
25. Nakagawa Y, Sumikawa Y, Nakamura T, Itami S, Katayama I, Aoki T. Urticarial reaction caused by ethanol. Allergol Int. 2006;55(4):411-4.
26. Ribeiro F, Sousa N, Carrapatoso I, Segorbe Luís A. Urticaria after ingestion of alcoholic beverages. J Invest Allergol Clin Immunol. 2014;24(2):122-3.
27. Sticherling M, Brasch J, Bruning H, Christophers E. Urticarial and anaphylactoid reactions following ethanol intake. Br J Dermatol. 1995;132(3):464-7.
28. Rehm J. The risks associated with alcohol use and alcoholism. Alcohol Res Health. 2011;34(2):135-43.
29. Adams KE, Rans TS. Adverse reactions to alcohol and alcoholic beverages. Ann Allergy Asthma Immunol. 2013;111(6):439-45.
30. Hadjieconomou S, Mughal A. Segmental urticaria triggered by alcohol consumption. JAAD Case Rep. 2020;6(2):144-5.
31. Quirce Gancedo S, Freire P, Rivas M, Dávila I, Losada E. Urticaria from caffeine. J Allergy Clin Immunol. 1991;88:680-1.
32. Caballero T, García-Ara C, Pascual C, Diaz-Pena JM, Ojeda A. Urticaria induced by caffeine. J Investig Allergol Clin Immunol. 1993;3:160-2.
33. Cornejo-García JA, Jagemann LR, Blanca-López N, Doña I, Flores C, Guéant-Rodríguez RM, et al. Genetic variants of the arachidonic acid pathway in non-steroidal anti-inflammatory drug-induced acute urticaria. Clin Exp Allergy 2012;42(12):1772-81.
34. Searing DA, Leung DY. Vitamin D in atopic dermatitis, asthma and allergic diseases. Immunol Allergy Clin N Am. 2010;30:397-409.
35. Chandrashekar L, Rajappa M, Munisamy M, Ananthanarayanan PH, Thappa DM, Arumugam B. 25-Hydroxy vitamin D levels in chronic urticaria and its correlation with disease severity from a tertiary care centre in South India. Clin Chem Lab Med. 2014;52:115-8.
36. Rather S, Keen A, Sajad P. Serum levels of 25-hydroxyvitamin D in chronic urticaria and its association with disease activity: a case control study. Indian Dermatol Online J. 2018;9:170-4.
37. Kelly C. Nickel, boron, vanadium, cobalt and other trace metal nutrients. In: Kelly C (Ed). The Nutritional Trace Metals. UK: Blackwell Publishing Ltd; 2004. pp. 211-33.
38. Sharma AD. Benefit of iron therapy in the management of chronic urticaria due to nickel sensitivity. Indian J Dermatol. 2010;55(4):407-8.4.
39. Oršolić N. Allergic inflammation: Effect of propolis and its flavonoids. Molecules. 2022; 27(19):6694.

CHAPTER 26

Antihistamines in Urticaria

Sunil Kumar Gupta

INTRODUCTION

Management of urticaria is difficult because of the abrupt onset of wheals and/or angioedema. H1 antihistamines are the cornerstone of treatment, addressing symptoms by antagonizing histamine receptors. This chapter synthesizes current evidence on the role of H1 antihistamines in urticaria management. Intramuscular first-generation H1-antihistamines, notably diphenhydramine, combined with ranitidine or cimetidine, show efficacy in acute urticaria, while second-generation counterparts are preferred for chronic cases due to their superior safety profile. However, in cases of inadequate response or intolerance, systematic progression through treatment options, including dosage adjustments and transitioning between second-generation agents, is warranted. Special considerations apply to vulnerable populations, such as pregnant and lactating women, where safety profiles must be carefully weighed. In conclusion, the judicious selection and utilization of H1 antihistamines are vital in effectively managing urticaria and optimizing patient outcomes.

PATHOPHYSIOLOGY OF URTICARIA

Although several cells are involved in the etiology of urticaria, mast cells and basophils play critical roles. Urticaria symptoms are caused by the activation of cutaneous mast cells and followed by the release of inflammatory mediators such as histamines and cytokines. FcεRI, G protein-coupled receptor X2, C5a receptor 1, protease-activated receptors (PAR1 and PAR2), and chemoattractant receptors are expressed by dermal mast cells.

Two mechanisms are involved in the activation of basophils and mast cells. IgE mediates the first pathway, which acts against various autoallergens. IgG that is directed toward the FcεRI IgE receptor or FcεRI-bound IgE mediates the second pathway. The two mechanisms that include the stimulation of downstream signaling pathways and the cross-linking of FcεRI overlap. BTK serves as the hub of this regulatory network. Mast cell activation and degranulation result from the phosphorylation of downstream targets caused by BTK activation. Strong inflammatory mediators, including prostaglandin D2, histamine, tryptase, platelet-activating factor, leukotrienes, TNF, IL-4, IL-5, IL-13, IL-17, and IL-31, are therefore produced.

PHARMACOLOGY OF ANTIHISTAMINES

Histamine is a heterocyclic amine that is obtained via the decarboxylation of l-histidine in mast cells and basophils. Its effects on inflammation are both pro- and anti-inflammatory, depending on the cells activated and the histamine receptor subtype. Histamine receptors are of four different varieties: H1, H2, H3, and H4. Histamine, after binding with H1 receptors, exerts inflammatory reactions. Numerous organs and cells express them, such as the hepatic cells, endothelial cells, vascular smooth muscle cells, respiratory epithelium, neurons, and lymphocytes.

Erythematous wheals are caused by histamine binding to H1 receptors on tiny capillary venules (angioedema). Vasodilation and increased vascular permeability lead to the leaking of large molecular weight proteins such as immunoglobulins into the interstitium from plasma. In addition to causing itching due to sensory nerve stimulation, histamine also attracts neutrophils, eosinophils, basophils, and other immune cells, as shown by the mixed cellular infiltration found in histopathological specimens of wheals.

H1 antihistamines work as inverse agonists by interacting with and stabilizing the H1 receptor's inactive conformation. This results into the lower expression of molecules involved in cell adhesion, chemotaxis, and antigen presentation, as well as proinflammatory cytokines. At a higher dose, antihistamines further reduce the release of inflammatory mediators via calcium ion channels.

Evolution of Antihistamines

H1 antihistamines are the main treatment of urticaria. The development of different generations of H1 antihistamines has taken a long time. At the Pasteur Institute, systematic searches for compounds that counteract histamine's physiological effects began in the 1930s. As early as 1911, thymoxy ethyldiethylamine was synthesized to make the first antihistamines. Fourneau and Bovet found that the best phenolic ether for blocking or neutralizing histamine's effects was 2-isopropyl-5-methyl phenoxyethyl diethylamine. This substance served as the basis for the ethanolamine series. The first antihistamine to be used clinically in humans was the chemical Antergan (N1N dimethyl-N1-benzyl-Nphenyl-ethylenediamine), which was introduced in 1942.

Following that, phenergan (1948) and diphenhydramine (1945) came into existence. The name H1 receptor was given by Ash and Schild in 1966.

Classification of H1 Antihistamines

The classification of antihistamines is given in **Table 1**.

TABLE 1: Classification of oral H1 antihistamines.		
First generation	**Chemical classification**	**Second generation**
• Brompheniramine, Chlorpheniramine	Alkylamines	Acrivastine
• Buclizine • Cyclizine • Hydroxyzine • Meclizine	Piperazines	• Cetirizine • Levocetirizine
• Azatadine • Cyproheptadine • Diphenylpyraline	Piperidines	• Astemizole • Bilastine • Desloratadine • Ebastine • Fexofenadine • Loratadine • Mizolastine • Olopatadine • Rupatadine • Terfenadine
• Carbinoxamine • Clemastine • Dimenhydrinate • Diphenhydramine • Doxylamine	Ethanolamines	
• Antazoline • Pyrilamine • Tripelennamine	Ethylenediamines	
• Methdilazine • Promethazine	Phenothiazines	

Pharmacokinetics and Pharmacodynamics of Oral H1 Antihistamine

Table 2 shows the pharmacokinetics and pharmacodynamics of different H1 antihistamines adopted from Simons.

First-generation H1 Antihistamines

Since these drugs are lipophilic and readily cross the blood–brain barrier, they have sedative and anticholinergic side effects. More than 20% of patients have significant drowsiness and performance impairment (e.g., fine motor skills, driving abilities, and response times).

Dry mouth, diplopia, impaired vision, urine retention, and vaginal dryness are among potential adverse effects of anticholinergic medications. It is recommended

TABLE 2: Pharmacokinetics and pharmacodynamics of oral H1 antihistamines.

H1 Antihistamines	Time to maximum plasma concentration (t_{max}) in hours	Onset of action (hours)	Duration of actions (hours)	Elimination half-life ($t_{1/2}$) in hours	Mean oral bio-availability
Chlorpheniramine	2.8 ± 0.8	3	24	27.9 ± 8.7	25–59%
Diphenhydramine	1.7 ± 1.0	2	12	9.2 ± 2.5	40–60%
Hydroxyzine	2.1 ± 0.4	2	24	20.0 ± 4.1	80%
Cetirizine	1.0 ± 0.5	1	24	6.5–10	70%
Levocetirizine	0.8 ± 0.5	1	24	7 ± 1.5	85%
Loratadine	1.2 ± 0.3	2	24	7.8 ± 4.2	40%
Desloratadine	1–3	2	24	27	83%
Ebastine	2.6–5.7	2	24	10.3–19.3	60–70%
Fexofenadine	2.6	2	24	14.4	33%
Mizolastine	1.5	1	24	12.9	65%
Rupatadine	0.75–1.0	2	24	4.3–13.0	25%
Bilastine	1.13	1	24	12–14.5	60%

TABLE 3: Parenterally used first-generation H1 antihistamines.

Drug	Dose in adults	Dose in children
Diphenhydramine	25–50 mg IV/IM QID	0.5–1.25 mg/kg IV/IM QID
Hydroxyzine	25–50 mg deep IM QID	0.5–1 mg/kg deep IM QID

that the drug should be taken at bedtime in order to avoid sedative side effects. Apart from their oral use, nowadays, the drugs of this group are increasingly being used parenterally to manage acute urticaria in an emergency. These are described in **Table 3**.

Second-generation H1 Antihistamines

These medications have few notable drug–drug interactions, need less frequent doses than first-generation medicines, have little sedative effects, and are almost devoid of anticholinergic effects. Higher than usual dosages may be necessary for certain people to treat their urticarial symptoms, and these higher doses may cause drowsiness. Therefore, prudence is advised until the effects on the person are known. The important drugs of this group are tabulated in **Table 4**.

ANTIHISTAMINES IN URTICARIA

The H1 antihistamines are often used as a first-line drug to manage acute or chronic urticaria with or without angioedema.

TABLE 4: Orally used second-generation antihistamines.

Drugs	Nature	Dose in adults	Dose in children	Safety in hepatic/Renal disorders	Drug/Food interaction
Cetirizine	• Mast cell stabilizer • Moderately sedative	10 mg OD	2–12 years—5 mg OD 6 months to 2 years—2.5 mg OD	Dose should be halved	–
Levocetirizine	• Active enantiomer of cetirizine • Mild sedative	5 mg OD	6–11 years—2.5 mg OD	Dose reduced in renal disease	–
Loratadine	• Selective H1 antihistamine • Longer duration of action	10 mg OD	>6 years—10 mg OD 2–5 years—5 mg OD	Alternate-day dosing in hepatic/renal disease	–
Desloratadine	Active metabolite of loratadine	5 mg OD	>12 years—5 mg OD 5–11 years—2.5 mg OD 1–5 years—1.25 mg OD 6 months to 1 year—1 mg OD	Alternate-day dosing in hepatic/renal disease	–
Fexofenadine	Minimally sedative	180 mg OD	>12 years—180 mg OD 2–11 years—30 mg BID 6 months to 2 years—15 mg BID	Not safe in renal disease, dose should be 60 mg OD in adults	Avoid with food, should be taken empty stomach
Bilastine	• A zwitterion, slightly passes the blood brain barrier • Minimally sedative	20 mg OD	>12 years—20 mg OD	No safety data	Avoid with food, grapefruit juice, ketoconazole and erythromycin
Rupatadine	Also block platelet activating factor receptor	10 mg OD	>12 years—10 mg OD		Avoid with grapefruit juice, ketoconazole and erythromycin

The systematic review and meta-analysis on the treatment of acute urticaria have given more weightage to the intramuscular first-generation H1-antihistamine in decreasing pruritus symptoms though sedation and drowsiness are prominent with this.

The newer second-generation antihistamines in standard doses are recommended by the experts as first-line therapy for the treatment of chronic spontaneous/inducible urticaria and strongly against the use of first-generation drugs, especially in children according to the international EAACI/GA²LEN/EuroGuiDerm/APAAACI guideline. Astemizole and terfenadine should also be avoided due to cardiotoxic effects in individuals treated with cytochrome P450 (CYP) 3A4 isoenzyme inhibitors such as ketoconazole or erythromycin.

The research indicates that certain individuals experiencing urticaria, who do not adequately respond to the standard dosage of a second-generation H1-antihistamine, may derive benefits from increasing the dosage, rather than combining different types of second-generation H1-antihistamines due to their distinct pharmacological properties. Guidelines advise considering an increase in dosage by up to four times in such cases. However, it is essential to note that informing patients about this practice is crucial, as it falls under off-label use. Furthermore, exceeding a four-fold dosage increment is not recommended, as it lacks sufficient testing and validation.

Consider transitioning to an alternative second-generation H1-antihistamine in individuals whose symptoms exhibit insufficient response or intolerance to the initial medication, whether at standard or escalated doses.

It is advisable to gradually raise the dose of second-generation H1 antihistamine medication every 2–4 weeks, in patients of severe and treatment-resistant illness.

H1 Antihistamines in Children

It is noteworthy that first-generation H1 antihistamines are not very safe in children. Conversely, second-generation H1-antihistamines (bilastine, cetirizine, desloratadine, fexofenadine, levocetirizine, loratadine, and rupatadine) are quite safe and effective in pediatric populations. In the selection of a second-generation H1-antihistamine for pediatric urticaria management, factors such as the child's age and the availability of appropriate formulations (e.g., syrup or fast-dissolving tablets) should be carefully considered, recognizing that not all formulations are universally accessible or suitable for pediatric use.

H1 Antihistamines in Pregnant and Lactating Women

The safety of urticaria treatment remains inadequately explored in pregnant women. The available evidence recommend the use of cetirizine and loratadine. Given the paramount importance of ensuring safety during pregnancy, the recommendation leans toward the use of loratadine and cetirizine. The consideration of increased dosages of modern second-generation H1-antihistamines during pregnancy warrants careful deliberation, given the absence of comprehensive safety studies. The first-generation antihistamines should be avoided during pregnancy.

It is interesting to note that breast milk contains very little amounts of all H1-antihistamines. Therefore, the utilization of second-generation H1-antihistamines is encouraged, as infants nursed by mothers occasionally exhibit sedation when exposed to older first-generation H1-antihistamines through breast milk.

CONCLUSION

H1 antihistamines are essential for the treatment of acute and chronic urticaria, with or without angioedema. They are the cornerstone of pharmacotherapy due to their ability to alleviate symptoms by blocking histamine receptors. In acute urticaria, first-generation H1-antihistamines, particularly when administered intramuscularly, demonstrate efficacy in reducing pruritus symptoms. For chronic urticaria, second-generation H1-antihistamines are recommended as first-line therapy, offering superior safety profiles and efficacy, especially in pediatric populations.

However, in cases where symptoms persist or intolerances arise, a systematic approach is advocated, including transitioning to alternative second-generation H1-antihistamines or considering dosage adjustments. It's essential to prioritize safety, particularly in vulnerable populations such as pregnant and lactating women, where the use of loratadine and cetirizine may be considered with caution.

Overall, the judicious selection and utilization of H1 antihistamines, guided by evidence-based recommendations and individual patient characteristics, are crucial in effectively managing urticaria and improving patient outcomes.

LEARNING POINTS

- In both acute and chronic urticaria, H1 antihistamines are often used as first-line treatment.
- Intramuscular first-generation H1-antihistamines have shown efficacy in relieving pruritus symptoms in acute urticaria.
- Second-generation antihistamines are safe in children and used as first-line therapy in urticaria.
- Modern second-generation H1-antihistamines, such as loratadine and cetirizine, are generally considered safe during pregnancy, with caution and careful consideration of dosage adjustments.
- Updosing of second-generation H1-antihistamines may benefit individuals with urticaria who do not respond adequately to standard dosages.
- Transitioning to alternative second-generation H1-antihistamines is recommended for individuals with insufficient response or intolerance to the initial medication.
- Systematic progression through first-line treatment options every 2–4 weeks is advised, with more frequent intervals in severe and treatment-resistant cases.

SUGGESTED READINGS

1. Giménez-Arnau AM, Manzanares N, Podder I. Recent updates in urticaria. Med Clin (Barc). 2023;161(10):435-44. [English, Spanish].
2. Liu X, Cao Y, Wang W. Burden of and trends in urticaria globally, regionally, and nationally from 1990 to 2019: Systematic analysis. JMIR Public Health Surveill. 2023;9:e50114.
3. Kolkhir P, Gimenez-Arnau AM, Kulthanan K, Peter J, Metz M, Maurer M. Urticaria. Nat Rev Dis Primers. 2022;8:61.
4. Alvarado D, Maurer M, Gedrich R, Seibel SB, Murphy MB, Crew L, et al. The anti-KIT monoclonal antibody CDX-0159 induces profound and durable mast cell suppression in a healthy volunteer study. Allergy. 2022;77:2393-403.
5. Bernstein JA, Maurer M, Saini SS. BTK signaling-a crucial link in the pathophysiology of chronic spontaneous urticaria. J Allergy Clin Immunol. 2024;153(5):1229-40.
6. Bolognia J, Schaffer JV, Cerroni L. Dermatology, 4th edition. Philadelphia: Elsevier; 2018.
7. Emanuel MB. Histamine and the antiallergic antihistamines: a history of their discoveries. Clin Exp Allergy. 1999;29(Suppl 3):1-11; discussion 12.
8. Simons FE. Advances in H1-antihistamines. N Engl J Med. 2004;351(21):2203-17.
9. Simons FE, Simons KJ. Histamine and H1-antihistamines: celebrating a century of progress. J Allergy Clin Immunol. 2011;128(6):1139-50.
10. Adelsberg BR. Sedation and performance issues in the treatment of allergic conditions. Arch Intern Med. 1997;157(5):494-500.
11. Badloe FMS, Grosber M, Ring J, Kortekaas Krohn I, Gutermuth J. Treatment of acute urticaria: A systematic review. J Eur Acad Dermatol Venereol. 2024;38(11):2082-92.
12. Sabroe RA, Lawlor F, Grattan CEH, Ardern-Jones MR, Bewley A, Campbell L, et al. British Association of Dermatologists guidelines for the management of people with chronic urticaria 2021. Br J Dermatol. 2022;186(3):398-413.
13. Zuberbier T, Abdul Latiff AH, Abuzakouk M, Aquilina S, Asero R, Baker D, et al. The international EAACI/GA²LEN/EuroGuiDerm/APAAACI guideline for the definition, classification, diagnosis, and management of urticaria. Allergy. 2022;77:734-66.
14. Weber-Schoendorfer C, Schaefer C. The safety of cetirizine during pregnancy. A prospective observational cohort study. Reprod Toxicol. 2008;26(1):19-23.
15. Schwarz EB, Moretti M, Nayak S, Koren G. Risk of hypospadias in offspring of women using loratadine during pregnancy: a systematic review and meta-analysis. Drug Saf. 2008;31(9):775-88.
16. Church MK, Maurer M, Simons FE, Bindslev-Jensen C, van Cauwenberge P, Bousquet J, et al. Risk of first-generation H(1)-antihistamines: A GA(2)LEN position paper. Allergy. 2010;65(4):459-66.

CHAPTER 27

Systemic Therapies in Urticaria

Aanchal Bansal, Geeti Khullar

INTRODUCTION

Urticaria is derived from the Latin word "*urtica*" meaning "to burn". It presents with transient well-demarcated, itchy, superficial wheals with surrounding erythema and dermal edema. Urticaria has been broadly classified into spontaneous urticaria and inducible urticaria. Spontaneous urticaria is further divided into acute urticaria, presenting with wheals or angioedema for less than 6 weeks and chronic urticaria of disease duration more than 6 weeks. Many etiological factors such as infections, food, drugs, and psychogenic factors are implicated, but mostly it is idiopathic. Inducible urticaria, on the other hand, is broadly classified into thermal, mechanical (pressure-/vibration-induced), cholinergic, solar, aquagenic, and contact urticaria.

The pathophysiologic mechanism involves cutaneous mast cells as predominant cells, with some evidence for the role of peripheral blood basophils relevant to delayed response in spontaneous urticaria. Immunologic and non-immunologic triggers lead to degranulation of mast cells and release of various inflammatory mediators such as histamine, tryptase and other cytokines causing recruitment of inflammatory cells such as neutrophils, basophils, eosinophils and lymphocytes, vasodilation, and increased vascular permeability. Eosinophils lead to degranulation of mast cells indirectly by release of major basic protein. The sustained release of histamine from influxed basophils with generation of cysteinyl leukotrienes (CysLTs) may prolong the wheal response. An immunopathologic mechanism involving immunoglobulin E (IgE) bound to high-affinity IgE receptor (FcεR1) on mast cells leads to intracellular signaling, inducing mast cell degranulation.

The definite treatment of urticaria is elimination of the inciting cause, avoidance of triggering factors, and treatment of acute symptoms with H1 antihistamines until remission occurs. Second-generation antihistamines are preferred as the first-line treatment due to their lower anti-cholinergic and central nervous system side effects. The dose can be uptitrated up to four times the standard dose if symptoms are not controlled and replaced with another second-generation H1 antihistamine, if symptoms still persist. In patients who do not achieve adequate control with antihistamines, GA²LEN/EAACI/EuroGuiDerm/APAAACI guidelines recommend addition of omalizumab as add-on therapy. However, inadequate control with either therapy necessitates consideration of other systemic treatment options. This chapter highlights important systemic agents and their evidence in literature in the treatment of urticaria.

IMPORTANT SYSTEMIC AGENTS

Leukotriene Antagonists

Leukotriene antagonists (LTAs) are selective competitive inhibitors of CysLT receptor. These are classically used in the treatment of allergic rhinitis and bronchial asthma due to their bronchodilator action. Montelukast is a leukotriene D4 (LTD4) antagonist and zafirlukast is a leukotriene C4 (LTC4) antagonist, used more specifically in the treatment of urticaria.

Mechanism of Action in Urticaria
- Arachidonic acid is released from membrane phospholipids by phospholipase A2 enzyme and further catabolized to LTA4 by the 5-lipooxygenase pathway.
- LTA4 is an unstable molecule, which is either converted to LTB4 (chemoattractant) or conjugated to glutathione-containing molecule LTC4, which is further converted to yield LTD4 and LTE4.
- CysLT 1 and 2 receptors are activated by CysLTs: LTC4, LTD4, and LTE4.
- CysLTs play a role in eosinophil recruitment and increased vascular permeability leading to wheal formation and inflammation.
- LTAs bind to G-coupled CysLT receptors exhibiting different expression patterns, thereby inhibiting inflammation as shown in **Figure 1**.

Use and Efficacy in Urticaria
- The British Association of Dermatologists (BAD) guidelines suggest addition of montelukast besides antihistamines as first line in chronic spontaneous urticaria (CSU), if control is not achieved with higher doses of antihistamines alone, in salicylates-induced urticaria, or when angioedema is the predominant symptom.
- Anecdotal evidence suggests the therapeutic role of LTAs in chronic idiopathic urticaria (CIU) associated with aspirin, food hypersensitivity, or autoreactivity to autologous serum skin testing, in addition to antihistamines.
- LTAs are also considered effective in primary cold urticaria, delayed-pressure urticaria, and dermographism.
- Rayner et al. conducted a systematic review and meta-analysis that showed the efficacy of combination of LTAs with antihistamines in improving urticaria, itch, and wheal severity and achievement of better quality of life as compared to antihistamines alone. The study recommended that addition of LTAs increased the absolute chance of improvement in urticaria activity by 12% (moderate evidence); however, their role in the treatment of angioedema remains uncertain.

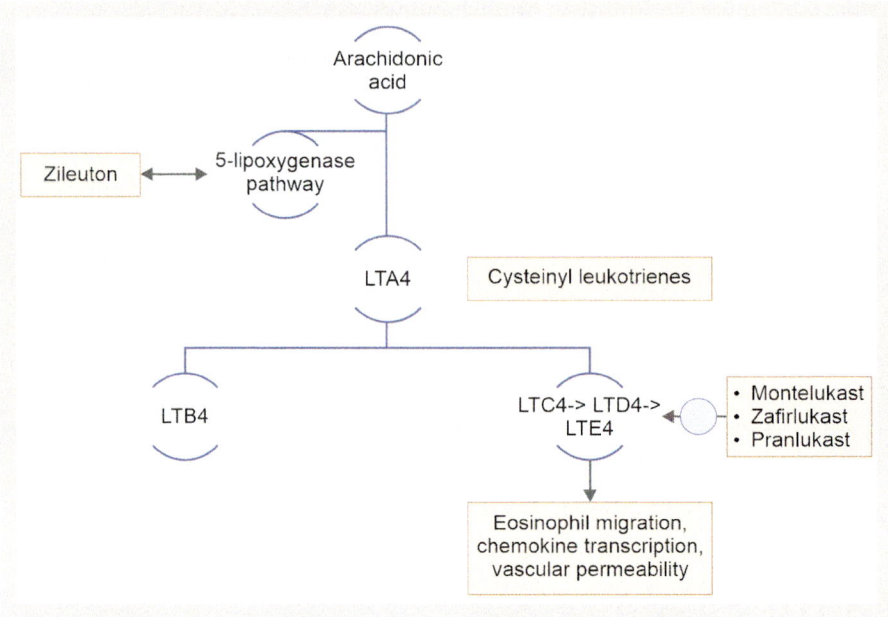

FIG. 1: Leukotriene pathway with 5-lipooxygenase cascade.

Dose
- *Montelukast*:
  - Adults (>15 years): 10 mg/day before bed
  - Children (6–14 years): 5 mg/day before bed; (2–5 years): 4 mg/day before bed
- *Zafirlukast*:
  - Age > 11 years: 20 mg twice daily
  - Age 7–11 years: 10 mg twice daily

Side Effects
- Montelukast has been reported to cause hepatobiliary and pancreatic dysfunction. Hepatotoxicity is reversible after discontinuation of medication.
- Neuropsychiatric features such as hyperactivity (most common), nervousness, nyctophobia, agitation, insomnia, and hallucinations were reported by Calapai et al.
- The Food and Drug Administration (FDA) has added a black-box warning regarding neuropsychiatric adverse events of LTAs; however, Rayner et al. claimed that no large-scale randomized controlled trials have been undertaken to evaluate these neuropsychiatric side effects. Studies on LTAs in asthma and allergic rhinitis have reported only 0.6% higher risk of these events; hence, further studies are warranted to confirm this.

Systemic Corticosteroids

Systemic corticosteroids are the mainstay of treatment in various dermatological conditions considering their vast anti-inflammatory and immunosuppressive actions exerted through both cytosolic and intranuclear receptors.

Mechanism of Action in Urticaria
- The known anti-inflammatory and vasoconstrictive activity leads to improvement in symptoms.
- Corticosteroids do not directly inhibit the mast cell activation and histamine release; instead, they modulate the immune response by reducing mast cell numbers and tissue histamine content.
- They also suppress autoantibody formation.

Use and Efficacy in Urticaria
- The GA^{2}LEN/EAACI/EuroGuiDerm/APAAACI guidelines recommend a short course of systemic steroids (maximum 10 days) for acute urticaria and acute severe exacerbations of CSU.
- Corticosteroids are preferred in low doses with rapid tapering when disease control is achieved.
- Many case reports mention efficacy of steroids in rapid control of disease in autoimmune urticaria; however, none of the studies reported long-term remission and complete disease control.
- Vas et al. reported use of low-dose steroid therapy (40 mg/day till symptoms subsided, followed by tapering) for an average period of 3.5 months with long-term remission and no relapse on follow-up in 35 out of 42 patients.

Dose
The starting dose is 0.5 mg/kg/day.

Side Effects
Long-term use of steroid therapy can be associated with systemic adverse events as summarized in **Table 1**.

Cyclosporine

Cyclosporine (CsA) is an oral calcineurin inhibitor derived from fungus *Tolypocladium inflatum*. It is used for its immunomodulatory and anti-inflammatory properties due to its action on T cells. It is approved by the FDA for the treatment of severe, recalcitrant psoriasis and used off-label in various inflammatory dermatoses.

Mechanism of Action in Urticaria
- Formation of complex between CsA and cyclophilin leads to inhibition of calcineurin enzyme **(Fig. 2)**.

TABLE 1: Side effects related to prolonged systemic corticosteroid treatment.	
System	Side effects
Metabolic	• Hyperglycemia, hypertension, cushingoid features • Weight gain, menstrual irregularities
Bone	• Osteoporosis • Osteonecrosis
Psychiatric	• Psychosis • Depression
Ocular	• Cataract • Glaucoma
Cutaneous	Delayed wound healing, acneiform eruptions, purpura, infections, hypertrichosis
Hypothalamic-pituitary axis suppression	• Steroid withdrawal syndrome • Addisonian crisis

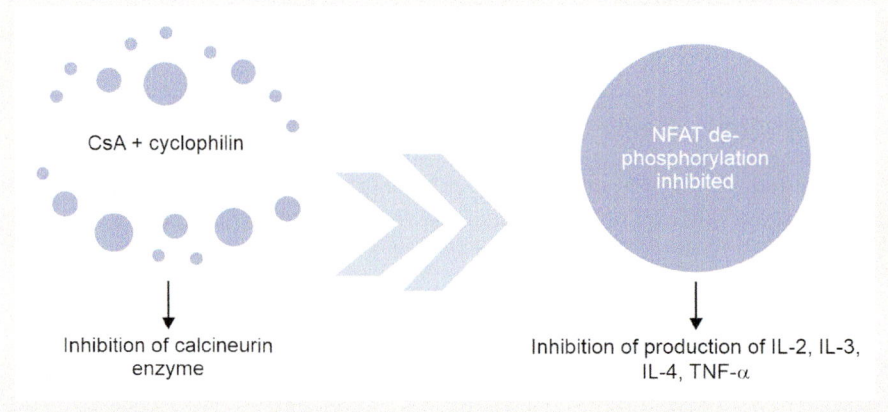

FIG. 2: Mechanism of action of cyclosporine (CsA).
(NFAT-1: nuclear factor of activated T cells; TNF: tumor necrosis factor)

- Calcineurin inhibition leads to reduced activity of transcription factor, nuclear factor of activated T cells (NFAT-1), which leads to impaired pro-inflammatory cytokine production [interleukin-2 (IL-2), IL-3, IL-4, tumor necrosis factor α (TNF-α)].
- This leads to decreased activation of T cells, basophils, and mast cells.
- Decline in IL-4 levels leads to decreased IgE production and mast-cell activation.
- Inhibits IgE-mediated release of histamine from mast cells in a concentration-dependent manner.

Use and Efficacy in Urticaria
- The GA²LEN/EAACI/EuroGuiDerm/APAAACI guidelines suggest treatment with CsA in severe CSU patients who do not respond to higher doses of antihistamines and omalizumab.
- The BAD guidelines recommend CsA as a second-line agent for CSU, besides omalizumab.
- LaCava et al. reported the efficacy of low-dose CsA (1–3 mg/kg/day) in omalizumab-refractory chronic urticaria in a series of five adult patients, with complete remission in four out of five patients with concomitant use of antihistamines and leukotriene receptor antagonists. Adverse effects were noted in two cases, raised serum creatinine levels in one, and new-onset hypertension in the other, which led to discontinuation of the drug.
- In India, CsA is used as a second-line agent in patients refractory to up-dosed use of antihistamines up to four times, due to affordability issues with omalizumab.
- Efficacy of CsA is dose-dependent and moderate dose (4–5 mg/kg/day) is found to be more effective with rapid response as compared to low dose (2 to <4 mg/kg/day). Low-dose CsA was found to improve the clinical severity significantly in 70% of CSU patients versus 84.3% with moderate dose at 12 weeks.
- Relapse rate is high with discontinuation of therapy in <3 months.
- It can also be considered as a third-line option for cold urticaria as per BAD guidelines.
- Positive basophil histamine release assay indicates a higher disease response to CsA.

Dose
3–5 mg/kg/day.

Side Effects (Box 1)
- Two most important factors contributing to an adverse effect profile are prolonged duration of therapy (>2 years) and high dose (>5 mg/kg/day).
- The important adverse events related to CsA therapy are nephrotoxicity and hypertension.

Box 1: Side effects and contraindications of CSA.

Side effects:
- Nephrotoxicity
- Hepatotoxicity
- Hypertension
- Hyperkalemia
- Hyperuricemia
- Gingival hyperplasia, hypertrichosis
- Myalgias, arthralgia
- Nausea/vomiting

Contraindications:
- Abnormal renal function
- Uncontrolled hypertension
- History of hypersensitivity reaction to its use
- Concomitant phototherapy

Dapsone

Dapsone is an antifolate sulfone drug (4,4'-diaminodiphenylsulfone) with antimicrobial and anti-inflammatory properties.

Mechanism of Action in Urticaria
- Inhibition of prostaglandin and leukotriene activity and metabolism
- Disruption of integrin-mediated neutrophil adhesion, interference with G-protein coupled signaling cascade of chemotactic stimuli, and inhibition of generation of second messengers essential for respiratory and secretory functions of neutrophils
- Interference with the function of neutrophil and eosinophil lysosomal enzymes such as myeloperoxidase

Use and Efficacy in Urticaria
- Dapsone is potentially beneficial as a second-line agent for CIU, CSU, and chronic autoimmune urticaria (CAU).
- It can be considered as a treatment option in delayed-pressure urticaria.
- BAD guidelines recommend dapsone as a third-line option (in addition to second-generation H1 antihistamines).

Dose
1–2 mg/kg/day (50–100 mg/day).

Side Effects (Box 2)
- Main adverse effects are anemia (fall in hemoglobin by 1 g/dL with 100–150 mg daily therapy) and methemoglobinemia (ferrous heme form oxidized to ferric form).
- Rare side effects include hemolytic anemia [glucose 6-phosphate dehydrogenase (G6PD) deficiency], agranulocytosis, peripheral neuropathy, nephritis, and hypothyroidism.
- *Idiosyncratic adverse reactions*: Dapsone hypersensitivity syndrome is characterized by maculopapular rash, high fever, hepatitis, lymphadenopathy, and lymphocytosis.

Box 2: Side effects and contraindications of dapsone.

Side effects:
- *Hepatic*: Hepatitis, cholestatic jaundice
- *Hematologic*: Hemolytic anemia, methemoglobinemia
- *Idiosyncratic*: Agranulocytosis, leukopenia
- *Neurologic*: Psychosis, peripheral neuropathy
- Cutaneous hypersensitivity reaction

Contraindications:
- Hypersensitivity to components
- G6PD enzyme deficiency
- Liver dysfunction

Methotrexate

Methotrexate (4-amino-N^{10}methyl pteroylglutamic acid) is a synthetic folic acid analog that competitively inhibits enzyme dihydrofolate reductase. Considering the strong immune-modulating properties of the drug, it is used widely as a steroid-sparing agent for various autoimmune inflammatory dermatoses. The wide array of modes of administration (oral, subcutaneous, intramuscular) of the drug makes it a convenient choice of treatment.

Mechanism of Action in Urticaria

Anti-inflammatory effects are exerted by T-cell dependent and independent actions.
- Dose-dependent suppression of T-cell activation
- Decreased expression of intercellular adhesion molecules, cutaneous lymphocyte-associated antigen, and E-selectin
- Reduction of neutrophils, leukotriene B4, and alteration of cytokine levels (suppression of release of IL-2 and IL-6)

Use and Efficacy in Urticaria

- Methotrexate is useful in chronic steroid dependent urticaria and should be considered as an alternative or a substitute for other third-line therapies, such as CsA, when they are contraindicated or ineffective.
- A meta-analysis by Sandhu et al. reported good response to methotrexate in steroid dependent urticaria due to its steroid sparing effect.
- Salmons et al. reported the efficacy of methotrexate in combination with omalizumab in a patient who achieved long-term remission of refractory urticaria.

Dose

10–20 mg/week (0.2 mg/kg/week; escalation by 0.25 mg/kg/week if no response).

Side Effects (Box 3)

- Gastrointestinal side effects occur most commonly with oral therapy and can be managed with parenteral route.
- Hematologic adverse effects and hepatic complications are noted with higher doses of methotrexate.
- Rare side effects include pulmonary fibrosis and pneumonitis.

Box 3: Side effects and contraindications of methotrexate.

Side effects:
- Hepatotoxicity
- Hematologic toxicity
- Acute pneumonitis
- Malignancy induction
- Infection reactivation

Contraindications:
- Pregnancy/lactation
- Significant anemia/leukopenia/thrombocytopenia
- Abnormal renal function
- Liver dysfunction

Azathioprine

Azathioprine is a prodrug that is rapidly converted to 6-mercaptopurine by the purine metabolism pathway. As a purine analog, it inhibits DNA production and exerts antiproliferative action. Classically approved in organ transplant recipient patients and rheumatoid arthritis, it is used off-label in various immunobullous disorders, connective tissue diseases, and vasculitis.

Mechanism of Action in Urticaria
- The exact mechanism is unknown.
- There is reduction in serum IgE levels.
- Impairment of gammaglobulin synthesis, T-cell function, and release of T-cell mediated IL-2.

Use and Efficacy in Urticaria
- Low-dose azathioprine therapy (50 mg/day) is similar in efficacy to low-dose CsA in antihistamine refractory urticaria.
- It is a valuable adjunct in patients with contraindications to CsA or affordability issues.
- There is paucity of data for recommendation of azathioprine efficacy in chronic urticaria. Bhanja et al. found that low-dose azathioprine for 8 weeks reduced disease severity and maintained remission till 36 weeks of follow-up compared to placebo in autologous serum skin test (ASST) positive chronic urticaria.

Dose
50–100 mg/day.

Side Effects (Box 4)
- Nausea and vomiting are the most common adverse events; however, myelosuppression is an important concern.
- Measurement of thiopurine methyltransferase enzyme levels and relative dose adjustment are necessary before initiating treatment.

Box 4: Side effects and contraindications of azathioprine.	
Side effects: • Gastrointestinal • Myelosuppression • Hypersensitivity syndrome • *Malignancy*: Squamous cell carcinoma, lymphomas • Infection reactivation	*Contraindications*: • Pregnancy/lactation • Active serious infections • History of hypersensitivity reaction to its use • Allopurinol use • Liver dysfunction

Hydroxychloroquine

Hydroxychloroquine (HCQ) is an antimalarial drug with a wide variety of uses due to its immunomodulatory, anti-inflammatory, photoprotective, and metabolic actions and low side-effect profile.

Mechanism of Action in Urticaria
- Immunomodulatory action by alkalinization of cytoplasmic vacuolar contents, altering the cleavage of peptides required for binding and presentation by major histocompatibility complex (MHC) class II molecules.
- HCQ limits wheal formation by stabilizing the lysosomes and inhibiting the synthesis of cytokines and prostaglandins that promote vasodilatation and vascular permeability.

Use and Efficacy in Urticaria
- The efficacy of HCQ is not as well-established as other therapies.
- It is considered a safer option compared to other immunosuppressant drugs or as an add-on therapy with other agents in refractory CSU.
- It is reported to be an efficacious steroid sparing agent in infants.

Dose
≤5 mg/kg/day.

Side Effects (Box 5)
- HCQ is a considerably safe option without requirement of significant laboratory monitoring.
- Irreversible retinal damage is very rare (<1%) when HCQ is used at low doses (≤5 mg/kg/day) for a duration of <5 years.

Box 5: Side effects and contraindications of hydroxychloroquine.

Side effects:
- *Ocular (reversible)*: Corneal deposits, premaculopathy, loss of accommodation; (irreversible): "Bull's eye maculopathy"
- *Hematologic*: Agranulocytosis, pancytopenia
- *Neuromuscular*: Psychosis, seizures, vertigo, tinnitus, nystagmus, rhabdomyolysis
- *Cutaneous*: Blue gray pigmentation, minor hypersensitivity reactions

Contraindications:
- Hypersensitivity to antimalarials
- Myasthenia gravis
- Pregnancy (relative contraindication)

Sulfasalazine

Sulfasalazine (antifolate drug) is an aminosalicylate disease-modifying antirheumatoid drug approved for use in ulcerative colitis, rheumatoid arthritis, and psoriatic arthritis. The sulfa-moiety of the drug has antibacterial properties, while the salicylate component acts as an anti-inflammatory agent. Owing to its wide array of action, it is used for the treatment of various dermatological disorders such as alopecia areata, lichen planus, immunobullous disorders, Behçet disease, systemic lupus erythematosus, and morphea.

Mechanism of Action in Urticaria
- The metabolite of sulfasalazine, 5-aminosalicylic acid, causes reduction of IgE-induced release of histamine from basophils and mast cells.
- Decreases the activity of prostaglandin synthetase.
- Antimicrobial properties (dihydropteroate synthetase) by eradication of *Helicobacter pylori* may play a role in autoimmune urticaria.

Use and Efficacy in Urticaria
- The efficacy and safety of sulfasalazine in CIU are comparable to those of CsA.
- Impressive action in severe and long-standing recalcitrant CIU indicates that sulfasalazine therapy should be considered for patients with CIU who do not respond adequately to antihistamines.
- Reported efficacy in delayed-pressure urticaria recalcitrant to steroids.

Dose
Sulfasalazine is clinically effective up to 3 g/day; however, weekly escalation to an initial therapeutic dose of 2 g/day is appropriate.

Side Effects
See **Box 6**.

Box 6: Side effects and contraindications of sulfasalazine.

Side effects:
- *Gastrointestinal*: Nausea, vomiting, dyspepsia, diarrhea
- *Hematologic*: Leukopenia, macrocytic anemia
- *Cutaneous hypersensitivity*: SJS/TEN, DRESS
- *Neurologic*: Headache, dizziness
- *Reproductive*: Infertility

Contraindications:
- Pregnancy/lactation
- Significant anemia/leukopenia/thrombocytopenia
- Hypersensitivity to sulfonamides/salicylate allergy
- Liver dysfunction
- Porphyria, G6PD deficiency

(DRESS: drug reaction with eosinophilia and systemic symptoms; G6PD: glucose 6-phosphate dehydrogenase; SJS: Stevens–Johnson syndrome; TEN: toxic epidermal necrolysis)

Colchicine

Colchicine is an alkaloid derived from plant *Colchicum autumnale*. The drug exhibits significant antimitotic property at high dose and anti-inflammatory action at low dose. It is useful in various neutrophilic disorders, vasculitis, and recurrent aphthous stomatitis and is currently being explored for other conditions.

Mechanism of Action in Urticaria
- Suppression of cell-mediated immune responses via inhibition of immunoglobulin secretion, IL-1 production, histamine release, and HLA-DR expression
- Inhibition of cyclooxygenase (COX) enzymes: COX-1 and COX-2

Use and Efficacy in Urticaria
- Effective in treatment-resistant urticaria (as a safer option compared to other immunosuppressants).
- Although colchicine did not result in statistically significant improvement among subgroups, it was helpful in the management of signs and symptoms in a case–control study by Nabazivadeh et al.
- However, large clinical studies are lacking in support of the drug for the treatment of chronic urticaria.

Dose
0.5–2 mg/day.

Side Effects
Refer to **Box 7**.

Box 7: Side effects and contraindications of colchicine.

Side effects:
- *Gastrointestinal*: Nausea, vomiting, abdominal pain, diarrhea
- *Hematologic*: Agranulocytosis, thrombocytopenia, aplastic anemia
- *Cutaneous*: Toxic epidermal necrolysis, precipitation of porphyria cutanea tarda, alopecia
- *Neurologic*: Myopathy, axonal neuropathy

Contraindications:
- Pregnancy/lactation
- Significant anemia/leukopenia/thrombocytopenia
- Concomitant use of CYP3A4 inhibitor, p-glycoprotein inhibitor

---

Mycophenolate Mofetil

Mycophenolate mofetil (MMF) is a semisynthetic 2-morpholinoethylester. It is a pro-drug of its active compound mycophenolic acid. It acts as a selective inhibitor of enzyme inosine monophosphate dehydrogenase in purine synthesis. MMF has been explored in various dermatological conditions due to its immunosuppressive action.

Mechanism of Action in Urticaria
- MMF reversibly blocks de novo synthesis of guanine nucleotides for DNA and RNA synthesis, affecting the synthesis of B and T lymphocytes.
- Reduces expression of adhesion molecules on endothelial cells and inhibits invasion of leukocytes into the skin.

Use and Efficacy in Urticaria
- Zimmer et al. concluded that MMF is a useful, well-tolerated, second-line therapy in patients with CIU and CAU, who fail therapy with antihistamines or other second-line agents.
- Combining MMF with oral steroids can be helpful in immediate control of symptoms, followed by reintroduction of antihistamines and gradual withdrawal of MMF to maintain long-term remission.

Dose
2–3 g/day.

Side Effects (Box 8)
Potential adverse effects include gastrointestinal (most common), hematologic, and increased predisposition to infections.

Box 8: Side effects and contraindications of mycophenolate mofetil.

Side effects:
- *Gastrointestinal*: Nausea, vomiting, abdominal cramps, diarrhea
- *Hematologic*: Neutropenia, thrombocytopenia, anemia
- *Genitourinary*: Urgency, frequency, dysuria, burning, sterile pyuria
- *Neurologic*: Weakness, fatigue, tinnitus, insomnia, depression

Contraindications:
- Pregnancy/lactation
- Hypersensitivity to any components of formulation
- Neutropenia, pure red cell aplasia
- Active infections

Intravenous Immunoglobulin

Intravenous immunoglobulin (IVIg) is a polyvalent antibody by-product derived from pooled plasma of healthy donors and contains IgG in supraphysiologic levels and traces of other immunoglobulins (IgA, IgE, IgM) and albumin, with other solvents. It exerts significant immune-modulating action by reducing antibody production, binding to complements, and inhibiting autoreactive T cells, thereby exhibiting its role in various disorders.

Mechanism of Action in Urticaria
IVIg acts as an immunomodulator due to the presence of anti-idiotypic antibodies. In chronic urticaria mediated by functionally significant autoantibodies, IVIg provides anti-idiotypic antibodies capable of suppressing histamine-releasing IgE autoantibodies.

Use and Efficacy in Urticaria
- The GA^{2}LEN/EAACI/EuroGuiDerm/APAAAACI guidelines mention IVIg at specialized centers as the last option, when other therapies fail as there is little

evidence in support, with only few case series published supporting its role in autoimmune urticaria.
- IVIg remains a viable alternative in patients with persistent urticaria with evidence of increased basophil CD203c expression, unresponsive to first-line therapies.
- IVIg can be considered as a therapeutic option in patients with severe, treatment resistant, anti-FcεR1 antibody-positive CSU.

Dose
0.4 g/kg/day for 5 consecutive days (2 g/kg over 2 days) every 4–6 weeks.

Side Effects (Box 9)
- Infusion-related adverse effects including myalgias, headache, chills, flushing, and nausea are usually mild and managed easily by slowing down the infusion.
- Anaphylactic reactions have been reported with IVIg, particularly in patients with IgA deficiency having anti-IgA antibodies.

Box 9: Side effects and contraindications of IVIg.

Side effects:
- Infusion-related reactions
- Anaphylaxis and cutaneous hypersensitivity reactions
- Fluid overload, acute renal failure
- Risk of thromboembolism
- *Hematologic*: Transient neutropenia, rarely hemolysis
- *Neurologic*: Headache, aseptic meningitis

Contraindications:
- Hypersensitivity to human immunoglobulin products
- Isolated IgA deficiency
- Acute renal impairment
- Risk of hypercoagulability

Danazol

Danazol is a synthetic steroid derivative with androgenic properties. It generally inhibits steroidogenesis in adrenals and gonads along with inhibition of gonadotropins. It also displays immunoregulatory effects and has been reported to be useful in low dose in livedoid vasculopathy and lipodermatosclerosis.

Mechanism of Action in Urticaria
Danazol increases the levels of C1 esterase inhibitor and other protease inhibitors like alpha-1 antitrypsin and antithrombin III. In cholinergic urticaria, serum levels of alpha-1 antichymotrypsin are found to be low, which have been proposed to be corrected by danazol therapy.

Use and Efficacy in Urticaria
- Wong et al. reported substantial reduction of exercise-induced whealing with danazol therapy in patients of cholinergic urticaria within 2 weeks.

- BAD guidelines recommend consideration of danazol, besides anticholinergics and propranolol, for the treatment of severe, refractory cholinergic urticaria.

Dose
100 mg once/twice per day.

Side Effects
- Side effects are reported with prolonged duration of therapy. Most frequent side effects include weight gain followed by menstrual irregularities like amenorrhea, acne, virilization changes including voice and hair changes, depression, headache, and myalgia.
- A rare side effect is hepatocellular adenoma.

Narrowband Ultraviolet B Phototherapy

Narrowband ultraviolet B phototherapy (NB-UVB) is a selective range of UVB spectrum from 311 to 313 nm. It is an effective treatment option for various dermatological conditions like psoriasis, vitiligo, atopic dermatitis, mycosis fungoides, and other inflammatory dermatoses due to its suppressive action on cell-mediated immunity.

Mechanism of Action in Urticaria
- The exact mechanism of action is unclear.
- The immunosuppressive effect can be attributed to inhibitory action on peripheral natural killer cell activity, lymphocyte proliferation and production of immune regulatory cytokines, both T-helper cell 1 (Th1) mediated: IL-2, interferon γ (IFN-γ) and T-helper cell 2 (Th2) mediated: IL-10.
- The effect on the number of mast cells and their depletion is still unclear. UVB primarily affects lesional T cells, thereby inhibiting T-cell-induced activation of mast cells and histamine release.

Use and Efficacy in Urticaria
- Sheikh et al. studied the role of NB-UVB in conjugation with loratadine in 80 patients of chronic urticaria and found significant reduction in urticaria activity score (UAS7) at 4 weeks (8 sessions of NB-UVB) and 8 weeks (16 sessions of NB-UVB) as compared to loratadine group alone.
- Other studies by Engin et al. and Berroeta et al. reported significant improvement in 10 sessions and 22 sessions, respectively.
- BAD guidelines recommend NB-UVB as a third-line option in CSU cases resistant to rest of the systemic therapies, in symptomatic dermographism, and as prophylactic therapy for solar urticaria after photoinvestigation.
- Recommended course is of around 30 treatments, repeated after 12 months, if necessary (not continuous treatment).
- GA²LEN guidelines mention consideration of phototherapy (NB-UVB/UV-A and PUVA) in resistant cases of CSU and symptomatic dermographism, in addition to antihistamines for 1–3 months.

Dose

The starting dose is 70% of minimal erythema dose with 10–20% increment, two to three sessions per week.

Side Effects

- Usually well-tolerated; mild erythema, burning, and pruritus may occur.
- Caution regarding carcinogenic properties of UVB therapy. However, these are rare with NB-UVB.

CONCLUSION

Urticaria is a chronic, debilitating disease with a recurrent and relapsing course. It causes significant physical and functional morbidity leading to reduced quality of life. Early identification of the type of urticaria and management is necessary to reduce the burden of disease. Although antihistamines and omalizumab are recommended therapies, many systemic treatment options have been proven to be effective in the treatment of urticaria and are currently under therapeutic trials for use in CSU. Further clinical studies are required for the assessment of these emerging therapies to demonstrate their efficacy in larger population.

SUGGESTED READINGS

1. Grattan C. The urticarias: pathophysiology and management. Clin Med. 2012;12:164-7.
2. Zuberbier T, Abdul Latiff AH, Abuzakouk M, Aquilina S, Asero R, Baker D, et al. The international EAACI/GA(2)LEN/EuroGuiDerm/APAAACI guideline for the definition, classification, diagnosis, and management of urticaria. Allergy. 2022;77:734-66.
3. Sabroe RA, Lawlor F, Grattan CEH, Ardern-Jones MR, Bewley A, Campbell L, et al. British Association of Dermatologists' Clinical Standards Unit. British Association of Dermatologists guidelines for the management of people with chronic urticaria 2021. Br J Dermatol. 2022;186:398-413.
4. Di Lorenzo G, D'Alcamo A, Rizzo M, Leto-Barone MS, Bianco CL, Ditta V, et al. Leukotriene receptor antagonists in monotherapy or in combination with antihistamines in the treatment of chronic urticaria: a systematic review. J Asthma Allergy. 2008;2:9-16.
5. Rayner DG, Liu M, Chu AWL, Chu X, Guyatt GH, Oykhman P, et al. Leukotriene receptor antagonists as add-on therapy to antihistamines for urticaria: Systematic review and meta-analysis of randomized clinical trials. J Allergy Clin Immunol. 2024;7:S0091-6749(24)00571-2.
6. Calapai G, Casciaro M, Miroddi M, Calapai F, Navarra M, Gangemi S. Montelukast-Induced Adverse Drug Reactions: A Review of Case Reports in the Literature. Pharmacology. 2014;94:60-70.
7. Vas K, Altmayer A, Mihályi L, Garaczi E, Kinyó Á, Jakobicz E, et al. Successful Treatment of Autoimmune Urticaria with Low-dose Prednisolone Therapy Administered for a Few Months: A Case Series of 42 Patients. Dermatology. 2017;233:419-24.
8. Harrison CA, Bastan R, Peirce MJ, Munday MR, Peachell PT. Role of calcineurin in the regulation of human lung mast cell and basophil function by cyclosporine and FK506. Br J Pharmacol. 2007;150:509-18.
9. LaCava AF, Fadugba OO. Cyclosporine for omalizumab-refractory chronic urticaria: a report of five cases. Allergy Asthma Clin Immunol. 2023;19:78.
10. Kulthanan K, Chaweekulrat P, Komoltri C, Hunnangkul S, Tuchinda P, Chularojanamontri L, et al. Cyclosporine for chronic spontaneous urticaria: A meta-analysis and systematic review. J Allergy Clin Immunol Pract. 2018;6:586-99.

11. Debol SM, Herron MJ, Nelson RD. Anti-inflammatory action of dapsone: inhibition of neutrophil adherence is associated with inhibition of chemoattractant-induced signal transduction. J Leukoc Biol. 1997;62:827-36.
12. Bozeman PM, Learn DB, Thomas EL. Inhibition of the human leukocyte enzymes myeloperoxidase and eosinophil peroxidase by dapsone. Biochem Pharmacol. 1992;44:553-63.
13. Liang SE, Hoffmann R, Peterson E, Soter NA. Use of Dapsone in the Treatment of Chronic Idiopathic and Autoimmune Urticaria. JAMA Dermatol. 2019;155:90-5.
14. Grundmann SA, Kiefer S, Luger TA, Brehler R. Delayed pressure urticaria—dapsone heading for first-line therapy? J Dtsch Dermatol Ges. 2011;9:908-12.
15. Sandhu J, Kumar A, Gupta SK. The therapeutic role of methotrexate in chronic urticaria: A systematic review. Indian J Dermatol Venereol Leprol. 2022;88:313-21.
16. Garbayo-Salmons P, Butt S, Dawe RS. Methotrexate combined with omalizumab for difficult to treat urticaria: a further step-up treatment? Clin Exp Dermatol. 2021;46:350-1.
17. Leducq S, Samimi M, Bernier C, Soria A, Amsler E, Staumont-Sallé D, et al. Efficacy and safety of methotrexate versus placebo as add-on therapy to H1 antihistamines for patients with difficult-to-treat chronic spontaneous urticaria: A randomized, controlled trial. J Am Acad Dermatol. 2020;82:240-3.
18. Pathania YS, Bishnoi A, Parsad D, Kumar A, Kumaran MS. Comparing azathioprine with cyclosporine in the treatment of antihistamine refractory chronic spontaneous urticaria: A randomized prospective active-controlled non-inferiority study. World Allergy Organ J. 2019;12:100033.
19. Fournier C, Bach MA, Dardenne M, Bach JF. Selective action of azathioprine on T cells. Transplant Proc. 1973;5:523-6.
20. Bhanja DC, Ghoshal L, Das S, Das S, Roy AK. Azathioprine in autologous serum skin test positive chronic urticaria: A case-control study in a tertiary care hospital of eastern India. Indian Dermatol Online J. 2015;6:185-8.
21. Reeves GE, Boyle MJ, Bonfield J, Dobson P, Loewenthal M. Impact of hydroxychloroquine therapy on chronic urticaria: chronic autoimmune urticaria study and evaluation. Intern Med J. 2004;34:182-6.
22. Mushtaq S, Sarkar R. Sulfasalazine in dermatology: A lesser explored drug with broad therapeutic potential. Int J Womens Dermatol. 2020;6:191-8.
23. Peppercorn MA. Sulfasalazine. Pharmacology, clinical use, toxicity, and related new drug development. Ann Intern Med. 1984;101:377-86.
24. McGirt LY, Vasagar K, Gober LM, Saini SS, Beck LA. Successful Treatment of Recalcitrant Chronic Idiopathic Urticaria with Sulfasalazine. Arch Dermatol. 2006;142:1337-42.
25. Orden RA, Timble H, Saini SS. Efficacy and safety of sulfasalazine in patients with chronic idiopathic urticaria. Ann Allergy Asthma Immunol. 2014;112:64-70.
26. Engler RJ, Squire E, Benson P. Chronic sulfasalazine therapy in the treatment of delayed pressure urticaria and angioedema. Ann Allergy Asthma Immunol. 1995;74:155-9.
27. Nabavizadeh SH, Babaeian M, Esmaeilzadeh H, Mortazavifar N, Alyasin S. Efficacy of the colchicine add-on therapy in patients with autoimmune chronic urticaria. Dermatol Ther. 2021;34:e15119.
28. Zimmerman AB, Berger EM, Elmariah SB, Soter NA. The use of mycophenolate mofetil for the treatment of autoimmune and chronic idiopathic urticaria: experience in 19 patients. J Am Acad Dermatol. 2012;66:767-70.
29. Raghavendran RR, Humphreys F, Kaur MR. Successful use of mycophenolate mofetil to treat severe chronic urticaria in a patient intolerant to ciclosporin. Clin Exp Dermatol. 2014;39:68-9.
30. Amar SM, Harbeck RJ, Dreskin SC. Effect of Intravenous Immunoglobulin in Chronic Urticaria with Increased Basophil CD203c Expression. J Allergy Clin Immunol. 2008;121(2):S98.
31. O'donnell BF, Barr RM, Black AK, Francis DM, Kermani F, Niimi N, et al. Intravenous immunoglobulin in autoimmune chronic urticaria. Br J Dermatol. 1998;138:101-6.
32. Dmowski WP. Danazol. A synthetic steroid with diverse biologic effects. J Reprod Med. 1990;35:69-74; discussion 74-5.

33. Wong E, Eftekhari N, Greaves MW, Ward AM. Beneficial effects of danazol on symptoms and laboratory changes in cholinergic urticaria. Br J Dermatol. 1987;116:553-6.
34. Sheikh G, Latif I, Lone KS, Hassan I, Jabeen Y, Keen A. Role of Adjuvant Narrow Band Ultraviolet B Phototherapy in the Treatment of Chronic Urticaria. Indian J Dermatol. 2019;64:250.
35. Engin B, Ozdemir M, Balevi A, Mevlitoğlu I. Treatment of chronic urticaria with narrowband ultraviolet B phototherapy: A randomized controlled trial. Acta Derm Venereol. 2008;88:247-51.
36. Berroeta I, Clark C, Ibbotson SH, Ferguson J, Dawe RS. Narrow-band (TL-01) ultraviolet B phototherapy for chronic urticaria. Clin Exp Dermatol. 2004;29:97-9.

CHAPTER 28

Biologicals in Urticaria

Priyadarshini Sahu, Sanjeev Gupta

INTRODUCTION

Urticaria is a skin disorder characterized by extremely itchy wheals, angioedema, or both. When symptoms persist for more than 6 weeks without an identifiable trigger, it is known as chronic spontaneous urticaria (CSU). Approximately 40–50% of CSU patients experience angioedema, with around 10% reporting it as their primary symptom. This condition places a considerable burden on patients and their family members. Recently, the advent of biological drugs has transformed disease management. This chapter aims to review the current available biological agents and their status.

PATHOGENESIS

The exact pathogenesis of urticaria is still not clear, but its understanding is very crucial to know the effect of various inflammatory markers and their site of action. Histamine release from mast cells is crucial in the development of urticarial lesions which can be mediated immunologically and nonimmunologically. Immunologically, there are two distinct endotypes of CSU, types I and IIb, based on the pathogenesis, disease markers, clinical progression, and responsiveness to treatment. Type I response (autoallergic) involves the cross-linking of IgE (immunoglobulin E) via autoallergen binding. In contrast, type IIb autoimmune responses are driven by autoantibodies that cross-link FcεRI (high-affinity IgE receptor), either through IgG or IgM binding to FcεRI or to FcεRI-bound IgE, leading to activation of mast cells. After IgE activation, mast cells and basophils in the skin and peripheral blood degranulate, resulting in release of histamine. This process attracts primarily vasoactive mediators like lymphocytes and eosinophils, as well as neutrophils, which are abundant in the affected skin of CSU. Mast cells, basophils, and eosinophils possess activated receptors for interleukin (IL)-4 and IL-5, which contribute to the development of CSU by extending the inflammatory symptoms. The pathogenesis is described in **Figure 1**. Thus, pathogenesis of urticaria is very important to understand and to identify the targets of biological agents in the treatment of CSU patients.

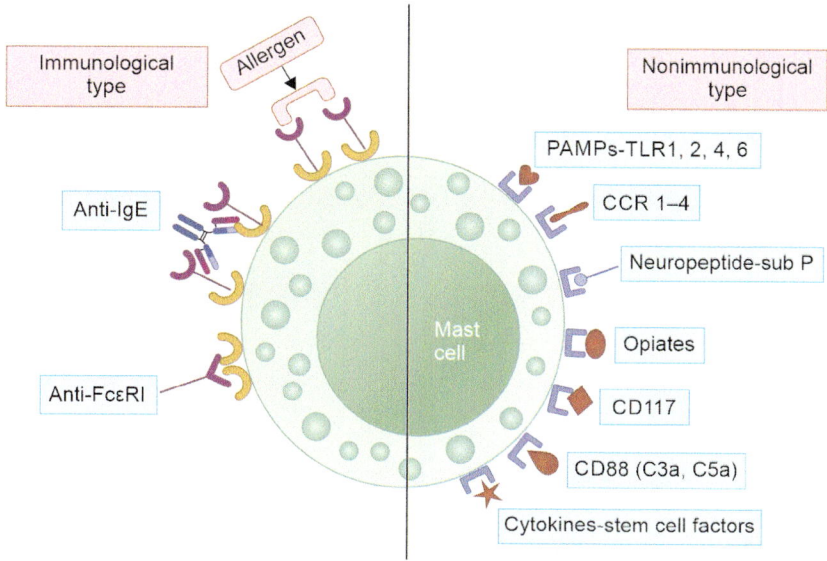

FIG. 1: Different mast cell receptors involved in immunological and nonimmunological mechanisms of urticaria.

Mechanism of all the biologicals is summarize in **Figure 2**. Various biological agents are listed below:
- *Anti-IgE monoclonal antibodies (mAbs)*: Omalizumab, Ligelizumab, UB-221
- *Anti-IL-4α mAb*: Duplimuab
- *Bruton's tyrosine kinase (BTK) inhibitors*: Remibrutinib, Rilzabrutinib, Fenebrutinib
- *C-kit inhibitor*: CDX-0159
- *Anti-Siglec-8 mAb*: Lirentelimab
- *Anti-IL-1β mAb*: Canakinumab
- *Anti-IL-5Rα mAb*: Benralizumab
- *Anti-IL-5 mAb*: Mepolizumab
- *Antitryptase mAb*: MTOS9579A
- *Anti-OSMRβ mAb*: Vixarelimab
- *JAK-STAT inhibitors*: Tofacitinib and Ruxolitinib

ANTI-IgE MONOCLONAL ANTIBODIES

Omalizumab

Mechanism of action: It is a recombinant humanized monoclonal IgG1 antibody against human IgE. By binding to free IgE in the blood and preventing it from attaching to its FcεRI on basophils and mast cells, omalizumab reduces the inflammatory response. It also promotes FcεRI receptor downregulation on basophils as a number of FcεRI receptors on basophils depend on the free serum IgE levels.

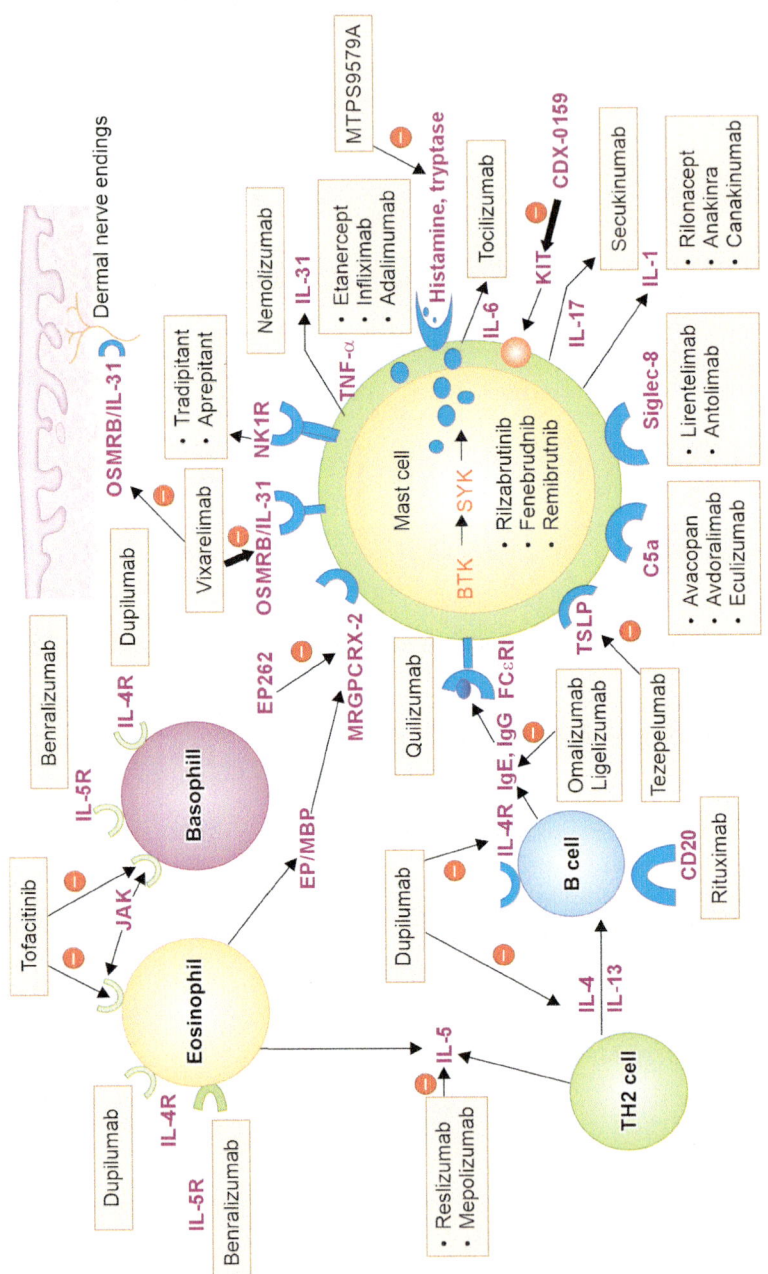

FIG. 2: Different biological drugs and their sites of action used in urticarias.

Dosage and route: The recommended dose is 150–300 mg administered subcutaneously every 4 weeks, depending on the patient's response to treatment. The medication comes in a lyophilized powder form, which must be reconstituted with sterile water prior to injection. Each vial contains 150 mg of the drug, which is administered per injection site. If the patient responds well, the treatment is continued for 6 months, followed by gradual tapering over 3–4 months. Approximately 30% of patients do not respond to the standard regimen and require higher dose or increased frequency of omalizumab. The dose can be increased to 300–600 mg every 2 weeks, depending on the severity of the condition. The maximum dose and duration of treatment have not been definitively established till now. The dose does not depend on the serum IgE (total or free) level or the patient's body weight. In addition, antihistamines can be given along with omalizumab. It is a safe and effective alternative to corticosteroids for refractory patients of urticaria. Systematic review and meta-analysis found no risk of malignancy on its long-term use.

Food and Drug Administration (FDA) approval: US FDA approved omalizumab for the treatment of CSU in patients ≥ 12 years of age since March 2014. It is not recommended for the management of other forms of urticaria.

Efficacy: Phase II–IV trials have shown efficacy of omalizumab ranging from 34 to 70%.

Based on the onset of response, patients can be divided into three types of responders:
1. *Early responders*: Respond within a week. Patients with high expression of FcεRI, negative autoimmune serum skin test (ASST), and normal to high IgE levels
2. *Late responders*: Respond after 12 weeks. Patients with positive basophil histamine-release assay, lower FcεRI expression, and positive ASST.
3. *Nonresponders*: Do not respond even after 3 months of treatment

Predictors of good response: Negative ASST, negative basophil activation test, high D-dimer, normal-to-high IgE, and very-high expression of FcεRI

Predictors of poor response: Positive ASST, positive basophil activation test and CD63, basopenia, eosinopenia, low IgE, lower expression of FcεRI, and high C-reactive protein (CRP)

Investigations prior to administration and monitoring:
- Before starting omalizumab treatment, it is essential to perform a complete blood count (CBC), random blood sugar test, and urine analysis with microscopy. Unlike other biologics, screening for tuberculosis is not required. Additionally, body weight measurement and baseline serum IgE levels are not needed before administering omalizumab for CSU.
- Omalizumab can be administered without hospital admission. Patients should be observed for 2 hours during the first three injections and for 30 minutes during subsequent injections.

Omalizumab in special situations:
Children: The efficacy and safety of omalizumab in children < 12 years with CSU have not been established. The safety and efficacy in patients between 12 and 17 years of age was tried in three randomized controlled trials (RCTs) and found to be similar to adults.

Pregnancy and lactation: Omalizumab is pregnancy category B drug according to FDA. It crosses placenta as pregnancy progresses in a linear fashion, so potential effects are likely to be greater in the second to third trimester. However, studies on monkey have not shown any evidence of adverse effects on fetal or neonatal growth. Omalizumab is secreted in a very small amount into the breast milk. So, omalizumab can be administered in breastfeeding women depending on the underlying maternal condition.

Elderly: There is not sufficient data available for patients over 65 years. There are no apparent age-related changes observed in various studies.

Adverse effects:
- *Skin manifestations*: Injection site reaction and rash, anaphylaxis, dermatitis with pruritus
- *Cardiovascular system*: Hypertension, cardiomyopathy, heart failure, myocardial infarction (MI), thrombosis, pericardial effusion
- *Respiratory manifestations*: Sinusitis, upper respiratory tract infection (URTI), pharyngitis, pulmonary hypertension with bronchospasm
- *Hematological manifestations*: Thrombocytopenia, eosinophilia
- *Respiratory manifestations*: URTI, sinusitis, pharyngitis, pulmonary hypertension, and bronchospasm
- *Musculoskeletal manifestations*: Arthralgia, fracture
- *Miscellaneous*: Headache, earache, dizziness, fatigue, viral infections

Omalizumab should not be used in patients with a known hypersensitivity to the drug or any of its ingredients. It is absolutely contraindicated in patients developing anaphylaxis with omalizumab, which presents as bronchospasm, hypotension, or syncope.

Main points:
- US FDA approved treatment for CSU in patients ≥ 12 years of age
- Typical dose is 150–300 mg administered subcutaneously every 4 weeks, with adjustments made based on the patient's response
- For nonresponders, the dose can be increased to 300–600 mg every 2 weeks.
- Maximum dose and duration of treatment have not been firmly established, necessitating individualized treatment plans.
- Generally well tolerated with a low risk of severe adverse effects
- Regular monitoring for allergic reactions, especially during the first few doses, is recommended.

Ligelizumab

Mechanism of action: This drug is a type of antibody called a second-generation humanized monoclonal IgG4 antibody. It works by precisely attaching to a specific part of the IgE antibody called the Cε3 domain. Compared to omalizumab, it has a significantly stronger affinity for IgE, approximately 40–50 times more, and a slower rate of dissociation from IgE. Therefore, unlike omalizumab, ligelizumab induces a more rapid, thorough, and prolonged reduction in free IgE levels. It has the ability to neutralize serum IgE and also seems to hinder the generation of IgE by inhibiting the binding activity of IgE-FcεRI, hence limiting the quantity of free IgE that can initiate the allergic reaction cascade.

Route of administration and preparations: It is available in dose of 72 mg/120 mg/240 mg given subcutaneously.

FDA approval: It is not yet FDA approved. It is currently in phase 3 clinical trial for CSU.

Efficacy: In a phase IIb RCT, it demonstrated a rapid onset of action, longer remission period, and superior efficacy compared to omalizumab while maintaining a similar safety profile.

Adverse effects: It is a well-tolerated drug and poses no serious adverse effects. Side effects like pain and discomfort at the injection site, nasopharyngitis, headache, and upper respiratory infection can be seen.

UB-221

UB-221 is a humanized IgG1 mAb that targets the Cε3 domain of IgE. UB-221 binds IgE with a higher affinity than omalizumab and is superior in IgE neutralization and prevention of basophil degranulation. Apart from this, it also binds with CD23 (FcεRII), which is expressed mainly in B lymphocytes, thereby inhibiting IgE synthesis. The prolonged suppression of urticaria symptoms and reduction of serum IgE levels suggest that a single dose can be administered every 3–6 months, providing long-lasting symptoms relief for CSU as compared to omalizumab. In 2022, Taiwan-based United BioPharma company has declared its approval for phase 2 clinical trial.

ANTI-IL-4α MONOCLONAL ANTIBODY

Dupilumab

Mechanism of action: It is a fully humanized mAb that blocks IL-4α receptor, leading to IL-4/IL-13 signaling. It plays a crucial role in promoting type 2 inflammation in various illnesses. Type 2 inflammatory cytokines directly and indirectly activate mast cells, basophils, and eosinophils, leading to an increase in their activity and production of cytokines. It also inhibits B-cell immunoglobulin and further reduces IgE production.

Dosage and route: Patients with a body weight exceeding 60 kg were administered a loading dosage of 600 mg of dupilumab, which consisted of two injections of 300 mg each. Subsequently, they received a maintenance dose of 300 mg of dupilumab every 2 weeks. Adolescents weighing < 60 kg and children weighing > 30 kg were administered a loading dose of 400 mg of dupilumab (two injections of 200 mg each), followed by a maintenance dosage of 200 mg of dupilumab every 2 weeks. Children weighing between 15 and 30 kg are administered a loading dosage of 600 mg of dupilumab, which consisted of two injections of 300 mg each. This is followed by a maintenance dose of 300 mg every 4 weeks. It is administered via subcutaneous injection.

FDA approval: It is not yet FDA approved for urticaria. It has now completed the phase 3 clinical trial.

Efficacy: In a phase-3, double-blind, placebo-controlled, multicenter, parallel-group study for the treatment of CSU, there were two groups in this study. In group A, those patients were included who remained symptomatic despite the use of antihistamines but were omalizumab naive. Group B included patients who were omalizumab-intolerant or were incomplete responders. This study revealed that at week 24, patients in group A showed clinical and statistically significant efficacy, in comparison to standard antihistamines. Dupilumab provides minimal improvement in patients who were either intolerant or incomplete responders to omalizumab.

Adverse effects: Nasopharyngitis, injection site erythema, eosinophilia, conjunctivitis, and keratitis arthralgia can be seen.

BRUTON'S TYROSINE KINASE INHIBITORS

Bruton's tyrosine kinase (BTK) is a cytoplasmic tyrosine kinase and is expressed in mast cells/basophils, B cells, macrophages, and platelets. Upon binding of IgE with FcεRI on mast cells, it leads to phosphorylation of BTK. This activated BTK activates phospholipase Cγ1, resulting in increased cytoplasmic calcium levels and further mast cells' degranulation and histamine release. Inhibiting of BTK prevents autoantibody production in B cells and inhibits mast cells and basophil activation or degranulation. This approach may be particularly effective for patients with CSU, especially those with type IIb CSU, who experience severe disease activity and inadequate control with current treatments. Further, all the drugs in this group are orally administered, offering the convenience of home administration.

Remibrutinib

Mechanism of action: It is a highly selective BTK inhibitor.

Dosage and route of administration: The drug is administered orally and can be prescribed in a dosage range of 10 mg once daily to 100 mg twice daily. *Dose of 25 mg/100 mg twice a day.*

FDA approval: Not yet FDA approved, currently in phase 3 trial.

Efficacy: The core phase 2b dose-finding study (NCT03926611) demonstrated the efficacy of this medication for CSU, with a rapid onset of action and a favorable safety profile lasting up to 12 weeks. This treatment was particularly helpful for individuals who had unsatisfactory control of their symptoms with H1 antihistamines. In a separate phase 2b extension study lasting up to 52 weeks, it was shown that the overall safety profile and the quick and sustained effectiveness were similar between the extension study and the core studies.

Adverse effects: Treatment-emergent adverse effects were respiratory tract infections (COVID-19 and nasopharyngitis) and gastrointestinal (GI) disorders.

Rilzabrutinib

Mechanism of action: It is a reversible, covalent BTK inhibitor.

Dose and route of administration: Given orally in dose of 400 mg once, twice, or thrice a day

FDA approval: It is not yet FDA approved. Currently, phase 2 results were released in a press conference. Phase 3 study was planned to start in 2024.

Efficacy: The phase 2 research yielded positive outcomes, demonstrating that rilzabrutinib effectively relieved itch and urticaria in patients with moderate-to-severe CSU, whose symptoms were not sufficiently managed by H1 antihistamines. Phase 2 involved a dose-ranging trial where several dosages of rilzabrutinib were assessed: 400 mg administered once a day in the evening (QPM), 400 mg taken twice daily (BID), and 400 mg consumed three times daily (TID). The most optimal outcome was observed while administering a dosage of 400 mg, three times a day.

Adverse effects: Treatment-emergent adverse effects were seen which include diarrhea, nausea, headache, and abdominal pain.

Fenebrutinib

Mechanism of action: It is an orally available BTK inhibitor.

Dosage and route of administration: Given orally in dose of 200 mg twice daily.

FDA approval: Not yet FDA approved. It is currently in phase 2 trial.

Efficacy: In a recent study conducted by Metz et al., a double-blind, placebo-controlled, phase 2 trial was conducted. The trial involved randomly administering fenebrutinib (at doses of 50 mg daily, 150 mg daily, or 200 mg twice a day) or a placebo to 93 persons with CSU who were unresponsive to increased doses of H1 antihistamines. The treatment period lasted for 8 weeks. Fenebrutinib showed superior efficacy compared to placebo in decreasing the urticaria activity score after 8 weeks. It achieved well-controlled illness rates of up to 57% when administered at a dose of 200 mg twice daily. Fenebrutinib reduced disease activity in individuals with CSU who did not respond to antihistamines, especially patients with type IIb autoimmunity.

Adverse effects: It is a well-tolerated drug, with minor side effects like nasopharyngitis, headache, periorbital cellulitis, and an increase in hepatic enzymes.

C-KIT INHIBITOR

Barzolvolimab (CDX-0159)

Mechanism of action: This is a humanized mAb that targets and binds to the tyrosine kinase KIT receptor with a high level of specificity, effectively blocking its function. KIT is a cell surface receptor that is found in various types of cells, such as mast cells. It plays a crucial role in facilitating inflammatory reactions in chronic urticaria.

Dosage and administration: It is given intravenously at a dose of 3 mg/kg.

FDA approval: Not yet FDA approved. Currently, phase 2 study is going on for CDX-0159.

Efficacy: The press release for the phase 1b research reported a favorable outcome, indicating a complete response rate of 95% in patients with chronic inducible urticaria, specifically cold urticaria and symptomatic dermographism, with single dosage of CDX-0159. The clinical response was associated with a decrease in serum tryptase levels and skin mast cells.

Adverse effects: It is generally well accepted without causing significant adverse effects. The predominant adverse effects seen were localized hair color alterations (small regions of hair color lightening), mild infusion responses, and temporary alterations in taste perception.

ANTI-Siglec-8 MONOCLONAL ANTIBODY

Lirentelimab (AK002)

Mechanism of action: It is a humanized nonfucosylated IgG1 mAb directed against sialic acid-binding immunoglobulin-like lectin 8 (Siglec-8). It is predominantly found on fully developed eosinophils and mast cells, with relatively lower expression on basophils. Blocking this receptor prevents mast cell activation and induces the death of eosinophils.

Dosage and administration: The drug is given intravenously at a dosage that varies between 0.3 and 3 mg/kg of body weight. Patients are administered six intravenous doses of lirentelimab every 6 months, with the initial dose being 0.3 mg/kg. If the patient tolerated the medication well, the dosage for the second and third doses was raised to 1 mg/kg and thereafter increased to 3 mg/kg for the remaining doses.

FDA approval: It is not yet FDA approved. Currently, phase 2b data has been published.

Efficacy: A recent study by Altrichter et al. showed that lirentelimab is efficacious in all types of patients who were omalizumab-naive and those who were refractory to omalizumab. Complete response rates were reached for those with cholinergic urticaria and with symptomatic dermographism.

Adverse effects: The most often reported negative effects were infusion-related responses, nasopharyngitis, and headache. There were no major adverse effects that were caused by the treatment.

Anti-TSLP mAb

Tezepelumab

Mechanism of action: It is first-in-class fully human mAb IgGλ that targets the interaction of thymic stromal lymphopoietin (TSLP) with TSLP receptors. It is an epithelial cytokine that promotes Th2 inflammation, which plays an important role in the pathogenesis of urticaria.

Dosage and route of administration: It is a formulated as prefilled syringes with 210 mg solution for subcutaneous administration. Dose adjusted is not required in renal and hepatic impairment as it is degraded by proteolytic enzymes, so it is not metabolized by hepatic enzymes.

FDA approval: Tezepelumab has been approved in the United States as an add-on therapy for adults, adolescents, and children aged 12 years and above who have severe, unmanageable asthma. It is not yet FDA approved in urticaria. Currently, it is in phase 2b INCEPTION study (NCT04833855).

Efficacy: The use of anti-TSLP drugs in patients who have not been previously treated with anti-IgE resulted in ongoing decreases in disease activity and biomarkers such as IL-5 and IL-13 even after stopping the drug. This sustained effect was not seen with omalizumab or placebo, indicating that anti-TSLP drugs have a lasting impact even after treatment is discontinued.

Adverse effects: Pain and redness at the injection site, tachycardia, infection, infestations, nasopharyngitis, URTI, nausea, headache, and GI disorders

ANTI-IL-5 MONOCLONAL ANTIBODY

Cutaneous eosinophilic infiltration, driven by mast cell recruitment through IL-5, plays an important role in the pathogenesis of CSU, as these patients exhibit higher eosinophil levels in both affected and unaffected skin areas compared to healthy controls. Mepolizumab and reslizumab inhibit IL-5 and benralizumab inhibits IL-5α receptor.

Mepolizumab

Mechanism of action: It is a monoclonal humanized antibody that targets interleukin IL-5. It binds to IL-5 and inhibits its binding to its receptor on the surface of eosinophils. By binding to eosinophils, it reduces the blood levels of IL-5.

Dosage and administration: It is available in two formulations, i.e., as lyophilized powder for reconstitution with sterile water and as a prefilled autoinjector or syringe. Both are available as 100 mg/mL, given subcutaneously.

FDA approval: It is first approved in 2015 for severe asthma with an eosinophilic phenotype in the United States. It is currently approved by US FDA as add-on maintenance for patients with chronic rhinosinusitis with nasal polyps. For urticaria, it is in phase 1 study.

Efficacy: Margerl et al. had first reported its therapeutic response in a female suffering from eosinophilic asthma and CSU. A phase 1 open-label, single-arm study is currently in progress to evaluate the efficacy of mepolizumab therapy given for 10 weeks in urticaria patients (NCT03494881).

Adverse effects: Headache and injection site reactions are the most common side effects observed. Other less common side effects are hypersensitivity reactions including anaphylaxis, abdominal pain, urinary tract infections, back pain, fatigue, and upper respiratory infection.

ANTI-IL-5Rα MONOCLONAL ANTIBODY

Benralizumab

Mechanism of action: It is a fucosylated monoclonal humanized antibody targeting anti–interleukin-5-receptor alpha (IL-5Rα), which causes nearly depletion of eosinophils as well as reduces the basophil counts, thereby showing efficacy in CSU.

Dosage and route of administration: 30–60 mg can be given to adults subcutaneously.

FDA approval: It is not yet FDA approved. Phase IIb ARROYO clinical trial (NCT04612725) has been published recently.

Efficacy: Phase IIb trial showed a decrease in the blood eosinophil counts, although there was no clinical benefit of benralizumab over placebo.

Adverse effects: Headache, pharyngitis, pyrexia, and hypersensitivity reactions can be seen in some cases.

ANTI-IL-1β MONOCLONAL ANTIBODY

Canakinumab

Mechanism of action: This is a recombinant mAb that specifically targets and attaches to IL-1β, a protein involved in immune responses. By doing so, it prevents IL-1β from interacting with IL-1 receptors and inhibits its biological effects.

Dosage and administration: It is available as lyophilized powder 180 mg/vial, which becomes 150 mg/mL after reconstitution with 1 mL sterile water. It is administered subcutaneously.

FDA approval: Currently, it is in phase II trial.

Efficacy: It has been found to be beneficial in treating cryopyrin-associated periodic syndromes that were characterized by urticarial symptoms and urticarial vasculitis. Therefore, there was a suspicion that it might also be effective in individuals with CSU. However, in a phase II clinical trial, a randomized, double-blind, placebo-controlled investigation was conducted at a single center, in 20 patients and it failed to show any significant superiority to the placebo.

Adverse effects: Nasopharyngitis, diarrhea, headache, injection-like pain, and gastroenteritis

OTHER DRUGS CURRENTLY IN DEVELOPMENT

- *Antitryptase mAb (MTPS9579A)*: It is humanized IgG4 antibody that binds with high affinity to human tryptase, secreted by mast cells and its activity. Currently, it is undergoing phase 2 clinical trials for patients with CSU who have not responded to antihistamines.
- *Anti-OSMRβ mAb: Vixarelimab (KPL-716)*: This is a mAb that specifically attaches to the oncostatin M receptor (OSMRβ), preventing the transmission of signals from both IL-31 and oncostatin M, which are involved in causing itching. Vixarelimab exhibited a swift decrease in itchiness and the attainment of clear or nearly clear skin in around one-third of prurigo nodularis patients by the eighth week of treatment. Vixarelimab is now undergoing a phase II trial to evaluate its effectiveness in treating CSU.
- JAK-STAT inhibitors are new in this field. JAK-STAT signaling is associated with interaction of interferon and IL networks, which play a vital role in the pathogenesis of urticaria. Ruxolitinib (JAK1/2 inhibitor) has demonstrated efficacy in a single case report involving a 61-year-old female. Similarly, tofacitinib (JAK1/3 inhibitor) has shown effectiveness in four cases of refractory chronic urticaria. These findings suggest that JAK-STAT inhibitors may downregulate inflammatory processes associated with mast cells, offering a potential new therapeutic option for patients with refractory chronic urticaria.

CONCLUSION

The complexity of CSU necessitates a comprehensive approach to diagnosis and management, involving a thorough patient history, identification of potential triggers, and a combination of symptomatic and immunomodulatory treatments. Advances in understanding the biological mechanisms of CSU hold promise for more targeted therapies and improved patient outcomes. There is no doubt that omalizumab is the game changer in the management of CSU. But there are many patients who do not respond to omalizumab. There are various newer biologicals targeting various other cells involved in the pathomechanism of CSU, as summarized in **Table 1** and **Figure 2**. Further research into the immunological and genetic aspects of CSU will be crucial in understanding the phenotype and endotype of each patient and in developing more effective and personalized treatment strategies.

TABLE 1: Summary of biologicals in urticaria.

Biological drug	Target site	Dose and route of administration	Status of drug	Efficacy	Adverse effects
Omalizumab	Anti-IgE mAb	• US FDA approved: 150 mg/300 mg every 4 weeks (dose can be increased in case the patient is not responding) • Given subcutaneously	FDA approved (2014)	Approved treatment of CSU in patients ≥ 12 years of age who remain symptomatic despite H1 antihistamine treatment	• Most common adverse effects are nausea, nasopharyngitis, sinusitis, URTI, arthralgia, headache, and injection site reaction • Black-box warning: Anaphylaxis
Ligelizumab	Anti-IgE mAb	Given subcutaneously in dose of 72 mg/120 mg/ 240 mg every 4 weeks	Phase 3 study NCT02649218	It is 40–50-fold increased affinity to Cε3 domain of IgE compared to the drug omalizumab	Nasopharyngitis, headache, URTI most prevalent treatment emergent side effects
UB-221	Targets both Cε3 domain of IgE and CD23-bound IgE	Dosing not yet finalized	Phase 1 study NCT03632291	Prolonged suppression of urticaria symptoms with a single dose	–
Dupilumab	Monoclonal antibody against IL-4/13Ra	Given subcutaneously with a loading dose of 600 mg which is followed by 300 mg every 2 weeks	Phase 3 study NCT05526521 and NCT04180488	Omalizumab-naive patients with uncontrolled CSU experienced a decrease in urticaria activity when treated with dupilumab, while improvement for omalizumab-incomplete responders was not achieved	Nasopharyngitis, injection site erythema, eosinophilia, conjunctivitis, keratitis arthralgia

Continued

Continued

Biological drug	Target site	Dose and route of administration	Status of drug	Efficacy	Adverse effects
Remibrutinib	BTK inhibitor	100 mg twice daily orally	Phase 3 trial NCT05513001 NCT05677451 NCT05048342 NCT05032157 NCT05030311	In both core phase 2b and extension study of phase 2b showed its rapid onset of action and favorable safety profile	Respiratory tract infection and gastrointestinal disorders
Rilzabrutinib	BTK inhibitor	400 mg three times a daily	Phase 2 NCT05107115	In phase 2 study, it showed favorable results at a dose of 400 mg TDS	Diarrhea, nausea, headache, and abdominal pain
Fenebrutinib	BTK inhibitor	200 mg thrice a day	Phase 2 NCT03693625	In phase 2 trial, it was found to be more effective as compared to placebo in reducing urticaria activity	Nasopharyngitis, headache, periorbital cellulitis, and increase in hepatic enzymes
Barzolvolimab (CDX-0159)	C-KIT inhibitor	Given intravenously at a dose of 3 mg/kg	Phase 2 NCT05368285	Both phase 2 and 3 showed encouraging results in patients suffering from chronic inducible urticaria	Hair color changes, infusion reactions, and temporary changes in perception of taste
Lirentelimab	Anti-Siglec-8 mAb	Administered intravenously in a dose of 0.3–3 mg/kg body weight every 4 weeks	Phase 2 NCT05528861	It is found to be efficacious in all patients who are refractory to omalizumab	Infusion-related reactions, nasopharyngitis, and headache
Tezepelumab	Anti-TSLP mAb	Given subcutaneously with 210 mg prefilled syringes	Phase 2b NCT04833855	This drug resulted in sustained decreases in CSU disease activity and biomarkers even after withdrawal of medication. This response was not seen with omalizumab	Pain and redness at injection site, tachycardia, nasopharyngitis, upper respiratory tract infection, nausea, headache, GI disorders

Continued

Continued

Biological drug	Target site	Dose and route of administration	Status of drug	Efficacy	Adverse effects
Mepolizumab	Anti-IL-5 mAb	Given 100 mg subcutaneously every 4 weeks	Phase 1 NCT03494881	Currently US FDA approved as an add-on maintenance for patients with chronic rhinosinusitis with nasal polyps. For urticaria, it is in phase 1 study	Most common side effects are headache and injection site reactions
Benralizumab	Anti-IL-5Rα mAb	30 mg subcutaneously every 4 weeks	Phase 2 NCT04612725	Phase IIb trial showed decrease in the blood eosinophil counts, although there was no clinical benefit of benralizumab over placebo	Headache, pharyngitis, pyrexia, and hypersensitivity reactions
Canakinumab	Anti-IL-1β mAb	150 mg subcutaneously every 4 weeks	Phase 2 NCT01635127	In phase II double-blind placebo-controlled randomized study, it failed to show any significant superiority to the placebo	Nasopharyngitis, diarrhea, headache, injection-like pain, and gastroenteritis

SUGGESTED READINGS

1. Maurer M, Costa C, Gimenez Arnau A, Guillet G, Labrador-Horrillo M, Lapeere H, et al. Antihistamine-resistant chronic spontaneous urticaria remains undertreated: 2-year data from the AWARE study. Clin Exp Allergy. 2020;50(10):1166-75.
2. Saini SS, Kaplan AP. Chronic spontaneous urticaria: the devil's itch. J Allergy Clin Immunol Pract. 2018;6(4):1097-106.
3. Kaplan A, Lebwohl M, Giménez-Arnau AM, Hide M, Armstrong AW, Maurer M. Chronic spontaneous urticaria: Focus on pathophysiology to unlock treatment advances. Allergy. 2023;78(2):389-401.
4. Holgate ST, Djukanovic R, Casale T, Bousquet J. Anti-immunoglobulin E treatment with omalizumab in allergic diseases: An update on anti-inflammatory activity and clinical efficacy. Clin Exp Allergy. 2005;35:408-16.
5. Poddighe D, Vangelista L. Effects of omalizumab on basophils: Potential biomarkers in asthma and chronic spontaneous urticaria. Cell Immunol. 2020;358:104215.
6. Mustari AP, Bishnoi A, Kumaran MS. Biologicals in treatment of chronic urticaria: A narrative review. Indian Dermatol Online J. 2023;14:9-20.
7. Busse W, Buhl R, Fernandez Vidaurre C, Blogg M, Zhu J, Eisner MD, et al. Omalizumab and the risk of malignancy: Results from a pooled analysis. J Allergy Clin Immunol. 2012;129:983-9.
8. Eghrari-Sabet J, Sher E, Kavati A, Pilon D, Zhdanava M, Balp MM, et al. Real-world use of omalizumab in patients with chronic idiopathic/spontaneous urticaria in the United States. Allergy Asthma Proc. 2018;39(3):191-200.
9. Gasser P, Tarchevskaya SS, Guntern P, Brigger D, Ruppli R, Zbaren N, et al. The mechanistic and functional profile of the therapeutic anti-IgE antibody ligelizumab differs from omalizumab. Nat Commun. 2020;11:165.
10. Maurer M, Gimenez-Arnau AM, Sussman G, Metz M, Baker DR, Bauer A, et al. Ligelizumab for chronic spontaneous urticaria. N Engl J Med. 2019;381:1321-32.
11. Kuo BS, Li CH, Chen JB, Shiung YY, Chu CY, Lee CH, et al. IgE-neutralizing UB-mAb, distinct from omalizumab and ligelizumab, exhibits CD23-mediated IgE downregulation and relieves urticaria symptoms. J Clin Invest. 2022;132:e157765.
12. Maloney NJ, Tegtmeyer K, Zhao J, Worswick S. Dupilumab in dermatology: potential for uses beyond atopic dermatitis. J Drugs Dermatol. 2019;18:S1545961619P1053X.
13. Maurer M, Casale TB, Saini SS, Ben-Shoshan M, Giménez-Arnau AM, Bernstein JA, et al. Dupilumab in patients with chronic spontaneous urticaria (LIBERTY-CSU CUPID): Two randomized, double-blind, placebo-controlled, phase 3 trials. J Allergy Clin Immunol. 2024;154(1):184-94.
14. Casale TB. Novel biologics for treatment of chronic spontaneous urticaria. J Allergy Clin Immunol. 2022;150(6):1256-9.
15. Maurer M, Berger W, Giménez-Arnau A, Hayama K, Jain V, Reich A, et al. Remibrutinib, a novel BTK inhibitor, demonstrates promising efficacy and safety in chronic spontaneous urticaria. J Allergy Clin Immunol. 2022;150(6):1498-506.e2.
16. Jain V, Giménez-Arnau A, Hayama K, Reich A, Carr W, Tillinghast J, et al. Remibrutinib demonstrates favorable safety profile and sustained efficacy in chronic spontaneous urticaria over 52 weeks. J Allergy Clin Immunol. 2024;153(2):479-86.e4.
17. Metz M, Sussman G, Gagnon R, Staubach P, Tanus T, Yang WH, et al. Fenebrutinib in H1 antihistamine-refractory chronic spontaneous urticaria: a randomized phase 2 trial. Nat Med. 2021;27(11):1961-9.
18. Alvarado D, Maurer M, Gedrich R, Seibel SB, Murphy MB, Crew L, et al. Anti-KIT monoclonal antibody CDX-0159 induces profound and durable mast cell suppression in a healthy volunteer study. Allergy. 2022;77(8):2393-403.
19. Molawi DT, Hawro T, Grekowitz E, Kiefer L. The Anti-KIT antibody, CDX-0159, reduces mast cell numbers and circulating tryptase and improves disease control in patients with chronic inducible urticaria (Cindu). J Allergy Clin Immunol. 2022;149:AB178.

20. Altrichter S, Staubach P, Pasha M, Singh B, Chang AT, Bernstein JA, et al. An open-label, proof-of-concept study of lirentelimab for antihistamine-resistant chronic spontaneous and inducible urticaria. J Allergy Clin Immunol. 2022;149(5):1683-90.e7.
21. Yosipovitch G, Biazus Soares G, Mahmoud O. Current and Emerging Therapies for Chronic Spontaneous Urticaria: A Narrative Review. Dermatol Ther (Heidelb). 2023;13(8):1647-60.
22. Licari A, Manti S, Leonardi S, Minasi D, Caffarelli C, Cardinale F, et al. Biologic drugs in chronic spontaneous urticaria. Acta Biomed. 2021;92(S7):e2021527.
23. Magerl M, Terhorst D, Metz M, Altrichter S, Zuberbier T, Maurer M, et al. Benefit of mepolizumab treatment in a patient with chronic spontaneous urticaria. J Dtsch Dermatol Ges. 2018;16(4):477-8.
24. Altrichter S, Giménez-Arnau AM, Bernstein JA, Metz M, Bahadori L, Bergquist M, et al. Benralizumab does not elicit therapeutic effect in patients with chronic spontaneous urticaria: results from the phase IIb multinational randomized double-blind placebo-controlled ARROYO trial. Br J Dermatol. 2024;191(2):187-99.
25. Kuemmerle-Deschner JB, Haug I. Canakinumab in patients with cryopyrin-associated periodic syndrome: an update for clinicians. Ther Adv Musculoskelet Dis. 2013;5(6):315-29.
26. Maul JT, Distler M, Kolios A, Maul LV, Guillet C, Graf N, et al. Canakinumab Lacks Efficacy in Treating Adult Patients with Moderate to Severe Chronic Spontaneous Urticaria in a Phase II Randomized Double-Blind Placebo-Controlled Single-Center Study. J Allergy Clin Immunol Pract. 2021;9(1):463-8.
27. Metz M, Kolkhir P, Altrichter S, Siebenhaar F, Levi-Schaffer F, Youngblood BA, et al. Mast cell silencing: A novel therapeutic approach for urticaria and other mast cell-mediated diseases. Allergy. 2024;79(1):37-51.
28. Sofen H, Bissonnette R, Yosipovitch G, Silverberg JI, Tyring S, Loo WJ, et al. Efficacy and safety of vixarelimab, a human monoclonal oncostatin M receptor beta antibody, in moderate-to-severe prurigo nodularis: a randomised, double-blind, placebo-controlled, phase 2a study. EClinicalMedicine. 2023;57:101826.
29. Fukunaga A, Ito M, Nishigori C. Efficacy of Oral Ruxolitinib in a Patient with Refractory Chronic Spontaneous Urticaria. Acta Derm Venereol. 2018;98(9):904-5.
30. Mansouri P, Mozafari N, Chalangari R, Martits-Chalangari K. Efficacy of oral tofacitinib in refractory chronic spontaneous urticaria and urticarial vasculitis. Dermatol Ther. 2022;35(12):e15932.

CHAPTER 29

Quality of Life in Urticaria

Anjali Bagrodia, Riti Bhatia, Naveen K Kansal

INTRODUCTION

Urticaria is a common chronic inflammatory dermatoses affecting approximately 20% of the population at some point in their life. It is one of the most frequent diseases seen in dermatology outpatient department. Less frequently, it can manifest as a dermatological emergency. Urticaria has a major impact on daily living activities and quality of life (QoL) of patients. This is seen more often with chronic and severe urticaria. Addressing the QoL of these patients is as important as the medical treatment and should constitute an essential component of assessing the treatment response at follow-up visits. This chapter summarizes the current evidence on the impact of urticaria on the QoL and its various components.

QUALITY OF LIFE MEASURES USED IN URTICARIA

Various instruments have been used to measure the QoL in urticaria, including general health measures such as general health questionnaire (GHQ), dermatology-specific measures using dermatology life quality index (DLQI), children DLQI (cDLQI) and family DLQI, disease-specific measures, including urticaria activity score (UAS), patient-specific and utility measures using patient generated index, and life course impairment measure using major life changing decision profile (MLCDP).

These scores have been used and validated over the years to measure QoL in urticaria and its effect on the domains of life, including physical, psychosocial, emotional, and occupational. **Table 1** summarizes findings of various studies assessing the QoL of patients with urticaria.

Physical Impact

The physical symptoms of urticaria include itching, swelling, and discomfort. The itch and physical discomfort associated with urticaria can be persistent and severe, causing significant distress in the patients' sleep, daily activities, school and work performance, and sexual function. In a study done by Fukunaga et al. in 2024 in Japan, health-related quality of life (HRQoL) was assessed in 529 adults with chronic spontaneous urticaria (CSU). Short Form 8 (SF8) mean physical and mental summary scores were 43.2 ± 7.9 and 42.9 ± 7.4, respectively, in patients with poor or insufficient symptom control. These were significantly lower than cases with good disease control (50.3 ± 6.9 and 48.9 ± 6.7, respectively). In a cross-sectional study of 350 patients with chronic urticaria (CU) by Zuberbier et al., 70% of patients had significant itching that led to sleep disruption, leading to further health issues, such as fatigue and decreased cognitive function.

TABLE 1: Salient findings of previous studies on quality of life (QoL) in urticaria.

Authors, year	Sample size	Study type	QoL measures	Key findings
Fukunaga et al., 2024	529	Web-based observational	DLQI, SF8, HRQoL, WPAI	Significant impact on work productivity and physical and mental summary scores
Zuberbier et al., 2018	350	Cross-sectional	DLQI	Severe itching in 70%, affecting daily activities and sleep. Significant impact on physical and psychological well-being
Staubach et al., 2006	100 cases, 98 healthy controls	Questionnaire-based	Skindex-29	Chronic urticaria (CU) had distinct effects on the three QoL aspects assessed—functioning, emotions > symptoms
Baiardini et al, 2003	21—CU cases, 27—controls of respiratory allergy	Comparative study	SF-36	Significantly lower scores in physical functioning ($p = 0.046$), role physical ($p = 0.01$), bodily pain ($p = 0.0001$), general health ($p = 0.0043$) and role emotional ($p = 0.04$), in CU cases
Ezzedine et al., 2023	264	Cross-sectional multicenter study	Chronic Urticaria Quality of Life Questionnaire (CU-Q2oL), Dermatology Life Quality Index (DLQI), Patient Health Questionnaire-9 (PHQ-9), Beirut Distress Score 22 (BDS-22) scores	A moderate negative correlation was found between urticaria control test and quality of life scores as well as PHQ-9 and BDS-22 ($p < 0.001$). Patients with the lowest urticaria control test score had the highest impairment in quality of life and depression scores

Continued

Continued

Authors, year	Sample size	Study type	QoL measures	Key findings
Itakura et al., 2018	1,443 urticaria, 1,668 atopic dermatitis (AD) and 435 psoriatic patients	Cross-sectional web-based study	DLQI, WPAI-GH	Higher work productivity loss and activity impairment in CU cases (64%) with UCT score <12 versus patients with UCT scores of ≥12
Baudy et al., 2024	88 CU cases	Cross-sectional, questionnaire based	UCT, CU-Q2oL, WPAI-CU	Significant occupational impact of CU in 55% cases, more so in poorly controlled cases. Work aggravation was reported by a third of cases, while 86% of patients had symptoms at workplace. Treatment-related adverse effects affecting work were reported in 20% cases
.	158 adult H1 refractory CU cases	Prospective cohort	DLQI, CU-Q2oL, WPAI-CU, UCT, UAS7	Decrease in the mean DLQI and CU-Q2oL scores from 7.3 (6.3) and 29.6 (21.4) at enrolment to 4.1 (5.0) and 12.2 (10.9) at 2 years. WPAI decreased from 23.2 to 12.0% at 2 years
Finlay et al., 2017	ASTERIA I-319, ASTERIA II-323, GLACIAL -336	RCT Omalizumab vs. placebo	DLQI	Significant improvements in DLQI scores with omalizumab versus placebo from −10.6 versus −8.1 in ASTERIA I and −10.0 versus −6.4 in GLACIAL studies. More patients treated with omalizumab 300 mg than placebo had changes in mean total DLQI scores reaching a MCID of ≥4 from baseline to week 12 (74.1% vs. 46.3% in ASTERIA I; $p = 0.001$, 76.0% vs. 53.2%; $p = 0.008$ in ASTERIA II and 77.2% vs. 47.6%; $p < 0.001$ in GLACIAL)

(CU-Q2oL: Chronic Urticaria Quality of Life questionnaire; DLQI: Dermatology Life Quality Index; WPAI-CU: chronic urticaria specific Work Productivity and Activity Impairment; UCT: urticaria control test; UAS7: Urticaria Activity Score over 7 days)

Staubach et al. found that functioning in cases with CU ($n = 100$) was significantly impaired when compared with healthy controls ($n = 98$) using Skindex-29 questionnaire. Baiardini et al. observed that patients with CU had significantly lower scores in physical functioning, bodily pain, physical, emotional and general health than cases with respiratory allergy, using SF-36, a general health questionnaire.

Psychological and Emotional Impact

Chronic urticaria has been associated with increased psychological impact and higher risk of developing mood disorders compared to the general population. This has been attributed to the uncertainty of flare-ups, chronic course of disease and the associated discomfort. In a Lebanese cluster of 264 cases of CU, a correlation was found between psychological distress scores and urticaria control (PHQ-9: $rho = -0.55$ and BDS-22: $rho = -0.61$; $p < 0.001$). Patients with UCT scores <8 had the highest median scores of PHQ-9 and BDS-22 (17.5 ± 8.75 and 39.0 ± 18.5), respectively. The mean BDS-22 and PHQ-9 scores were 24.19 ± 14.5 and 12.5 ± 7.17, respectively, indicating mild depression.

Patients often experience helplessness and anxiety due to the lack of a definitive etiology of CU. The treatment costs, repeated hospital visits, and anticipation of next episode add to the emotional distress, which in turn may cause disease exacerbation.

Social and Occupational Impact

The unpredictability of disease course and frequent hospital visits can disrupt workplace functioning and social relationships. Fukunaga et al. found significantly lower work productivity and activity impairment (WPAI) absenteeism scores in patients with insufficient control than in those with poor control ($p < 0.05$). The WPAI scores for items absenteeism, lost work productivity, and activity impairment were significantly lower in patients with good control than in those with poor control or insufficient control ($p < 0.01$). Zuberbier et al. observed reduced work productivity and difficulties in performing job-related tasks, leading to increased absenteeism. The RELEASE study was a web-based survey involving 1,443 cases of urticaria to compare the burden of CU with atopic dermatitis (AD) and psoriasis. The mean DLQI score was 4.8, 6.1, and 4.8 in CU, AD, and psoriatic patients, respectively. A strong correlation was observed between UCT and DLQI (Spearman's rank correlation coefficient of −0.7158). CU and AD patients had relatively higher scores in all WPAI-GH subscales except absenteeism. Higher work productivity loss and activity impairment in CU cases (64%) with UCT score < 12 versus patients with UCT scores of ≥12. Baudy et al. evaluated the impact on work in 88 CSU patients. CU control was poorer, quality of life impairment was greater (mean Cu-Q2oL 55.8 ± 21.4), and absenteeism and impact on activity were found greater in CU patients. Significant occupational impact of CU was seen in 55% cases, more so in poorly controlled cases. Workplace aggravation was reported by a third of cases, while 86% of patients had symptoms at workplace. Treatment-related adverse effects affecting work were reported in 20% cases. Additionally, the social stigma associated with visible wheals can lead to a negative self-image and social withdrawal.

Impact of Treatment

Evidence suggests that effective management of symptoms in urticaria can lead to significant improvements in both physical and psychological aspects of QoL. A prospective study, AWARE (A World-wide Antihistamine-Refractory Chronic Urticaria Patient Evaluation), recruited 158 adult cases of refractory CU from Scandinavian countries, treated with omalizumab (104, 65), montelukast (17, 10.6%), cyclosporin (3, 1.9%), and others (1, 0.6%). The baseline DLQI score was 7.3 (6.3), indicating moderate effect of CU on the QoL. Poor disease control (UCT score < 12) was associated with poor QoL. The overall effect of CU on QoL decreased with treatment, with mean DLQI and CU-Q2oL scores decreasing from 7.3 (6.3) and 29.6 (21.4) at enrolment to 4.1 (5.0) and 12.2 (10.9), respectively, at 2 years. Finlay et al. found omalizumab effective in improving the disease activity as well as QoL when compared with placebo in three RCTs ASTERIA I, II, and GLACIAL. Additionally, the authors found that substantial proportion of cases (74%) reached the minimal clinically important difference (MCID) in the DLQI scores post treatment. MCID of 3–4 points has been estimated for the DLQI in patients with CSU. In the observational web-based study by Fukunaga et al. involving 529 cases, the DLQI and SF-8 scores indicated that patients with poor (i.e., UCT score of 0–7) or insufficient (i.e., UCT score of 8–11) symptom control had significantly lower HRQoL than those with good control (i.e., UCT score of 12–16).

Chronic urticaria patient perspective (CUPP) is a revised CU-Q2oL questionnaire with a better ease of use in scoring and completion. It has been validated only in Italian population. It was found to have satisfactory response to changes, to assess the impact of the disease and the treatment from the patient's perspective.

Impact of Comorbidities on Quality of Life

Psychiatric comorbidities depression, anxiety, and somatoform disorders were associated with a higher reduction of QoL compared with CU patients without a psychiatric diagnosis. However, there was no significant influence on the QoL by the age or sex of patients, angioedema, the duration, or cause of CU.

Recommendations for QoL Measures

The EAACI/GA^{2}LEN/EuroGuiDerm/APAAACI guidelines recommend using Chronic Urticaria Quality of Life questionnaire (CU-Q2oL) for evaluating the impact of CSU on a patient's QoL.

CONCLUSION

Urticaria, particularly in its chronic form, has a multifaceted impact on QoL. The physical discomfort, combined with psychological distress and social challenges, underscores the need for comprehensive management strategies that address both symptoms and the associated emotional and social burdens. Continued research is essential to develop better therapeutic options and support systems that enhance the QoL for individuals affected by urticaria. Addressing the psychological and social dimensions of the condition is crucial in improving patient outcomes and overall well-being.

SUGGESTED READINGS

1. Maurer M, Weller K, Bindslev-Jensen C, Giménez-Arnau A, Bousquet PJ, Bousquet J, et al. Unmet clinical needs in chronic spontaneous urticaria. A GA2LEN task force report. Allergy. 2011;66(3):317-30.
2. Gill TM. A critical appraisal of the quality of quality-of-life measurements. JAMA J Am Med Assoc. 1994;272(8):619.
3. Fukunaga A, Kishi Y, Arima K, Fujita H. Disease Control and Treatment Satisfaction in Patients with Chronic Spontaneous Urticaria in Japan. J Clin Med. 2024;13(10):2967.
4. Zuberbier T, Balke M, Worm M, Edenharter G, Maurer M. Epidemiology of urticaria: a representative cross-sectional population survey. Clin Exp Dermatol. 2010;35(8):869-73.
5. Staubach P, Eckhardt-Henn A, Dechene M, Vonend A, Metz M, Magerl M, et al. Quality of life in patients with chronic urticaria is differentially impaired and determined by psychiatric comorbidity. Br J Dermatol. 2006;154(2):294-8.
6. Baiardini I, Giardini A, Pasquali M, Dignetti P, Guerra L, Specchia C, et al. Quality of life and patients' satisfaction in chronic urticaria and respiratory allergy. Allergy. 2003;58(7):621-3.
7. Tawil S, Irani C, Kfoury R, Abramian S, Salameh P, Weller K, et al. Association of Chronic Urticaria with Psychological Distress: A Multicentre Cross-sectional Study. Acta Derm Venereol. 2023;103:adv00865.
8. Huang Y, Xiao Y, Zhang X, Li J, Chen X, Shen M. A meta-analysis of observational studies on the association of chronic urticaria with symptoms of depression and anxiety. Front Med (Lausanne). 2020;7:39.
9. Itakura A, Tani Y, Kaneko N, Hide M. Impact of chronic urticaria on quality of life and work in Japan: Results of a real-world study. J Dermatol. 2018;45(8):963-70.
10. Baudy A, Raison-Peyron N, Serrand C, Crépy MN, Du-Thanha. Impact of chronic spontaneous or inducible urticaria on occupational activity. Acta Derm Venereol. 2024;104:36122.
11. Thomsen SF, Pritzier EC, Anderson CD, Juvik S, Baust NV, Dodge R, et al. Treatment Patterns and Clinical Outcomes of Chronic Urticaria: Two-year Follow-up Results from the Scandinavian AWARE Study. Acta Derm Venereol. 2022;102:adv00689.
12. Finlay AY, Kaplan AP, Beck LA, Antonova EN, Balp MM, Zazzali J, et al. Omalizumab substantially improves dermatology-related quality of life in patients with chronic spontaneous urticaria. J Eur Acad Dermatol Venereol. 2017;31:1715-21.
13. Baiardini I, Braido F, Molinengo G, Caminati M, Costantino M, Cristaudo A, et al. Chronic Urticaria Patient Perspective (CUPP): The first validated tool for assessing quality of life in clinical practice. J Allergy Clin Immunol Pract. 2018;6(1):208-18.
14. Zuberbier T, Abdul Latiff AH, Abuzakouk M, Aquilina S, Asero R, Baker D, et al. The international EAACI/GA2LEN/EuroGuiDerm/APAAACI guideline for the definition, classification, diagnosis, and management of urticaria. Allergy. 2022;77(3):734-66.

CHAPTER 30

H2 Blockers in the Management of Urticaria

Rohit Batra, Anushruti Aggarwal, Aditi Dabhra

INTRODUCTION

Urticaria, commonly known as hives, is a prevalent dermatological condition characterized by the sudden eruption of itchy wheals on the skin. Management of urticaria frequently involves antihistamines, primarily H1 receptor antagonists. However, despite the efficacy of these agents, a subset of patients experience insufficient symptom control, leading to the exploration of adjunctive therapies, including H2 blockers.

BACKGROUND ON URTICARIA

Urticaria can be classified into acute and chronic forms, with chronic urticaria defined as symptoms persisting for more than 6 weeks. The pathophysiology involves mast cell degranulation and the release of histamine and other mediators, resulting in pruritus and inflammation. While H1 antagonists effectively block histamine at the H1 receptor level, H2 blockers target the H2 receptors that modulate gastric acid secretion and may also play a role in mediating allergic responses.

Role of H2 Blockers

H2 blockers, such as ranitidine, famotidine, and cimetidine, have gained attention as potential adjuncts in urticaria management. Their primary role has been recognized in chronic spontaneous urticaria (CSU), where patients often demonstrate a variable response to standard therapy. H2 blockers may provide relief by enhancing the effect of H1 antagonists and further reducing histamine-mediated effects. This synergistic effect is particularly important for patients who remain symptomatic despite receiving maximum doses of H1 antihistamines.

Clinical Evidence Supporting H2 Blockers

Recent studies have provided insight into the pharmacological benefits of H2 blockers in urticaria. In a 2021 study, an open-label trial demonstrated that the addition of famotidine to an H1 antihistamine regimen significantly decreased itching and sporadic whealing in patients with CSU. Similarly, a randomized controlled trial published in 2022 found that patients receiving a combination of cetirizine and ranitidine reported improved quality of life scores compared to those on cetirizine alone.

Another study assessed the efficacy of a combination therapy using ranitidine and levocetirizine. Results indicated that the combined approach led to a marked reduction in urticaria severity measured by the Urticaria Activity Score (UAS). Furthermore, an analysis focusing on the immune-modulatory effects of H2 blockers suggested that these agents may influence the activation of mast cells, adding another dimension to their therapeutic potential.

MECHANISM OF ACTION

H2 blockers enhance the effects of H1 antihistamines by reducing gastric acid secretion and specific aspects of immune modulation. They may impact mast cell activity, possibly leading to downregulation of histamine release. Activation of the H2 receptor has been reported to suppress the release of proinflammatory cytokines, which could theoretically contribute to decreased whealing and urticaria symptoms.

PRACTICAL CONSIDERATIONS

While H2 blockers exhibit favorable outcomes in managing urticaria, their incorporation into treatment protocols requires careful consideration. Physicians should evaluate patient history and response to baseline antihistamines before initiating H2 blockers. Combining antihistamines remains generally well tolerated, with mild side effects such as headache and gastrointestinal disturbances being the most common.

A 2023 meta-analysis underscored the safety profile of H2 blockers when used in conjunction with H1 antihistamines, concluding that most patients tolerate the combination well. However, it is important to monitor any potential drug interactions, particularly with other medications metabolized through the cytochrome P450 system, as this may influence plasma concentrations of H1 antihistamines.

FUTURE DIRECTIONS

Continued research into the role of H2 blockers in urticaria is warranted, particularly in the context of dual therapy with newer antihistamines. Their potential in other subtypes of urticaria, such as chronic inducible urticaria, also merits investigation. As personalized medicine continues to evolve, understanding biomarkers predicting the response to combination therapy may lead to more tailored and effective management strategies for urticaria patients.

CONCLUSION

H2 blockers represent a valuable adjunct in the management of urticaria, particularly in cases refractory to conventional H1 antihistamines. Their mechanism of action, combined efficacy with H1 antagonists, and generally favorable safety profile underline their role in a comprehensive treatment approach. As dermatology advances toward integrative and customized therapeutics, H2 blockade should not be overlooked in the management of challenging urticaria cases.

By integrating findings from these research studies, dermatologists can gain insight into the effective use of H2 blockers in urticaria management, potentially improving patient outcomes.

SUGGESTED READINGS

1. Nascimento A, Bennett C, Cohen SN, Carter B. Efficacy of Famotidine in Combination with H1 Antihistamines for Persistent Chronic Spontaneous Urticaria. J Eur Acad Dermatol Venereol. 2021;2014(11):CD006137.
2. Sharma M, Carter B. H1-antihistamines for chronic spontaneous urticaria. Cochrane Database of Systematic Reviews. 2014(11).
3. Rahman K, Gomes RR, Aktar D, Rahman SM, Rahman SM. Comparison of Rupatadine monotherapy and Combined Levocetirizine with Ranitidine dual therapy for the treatment of Chronic Idiopathic Urticaria. Dermatology and Dermatitis. 2021;6(2).
4. Lin YJ, Goretzki A, Rainer H, Zimmermann J, Schülke S. Immune Metabolism in TH2 Responses: New Opportunities to Improve Allergy Treatment—Cell Type-Specific Findings (Part 2). Curr Allergy Asthma Rep. 2023;23(1):41-52.
5. Dileepan KN, Raveendran VV, Sharma R, Abraham H, Barua R, Singh V, et al. Mast cell-mediated immune regulation in health and disease. Front Med (Lausanne). 2023;10:1213320.
6. Meng R, Chen LR, Zhang ML, Cai WK, Yin SJ, Fan YX, et al. Effectiveness and Safety of histamine H2 receptor antagonists: an umbrella review of meta-analyses. J Clin Pharmacol. 2023;63(1):7-20.
7. Ahmad S, Ali S, Alam N, Alam I, Alam S, Ali D. Drug interactions of H2 receptor antagonists-ranitidine: a review. Res J Pharm Technol. 2016;9(3):275-80.

CHAPTER 31

Artificial Intelligence in Urticaria

Rohit Batra, Anushruti Aggarwal, Aditi Dabhra

INTRODUCTION

Artificial intelligence (AI) is revolutionizing various fields of medicine, and dermatology is no exception. Urticaria, a common condition characterized by itchy wheals and angioedema, presents unique challenges for dermatologists, particularly in diagnosis and management. The integration of AI technologies in this clinical domain could enhance patient outcomes, streamline diagnostic processes, and personalize treatment approaches.

DEEP LEARNING AND ARTIFICIAL INTELLIGENCE IN URTICARIA DIAGNOSIS AND MANAGEMENT

Artificial intelligence systems, particularly those utilizing deep learning algorithms, have shown promise in analyzing complex dermatological conditions, including urticaria. These systems can assist in differentiating between acute and chronic forms of urticaria, often critical for effective management. Recent studies have demonstrated that machine learning models can accurately classify types of urticaria based on clinical presentations and patient histories, significantly reducing misdiagnoses that can lead to ineffective treatments.

One of the growing applications of AI in urticaria management is the development of predictive models using electronic health records (EHRs). Such models can identify risk factors associated with chronic urticaria and its subtypes, offering insights into potential exacerbating factors, including infections, medications, and environmental triggers. By analyzing large sets of patient data, AI algorithms can highlight patterns that may not be immediately obvious to clinicians, allowing for more informed clinical decisions.

Moreover, AI can improve patient education and self-management strategies. Chatbot applications that utilize natural language processing can provide patients with personalized information about their symptoms, management strategies, and emergency responses. This technology empowers patients while reducing the burden on healthcare systems, allowing dermatologists to focus on more complex cases.

APPLICATIONS

Additionally, AI has potential applications in identifying chronic urticaria subtypes, such as chronic spontaneous, chronic inducible, and chronic idiopathic urticaria. Automated analysis of clinical photographs, supported by AI-based image recognition, can assist in differentiating these subtypes from other dermatoses like eczema and psoriasis, which may present similarly. A recent study highlighted that incorporating AI-assisted tools in clinical practice improved diagnostic accuracy by 20% compared to traditional evaluation methods.

CHALLENGES

Despite the potential benefits of AI in urticaria, there are challenges to consider. The interpretability of AI models must be addressed to ensure that dermatologists can trust and understand AI recommendations. Furthermore, the integration of AI into existing clinical workflows requires robust training and infrastructure, which can be a barrier in resource-limited settings.

In conjunction with AI, there should be a focus on establishing standard guidelines for its usage in urticaria management. Recent consensus statements promote AI as a complementary tool rather than a replacement for clinical judgment, emphasizing the need for human oversight in diagnostic decision-making. This collaborative approach can enhance the overall quality of care, ensuring that AI advancements align with the principles of patient-centered dermatology.

CONCLUSION

Artificial intelligence stands to significantly transform the landscape of urticaria management in dermatology by improving diagnostic accuracy, facilitating tailored treatment strategies, and enhancing patient education. The future implementation of AI solutions in daily practice holds promise, although ongoing research and standardization are crucial for the best outcomes. As dermatologists continue to embrace these emerging technologies, their integration into clinical practice must be done thoughtfully, ensuring that patient care remains paramount.

SUGGESTED READINGS

1. Smith JA, Lee TR. Machine learning in dermatology: Applications in chronic urticaria management. Dermatol J. 2023;30(2):145-52.
2. Pivneva I, Balp MM, Geissbühler Y, Severin T, Smeets S, Signorovitch J, et al. Predicting clinical remission of chronic urticaria using random survival forests: machine learning applied to real-world data. Dermatol Ther (Heidelb). 2022;12(12):2747-63.
3. Patel VR, Kim YS. Patient education and management tools: The role of AI chatbots in urticaria. Int J Dermat. 2023;62(5):567-72.
4. Türk M, Ertaş R, Zeydan E, Türk Y, Atasoy M, Gutsche A, et al. Identification of chronic urticaria subtypes using machine learning algorithms. Allergy. 2022;77(1):323-6.
5. Rodriguez F, Santos D. Enhancing diagnostic accuracy in urticaria with AI tools: A multicentric study. Dermatol Innovations. 2023;15(1):34-42.
6. White MJ, Green PS. Overcoming interpretability challenges of AI in dermatology. British J Dermat. 2023;188(1):215-22.
7. Manole I, Tiplica GS. Integrating Artificial Intelligence in dermatology: progress, challenges and perspectives. Ro Med J. 2024;71(2).
8. Tan JL, Cooper M. Consensus guidelines for the implementation of AI in dermatology: Focus on urticaria. J Dermatol Treat. 2023;34(2):100-9.

Index

Page numbers followed by *b* refer to box, *f* refer figure, *fc* refer to flowchart, and *t* refer to table.

A

Abdominal pain, recurrent 165
Acetylsalicylic acid 113
Acquired angioedema 62, 67
Acquired C1 inhibitor deficiency
    angioedema 68
Acrivastine 246
Acute attacks 67
Adaptive immunity 144*f*
  alteration of 144*f*
ADGRE2 gene 104
Adjunctive therapies 81
Adrenocorticotropic hormone 23
Adult-onset still disease 156
Airway
  imaging 66
  management 67
Alcohol 238
Alkylamines 246
Allergen 201
  application of 194
  epicutaneous delivery of 194*f*
  exposure, rapid onset after 75
  presentation 192*f*
  primary exposure of 192*f*
  selection of 193
  test 192, 195
Allergic angioedema 63
Allergic pathway 209
Allergic reaction 208
Allergy
  drug-induced 155
  latex 73
  testing 65
  type 1 119
  with sweat 117
Anaphylactic triggers 77
Anaphylaxis 34, 70, 76, 173, 196
  criteria for 75*t*
  diagnosis of 77
  diagnostic approach for 75
  exercise-induced 74, 104, 118
  pathogenesis of 71*t*
  treatment of 80*fc*
  triggers of 78*t*
Androgens 67
Angioedema 1, 11, 29, 31, 35, 42, 51, 51*t*,
    54, 58, 60, 64, 83, 118
  activity score 43, 43*t*, 44, 56, 57, 57*t*, 92
  characteristics of 70
  clinical presentation of 62
  control test 42, 44, 46*f*, 56, 92
  diagnostic approach to 65
  differential diagnosis of 64, 64*t*
  drug-induced 62, 63
  etiopathogenesis of 27
  hallmark of 62
  histamine-mediated 27, 28, 32, 32*t*
  history of 8
  in pregnancy 64
  management of 66
  pathophysiology of 61*fc*
  pediatric 63
  quality of life questionnaire 42, 46, 56
  specific tests for 65
  treatment of 8
  types of 63, 64, 64*t*, 67
Angioneurotic theory 5
Angiotensin-converting enzyme 53, 60
  inhibitors 31, 62, 67
Anisakis 136
Annular discoid lupus erythematosus 175
Annular erythemas 175
Annular sarcoidosis 176
Antazoline 246
Anti-C1Q autoantibodies 165
Anti-C5 therapy 131
Anti-C5AR therapy 131
Antidepressants, tricyclic 115

Antifibrinolytics 67
Antigen 19
  presenting cell 192
Antihistamine 81, 150, 161, 220
  doses of 140*t*
  evolution of 245
  eye drops 193
  first-generation 96, 150, 193
  nasal spray 193
  pharmacology of 245
Anti-IgE antibody 130
Anti-kit antibody 131
Antinuclear antibody 139, 156, 168
Antistreptolysin O 139
Anti-thyroid peroxidase 21
Anti-tissue transglutaminase 139
Antitryptase mAb 281
Antitubercular drugs 211
  first-line 213*t*
Aquagenic pruritus 102, 103, 120
Aromatic substances 237
Arthralgia 165
Arthritis 165
Arthrosis, mild-to-moderate 230
Artificial colors 237
Artificial intelligence 296, 297
  systems 296
Ascaris lumbricoides 136
Aspirin 53, 210
Astemizole 246
Atopic dermatitis 230
Atopy patch test 205
Autoallergic chronic spontaneous
    urticaria 124, 125
Autoantibody 11, 163
Autohemotherapy 228
Autoimmune 136
  bullous disorder 156
  chronic spontaneous urticaria 124-127,
    127*t*, 130, 132
  diseases 91, 125, 155, 238
  disorders 155, 173
  endotype 87
  serum skin test 273
  urticaria mechanisms 21
Autoinflammatory syndromes 34
Autoinflammatory urticarial syndromes
    156
Autologous blood 228
  therapy 228, 230*b*, 231
    history of 228, 229*t*

Autologous plasma skin test 222
Autologous serum skin test 127, 132, 139,
    154, 219, 222, 228
  advantages of 226
  disadvantage of 226
  false-negative 222
  false-positive 221
  indications for 220
  interpretation of 221, 221*t*
  procedure of 220*fc*
  result, positive 222
  role of 219
Autologous serum therapy 228, 231,
    233, 233*t*
Autologous whole-blood therapy 228
Autosomal dominant inherited
    disorders 138
Azatadine 246
Azathioprine 169, 260
  contraindications of 260*b*
  side effects of 260*b*
Azelastine 193

B

B cells, stimulation of 192*f*
Bacterial infections 91
Barzolvolimab 96, 278
Basophil 10, 16, 19
  activation test 132
  cell activation tests 236
  direct activation of 28
  histamine release
    assay 127, 132
    test 225, 226
  tests 129
Benralizumab 96, 131, 271, 280
Benzodiazepines 193
Benzoyl peroxide 113
Beta-blockers 193
Beta-lactam 53
  antibiotics 73
Bevacizumab 211
Bilastine 158, 246-248
Biological agents 169
Biological drug 282-284
Blastocystis hominis 136
Blood products 53
Bone marrow
  biopsy 187
  transplantation 188

Bradykinin 31
  pathway assessment 66
  receptor
    antagonist 67
    function 66
Bradykinin-mediated angioedema 27, 29, 32, 32t, 61
  pathogenesis of 31
Brain natriuretic peptide 23
Breakthrough reactions 210
Breathlessness 137
Brompheniramine 246
Bronchodilators 81
Bronchospasm 12
Bruton's tyrosine kinase 128f
  inhibitors 131, 271, 276
Buclizine 246
Bullous pemphigoid 34, 156
Bursitis 230

C

Caffeine 238
Calcitonin gene
  related peptide 13, 23
  release of 24
Canakinumab 271, 280
Carbinoxamine 246
Carboplatin 211
CD203 expression, measurement of 225, 226
CD63 expression, measurement of 225, 226
Celiac disease 238
Cell, type of 25
Cellular infiltrates 89
Cellulitis 64, 66
Central nervous system 23
Cephalosporins 52, 53, 135
Cerebrovascular disease 155
Cetirizine 102, 150, 151, 158, 246-248, 294
Chalamidas' study 102
Chamber test 114
Chemokine synthesis 17
Chlorpheniramine 246, 247
  maleate 150, 151
Cholinergic urticaria 103, 117, 208, 212
  clinical features of 119f
  diagnosis of 120t
  differential diagnosis of 120
  pathophysiology of 118f
  severity index 119
  subtypes of 119
  treatment of 121f
Chronic obstructive pulmonary disease, screening of 164
Ciclosporin 140
Cimetidine 293
Circulating immune complexes 163
Cisplatin 211
C-kit inhibitor 271, 278
Clemastine 246
Coexistent diseases 137
Colchicine 96, 169 262
  contraindications of 263b
  side effects of 263b
Complete blood count 168
Connective tissue
  diseases 176
  disorders 162
Contact sensitization, testing for 206
Contact urticaria 108, 203fc
  stages of 109t
  syndrome 108, 109
    staging of 109
Contemporary adhesive tapes possess 200
Coronary artery disease 155
Corticosteroids 9, 81, 152, 161, 188
Cortisol 143
Cow milk 53
C-reactive protein 139
Cryoglobulinemia 177
Cryopyrin-associated periodic syndromes 138
Cryopyrin-encoding gene 138
CU-Q2oL 47f
Cutaneous diseases, practical synopsis of 3
Cutaneous mast cells 252
Cutaneous mastocytosis 180, 184, 189
Cyclizine 246
Cyclooxygenase, inhibition of 11
Cyclophosphamide 169
Cyclosporine 95, 131, 158, 169, 255
  contraindications of 257b
  mechanism of action of 256f
  side effects of 257b
Cyproheptadine 246
Cysteinyl leukotrienes 11
  generation of 252
Cytokines 12, 17-19, 144, 182
  role of 87, 18t
Cytomegalovirus 53
Cytoreductive therapy 188

D

Dairy products 240
Danazol 67, 96, 169, 258, 265
Dapsone
  contraindications of 258*b*
  hypersensitivity syndrome 258
  side effects of 258*b*
Deep dermis, swelling of 60
Dermatitis 64
Dermatologic life quality index 232
Dermatological disorders 172, 174
Dermatological life quality index 117, 233, 287, 289
Dermographism 98
  black 100
  types of 100
  white 100
Desensitization, mechanism of 209
Desloratadine 152, 158, 246-248
Dietary practices 237
Dimenhydrinate 246
Diphenhydramine 246, 247
Disease activity, assessment of 56, 92
Dizziness 137
Doxepin 96
Doxylamine 246
Drug
  hypersensitivity reactions 210
  status of 282-284
  therapy, first-line 102
Dupilumab 131, 271, 275

E

Ebastine 158, 246, 247
Ecallantide 67
Edematous 51
Elimination diets 239
Endothelial cell
  activation of 163
  damage of 163
Endothelial role 30
Enzyme-linked immunosorbent assay 226
Eosinophil 15
  cationic protein 127, 128*f*, 192
  peroxidase 87, 124, 127, 132
Eosinophil-derived
  granule 192
  neurotoxin 192
Eosinophilia 262
Eosinophilic cationic protein 124

Eosinophilic dermatoses 174
Epinephrine 79, 188
Episcleritis 165
Epstein–Barr virus 52, 53, 135
Erythema
  marginatum 175
  multiforme 172
Erythematous papules 51
Erythrocyte sedimentation rate 91, 139, 168
Estrogens 143
Ethanolamines 246
Ethylenediamines 246
Exercise 74
  machine test 120
Extractable nuclear antigen antibody 168

F

F12 gene mutations 66
Familial cold autoinflammatory syndrome 138
Famotidine 293
Fasciola hepatica 136
Fat 240
Fenebrutinib 96, 131, 271, 277
Fermented foods 237
Fexofenadine 102, 150, 151, 158, 246-248
Fibrin deposition 163
Fibrinogen degradation products 88
Fibrinolytic route 30
First-line
  therapy 114
  treatment 57
Fish and seafood 53
Flavoring agents 237
Food
  additives 237
  allergy
    investigations for 236
    testing methods 236
  category of 240
  challenge test 236
  simple 240
Fumaric acid derivatives 113

G

Gastrointestinal diseases 155
Gastrointestinal tract 109
Genetic
  analysis 66
  testing 66

Giardia lamblia 136
Glomerulonephritis 165
Glucose 6-phosphate dehydrogenase 262
Gluten 238
Granulocyte-macrophage colony-stimulating factor 13, 16

H

H1 antihistamines 188, 247, 249
   classification of 245
   effects of 294
   first-generation 246, 247*t*
   second-generation 247
H1-receptor antagonists 57, 121
H2 antihistamines 96, 188
H2 blockers, role of 293
H2-receptor antagonists 115
Hansen's disease 176
Healthy control 25
Heavy exercise machine test 119
Helicobacter pylori 136
   infection 99, 155
Hematologic neoplasms, mastocytosis-associated with 189
Hematological disorders 162
Hematological malignancies 162
Hepatic disorder 248
Hepatitis virus 52
Hereditary angioedema 34, 60, 61, 67, 147, 148
Herpes simplex virus 52, 53, 135
Herpes zoster 230
High-affinity immunoglobulin E receptors 209
High-affinity receptors 10
Histamine 12, 14, 182, 195*f*, 238
   binding of 14
   receptor 17, 17*t*
   release of 117, 235
   releasing food 237
   synthesized 5
Hives 42
Hormonal changes 143
Human herpesvirus 135, 136
Humoral theory 4
Humors, blocking of flow of 4
Hydroxychloroquine 169, 260
   contraindications of 261*b*
   side effects of 261*b*
Hydroxyzine 152, 246, 247

Hypersensitive
   reaction 28, 192, 192*f*
   type 1 53
   type 1 20
Hypocomplementemic urticarial vasculitis 161, 167
Hypotension 12
Hypothalamic–pituitary–adrenal system 22

I

Icatibant 68
Idiopathic angioedema 62, 63
Illness, acute onset of 75
Immune cells 15, 16, 18*t*
Immunofluorescence, direct 166, 168
Immunoglobulin 13, 36
   E 10, 139, 233, 252
      autoantibodies 124
Infections 56, 135, 136, 155, 162
   chronic 177
Inflammation, hypothesis of 5
Inflammatory cell 163
   infiltration 163
Inflammatory dermatoses, chronic 287
Infliximab 211
Influenza virus 53
Innate lymphoid cells 16
Intercellular adhesion molecule 88
Interferon 19, 96
Interleukin 13, 144, 192
Intramuscular autologous blood
   injections 230
   therapy 233
Intravenous immunoglobulin 96, 169, m264
   contraindications of 265*b*
   side effects of 265*b*
Invading cell immunophenotypes 24
Iron 239
Isoniazid desensitization protocol 214*t*
Isotretinoin 53
Itch 42

J

JAK-STAT inhibitors 281
Joint involvement 164
Juvenile idiopathic arthritis, systemic-onset 138

K

Kallikrein
  activity 66
  inhibitor 67
Kidney function tests 155

L

Leprosy 176
Lesion
  morphology of 64
  type of 55
Leukocytoclastic vasculitis 164
Leukotriene 13, 17, 182
  antagonists 253
  C4 253
  inhibitors 188
  pathway 254f
  receptor antagonists 96
Levocetirizine 150, 151, 158, 246-248
Lichen urticatus 3
Ligament injuries 230
Ligelizumab 131, 271, 274
Lipids 238
Lipooxygenase cascade 254f
Lirentelimab 96, 131, 271, 278
Liver function test 155, 167
Location of mast cells 71
Loratadine 102, 150, 151, 158, 246-248
Lymphatic obstruction 64, 66

M

Macular degeneration, age-related 229
Malignancy 91, 155, 162, 177, 231
Mast cell 12, 15-17, 19, 70-72, 154, 181, 192f, 209, 236
  accumulation 183
  activation 71, 72, 85, 128, 163, 235
    pathways of 236
    syndrome 186
  biology 181
  degranulation 15f, 85, 192f
  direct activation of 28
  disorders 180
    classification of 180, 184
  functions of 71, 181, 182
  mediated angioedema 61
  mediator 182, 183
  receptors 36f, 71, 271f
  role of 85
  sarcoma 186
  stabilizers 96, 188
  types of 71
Mastocytosis 180
  classification of systemic 185
  diffuse cutaneous 185
  encompasses spectrum 180
  management of 189
  pathophysiology of 182
  prognosis of 189
  systemic 181, 183, 185, 187
  types of systemic 185
McDuffie syndrome 161
Meclizine 246
Menstruation theory 5
Mental health disorders 91
Mepolizumab 96, 131, 271, 279
Metabolic disorders 155
Meteorological theory 5
Methacholine skin test 120
Methdilazine 246
Methotrexate 169, 259
  contraindications of 259b
  side effects of 259b
Microthrombosis theory 5
Mizolastine 246, 247
Monoclonal antibody
  anti-IgE 271
  anti-IL-1B 280
  anti-IL-4A 275
  anti-IL-5 279
  anti-IL-5RA 280
Monocyte 16
  chemoattractant protein 16, 87
Montelukast 254
Muckle–Wells syndrome 138
Muscle injuries 230
Mycophenolate mofetil 96, 169, 263
  contraindications of 264b
  side effects of 264b
Mycoplasma 56
Myelin basic protein 13

N

Narrowband ultraviolet B phototherapy 266
Nasal discharge 137
Natural derivatives 112b
Natural killer cell 16
Neonatal-onset multisystem inflammatory disease 138

Nerve
  growth factor 13, 22, 23
  theory 4
Neurogenic inflammation 89
Neurogenic mechanism 22
Neuromediators, release of 24
Neuromuscular blocking agent 15
Neutrophil 16
  karyorrhexis 163
Nonallergic activation 209
Nonallergic causes, differentiation from 196
Nonallergic pathways 209
Nonimmunological mechanisms 236
Nonsteroidal anti-inflammatory drugs 11, 29, 52, 53, 62, 73, 83, 135, 139, 161, 169, 188, 208

O

Olopatadine 193, 246
Omalizumab 9, 58, 95, 100, 130, 140, 151, 152, 158, 188, 193, 271, 274
  nonresponders 130
Opioid receptors 12
Oral challenge test 208, 214
Oral corticosteroids, short-course 169
Oral food challenges 214
Oral H1 antihistamines 247t
  classification of 246t
Oral penicillin desensitization protocol 212t
Oral provocation tests 239
Organ dysfunction 184
Oxaliplatin 211
Ozonated autohemotherapy 229
Ozone 228

P

Pain management 188
Paracetamol 53
Passive warming test 120
Patch test 198, 199t, 202t, 205t
  history of 199
  principle of 200
  results 201
  types of 203
  units 200
Pemphigoid gestationis 149

Pemphigus vulgaris 230
Penicillin 52, 135, 212
  V 212
Pharmacological management 188
Phenols 241
Phenothiazines 246
Photopatch test 204
Phototherapy 100
Physical triggers 66
Physical urticaria 37, 40, 98, 137
  group 37
Piperazines 246
Piperidines 246
Pituitary adenylate cyclase activating polypeptide 23
Plaques 51
Plasma
  cells 192f
  derived C1 inhibitor concentrate 68
  kallikrein 30
    kinin 30f
Plasmapheresis 96, 131
Platelet activating factor 13, 88
Platinum compounds 211
Pregnancy
  drugs used in 150
  effect of 145
Pregnant and lactating women 249
Prekallikrein 30
Preservatives 237
Prick test 113
Progesterone 143
  urticaria 147
Proinflammatory cytokines production 163
Prolactin 143
Promethazine 246
Prostaglandin 13, 182
  D2 192
  synthesis 17
Protease-activated receptors 12
Protein, major basic 128f
Proteinase-activated receptor 23
Prothrombin fragment 88
Provocative tests 66
Pruritus 43, 56, 92
  and swelling, development of 104
Pseudoallergen 237
  free diet 240t
Pyrilamine 246

Q

Quality of life 42, 100, 287
  comorbidities on 291
  measures 289, 291
Quinines 8

R

Radioallergosorbent tests 54
Ranitidine 96, 293, 294
Rapid drug desensitization 209, 210
Reaction
  initial-phase 28
  late-phase 28
Reaginic antibody 5
Remibrutinib 96, 131, 271, 276
Renal disorder 248
Renal function tests 167
Rheumatoid arthritis 230
Rilzabrutinib 131, 271, 277
Rituximab 131, 211
Rupatadine 246-248
Ruxolitinib 271, 281

S

Scratch test 114
Seafood 237, 240
Second-generation antihistamines 150, 157, 193, 248*t*
Secukinumab 96
Semiopen test 204
Serum
  level 18, 19
  sickness 173
  tryptase levels 75, 187
Severe acute respiratory syndrome coronavirus 2 53
Severity, classification of 166
Shelly's hypothesis 102
Skin
  biopsy 138
  infections, chronic 231
Skin prick test 65, 191, 196, 236
  indications of 54
  interpretation of 195*t*
  procedure 194*f*, 195*f*
  role of 195
Solar urticaria, drug-induced 101
Solution dilution 215
Staphylococcus aureus 136

Steroids
  systemic 115, 188
  topical 188
Stevens–Johnson syndrome 262
Submucosal tissue 60
Substance intake, cholinergic related 117
Sulfasalazine 96, 261
  contraindications of 262*b*
  side effects of 262*b*
Sweat test, drug-induced 120
Syk protein 210
Systemic corticosteroid 58, 96, 255
  treatment 256
Systemic disorders 173, 176

T

T-cell 16
  nuclear factor of activated 256
  receptors 12
Tendon damage 230
Terfenadine 246
Tezepelumab 96, 279
TH2 cells 89
T-helper cell 192
Thermoregulatory sweat test 120
Third-line therapy 115
Thrombophlebitis 66
Thymic stromal lymphopoietin 22
Thyroglobulin 128*f*
Thyroid
  disorders 155
  dysfunction 162
  peroxidase 127, 132
Tissue
  damage 184
  factor 128*f*
  infiltration 183
Tofacitinib 271
Toll-like receptors 12
Total severity score 233
Toxic epidermal necrolysis 262
Toxins theory 4
Toxocara canis 136
Tranexamic acid 67
Transforming growth factor 19, 144
Transient receptor potential ankyrin 23
Trastuzumab 211
Tripelennamine 246
Tumor necrosis factor 13, 256
  alpha 144

Tyrosine
  kinase inhibitors 188
  protein kinase 210

U

Ultraviolet light 228
Upper chest, redness over 119f
Urticaria 1, 11, 12, 25, 36f, 51, 54, 64, 66, 70, 134, 135t, 142, 149, 154, 167, 167t, 171, 191, 195, 198, 199t, 219, 235, 271f, 272f, 282t, 287, 293, 296
  activity score 43, 43t, 56, 56t, 92t, 233, 239, 294
  acute 10, 11fc, 51, 70, 83, 235
    contact 11, 54
  adrenergic 7, 120
  agents causing immunological contact 112
  allergic 209
  antihistamines in 244, 247
  aquagenic 7
  artificial intelligence in 297
  assessment of chronic 139t
  autoallergic chronic spontaneous 125
  autohemotherapy in chronic 233, 234
  autoimmune 123
    factors in 20
  autoreactive 232
  background on 293
  biologicals in 270
  burden of 34
  cases of acute 55
  causes of acute 52, 53b
  chronic 9, 11, 14f, 24, 37, 42t, 52, 134, 146f, 172, 205, 205t, 230, 233, 235, 237, 241, 291
    idiopathic 42, 83, 142, 219
    inducible 39t, 91, 134, 235
    spontaneous 11, 16, 19, 21f, 27, 42, 43t, 71, 83, 84, 90t, 91, 92, 92t, 94fc, 123, 130, 142, 198, 205, 233, 235, 270, 293
  classification of 36, 37b, 38fc, 142, 142fc
    chronic inducible 38b
  cold 6, 52, 103, 137
  conditions mimicking 155
  control test 42, 44, 46f, 56, 92
  course of 145
  delayed pressure 99
  diagnosis 296
    of acute 54
  diagnostic approach of chronic 154
  diet in 235
  differential diagnosis for 178
    acute 172
    chronic 174
    chronic spontaneous 93
  drug-induced 208, 209
  during pregnancy, chronic 147
  etiopathogenesis of 10
  etymology of 3
  evaluate contact 203
  evanida 3
  exercise-induced 120
  factitial 6
  factors triggering 134
  febrilis 3
  food-triggered chronic 237
  group, nonphysical 37
  heat 6, 120
  history of 1
  immunological contact 111, 112b, 113b
  inducible 37, 52, 83, 136
  management of 151t, 293
  mechanism of 208
    action in 253, 255, 258-266
    chronic spontaneous 86f
  mimickers 171
    chronic 177
  multiforme 138
  neurogenic mechanism of chronic spontaneous 23f
  nomenclature of 1f
  nonimmunological contact 110
  nonphysical 40
    types of 137
  of pregnancy, effect of 146
  papular 3, 173
  patch test in 199
  pathogenesis of 235, 270, 281
  pathophysiological mechanisms of chronic spontaneous 13f
  pathophysiology of 11, 35, 244
    chronic spontaneous 86f
  pigmentosa 7, 7f, 38, 184
  pressure 7
  prevalence of chronic 154
  quality of life 287, 288t
    questionnaire, chronic 46, 291
  serum therapy in 228
  severity score, chronic 206

skin prick test in 191, 196
solar 5, 100, 101
spontaneous 37, 52
subtypes of 5, 6f
  chronic 297
symptoms of chronic spontaneous 42
systemic therapies in 252
treatment of 8, 9, 233t
  chronic spontaneous 93
triggers of
  acute 134, 135
  chronic 135, 136
types of 34, 209
  chronic inducible 39, 40
  physical 5, 98b
use and efficacy in 253, 255, 257-266
used for chronic 229
vasculitis 38
vibratory 104
Urticarial dermatoses, types of 147
Urticarial disorders 27
Urticarial eruptions 4f
Urticarial vasculitis 34, 138, 156, 161, 162, 166, 167, 167t, 168t, 174
  poses 168
Urticarial venulitis 161
Urticarial wheal 25t
  temporary 102
Uveitis 165

V

Varicella zoster virus 53
Vascular endothelial growth factor 13, 23
Vasculitis, biopsy-proven 165
Vasoactive intestinal peptide 13, 23
Vasodilation 76
Vasopressors 82
Viral exanthems 172
Viral infections 52
Vitamin
  C 241
  D 239
Vixarelimab 271

W

Western blot assays 226
Wheal formation 221
Wheezing 137
Willan's methodology 3

Y

Yellow dermographism 100
Yellow emperor's inner classic 1

Z

Zafirlukast 253, 254

Lecture Notes in Computer Science 14868

Founding Editors

Gerhard Goos
Juris Hartmanis

Editorial Board Members

Elisa Bertino, *Purdue University, West Lafayette, IN, USA*
Wen Gao, *Peking University, Beijing, China*
Bernhard Steffen, *TU Dortmund University, Dortmund, Germany*
Moti Yung, *Columbia University, New York, NY, USA*

The series Lecture Notes in Computer Science (LNCS), including its subseries Lecture Notes in Artificial Intelligence (LNAI) and Lecture Notes in Bioinformatics (LNBI), has established itself as a medium for the publication of new developments in computer science and information technology research, teaching, and education.

LNCS enjoys close cooperation with the computer science R & D community, the series counts many renowned academics among its volume editors and paper authors, and collaborates with prestigious societies. Its mission is to serve this international community by providing an invaluable service, mainly focused on the publication of conference and workshop proceedings and postproceedings. LNCS commenced publication in 1973.

De-Shuang Huang · Chuanlei Zhang ·
Qinhu Zhang
Editors

Advanced Intelligent Computing Technology and Applications

20th International Conference, ICIC 2024
Tianjin, China, August 5–8, 2024
Proceedings, Part VII

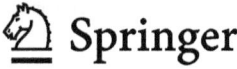

Editors
De-Shuang Huang
Eastern Institute of Technology
Ningbo, China

Chuanlei Zhang
Tianjin University of Science and Technology
Tianjin, China

Qinhu Zhang
Eastern Institute of Technology
Ningbo, China

ISSN 0302-9743　　　　　　ISSN 1611-3349 (electronic)
Lecture Notes in Computer Science
ISBN 978-981-97-5599-8　　　ISBN 978-981-97-5600-1 (eBook)
https://doi.org/10.1007/978-981-97-5600-1

© The Editor(s) (if applicable) and The Author(s), under exclusive license to Springer Nature Singapore Pte Ltd. 2024

This work is subject to copyright. All rights are solely and exclusively licensed by the Publisher, whether the whole or part of the material is concerned, specifically the rights of translation, reprinting, reuse of illustrations, recitation, broadcasting, reproduction on microfilms or in any other physical way, and transmission or information storage and retrieval, electronic adaptation, computer software, or by similar or dissimilar methodology now known or hereafter developed.
The use of general descriptive names, registered names, trademarks, service marks, etc. in this publication does not imply, even in the absence of a specific statement, that such names are exempt from the relevant protective laws and regulations and therefore free for general use.
The publisher, the authors and the editors are safe to assume that the advice and information in this book are believed to be true and accurate at the date of publication. Neither the publisher nor the authors or the editors give a warranty, expressed or implied, with respect to the material contained herein or for any errors or omissions that may have been made. The publisher remains neutral with regard to jurisdictional claims in published maps and institutional affiliations.

This Springer imprint is published by the registered company Springer Nature Singapore Pte Ltd.
The registered company address is: 152 Beach Road, #21-01/04 Gateway East, Singapore 189721, Singapore

If disposing of this product, please recycle the paper.

Preface

The International Conference on Intelligent Computing (ICIC) was started to provide an annual forum dedicated to emerging and challenging topics in artificial intelligence, machine learning, pattern recognition, bioinformatics, and computational biology. It aims to bring together researchers and practitioners from both academia and industry to share ideas, problems, and solutions related to the multifaceted aspects of intelligent computing.

ICIC 2024, held in Tianjin, China, August 5–8, 2024, constituted the 20th International Conference on Intelligent Computing. It built upon the success of ICIC 2023 (Zhengzhou, China), ICIC 2022 (Xi'an, China), ICIC 2021 (Shenzhen, China), ICIC 2020 (Bari, Italy), ICIC 2019 (Nanchang, China), ICIC 2018 (Wuhan, China), ICIC 2017 (Liverpool, UK), ICIC 2016 (Lanzhou, China), ICIC 2015 (Fuzhou, China), ICIC 2014 (Taiyuan, China), ICIC 2013 (Nanning, China), ICIC 2012 (Huangshan, China), ICIC 2011 (Zhengzhou, China), ICIC 2010 (Changsha, China), ICIC 2009 (Ulsan, South Korea), ICIC 2008 (Shanghai, China), ICIC 2007 (Qingdao, China), ICIC 2006 (Kunming, China), and ICIC 2005 (Hefei, China).

This year, the conference concentrated mainly on the theories and methodologies as well as the emerging applications of intelligent computing. Its aim was to unify the picture of contemporary intelligent computing techniques as an integral concept that highlights the trends in advanced computational intelligence and bridges theoretical research with applications. Therefore, the theme for this conference was "Advanced Intelligent Computing Technology and Applications". Papers that focused on this theme were solicited, addressing theories, methodologies, and applications in science and technology.

ICIC 2024 received 2189 submissions from 15 countries and regions. All papers went through a rigorous single-blind peer-review procedure and each paper received at least three review reports. Based on the review reports, the Program Committee finally selected 863 high-quality papers for presentation at ICIC 2024, included in twenty-one volumes of proceedings published by Springer: thirteen volumes of Lecture Notes in Computer Science (LNCS), six volumes of Lecture Notes in Artificial Intelligence (LNAI), and two volumes of Lecture Notes in Bioinformatics (LNBI).

In addition, this year we selected 134 Poster papers from the remaining papers, which will be made accessible on the open access website http://poster-openaccess.com/.

This volume of LNCS_14868 includes 41 papers.

The organizers of ICIC 2024, including Eastern Institute of Technology, Ningbo, China; Tianjin University of Science and Technology, China; China University of Mining & Technology (Beijing), China; China University of Mining and Technology (Xuzhou), China; and North China University of Science and Technology, China, made an enormous effort to ensure the success of the conference. We hereby would like to thank the members of the Program Committee and the referees for their collective effort in reviewing and soliciting the papers. In particular, we would like to thank all the authors for contributing their papers. Without the high-quality submissions from the authors, the success of the conference would not have been possible. Finally, we are especially grateful to the International Neural Network Society and the National Science Foundation of China for their sponsorship.

De-Shuang Huang
Fuping Lu

Organization

General Co-chairs

De-Shuang Huang   Eastern Institute of Technology, China
Fuping Lu   Tianjin University of Science and Technology, China

Program Committee Co-chairs

Prashan Premaratne   University of Wollongong, Australia
Xiankun Zhang   Tianjin University of Science and Technology, China
Chuanlei Zhang   Tianjin University of Science and Technology, China
Wei Chen   China University of Mining and Technology, China
Jair Cervantes Canales Autonomous University of Mexico State, Mexico
Yijie Pan   Eastern Institute of Technology, China
Qinhu Zhang   Eastern Institute of Technology, China
Jiayang Guo   Xiamen University, China

Organizing Committee Co-chairs

Zhanjun Si   Tianjin University of Science and Technology, China
Xiaoyue Liu   North China University of Science and Technology, China
Fan Zhang   China University of Mining and Technology (Beijing), China

Organizing Committee Members

Yarui Chen   Tianjin University of Science and Technology, China
Jing Su   Tianjin University of Science and Technology, China

Shuo Yang	Tianjin University of Science and Technology, China
Jing Han	Tianjin University of Science and Technology, China
Yiying Zhang	Tianjin University of Science and Technology, China
Jucheng Yang	Tianjin University of Science and Technology, China
Qian Long	Tianjin University of Science and Technology, China
Yongjun Ma	Tianjin University of Science and Technology, China
Lin Sun	Tianjin University of Science and Technology, China
Guoliang Gong	Tianjin University of Science and Technology, China

Award Committee Chair

Kang-Hyun Jo	University of Ulsan, South Korea

Tutorial Co-chairs

Abir Hussain	Liverpool John Moores University, UK
Michal Choras	Bydgoszcz University of Science and Technology, Poland

Publication Co-chairs

Jair Cervantes Canales	Autonomous University of Mexico State, Mexico
Chenxi Huang	Xiamen University, China

Special Session Co-chairs

Valeriya Gribova	Far Eastern Branch of Russian Academy of Sciences, Russia
M. Michael Gromiha	Indian Institute of Technology Madras, India

Special Issue Co-chairs

Yu-Dong Zhang — University of Leicester, UK
Yoshinori Kuno — Saitama University, Japan
Phalguni Gupta — Indian Institute of Technology Kanpur, India

International Liaison Chair

Prashan Premaratne — University of Wollongong, Australia

Workshop Co-chairs

Kyungsook Han — Inha University, South Korea
Laurent Heutte — Université de Rouen Normandie, France

Publicity Co-chairs

Chun-Hou Zheng — Anhui University, China
Dhiya Al-Jumeily — Liverpool John Moores University, UK
Han Huang — Nanjing University of Information Science and Technology, China

Program Committee Members

Antonio Brunetti — Polytechnic University of Bari, Italy
Bin Liu — Beijing Institute of Technology, China
Bin Qian — Kunming University of Science and Technology, China
Bin Yang — Zaozhuang University, China
Bing Wang — Anhui University of Technology, China
Bingqiang Liu — Shandong University, China
Binhua Tang — Hohai University, China
Bo Li — Wuhan University of Science and Technology, China
Caihong Mu — Xidian University, China
Changqing Shen — Soochow University, China
Chao Song — University of South China, China
Cheng Tang — Kyushu University, Japan

Chin-Chih Chang	Chung Hua University, Taiwan, RoC
Chuanlei Zhang	Tianjin University of Science and Technology, China
Chunhou Zheng	Anhui University, China
Chunmei Liu	Howard University, USA
Chunquan Li	University of South China, China
Cong Shen	Tianjin University of Technology, China
Daowen Qiu	Sun Yat-sen University, China
Delong Yang	First People's Hospital of Foshan, China
Dian Ding	Shanghai Jiao Tong University, China
Dong Wang	University of Jinan, China
Duo Chen	Nanjing University of Chinese Medicine, China
Eros Gian Alessandro Pasero	Politecnico di Torino, Italy
Fa Zhang	Beijing Institute of Technology, China
Fei Guo	Central South University, China
Fei Luo	Wuhan University, China
Fei Shen	Nanjing University of Science and Technology, China
Feng Liu	East China Normal University, China
Feng Zou	Huaibei Normal University, China
Fengfeng Zhou	Jilin University, China
Fudong Nian	Hefei University, China
Fuxue Li	Yingkou Institute of Technology, China
Gang Li	Qilu University of Technology, China
Gaoxiang Ouyang	Beijing Normal University, China
Guanghui Gong	Eastern Institute of Technology, Ningbo, China
Guohui Ding	Shenyang Aerospace University, China
Guoliang Li	Huazhong Agricultural University, China
Han Zhang	Nankai University, China
Hao Huang	Hubei University, China
Hao Lin	University of Electronic Science and Technology of China, China
Haodi Feng	Shandong University, China
Haodong Zhu	Zhengzhou University of Light Industry, China
Heng Li	Southern University of Science and Technology, China
Hoang-Anh Ngo	The University of Waikato, New Zealand
Hongjie Wu	Suzhou University of Science and Technology, China
Hongmin Cai	South China University of Technology, China
Hulin Kuang	Central South University, China
Jiahui Pan	South China Normal University, China

Jian Huang	University of Electronic Science and Technology of China, China
Jian Shen	Beijing Institute of Technology, China
Jiang Xie	Shanghai University, China
Jianrong Li	Tianjin University of Science and Technology, China
Jiawei Luo	Hunan University, China
Jiayang Guo	Xiamen University, China
Jing Chen	Suzhou University of Science and Technology, China
Jing Hu	Wuhan University of Science and Technology, China
Jintian Lu	Jishou University, China
Jin-Xing Liu	University of Health and Rehabilitation Sciences, China
Jipeng Wu	First People's Hospital of Foshan, China
Joaquin Torres-Sospedra	Universidade do Minho, Portugal
Juan Liu	Wuhan University, China
Junfeng Xia	Anhui University, China
Jungang Lou	Huzhou University, China
Junqing Li	Yunnan Normal University, China
Junyi Li	Harbin Institute of Technology (Shenzhen), China
Ka-Chun Wong	City University of Hong Kong, China
Kangning Zhang	Academy of Mathematics and Systems Science, CAS, China
Ke Niu	Beijing Information Science and Technology University, China
Laurent Heutte	Université de Rouen Normandie, France
Le Zhang	Sichuan University, China
Lei Wang	Guangxi Academy of Sciences, China
Lejun Gong	Nanjing University of Posts and Telecommunications, China
Liang Gao	Huazhong University of Science & Technology, China
Lida Zhu	Huazhong Agriculture University, China
Lin Wang	University of Jinan, China
Lin Yuan	Qilu University of Technology, China
Liqiang Liu	Xi'an Technological University, China
Li-Wei Ko	National Yang Ming Chiao Tung University, Taiwan, RoC
Long Shao	Beijing Institute of Technology, China
Long Xu	Ningbo University, China
Meiyan Xu	Minnan Normal University, China

xii   Organization

Meng Liu	National University of Defense Technology, China
Michael Gromiha	Indian Institute of Technology Madras, India
Michal Choras	Bydgoszcz University of Science and Technology, Poland
Mingyong Li	Chongqing Normal University, China
Mohd Helmy Abd Wahab	Universiti Tun Hussein Onn Malaysia, Malaysia
Nicola Altini	Polytechnic University of Bari, Italy
Nier Wu	Inner Mongolia University of Technology, China
Peipei Gu	Zhengzhou University of Light Industry, China
Peng Chen	Anhui University, China
Pengjiang Qian	Jiangnan University, China
Pengwei Hu	Xinjiang Technical Institute of Physics and Chemistry, CAS, China
Prashan Premaratne	University of Wollongong, Australia
Pu-Feng Du	Tianjin University, China
Qi Sun	Hangzhou Nuowei Information Technology Co., Ltd., China
Qi Zhao	University of Science and Technology Liaoning, China
Qifang Luo	Guangxi University for Nationalities, China
Qinhu Zhang	Eastern Institute of Technology, Ningbo, China
Qiuzhen Lin	Shenzhen University, China
Quan Zou	University of Electronic Science and Technology of China, China
Rong Wang	Sichuan Normal University, China
Rong-Qiang Zeng	Chengdu University of Information Technology, China
Rui Wang	National University of Defense Technology, China
Saiful Islam	Aligarh Muslim University, India
Shanfeng Zhu	Fudan University, China
Shitong Wang	Jiangnan University, China
Shixiong Zhang	Xidian University, China
Sungshin Kim	Pusan National University, South Korea
Taisong Jin	Xiamen University, China
Tian Wu	Nanchang University, China
Tieshan Li	University of Electronic Science and Technology of China, China
Valeria Gribova	Far Eastern Branch of Russian Academy of Sciences, Russia
Wangren Qiu	Jingdezhen Ceramic University, China
Waqas Haider Bangyal	Kohsar University Murree, Pakistan

Wei Chen	China University of Mining and Technology (Xuzhou), China
Wei Chen	Chengdu University of Traditional Chinese Medicine, China
Wei Jiang	Fujian Medical University, China
Wei Wang	Henan Normal University, China
Wei Xu	East China Normal University, China
Weichao Wu	Beijing Institute of Technology, China
Weiwei Kong	Xi'an University of Posts and Telecommunications, China
Weixiang Liu	Shenzhen University, China
Wen Jiang	Ctrip Computer Technology (Shanghai) Co., Ltd., China
Wen-Sheng Chen	Shenzhen University, China
Wenzheng Bao	Xuzhou University of Technology, China
Xiangtao Li	Jilin University, China
Xiaodi Li	Shandong Normal University, China
Xiaofeng Wang	Hefei University, China
Xiaoke Ma	Xidian University, China
Xiaolei Zhu	Anhui Agricultural University, China
Xiaoli Lin	Wuhan University of Science and Technology, China
Xiaoqing Li	Capital University of Economics and Business, China
Xin Zhang	Jiangnan University, China
Xingjian Xu	Inner Mongolia Normal University, China
Xingquan Cai	North China University of Technology, China
Xingtao Wang	Harbin Institute of Technology, China
Xinguo Lu	Hunan University, China
Xingyu Feng	City University of Hong Kong, China
Xinlu Li	Hefei University, China
Xinzheng Xu	China University of Mining and Technology (Xuzhou), China
Xiufen Zou	Wuhan University, China
Xiujuan Lei	Shaanxi Normal University, China
Xiwei Liu	Tongji University, China
Xiyuan Chen	Southeast University, China
Xizhao Luo	Soochow University, China
Xulong Zhang	Ping An Technology (Shenzhen) Co., Ltd., China
Yang Yang	Hubei University, China
Yansen Su	Anhui University, China
Yijie Pan	Eastern Institute of Technology, Ningbo, China
Yiming Tang	Hefei University of Technology, China

Yizhang Jiang	Jiangnan University, China
Yong Wang	Academy of Mathematics and Systems Science, CAS, China
Yong Wu	Anhui Normal University, China
Yonggang Lu	Lanzhou University, China
Yu Lu	Shenzhen Technology University, China
Yu Xue	Huazhong University of Science and Technology, China
Yunxia Liu	Zhengzhou Normal University, China
Yupei Zhang	Northwestern Polytechnical University, China
Yushan Qiu	Shenzhen University, China
Yuyan Zheng	Shandong Normal University, China
Zhan-Li Sun	Anhui University, China
Zhen Shen	Nanyang Institute of Technology, China
Zhendong Liu	Shandong Jianzhu University, China
Zhenran Jiang	East China Normal University, China
Zhenyi Shen	Zhejiang University, China
Zhi-Hong Guan	Huazhong University of Science and Technology, China
Zhi-Ping Liu	Shandong University, China
Zhong-Qiu Zhao	Heifei Institute of Technology, China
Zhuangzhuang Chen	Hong Kong University of Science and Technology, China
Zhuo Lei	City Cloud Technology China Co., Ltd., China
Zixiao Kong	University of International Relations, China

Contents – Part VII

Image Processing

Light-Dark: A Novel Lightweight Self-supervised Monocular Depth
Estimation in the Dark 3
   Qi Liang, Lizhe Wang, Lanmei Wang, Xiang Liu, and Guibao Wang

Non-homogeneous Image Dehazing with Edge Attention Based
on Relative Haze Density 15
   *Ruting Deng, Zhan Li, Yifan Deng, Hang Long, Zhanglu Chen,
Zhiqing Kang, and Zhichao Qiu*

Contrastive Learning for Silent Face Liveness Detection Based
on A Hybrid Framework 29
   *Ying Tang, Zhongyue Chen, Minchao Ye, Zhaojuan Zhang, Yaping Qi,
Huijuan Lu, and Wanli Huo*

BS2CL: Balanced Self-supervised Contrastive Learning for Thyroid
Cytology Whole Slide Image Multi-classification 41
   *Wensi Duan, Juan Liu, Lang Wang, Yu Jin, Peng Jiang, Cheng Li,
Dehua Cao, and Baochuan Pang*

Unsupervised Domain Adaptation Method for Medical Image
Segmentation Using Fourier Feature Decoupling and Multi-scale Feature
Fusion 53
   *Wei Hu, Qiaozhi Xu, Zhe Lian, Yanjun Yin, Min Zhi, Na Yang,
Wentao Duan, and Lei Yu*

LVMUM: Toward Open-World Object Detection with Large Vision
Models and Unsupervised Modeling 65
   Yangyang Huang, Xing Xi, Weiye Wu, and Ronghua Luo

Implementation and Application of Violence Detection System Based
on Multi-head Attention and LSTM 77
   Fengping Cao, Yi Miao, and Wangyi Zhang

GFFNet: An Efficient Image Denoising Network with Group Feature Fusion ... 89
   Lijun Gao, Youzhi Zhang, Xiao Jin, Qin Xin, Zeyang Sun, and Suran Wang

End-to-End Object Detection with YOLOF 101
   Xing Xi, Yangyang Huang, Weiye Wu, and Ronghua Luo

BiRGAN: Bi-directional Deep Image Retargeting 113
   Di Sun, Yunxiang Wang, Tingting Yang, Yijing Mei, and Gang Pan

MulTIR: Deep Multi-Target Image Retargeting 124
   Di Sun, Yitong Guo, Chaojie Yao, Yijing Mei, Dufeng Chen, and Gang Pan

PAAM (Parameter-free Attentional Aggregation Model) 134
   Xuan-Hao Qi, Min Zhi, Zeng Mi, Wei Hu, Yan-Jun Yin, Yue-Ning Zhang, Wen-Tao Duan, and Zhe Lian

FRFT Domain Watermarking Algorithm Based on GA Adaptive
Optimization 147
   Qiaoqiao Du, Yanchen Zhao, Weijie Hao, and Wenyin Zhang

Joint Semantic Feature and Optical Flow Learning for Automatic
Echocardiography Segmentation 160
   Juan Lyu, Jinpeng Meng, Yu Zhang, Sai Ho Ling, and Lin Sun

FMUnet: Frequency Feature Enhancement Multi-level U-Net
for Low-Dose CT Denoising with a Real Collected LDCT Image Dataset 172
   Yu Zhang, Xinqi Yang, Guoliang Gong, Xianghong Meng, Xiaoliang Wang, and Zhongwei Zhang

Research on Intelligent Recognition Algorithm of Container Numbers
in Ports Based on Deep Learning 184
   Zhehao Lin, Chen Dong, and Yuxuan Wan

Dr-SAM: U-Shape Structure Segment Anything Model for Generalizable
Medical Image Segmentation 197
   Xiangzuo Huo, Shengwei Tian, Bingming Zhou, Long Yu, and Aolun Li

Aerial Multi-object Tracking via Information Weighting 208
   Pengnian Wu, Bangkui Fan, Ruiyu Zhang, Yulong Xu, and Dong Xue

Optimization Method for Fractal Image Compression Based
on Self-similarity Evaluation and Gradient Bisection Algorithm 218
   Caixu Xu, Di Xie, Hui Guo, Jie He, and Minglang Chen

DiffGIC: Diffusion Prior Based Null-Space Correction for High
Resolution Grayscale Image Colorization 234
   Yachao Li, Yutian Fu, Feng Dong, and Dong Liang

Chinese Character Image Inpainting with Skeleton Extraction
and Adversarial Learning 246
   Di Sun, Tingting Yang, Xiangyu Pan, Jiahao Wang, and Gang Pan

The Weakly Supervised Network of Hierarchical Attention Mechanism
for Fine-Grained Classification 257
  Qian Long, Gaihua Wang, Hongwei Qu, Jingxuan Yao, and Bolun Zhu

CS-KD: Confused Sample Knowledge Distillation for Semantic
Segmentation of Aerial Imagery 266
  Yue Sun, Lingfeng Huang, Qi Zhu, and Dong Liang

CD-Font: One-Shot Font Generation via Conditional Diffusion Model
with Disentangled Guidance 279
  Siyi Chen, Zhenhua Li, and Dong Liang

Image Super-Resolution Reconstruction Based on Dual-Branch Channel
Attention 291
  Jinyu Shi, Zhanjun Si, Yingxue Zhang, and Xinbin Yang

A Flipped Reversible Information Hiding Method Based on AMP 300
  Yaowen Fu, Haoshan Shi, Tianyang Qi, Xueyan Gao, and Yifei Zou

Decoupling Control in Text-to-Image Diffusion Models 312
  Shitong Cao, Xuejie Zhang, Jin Wang, and Xiaobing Zhou

Arbitrary Scale Texture Synthesis with Feature Map Swapping 323
  *Di Sun, Yangde Lin, Sheng Shen, Zhiliang Zeng, Shizhao Zhang,
  and Qihang Wang*

A 3D-2D Hybrid Network with Regional Awareness and Global Fusion
for Brain Tumor Segmentation 333
  Wenxiu Zhao, Changlei Dongye, and Yumei Wang

GLAD: A Global-Attention-Based Diffusion Model for Infrared
and Visible Image Fusion 345
  Haozhe Guo, Mengjie Chen, Kaijiang Li, Hao Su, and Pei Lv

An Approach for Extracting Road Network from Remote Sensing Images 357
  Zhihui Wang, Yu Wang, and Yuliang Ni

Sparse Point Cloud Upsampling Based on Neural Implicit Functions 369
  Wenjun Wang, Xiangyu Kong, Daole Wang, and Xiuyang Zhao

Adaptive Non-local Means Filter Based on Multi-kernel for Complicated
Noise 381
  Qian long, Hongwei Qu, Yiping Wang, Gaihua Wang, and Bolun Zhu

One-Stage Lightweight Network of Object Detection for Rectangular
Panoramic Images 390
  Yingying Lu, Yun Tie, and Lin Qi

ISE-UFDS: A Dataset for Detecting the Degree of Danger to Vehicles
in Urban Flooding and Performance Assessment 402
  Jiwu Sun, Cheng Zhang, Cheng Xu, Pengfei Wang, and Hongzhe Liu

Convergence and Divergence: A New Paradigm for Pedestrian Detection 414
  Yueyan Zhu, Hai Huang, Shan Yue, Shu Zhang, and Aoran Chen

Improved YOLOv8-Based Lightweight Object Detection on Drone Images 426
  Maoxiang Jiang, Zhanjun Si, Ke Yang, and Yingxue Zhang

A Multi-dimensional Camera Image Stitching Method Under Large
Parallax Conditions 435
  Chuanlei Zhang, Yubo Li, Tianxiang Cheng, Jianrong Li, Haifeng Fan,
  Zhiqiang Zhao, Zhanjun Si, and Hui Ma

Harmonizing Stable Diffusion and GPT-4 for Mural Expansion
with ArtExtend 446
  Dufeng Chen, Yuqing Yang, Zehua Wang, Zishan Xu, Jueting Liu,
  Tingting Xu, and Wei Chen

MuralRescue: Advancing Blind Mural Restoration via SAM-Adapter
Enhanced Damage Segmentation and Integrated Restoration Techniques 456
  Zishan Xu, Dufeng Chen, Qianzhen Fang, Wei Chen, Tingting Xu,
  Jueting Liu, and Zehua Wang

Full-Range Fusion Network with Local-Global Attention for Change
Detection in Remote Sensing Images 464
  Shuting Niu, Yingxue Zhang, and Zhanjun Si

Author Index 473

Image Processing

Light-Dark: A Novel Lightweight Self-supervised Monocular Depth Estimation in the Dark

Qi Liang[1], Lizhe Wang[1], Lanmei Wang[1(✉)], Xiang Liu[2], and Guibao Wang[3]

[1] School of Physics, Xidian University, Xi'an 710071, China
lmwang@mail.xidian.edu.cn
[2] Institute of Science and Technology Innovation, Dongguan University of Technology, Dongguan 523808, China
[3] School of Electronic Information and Artificial Intelligence, Shaanxi University of Science and Technology, Xi'an 710021, China

Abstract. Self-supervised monocular depth estimation has been widely studied in recent years. In nighttime scenes where the photometric consistency assumption is not met, several solutions have emerged to address this challenge. However, existing monocular depth estimation algorithms for nighttime often require a large-scale model and a significant number of floating-point operations, making it challenging to apply them to practical problems such as autonomous driving. In this paper, we propose a lightweight monocular depth estimation algorithm tailored for nighttime scenes, named Light-Dark. Specifically, we design a lightweight Depth-Net incorporating Feature-Fusion blocks and Cross-connections. Additionally, in response to the low-light and high-noise issues in nighttime scenes, we introduce a Noise-Constrained Adaptive Image Enhancement (NCAIE) module. We deploy our model on the edge device Jetson AGX Orin to validate its real-world performance. A series of experiments conducted on nighttime datasets, Robot-Car and nuScenes, indicate the effectiveness of our proposed Light-Dark and the equilibrium between lightweight design and accuracy.

Keywords: Monocular depth estimation · Lightweight · Nighttime

1 Introduction

Monocular depth estimation is a vital task in the field of computer vision and essential for applications such as autonomous driving, robotic navigation and 3D reconstruction [1]. Self-supervised monocular depth estimation, which leverages photometric constraints between monocular image sequences without the need for collecting real depth maps, is gaining increasing attention. In addition to research on daytime datasets such as KITTI [2] and Make 3D [3], some self-supervised methods are attempting to be applied in nighttime scenarios [4, 5]. Meanwhile, lightweighting of models in monocular depth estimation has garnered attention. Recent researches often focus on reducing model parameters through techniques such as knowledge distillation [6] and exploring new convolution operations [7]. This allows models to be deployed on edge devices to solve real-world problems.

However, few lightweight methods are proposed to address the challenges posed in more complex nighttime scenarios. The DepthNet in current nighttime methods is primarily adapted from Monodepth2 [8], exhibiting a relatively high model complexity. Existing lightweight methods are primarily trained and evaluated on daytime scenes. Nighttime scenes disrupt the photometric consistency between adjacent frames, making the reconstruction of the target frame challenging and resulting in higher training loss. Meanwhile, in low-light and high-noise environments, depth prediction maps may exhibit irregularities such as non-smooth regions and large holes [4].

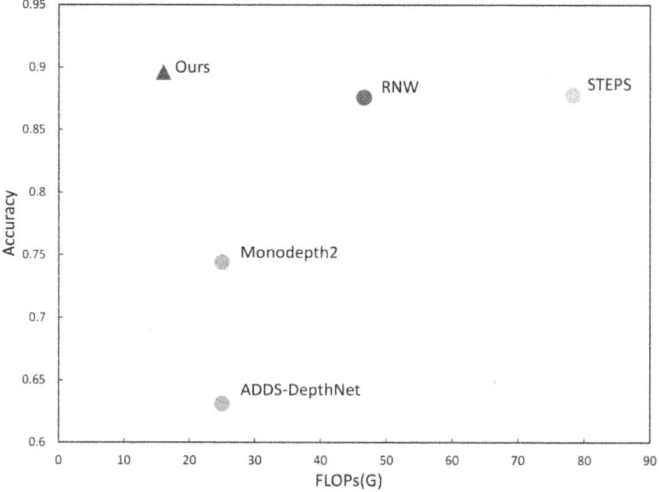

Fig. 1. Comparison graph of FLOPs (Floating Point Operations) and Accuracy(δ_1) for different models. All models were tested on the 576 × 320 RobotCar dataset. Smaller FLOPs is better, and higher Accuracy(δ_1) is better.

To address the aforementioned issues, this paper propose a lightweight self-supervised monocular depth estimation method tailored for nighttime scenes. Firstly, we design a lightweight depth estimation network by adopting a shallower network to reduce model complexity. To better capture and process both local and global features of the images, we introduce Feature-Fusion blocks by combining CNNs and Transformers. Within these blocks, cross-covariance attention (XCA) [9] is employed to reduce computational complexity. We also utilize Cross-connections to enhance the propagation of features. Secondly, we introduce a Noise-Constrained Adaptive Image Enhancement (NCAIE) module, which enhances image contrast while suppressing noise. Finally, we test our model on edge devices at different power levels to demonstrate its real-time inference performance. In summary, our model achieves a favorable equilibrium between lightweight design and accuracy compared to other nighttime methods (see Fig. 1). Our contributions can be summarized in three aspects:

(1) We propose a lightweight DepthNet and fuse it into the nighttime self-supervised depth estimation architecture.

(2) We employ the Noise-Constrained Adaptive Image Enhancement module to address the low-light and high-noise problem in nighttime scenes.
(3) We test the inference speed of our model on Nvidia Titan V and an edge device Jetson AGX Orin to confirm the practicality of our lightweight model.

2 Method

2.1 Nighttime Self-supervised Depth Estimation Architecture

In self-supervised monocular depth estimation, the system is primarily composed of a depth estimation network Φ_d and a pose network Φ_p [8]. However, due to the specificity of nighttime scenes, relying solely on the above methods can result in numerous abnormal depth values. To address this issue, we follow [4] by pretraining DepthNet $\Phi_{d'}$ on the daytime dataset and then utilizing an adversarial neural network to guide nighttime training. We utilize a Patch-GAN discriminator to differentiate between the nighttime depth map D_t generated by Φ_d and the daytime depth map D_d generated by Φ'_d. Figure 2 illustrates the fundamental architecture of our proposed Light-Dark model.

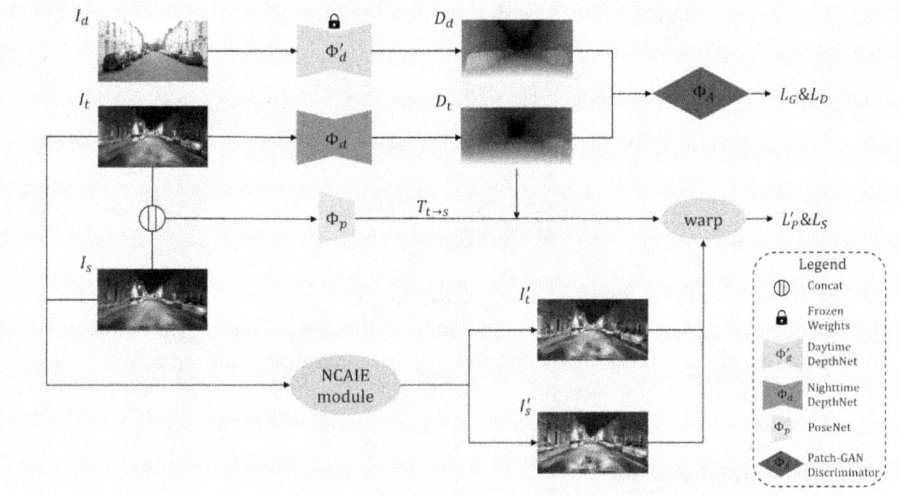

Fig. 2. Overview of our Light-Dark architecture. DepthNet Φ_d and Φ'_d share the same network, which serves as the core module in our lightweight approach. The NCAIE module represents the image enhancement module in our work.

Given a RGB image I_t, a depth map D_t can be predicted using a trainable network Φ_d: $D_t = \Phi_d(I_t)$. To achieve self-supervision, it's necessary to reconstruct the target frame I_t from the source frame I_s using geometric relationships: $T_{t \to s} = \Phi_p(I_t, I_s)$. The reconstruction process involves using the pose network to obtain the relative pose $T_{t \to s}$ between I_s and I_t. Then, we can project the point p_t in D_t onto the point p_s in I_s:

$$p_s \sim K T_{t \to s} D_t(p_t) K^{-1} p_t \tag{1}$$

where $\sim$ represents a homogeneous equivalence relationship, and K denotes the camera intrinsics. Then, I_s obtains the reconstructed target frame $\hat{I}_t$ through the differentiable bilinear sampling operation $s(\cdot, \cdot)$:

$$\hat{I}_t = s(I_s, p_s) \quad (2)$$

Following [8], we combine l_1 and SSIM (structural similarity) loss as the photometric loss L_P, the formula is:

$$L_P(I_t, \hat{I}_t) = \frac{\alpha}{2}(1 - SSIM(I_t, \hat{I}_t)) + (1-\alpha)\|I_t - \hat{I}_t\|_1 \quad (3)$$

where $\|\cdot\|_1$ represents the L1 norm, and the parameter α is set to 0.85 in all experiments. In addition, we apply edge-aware smoothness loss to reduce the noise and discontinuity of the depth map or surface normal vector, making the depth estimation results more accurate and stable. The expression is as follows:

$$L_S = |\partial_x D_t| e^{-|\partial_x I_t|} + |\partial_y D_t| e^{-|\partial_y I_t|} \quad (4)$$

where ∂_x and ∂_y are the image gradients in the horizontal and vertical directions respectively. Finally, we train the generator Φ_d and the discriminator Φ_A by minimizing the loss function of LSGAN, expressed as:

$$L_D = \frac{1}{2|I_d|} \sum_{D_d} (\Phi_A(D_d) - 1)^2 + \frac{1}{2|I_t|} \sum_{D_t} (\Phi_A(D_t))^2 \quad (5)$$

$$L_G = \frac{1}{2|I_t|} \sum_{D_t} (\Phi_A(D_t) - 1)^2 \quad (6)$$

where $|I_d|$ represents the number of daytime training images, and $|I_t|$ represents the number of nighttime training images. It's important to note that I_t and I_d do not correspond one-to-one to daytime and nighttime images, so the generated depth maps $D_d = \Phi'_d(I_d)$ and $D_t = \Phi_d(I_t)$ are not required to be paired.

2.2 Lightweight DepthNet

After training with the Light-Dark architecture, our subsequent inference only requires the use of the DepthNet. Therefore, designing a lightweight DepthNet can help us effectively reduce the model's complexity and inference speed. Inspired by recent research [10], we design a lightweight depth estimation network that incorporates Feature-Fusion blocks and Cross-connections, as shown in Fig. 3.

Depth Encoder. Using a shallower network can effectively reduce model complexity, hence we adopted a four-stage encoder. The Conv-stem consists of a 3 × 3 convolution with a stride of 2 followed by two 3 × 3 convolutions with a stride of 1, and the downsample module is a 3 × 3 convolution with a stride of 2. Due to the high requirements of depth estimation tasks for perceiving local details and scene structure, we introduce a Feature-Fusion block that can simultaneously integrate both local and global image features. First, the Feature-Fusion block utilizes a 3 × 3 dilated convolution to expand the receptive field, achieving the extraction of local features. Assuming a feature map x with dimensions $H \times W \times C$, this process can be represented as:

$$L(x) = Pw_2(Pw_1(BN(Dconv(x)))) + x \quad (7)$$

where $Dconv(\cdot)$ represents dilated convolution, BN stands for batch normalization, and $Pw1(\cdot)$ and $Pw2(\cdot)$ respectively signify the pointwise operations for dimensionality expansion and reduction. In the Feature-Fusion blocks of the encoder, the operation of extracting local features $L(\cdot)$ is repeated N times, with the respective counts being 3, 3 and 9 from top to bottom.

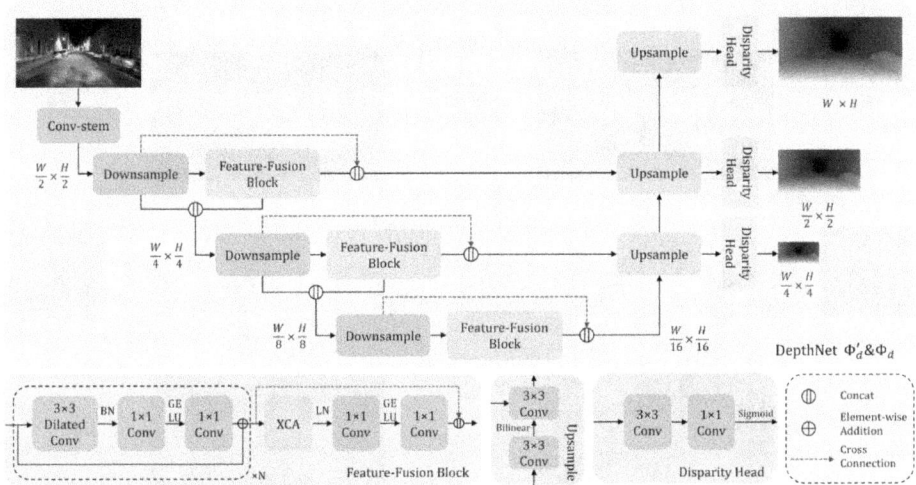

Fig. 3. DepthNet used in Light-Dark. The DepthNet adopts an encoder-decoder structure, where the encoder utilizes Feature-Fusion blocks and Cross-connections to merge local and global features.

Then, we replace the original self-attention [11] with the lower computational complexity Cross-Covariance Attention (XCA) [9] to model global context more efficiently. We denote this operation as $G(\cdot)$, and its expression is given by:

$$G(x') = Pw_2(Pw_1(LN(XCA(x')))) \quad (8)$$

where x' is the input feature, and LN represents layer normalization. To enhance the integration and propagation of local and global features, we utilized Cross-connections in both the Downsample module and Feature-Fusion blocks. The final output y of the Feature-Fusion block can be expressed as:

$$y = Concat[N \cdot L(x), G(N \cdot L(x))] \quad (9)$$

Depth Decoder. To reduce the complexity of the model, we follow [10] by using a decoder consisting only of convolutional layers, as illustrated in Fig. 3. The upsample module employs bilinear interpolation for upsampling, followed by a disparity head connected to each output. These outputs are generated at $\frac{1}{4}$, $\frac{1}{2}$, and full resolution, respectively.

2.3 Noise-Constrained Adaptive Image Enhancement

In nighttime images, the photometric consistency between the target frame I_t and the source frame I_s often does not hold, accompanied by low-light and high-noise levels. Therefore, inspired by Adaptive Histogram Euqalization, we propose the Noise-Constrained Adaptive Image Enhancement (NCAIE) module. This avoids the use of additional image enhancement networks, aligning with the goal of model lightweight design. Figure 4 illustrates the processing flow of NCAIE.

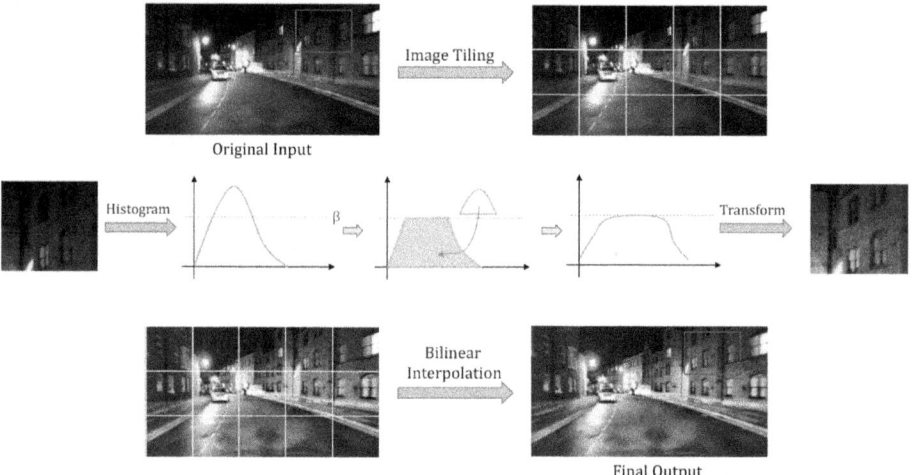

Fig. 4. Flowchart of Noise-Constrained Adaptive Image Enhancement (NCAIE). The main steps include image block tiling, histogram equalization for each block, and concatenation of blocks using interpolation methods.

We initially divide the target frame I_t and the source frame I_s into $I \times J$ small blocks. Each block from the partition of I_t is denoted as $t_{i,j}$, and each block from the partition of I_s is represented as $s_{i,j}$. Assuming each block has M pixels and N grayscale levels, we calculate the histogram $h_{i,j}(n)$ for each small block, where $n = 1, 2, \ldots, N-1$. Simultaneously, to control the noise amplification resulting from excessive contrast, we introduce a contrast limitation parameter β, obtaining the clipped histogram $h'_{i,j}(n)$. Then, we compute the cumulative distribution function (CDF) of the histogram as follows:

$$f_{i,j}(n) = \frac{(N-1)}{M} \cdot \sum_{k=0}^{n} h'_{i,j}(k) \tag{10}$$

The above expression represents the histogram equalization operation for each small block. Finally, we use bilinear interpolation to smoothly concatenate the processed blocks, obtaining the enhanced target frame I'_t and source frame I'_s. In our experiments, the size of each small block $I \times J$ is set to 8×8, and the contrast limitation parameter β is set to 4. The entire enhancement process can be expressed as:

$$I'_t = \varepsilon(I_t), I'_s = \varepsilon(I_s) \tag{11}$$

Here, ε represents the mapping function for image enhancement. Therefore, we can obtain the reconstructed frame $\hat{I'_t}$ from I'_s:

$$\hat{I'_t} = s(I'_s, p_s) \tag{12}$$

In conclusion, our photometric loss function is modified as follows:

$$L'_P(I'_t, \hat{I'_t}) = \frac{\alpha}{2}(1 - SSIM(I'_t, \hat{I'_t})) + (1 - \alpha)\|I'_t - \hat{I'_t}\|_1 \tag{13}$$

From Fig. 4, it is visually evident that there is a significant improvement in the contrast of the final output image, especially in the region highlighted in the red box. Additionally, the background noise in the enhanced image is effectively constrained.

2.4 Loss Function

In summary, the expression for the total loss function is:

$$L_{total} = mL'_P + \rho L_S + \sigma L_D + \varsigma L_G \tag{14}$$

where ρ, σ and ς are hyperparameters. The parameter m is the auto-mask introduced following the approach proposed by Wang et al. [4].

3 Experiments

3.1 Datasets

Robotcar. The Oxford RobotCar Dataset [12] is a large autonomous driving dataset that includes driving videos captured under various environmental conditions. Following the setup in [4], we selected a portion of the '2014–12-09-13-21-02' and '2014–12-16-18-44-24' datasets as daytime and nighttime data, respectively. This resulted in approximately 41,000 images for training and 570 images for testing. To eliminate the influence of the car hood, we cropped the images to 1152×672.

nuScenes. nuScenes [13] is a large-scale outdoor autonomous driving dataset that comprises 1000 video clips captured in diverse road and weather conditions. This dataset is more challenging than RobotCar. We selected daytime and nighttime scenes from nuScenes, cropped the images to 1536×768, and utilized them for both training and testing.

3.2 Implementation Detail

Our model is trained for 50 epochs using the Adam optimizer on a single Nvidia Titan V. Our training process consists of two steps. Initially, we train the DepthNet Φ'_d using the daytime dataset. Subsequently, we train the entire network using the nighttime dataset, during which the DepthNet Φ'_d trained in the first step is frozen. The batch size is set to 4, and the learning rate is set to $1e^{-4}$. When training with the RobotCar dataset, the hyperparameters in the total loss are set as follows: $\rho = 1e^{-3}, \sigma = 2.5e^{-4}, \varsigma = 2.5e^{-4}$. When using the nuScenes dataset, they are set as: $\rho = 1e^{-3}, \sigma = 4e^{-4}, \varsigma = 4e^{-4}$. The input resolutions for RobotCar and nuScenes are 576×320 and 768×384, respectively.

3.3 Evaluation Results

Comparison with Prior Work. Table 1 presents the comparison results between our model and previous nighttime depth estimation methods. Figure 5 illustrates more visualization results. In the evaluation, the maximum depths for the RobotCar and nuScenes datasets are set to 40 m and 60 m, respectively. We reproduced the latest models RNW [4] and STEPS [5] on our own device, while the quantitative results for the remaining models follow those reported in previous papers [14]. Quantitative results (see Table 1) show that our model achieved SOTA performance on the RobotCar dataset and outperformed most competitors on the nuScenes dataset. Below, we select the Sq Rel metric as a representative error measure for analysis. In the RobotCar and nuScenes datasets, our method reduced the error of Monodepth2 [8] by 91.4% and 88.6%, while achieving a reduction of 15.5% and 0.7% compared to STEPS. Moreover, our model maintains a comparable level of accuracy to STEPS while exhibiting significantly lower complexity (see Fig. 1).

Figure 5 illustrates the qualitative comparison results between our model and others. All methods are trained on the same dataset, and the best checkpoints are utilized to generate depth maps. The red boxes highlight some regions with low-light conditions or overexposure, as well as moving cars. It can be observed that our model performs well

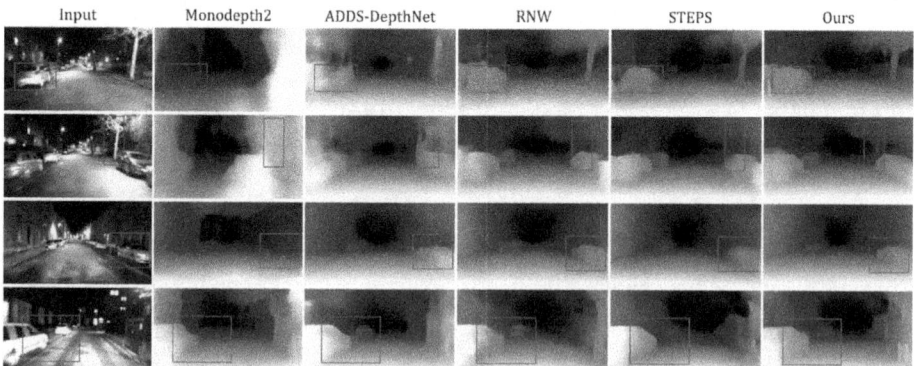

Fig. 5. Visualization results of the RobotCar dataset. Our model is compared with Monodepth2 [8], ADDS-DepthNet [14], RNW [4], and STEPS [5]. The leftmost column represents the RGB input image to the model.

Table 1. Quantitative results. We compare our model with previous SOTA methods on the RobotCar and nuScenes datasets. Smaller Depth Error is better, and higher Depth Accuracy is better.

Method	Depth Error($\downarrow$)				Depth Accuracy($\uparrow$)		
	Abs Rel	Sq Rel	RMSE	RMSE log	δ_1	δ_2	δ_3
RobotCar(Max Depth = 40m)							
Monodepth2 [8]	0.400	7.451	6.642	0.443	0.744	0.892	0.928
DeFeat-Net [15]	0.393	4.896	6.343	0.424	0.626	0.829	0.899
ADFA [16]	0.201	2.575	7.172	0.278	0.735	0.883	0.942
ADDS-DepthNet[14]	0.233	2.344	6.859	0.270	0.631	0.908	0.962
RNW [4]	0.124	0.712	3.368	0.172	0.876	0.961	**0.987**
STEPS [5]	0.121	0.757	3.321	0.173	0.878	0.959	0.983
Light-Dark(Ours)	**0.118**	**0.640**	**3.136**	**0.165**	**0.896**	**0.962**	**0.987**
nuScenes (Max Depth = 60m)							
Monodepth2 [8]	1.185	42.306	21.613	1.567	0.184	0.360	0.504
FeatDepth [17]	1.138	41.617	20.848	1.148	0.238	0.425	0.565
RNW [4]	0.371	5.956	11.261	0.432	0.499	0.767	0.879
STEPS [5]	0.348	4.873	**9.980**	0.425	**0.531**	0.765	0.886
Light-Dark(Ours)	**0.340**	**4.838**	10.136	**0.414**	0.526	**0.772**	**0.889**

in estimating the depth of objects in regions with low-light conditions or overexposure. Additionally, when facing moving objects like cars, our model can generate detailed contours.

Complexity and Speed Evaluation. We compared the complexity of the models, which includes the number of parameters and floating point operations (FLOPs). Table 2 illustrates that our model has significantly reduced the number of parameters by approximately 85% compared to previous models. Simultaneously, compared to recent nighttime models RNW and STEPS, our model achieves a significant reduction in FLOPs by 65.5% and 79.5%, respectively.

Considering limited computing resources in practical aplications, we ran our model on the edge device Jetson AGX Orin. Jetson AGX Orin is an embedded computing module introduced by Nvidia, offering various power modes. Generally, lower power consumption results in lower GPU and CPU frequencies, leading to slower inference speeds. We evaluated the average inference speed and frame rate of the model at different power levels and compared the results with those on Titan V. Table 3 displays the evaluation results on the nighttime test set of 411 images from RobotCar, where the first 10 images were used for warm-up and are not included in the statistics. Experiments indicate that our model achieves rapid inference across various power modes on edge

Table 2. Model complexity assessment. We compared the parameters and FLOPs during inference for each model, including the encoder, decoder, and full model. The input size is 576 × 320.

Method	Encoder		Decoder		Full Model	
	Params	FLOPs	Params	FLOPs	Params	FLOPs
Monodepth2 [8]	23.51M	15.18G	9.01M	9.82G	32.52M	25.00G
ADDS-DepthNet [14]	23.51M	15.18G	9.01M	9.82G	32.52M	25.00G
RNW [4]	23.51M	15.33G	9.33M	31.25G	32.84M	46.58G
STEPS[5]	23.52M	46.99G	9.33M	31.25G	32.85M	78.24G
Light- Dark(Ours)	**2.84M**	**6.47G**	**2.03M**	**9.60G**	**4.87M**	**16.07G**

Table 3. The evaluation of the average inference speed and frame rate for our model. The first three rows show the results under different power modes on Jetson AGX Orin, and the last row displays the results on Titan V. The batch size is set to 1.

Platform(Power Mode)	Input Size	Inference Speed	Frame Rate
Jetson AGX Orin (30W)	576 × 320	42.9ms	23.3 fps
Jetson AGX Orin (50W)	576 × 320	37.1ms	27.0 fps
Jetson AGX Orin (MaxN)	576 × 320	25.5ms	39.2 fps
Titan V	576 × 320	9.1ms	110.3 fps

devices. Even in the 30W mode, which operates at less than half of the maximum power consumption, the frame rate still meets the real-time requirement of 20 fps.

3.4 Ablation Study

We conducted ablation experiments on the RobotCar and nuScenes datasets, removing Feature-Fusion blocks, Cross-connections, and NCAIE modules from the Light-Dark model. The results in Table 4 show that each component enhances performance. Feature-Fusion blocks are crucial, as their removal increases Sq Rel by 18.8% (RobotCar) and 20.2% (nuScenes), highlighting their role in feature integration. The NCAIE module reduces the impact of inconsistent photometry and complex lighting, with Sq Rel increasing by 15.2% and 18.7% upon removal. Cross-connections facilitate feature propagation, with their removal leading to a 10.9% and 6.9% increase in Sq Rel.

Table 4. Quantitative results of ablation experiments on the RobotCar and nuScenes datasets.

Method	Depth Error(↓)				Depth Accuracy(↑)		
	Abs Rel	Sq Rel	RMSE	RMSE log	δ_1	δ_2	δ_3
RobotCar(Max Depth = 40 m)							
Light-Dark(Ours)	**0.118**	**0.640**	**3.136**	**0.165**	**0.896**	**0.962**	**0.987**
w/o Feature-Fusion	0.146	0.760	3.522	0.194	0.828	0.953	0.985
w/o Cross-conn	0.119	0.710	3.279	0.169	0.883	0.959	0.985
w/o NCAIE	0.138	0.737	3.418	0.189	0.850	0.956	0.983
nuScenes(Max Depth = 60 m)							
Light-Dark(Ours)	**0.340**	**4.838**	**10.136**	**0.414**	**0.526**	**0.772**	**0.889**
w/o Feature-Fusion	0.412	5.816	11.580	0.508	0.419	0.678	0.807
w/o Cross-conn	0.361	5.170	10.572	0.430	0.500	0.749	0.868
w/o NCAIE	0.374	5.741	10.578	0.429	0.498	0.758	0.882

4 Conclusions

In this paper, we propose a lightweight architecture for monocular depth estimation in nighttime conditions, named Light-Dark. We design a shallow DepthNet with low computational Feature-Fusion blocks and Cross-connections responsible for facilitating feature propagation. Considering the characteristics of nighttime scenes, we introduce the Noise-Constrained Adaptive Image Enhancement (NCAIE) module. Experiments demonstrate that Light-Dark achieves an excellent balance between model complexity and accuracy, making it particularly suitable for application on resource-constrained edge devices.

Acknowledgments. This work was supported by the National Natural Science Foundation of China under Grant 62071122, the Outstanding Youth Project of Guangdong Basic and Applied Basic Research Foundation under Grant 2023B1515020064, and the Key Research and Development Program Projects of Shaanxi Province under Grant 2024QCY-KXJ-168.

References

1. Ming, Y., Meng, X., Fan, C., Yu, H.: Deep learning for monocular depth estimation: a review. Neurocomputing **438**, 14–33 (2021)
2. Geiger, A., Lenz, P., Stiller, C., Urtasun, R.: Vision meets robotics: the kitti dataset. The Int. J. Robot. Res. **32**(11), 1231–1237 (2013)
3. Saxena, A., Sun, M., Ng, A.Y.: Make3d: Learning 3d scene structure from a single still image. IEEE Trans. Pattern Anal. Mach. Intell. **31**(5), 824–840 (2008)
4. Wang, K., Zhang, Z., Yan, Z., Li, X., Xu, B., Li, J., Yang, J.: Regularizing nighttime weirdness: efficient self-supervised monocular depth estimation in the dark. In: Proceedings of the IEEE/CVF International Conference on Computer Vision, pp. 16055–16064 (2021)

5. Zheng, Y., Zhong, C., Li, P., Gao, H.a., Zheng, Y., Jin, B., Wang, L., Zhao, H., Zhou, G., Zhang, Q., et al.: Steps: Joint self-supervised nighttime image enhancement and depth estimation. arXiv preprint arXiv:2302.01334 (2023)
6. Hu, J., Fan, C., Jiang, H., Guo, X., Gao, Y., Lu, X., Lam, T.L.: Boosting lightweight depth estimation via knowledge distillation. In: Jin, Z., Jiang, Y., Andrei Buchmann, R., Bi, Y., Ghiran, A.-M., Ma, W. (eds.) Knowledge Science, Engineering and Management: 16th International Conference, KSEM 2023, Guangzhou, China, August 16–18, 2023, Proceedings, Part I, pp. 27–39. Springer Nature Switzerland, Cham (2023). https://doi.org/10.1007/978-3-031-40283-8_3
7. Wofk, D., Ma, F., Yang, T.J., Karaman, S., Sze, V.: Fastdepth: Fast monocu- lar depth estimation on embedded systems. In: 2019 International Conference on Robotics and Automation (ICRA), pp. 6101–6108. IEEE (2019)
8. Godard, C., Mac Aodha, O., Firman, M., Brostow, G.J.: Digging into self-supervised monocular depth estimation. In: Proceedings of the IEEE/CVF international conference on computer vision, pp. 3828–3838 (2019)
9. Ali, A., et al.: Xcit: Cross-covariance image transformers. Adv. Neural. Inf. Process. Syst. **34**, 20014–20027 (2021)
10. Zhang, N., Nex, F., Vosselman, G., Kerle, N.: Lite-mono: A lightweight cnn and transformer architecture for self-supervised monocular depth estimation. In: Proceedings of the IEEE/CVF Conference on Computer Vision and Pattern Recognition, pp. 18537–18546 (2023)
11. Dosovitskiy, et al.: An image is worth 16x16 words: Transformers for image recognition at scale. arXiv preprint arXiv:2010.11929 (2020)
12. Maddern, W., Pascoe, G., Linegar, C., Newman, P.: 1 year, 1000 km: the ox-ford robotcar dataset. Int. J. Robot. Res. **36**(1), 3–15 (2017)
13. Caesar, H., et al.: nuscenes: A multimodal dataset for autonomous driving. In: Proceedings of the IEEE/CVF conference on computer vision and pattern recognition, pp. 11621–11631 (2020)
14. Liu, L., Song, X., Wang, M., Liu, Y., Zhang, L.: Self-supervised monocular depth estimation for all day images using domain separation. In: Proceedings of the IEEE/CVF International Conference on Computer Vision, pp. 12737–12746 (2021)
15. Spencer, J., Bowden, R., Hadfield, S.: Defeat-net: General monocular depth via simultaneous unsupervised representation learning. In: Proceedings of the IEEE/CVF Conference on Computer Vision and Pattern Recognition, pp. 14402–14413 (2020)
16. Vankadari, M., Garg, S., Majumder, A., Kumar, S., Behera, A.: Unsupervised monocular depth estimation for night-time images using adversarial domain feature adaptation. In: Computer Vision–ECCV 2020: 16th European Conference, Glasgow, UK, 23–28 Aug 2020, Proceedings, Part XXVIII 16, pp. 443–459. Springer (2020)
17. Shu, C., Yu, K., Duan, Z., Yang, K.: Feature-metric loss for self-supervised learning of depth and egomotion. In: Vedaldi, A., Bischof, H., Brox, T., Frahm, J.-M. (eds.) Computer Vision – ECCV 2020: 16th European Conference, Glasgow, UK, 23–28 Aug 2020, Proceedings, Part XIX, pp. 572–588. Springer International Publishing, Cham (2020). https://doi.org/10.1007/978-3-030-58529-7_34

Non-homogeneous Image Dehazing with Edge Attention Based on Relative Haze Density

Ruting Deng[1], Zhan Li[1(✉)] [iD], Yifan Deng[1], Hang Long[1], Zhanglu Chen[1], Zhiqing Kang[2], and Zhichao Qiu[3]

[1] Department of Computer Science, Jinan University, Guangzhou 510632, China
lizhan@jnu.edu.cn
[2] KingSoft Office Software, Wuhan, China
[3] Fesco Adecco Co. Ltd, Shenzhen, China

Abstract. Image dehazing is a widely used technology for recovering clear images from hazy inputs. However, most dehazing methods are designed to target a specific haze concentration, without considering the varying degrees of image degradation. Removing non-homogeneous haze from real-world images is challenging. To address this issue, this study proposes a dual-cycle framework based on relative haze density, in which inputs are regarded as both hazy images to be recovered by a restoration network (RNet) and clear images to be deteriorated by a degradation network (DNet). Edge attention blocks and multi-order derivative loss are proposed for RNet to enhance the details and colors. Furthermore, two multi-class discriminators are designed to distinguish between relative levels of haze density. Extensive experiments on both real-world and synthetic datasets demonstrate that the proposed method is superior to state-of-the-art approaches for non-homogeneous image dehazing using either supervised or unsupervised learning. This code is available at https://github.com/lizhangray/EARHD.

Keywords: Image Dehazing · Haze Density · Edge Attention · Multi-class Discriminator

1 Introduction

Images captured in hazy and foggy weather often suffer from color attenuation, limited visibility, and blurry edges, which adversely affect subsequent high-level computer vision tasks such as object detection, recognition, tracking, and semantic segmentation. Aiming to recover clear images from hazy inputs, image dehazing technology has broad application prospects.

Traditional prior-based methods approximate dehazed images according to the atmospheric scattering model [1] by incorporating handcrafted priors, such as the dark channel prior (DCP) [2] and non-local prior (NLP) [3]. However, these physical priors frequently result in inaccurate parameter estimation and unsatisfactory results [4, 5]. Recent advancements in deep learning have led to the development of learning-based methods [5–11] that have demonstrated remarkable performance in image dehazing challenges.

However, most networks have limitations in removing haze from real-world images with non-homogeneous haze [5, 10] because of their uniform processing of different haze densities without considering the diversity of image degradation.

In this study, we propose a dual-cycle framework for non-homogeneous image dehazing based on relative haze density. Because the haze concentrations are comparative, an input image is regarded as both a hazy image compared with clearer images, and a clear image compared with images with denser haze. As illustrated in Fig. 1, an image is always dehazed using a restoration network (RNet) and degraded using a degradation network (DNet). In cycle learning, image I_{in} is restored to a clear image I_{de}^A and then degraded to I_{cyc} in the upper branch, whereas it is degraded to an image with dense haze I_{add} and subsequently restored to a clear image I_{de}^B in the lower branch. Moreover, two multi-class discriminators, D_{clear} and D_{dense}, are designed to distinguish images with different haze levels generated by RNet or DNet, relative to clear or dense reference images. Furthermore, to recover details and colors, edge attention blocks and a multi-order derivative loss are proposed to construct and train the RNet, respectively. Guided by the dual-cycle framework, the RNet learns the image features of different degrees of degradation to remove thin or dense haze from the images.

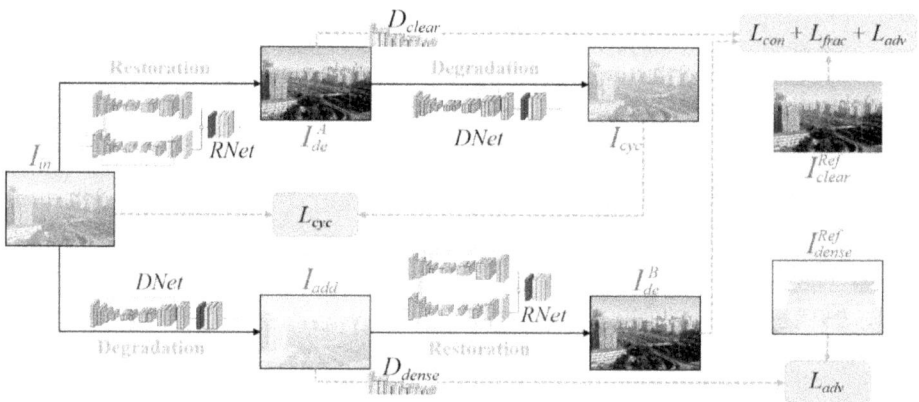

Fig. 1. Dual-cycle framework based on relative haze density.

The contributions of this study can be summarized as follows:

- We propose a dual-cycle framework based on relative haze density for non-homogeneous image dehazing, in which an input image is both dehazed by the RNet and added with haze by the DNet. The proposed framework is applicable for both supervised and unsupervised learning.
- We design an edge attention branch and a super-resolution branch to enhance details covered by haze. Moreover, we introduce a multi-order derivative loss to constrain dehazed images for recovering rich textures and bright colors.
- Distinguished from typical binary discriminators that determine if samples are real or fake, we design two novel multi-class discriminators to differentiate relative levels of haze density, which guide the RNet and DNet to produce haze-removed and haze-added images, respectively.

2 Related Works

Learning-based methods train neural network models to map hazy inputs to dehazed outputs in an end-to-end manner, divided into supervised and unsupervised dehazing.

Supervised dehazing networks learn from paired hazy and haze-free images to achieve an impressive performance. An all-in-one network for dehazing (AOD) [6] has been proposed to directly output clear images instead of estimating the parameters of the atmospheric scattering model [1]. A gated context aggregation network (GCA) [12] incorporates a gated sub-network for multi-scale feature fusion, which eliminates grid artifacts. A feature fusion attention network (FFA) [13] and an end-to-end network (T-Net) [7] have been proposed to overcome the bottleneck of conventional dehazing models using attention mechanisms. A fast dehazing model for 4K resolution images (4Kdehazing) [8] and a Laplacian pyramid dehazing network (LDN) [9] have been proposed to restore high-definition dehazed images. A trident dehazing network (TDN) [5] has been proposed as a coarse-to-fine model for automatic haze-density recognition. A knowledge transfer dehazing network (KTDN) [10] utilizes the teacher–student framework to calculate high-frequency features from hazy images. A principled synthetic-to-real dehazing (PSD) [4] network was pre-trained on synthetic datasets and fine-tuned to real-world images. A self-paced semi-curricular attention network (SCANet) [14] has been proposed to learn features between non-homogeneous haze and underlying scenes. An additional self-attention transformer (ASAT) [11] and a detail-enhanced attention network (DEA) [15] helps the model acquire more detailed information.

Dehazing methods based on unsupervised learning do not require paired haze-free images for training. Inspired by the CycleGAN [16], Cycle-Dehaze [17] employs a cycle structure and a perceptual loss constraint to train two generators. A deep DCP [18] network was trained by minimizing DCP-based loss. Visual quality-driven dehazing (VQDD) [19] combines deep and shallow features to compensate for the missing information. A zero-shot dehazing network named "you only look yourself" (YOLY) [20] combines three sub-networks to disentangle the parameters of the atmospheric scattering model. A self-guided disentangled representation learning (SGDRL) [21] model has been proposed to evaluate the degree of feature decomposition and guide the feature fusion for reconstruction. Although these models make improvements, they do not consider the impact of haze concentrations on image dehazing.

3 Proposed Method

3.1 Dual-Cycle Framework Based on Relative Haze Density

To learn image features with different degradation levels, this study proposes a dual-cycle framework that incorporates both supervised dehazing and unsupervised haze addition based on relative haze density. Considering the haze density as a relative variable, an image is recovered to a dehazed image by supervised learning, constrained by its corresponding clear reference image. Simultaneously, the image is degraded to a state containing dense haze through unsupervised learning using an unpaired reference image with dense haze, as illustrated in Fig. 1. In this dual-cycle framework, two networks, RNet and DNet, are employed for the restoration and degradation of images, respectively, and are trained and refined simultaneously.

Restoration Network. Figure 2 illustrates the architecture of the RNet, which consists of an edge attention (EA) branch, a super-resolution (SR) branch, and a feature compression (FC) module.

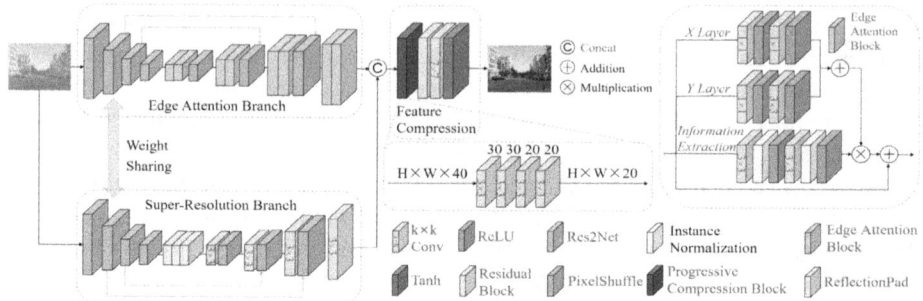

Fig. 2. Architecture of the restoration network RNet.

Edge Attention Branch. High-frequency components of images generally receive more attention, because they are related to rich and intricate details. Inspired by the Sobel edge detection operator [22] and attention mechanisms [13], we designed EA branch to capture more edges from hazy inputs. As illustrated in Fig. 2, an EA block comprises the X layer, Y layer, and information extraction layer with a residual connection. The X and Y layers are designed to learn the edge weights of the images in the X- and Y-directions, respectively. An EA map is produced by pixel-wise addition and multiplication of the outputs of the three layers. Composed of several EA blocks, the RNet is guided to focus on the edges.

Super-Resolution Branch. When training with high-resolution images, preprocessing steps including cropping and downsampling are commonly conducted to reduce the image size. However, these routines generally result in coarse textures and degrade the visual quality. To address this issue, we designed an SR branch to improve the resolution of the images and recover lost details. The SR branch adopts an encoder–decoder structure, wherein the encoder shares weights with Res2Net blocks in the EA branch, and the decoder incorporates three residual blocks and pixel shuffle layers [23].

Feature Compression Module. An FC module was designed to concatenate the feature maps produced by the EA and SR branches, producing a dehazed image. The progressive compression block is depicted in Fig. 2, where H and W are the height and width of the feature maps, respectively, and the number of convolution kernels is marked above each convolution layer, which has a stride of 1 and a padding of 1. Distinguished from commonly used post-processing blocks that compress channels of feature maps through a single convolution layer, the FC module compresses and merges features by progressive convolutions, which reduces information loss and enhances the capability of the feature representation of the RNet.

Degradation Network. Considering the function of the DNet, we constructed it as a simplified version of the RNet, which is composed of only the EA branch and the FC module of the RNet. DNet is trained to add haze to images, causing them to deteriorate from clear to containing thin haze or from containing thin haze to dense haze. The DNet is jointly trained with the RNet to enhance its performance, which removes haze at various concentrations from images.

3.2 Multi-class Discriminator

A discriminator was employed in the GAN to distinguish the real data from the results created by the generator. However, these binary classifiers are insufficient for categorizing images with different haze levels. To address this issue, we propose two multi-class discriminators: a clear image discriminator D_{clear} and a dense haze discriminator D_{dense}. Using adversarial learning, D_{clear} guides the RNet to generate clear images with lower haze concentrations and richer details. Conversely, D_{dense} guides the DNet to produce degraded images with higher haze density and lower clarity.

Figure 3 illustrates the structure of the D_{clear}. As the discriminator of the RNet, D_{clear} outputs the probabilities of four types of images: clear reference, input, dense haze reference, and dehazed image. Correspondingly, the discriminator of DNet, D_{dense} has the same structure as D_{clear}; however, it classifies the dense haze reference, input, clear reference, and haze-added images generated by DNet. Our ablation study demonstrates that employing multi-class discriminators improves the dehazing results because the capabilities of RNet and DNet are boosted.

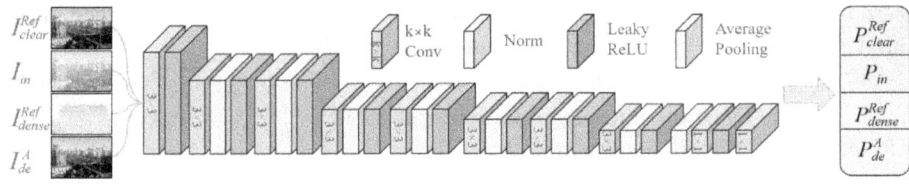

Fig. 3. The structure of a multi-class discriminator D_{clear}, which outputs the predicted probabilities of four types of input images.

3.3 Loss Function

In the proposed dual-cycle framework, our networks are trained by minimizing a total loss, which is a combination of the content (L_{con}), cycle-consistency (L_{cyc}), adversarial (L_{adv}), and multi-order derivative (L_{frac}) losses:

$$L_{total} = \lambda_1 L_{con} + \lambda_2 L_{cyc} + \lambda_3 L_{adv} + \lambda_4 L_{frac}, \tag{1}$$

where $\lambda_1, \lambda_2, \lambda_3, \lambda_4$ are the hyperparameters that balance the different losses.

Content Loss. The content loss is computed as the mean absolute errors between the clear reference image I_{clear}^{Ref} and the two dehazed images I_{de}^{A} and I_{de}^{B} generated by RNet, which are dehazed from the input and haze-added images, respectively. In this section, the images are labeled as shown in Fig. 1. N represents the number of training images.

$$L_{con} = \frac{1}{N} \sum_{i=1}^{N} (|I_{clear}^{Ref} - I_{de}^{A}| + |I_{clear}^{Ref} - I_{de}^{B}|). \tag{2}$$

Cycle-Consistency Loss. As illustrated in Fig. 1, $I_{in} \to I_{de}^{A} \to I_{cyc} \approx I_{in}$, where I_{cyc} is the hazy image degraded from dehazed image I_{de}^{A}. Therefore,

$$L_{cyc} = \frac{1}{N} \sum_{i=1}^{N} |I_{in} - I_{cyc}|. \tag{3}$$

Adversarial Loss. To distinguish clear images, the ratio of the clear image class is increased compared with the other three classes for training the multi-class discriminator D_{clear}, which is set as 3:1:1:1. Similarly, to train D_{dense}, the ratio is set to 1:1:3:1 to highlight the class of images with dense haze. For these two multi-class discriminators, cross-entropy (CE) loss is applied:

$$\begin{aligned}L_{adv}(D_{clear}) = &\tfrac{3}{4} CE(D_{clear}(I_{clear}^{Ref}), C_{clear}^{Ref}) + \tfrac{1}{4} CE(D_{clear}(I_{in}), C_{in}) \\ &+ \tfrac{1}{4} CE(D_{clear}(I_{dense}^{Ref}), C_{dense}^{Ref}) + \tfrac{1}{4} CE(D_{clear}(I_{de}^{A}), C_{de}^{A}),\end{aligned} \tag{4}$$

$$\begin{aligned}L_{adv}(D_{dense}) = &\tfrac{1}{4} CE(D_{dense}(I_{clear}^{Ref}), C_{clear}^{Ref}) + \tfrac{1}{4} CE(D_{dense}(I_{in}), C_{in}) \\ &+ \tfrac{3}{4} CE(D_{dense}(I_{dense}^{Ref}), C_{dense}^{Ref}) + \tfrac{1}{4} CE(D_{dense}(I_{add}), C_{add}),\end{aligned} \tag{5}$$

where C_x denotes the class of the corresponding image I_x; I_{dense}^{Ref} is the reference image with dense haze; and I_{add} is the image added with haze by DNet.

During the adversarial training process, RNet aims to generate I_{de}^{A} that approaches class C_{clear}^{Ref}, and DNet generates I_{add} that approaches class C_{dense}^{Ref}. The adversarial losses of RNet and DNet are defined as follows:

$$L_{adv}(RNet) = CE\left(D_{clear}\left(I_{de}^{A}\right), C_{clear}^{Ref}\right), L_{adv}(DNet) = CE(D_{dense}(I_{add}), C_{dense}^{Ref}). \tag{6}$$

Multi-order Derivative Loss. The integer-order derivatives of an image, such as Sobel (first-order) and Laplacian (second-order) operators, are commonly used for edge detection. By capturing both the edges and other information, fractional-order derivatives extract rich nonlinear features from images related to their contrasts, colors, and edges.

To better match dehazed images with clear images, we propose a multi-order derivative loss function based on the fractional-order derivative [24], which improves the visual quality of the dehazed outputs. The multi-order derivatives are computed using Tiansi convolution templates [25]. In addition, the fractional-order features of the dehazed images are constrained to be consistent with the clear images as follows:

$$L_{frac} = \frac{1}{N} \sum_{i=1}^{N} \sum_{v \in V}^{V} \left(\left| F_v\left(I_{clear}^{Ref}\right) - F_v\left(I_{de}^{A}\right) \right| + \left| F_v\left(I_{clear}^{Ref}\right) - F_v\left(I_{de}^{B}\right) \right| \right), \tag{7}$$

where N is the number of images; v represents the order of the derivative in the list of selected orders V; and F_v is the v th-order derivative convolution.

4 Experiments

4.1 Experimental Setup

Training Details. All the experiments were performed on an NVIDIA RTX3090 GPU using PyTorch 1.12.1. For data augmentation, rotations (90, 180, or 270°), horizontal flips, and cropping to a size of 512 × 512 were performed randomly for the training images. An Adam optimizer with settings $\beta_1 = 0.9$ and $\beta_2 = 0.999$ was employed to optimize the framework. The initial learning rate was set to 0.0001 and halved every 50 epochs. The parameters of the loss function were $\lambda_1 = 1.0$, $\lambda_2 = \lambda_3 = \lambda_4 = 0.1$.

Datasets. To test the dual-cycle framework by supervised learning, datasets NH-HAZE20, NH-HAZE21, and NH-HAZE23 [32] were used for non-homogeneous dehazing, which contain 55, 30, and 40 real-world image pairs of hazy and haze-free outdoor scenes, respectively. In addition to the original size, bicubic downsampling of 2× and 4× was also applied to the input images to evaluate the performance in dehazing for low-resolution hazy images. In particular, NH-HAZE23 is a high-definition image set containing images of extremely large size (6000 × 4000), which cannot be processed directly by most dehazing methods with the original size. Therefore, we only trained and tested the models on this dataset by downsampled images. To evaluate our method for unsupervised learning, we use three subsets of the benchmark dataset RESIDE [26]: the outdoor training set (OTS), synthetic objective testing set (SOTS), and hybrid subjective testing set (HSTS). Similar to most dehazing methods [4, 19, 21], our networks were trained on OTS and tested on outdoor scenes from SOTS and synthetic images from HSTS, which contain 500 and 10 hazy and haze-free image pairs, respectively.

4.2 Evaluation of Supervised Learning

Our method was compared with several state-of-the-art dehazing approaches, including DCP [2], AOD [6], GCA [12], FFA [13], KTDN [10], TDN [5], 4Kdehazing [8], SCANet [14], T-Net [7], LDN [9], ASTA [11], and DEA [15]. Two commonly used full-reference metrics were calculated: the peak signal-to-noise ratio (PSNR) [27] and structural similarity (SSIM) [28], which evaluate the recovery accuracy compared with the corresponding haze-free images. Meanwhile, no-reference indexes, namely the learned perceptual image patch similarity (LPIPS) [29] and fog aware density evaluator (FADE) [30], were used to measure the visual quality for real-world hazy images.

For a quantitative evaluation for real-world images with non-homogeneous haze, Tables 1 and 2 report the average metrics on the NH-HAZE series datasets. For a fair comparison, all the networks were retrained on the three NH-HAZE datasets. Notably, as indicated by the highest values in Table 2 and the best metrics in Table 1, our network generally outperforms other dehazing models for low-resolution images (sizes of 2× and 4× downsampling) with degradation introduced by both haze and downsampling. These experimental results demonstrate that our model is superior to its competitors in terms of dehazing performance, as measured by the FADE, recovery accuracy, as reflected by PSNR and SSIM values, and the perceptual quality as indicated by the LPIPS.

Table 1. Quantitative comparison of dehazing methods. **Bold** and underline indicate the rankings of 1st and 2nd, respectively. "↑" ("↓") indicates the larger (smaller) the better.

Method			DCP '10	AOD '17	GCA '19	FFA '20	4Kdehazing '21	T-Net '22	SCANet '23	LDN '24	ASTA '24	DEA '24	Ours
NH-HAZE20	1×	PSNR↑	13.28	16.00	17.00	18.16	17.37	19.06	19.50	17.79	18.85	19.39	**19.79**
		SSIM↑	0.479	0.533	0.559	0.638	0.469	0.644	0.650	0.618	0.652	0.656	**0.663**
		LPIPS↓	0.517	0.481	0.336	0.359	0.683	0.329	0.422	0.392	0.338	0.324	**0.304**
		FADE↓	0.358	0.595	0.492	0.298	0.530	0.331	0.306	0.318	0.311	0.318	**0.296**
	2×	PSNR↑	13.41	15.88	17.00	18.29	17.48	17.46	18.82	17.99	18.25	18.54	**19.66**
		SSIM↑	0.430	0.465	0.558	0.586	0.472	0.575	0.501	0.594	0.578	0.566	**0.607**
		LPIPS↓	0.643	0.634	0.507	0.555	0.682	0.526	0.602	0.505	0.585	0.537	**0.454**
		FADE↓	0.519	0.790	0.472	0.488	0.631	0.555	0.493	0.518	0.495	0.539	**0.459**
	4×	PSNR↑	13.22	15.61	17.63	16.96	17.21	16.35	16.97	16.15	16.57	16.52	**18.83**
		SSIM↑	0.337	0.362	0.447	0.432	0.406	0.424	0.343	0.437	0.416	0.395	**0.470**
		LPIPS↓	0.794	0.787	0.689	0.767	0.812	0.770	0.834	0.744	0.779	0.784	**0.666**
		FADE↓	0.819	1.167	0.736	0.839	0.875	0.911	0.955	0.719	0.885	1.017	**0.637**
NH-HAZE21	1×	PSNR↑	11.68	16.08	18.47	20.27	18.28	18.98	**21.12**	17.85	20.15	19.71	19.82
		SSIM↑	0.647	0.698	0.738	0.800	0.652	0.786	0.769	0.772	0.803	0.794	**0.814**
		LPIPS↓	0.448	0.378	0.327	0.264	0.548	0.259	0.364	0.310	0.275	0.281	**0.255**
		FADE↓	0.395	0.578	0.441	0.454	0.630	0.479	0.442	0.395	**0.355**	0.389	0.394
	2×	PSNR↑	11.80	15.83	18.55	19.29	18.00	18.60	**20.20**	17.77	19.53	19.22	19.56
		SSIM↑	0.564	0.597	0.672	0.690	0.600	0.678	0.555	0.614	0.694	0.660	**0.722**
		LPIPS↓	0.583	0.551	0.506	0.491	0.616	0.453	0.572	0.484	0.514	0.507	**0.439**
		FADE↓	0.491	0.725	0.592	0.519	0.702	0.583	0.651	0.517	**0.447**	0.439	0.473
	4×	PSNR↑	11.56	15.37	18.05	18.06	17.44	17.16	18.27	16.23	18.27	17.91	**18.80**
		SSIM↑	0.417	0.442	0.507	0.507	0.471	0.477	0.373	0.514	0.491	0.449	**0.530**
		LPIPS↓	0.761	0.756	0.711	0.748	0.792	0.742	0.868	0.721	0.775	0.791	**0.662**
		FADE↓	0.727	1.059	0.799	0.793	0.948	0.848	1.171	0.779	0.712	0.888	**0.693**

Table 2. Quantitative comparison of dehazing methods on NH-HAZE23 dataset.

Method		DCP '10	AOD '17	GCA '19	KTDN '20	TDN '20	4Kdehazing '21	T-Net '22	LDN '24	DEA '24	Ours
2×	PSNR↑	11.11	14.31	16.45	<u>18.18</u>	14.28	14.32	18.13	17.85	18.12	**18.19**
	SSIM↑	0.496	0.584	0.535	0.590	0.562	0.532	<u>0.614</u>	0.613	0.604	**0.620**
4×	PSNR↑	11.15	14.16	16.70	17.34	16.96	14.25	<u>17.57</u>	17.26	17.27	**17.79**
	SSIM↑	0.470	0.544	0.559	0.549	0.532	0.507	0.544	<u>0.563</u>	0.538	**0.565**

Figure 4 illustrates the dehazed images of the various methods when the input hazy image is downsampled by a factor of 2 (first two rows) and 4 (the 3rd and 4th rows), in which local regions in red boxes are enlarged below the global images. As shown in Fig. 4, DCP, 4Kdehazing, and LDN restores images with significant color distortions of the overall bluish, greenish, and reddish colors, respectively, whereas DCP, AOD, 4Kdehazing, and LDN suffer from insufficient haze removal. Generally, learning-based networks generate dehazed images of higher quality than prior-based models such as DCP. By employing the EA blocks, SR branch, and multi-order derivative loss, our RNet recovers the finest details and most vivid colors when the input images are degraded by both haze effects and downsampling.

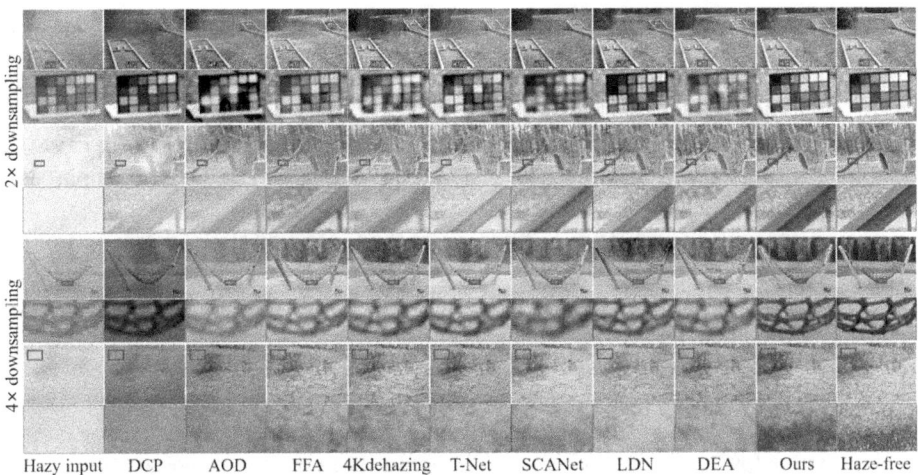

Fig. 4. Comparison of visual quality on the NH-HAZE20 and NH-HAZE21 datasets.

4.3 Ablation Study

To demonstrate the effectiveness of the components introduced in the proposed method, we conducted ablation experiments on the NH-HAZE20 dataset. The results are summarized in Table 3. Replacing the traditional channel attention (CA) or pixel attention (PA) with our EA blocks in RNet increases both PSNR and SSIM significantly, indicating a better quality of image recovery. Meanwhile, by gradually adding the SR branch, multi-class discriminator, and multi-order derivative loss, both metrics were further increased. The multi-class discriminator better constrains the types of output images, while the SR branch recovers lost details, resulting in better image quality restored by the RNet. Therefore, all the proposed components contribute to the performance improvement for haze removal from real-world images.

Table 3. Ablation study of components in our framework on the NH-HAZE20 dataset.

Components	Alternatives					
Attention block (CA/PA/EA)	CA	PA	EA	EA	EA	EA
SR branch	✓	✓	✗	✓	✓	✓
Classification of discriminator	multi	multi	multi	binary	multi	multi
Multi-order derivative loss	✓	✓	✓	✓	✗	✓
PSNR↑	18.12	17.66	19.08	19.36	19.51	**19.79**
SSIM↑	0.619	0.618	0.648	0.645	0.643	**0.663**

4.4 Evaluation of Unsupervised Learning

Based on prior knowledge, the proposed dual-cycle framework can be adapted for unsupervised learning by replacing the clear reference images. In our experiments, a simple yet effective linear function, i.e., Z-score normalization [31], was applied to the intensity of the pixels in a hazy image to produce a contrast-enhanced version of theinput, as a substitute for the clear reference image in supervised learning.

Table 4 presents a quantitative comparison of the SOTS and HSTS datasets. Trained using hazy images with unpaired dense reference images, our network was compared with several prior-based, supervised, and unsupervised methods. The proposed method outperforms all others on the HSTS dataset and is the second best on the SOTS dataset for outdoor scenes, achieving impressive performance in terms of PSNR and SSIM.

Figure 5 presents an example in HSTS dataset, in which local regions are enlarged below. As shown in Fig. 5, methods of DCP, AOD, YOLY, and SGDRL output images too dark with a low saturation, whereas PSD produces a dehazed image too bright with significant color distortions. Notably, the output of ours is most approximate to the ground-truth haze-free image with clear edges and color fidelity.

Table 4. Quantitative comparison of dehazing methods on SOTS and HSTS datasets.

Method		Prior			Supervised		Unsupervised					
		Z-score '07	DCP '10	NLP '16	AOD '17	PSD '21	Cycle GAN'18	Cycle-Dehaze'20	Deep DCP'20	YOLY '21	VQDD '23	SGDRL '24	Ours
SOTS	PSNR↑	14.57	18.38	18.07	20.08	20.49	17.38	18.60	20.99	20.39	22.25	**23.28**	22.76
	SSIM↑	0.527	0.819	0.802	0.861	0.844	0.706	0.797	0.893	0.889	0.847	**0.919**	0.912
HSTS	PSNR↑	15.27	17.01	17.62	19.68	19.37	16.05	17.96	21.21	21.02	22.53	22.01	**22.91**
	SSIM↑	0.567	0.803	0.798	0.835	0.824	0.703	0.777	0.871	0.905	0.875	0.888	**0.909**

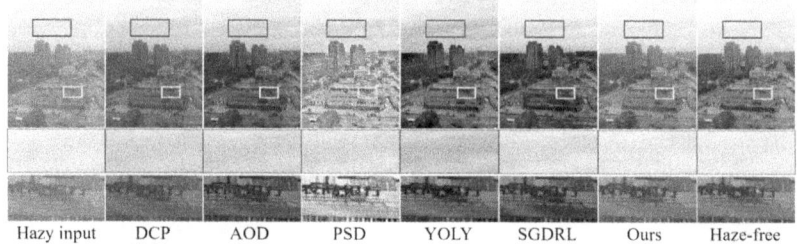

Fig. 5. Comparison of visual quality by unsupervised learning on the HSTS dataset.

5 Conclusion

This study proposes a dual-cycle framework based on relative haze density for non-homogeneous image dehazing, in which RNet and DNet are designed to remove and add haze. Composed of EA and SR branches and guided by multi-order differential loss, RNet recovers sharp edges and bright colors for haze scenes. Multi-classification discriminators are designed to distinguish the relative levels of haze density, helping RNet and DNet gradually learn the image features of different haze concentrations. Qualitative and quantitative evaluations of both supervised and unsupervised learning demonstrate the superiority of our method for image dehazing. In future work, we will extend the dual-cycle framework to other tasks such as low-light image enhancement.

Acknowledgments. This work was supported by the National Natural Science Foundation of China (No. 62071201), and the Guangdong Basic and Applied Basic Research Foundation (No. 2024A1515011762, No. 2022A1515010119).

References

1. Narasimhan, S.G., Nayar, S.K.: Chromatic framework for vision in bad weather. In: Proceedings of the IEEE Conference on Computer Vision and Pattern Recognition (CVPR), pp. 598–605. IEEE (2000)
2. He, K., Sun, J., Tang, X.: Single image haze removal using dark channel prior. IEEE Trans. Pattern Anal. Mach. Intell. **33**(12), 2341–2353 (2010)
3. Berman, D., Treibitz, T., Avidan S.: Non-local image dehazing. In: Proceedings of the IEEE Conference on Computer Vision and Patter Recognition (CVPR), pp. 1674–1682. IEEE (2016)
4. Chen, Z., Wang, Y., Yang, Y., Liu, D.: PSD: principled synthetic-to-real dehazing guided by physical priors. In: Proceedings of the IEEE/CVF Conference on Computer Vision and Pattern Recognition (CVPR), pp. 7180–7189. IEEE (2021)
5. Liu, J., Wu, H., Xie, Y., Qu, Y., Ma, L.: Trident dehazing network. In: Proceedings of the IEEE/CVF Conference on Computer Vision and Pattern Recognition Workshops (CVPRW), pp. 430–431. IEEE (2020)
6. Li, B., Peng, X., Wang, Z., Xu, J., Feng, D.: AOD-Net: all-in-one dehazing network. In: Proceedings of the IEEE International Conference on Computer Vision (ICCV), pp. 4770–4778. IEEE (2017)

7. Zheng, L., Li, Y., Zhang, K., Luo, W.: T-Net: deep stacked scale-iteration network for image dehazing. IEEE Trans. Multimedia **25**, 6794–6807 (2023)
8. Zheng, Z., Ren, W., Cao, X., Hu, X., Wang, T., Song, F., et al.: Ultra-high-definition image dehazing via multi-guided bilateral learning. In: Proceedings of the IEEE/CVF Conference on Computer Vision and Pattern Recognition (CVPR), pp. 16180–16189. IEEE (2021)
9. Xiao, B., Zheng, Z., Zhuang, Y., Lyu, C., Jia, X.: Single UHD image dehazing via interpretable pyramid network. Signal Process. **214**, 109225 (2024)
10. Wu, H., Liu, J., Xie, Y., Qu, Y., Ma, L.: Knowledge transfer dehazing network for nonhomogeneous dehazing. In: Proceedings of the IEEE/CVF Conference on Computer Vision and Pattern Recognition Workshops (CVPRW), pp. 478–479. IEEE (2020)
11. Cai, Z., Ning, J., Ding, Z., Duo, B.: Additional self-attention transformer with adapter for thick haze removal. IEEE Geosci. Remote Sens. Lett. **21**, 1–5 (2024)
12. Chen, D., He, M., Fan, Q., Liao, J., Zhang, L., Hou, D., et al.: Gated context aggregation network for image dehazing and deraining. In: Winter Conference on Applications of Computer Vision (WACV), pp. 1375–1383. IEEE (2019)
13. Qin, X., Wang, Z., Bai, Y., Xie, X., Jia, H.: FFA-Net: feature fusion attention network for single image dehazing. In: Proceedings of the AAAI Conference on Artificial Intelligence, vol. 34, pp. 11908–11915. AAAI (2020)
14. Guo, Y., Gao, Y., Liu, W., Lu, Y., Qu, J., He, S., et al.: SCANet: self-paced semi-curricular attention network for non-homogeneous image dehazing. In: Proceedings of the IEEE/CVF Conference on Computer Vision and Pattern Recognition Workshops (CVPRW), pp. 1884–1893. IEEE (2023)
15. Chen, Z., He, Z., Lu, Z.M.: DEA-Net: single image dehazing based on detail-enhanced convolution and content-guided attention. IEEE Trans. Image Process. **33**, 1002–1015 (2024)
16. Zhu, J.Y., Park, T., Isola, P., Efros, A.A.: Unpaired image-to-image translation using cycle-consistent adversarial networks. In: Proceedings of the IEEE International Conference on Computer Vision (ICCV), pp. 2223–2232. IEEE (2017)
17. Engin, D., Genç, A., Kemal Ekenel, H.: Cycle-Dehaze: enhanced CycleGAN for single image dehazing. In: Proceedings of the IEEE Conference on Computer Vision and Pattern Recognition Workshops (CVPRW), pp. 825–833. IEEE (2018)
18. Golts, A., Freedman, D., Elad, M.: Unsupervised single image dehazing using dark channel prior loss. IEEE Trans. Image Process. **29**, 2692–2701 (2019)
19. Yang, A., Liu, Y., Wang, J., Li, X., Cao, J., Ji, Z., et al.: Visual-quality-driven unsupervised image dehazing. Neural Netw. **167**, 1–9 (2023)
20. Li, B., Gou, Y., Gu, S., Liu, Z., Zhou, T., Peng, X.: You Only Look Yourself: unsupervised and untrained single image dehazing neural network. Int. J. Comput. Vision **129**, 1754–1767 (2021)
21. Jia, T., Li, J., Zhuo, L., Zhang, J.: Self-guided disentangled representation learning for single image dehazing. Neural Netw. **172**, 106107 (2024)
22. Gao, W., Zhang, X., Yang, L., Liu, H.: An improved Sobel edge detection. In: International Conference on Computer Science and Information Technology, vol. 5, pp. 67–71. IEEE (2010)
23. Shi, W., Caballero, J., Huszár, F., Totz, J., Aitken, A.P., Bishop, R., et al.: Real-time single image and video super-resolution using an efficient sub-pixel convolutional neural network. In: Proceedings of the IEEE Conference on Computer Vision and Pattern Recognition (CVPR), pp. 1874–1883. IEEE (2016)
24. Podlubny, I., Chechkin, A., Skovranek, T., Chen, Y., Jara, B.M.V.: Matrix approach to discrete fractional calculus ii: partial fractional differential equations. J. Comput. Phys. **228**(8), 3137–3153 (2009)
25. Yang, Z., Zhou, J., Huang, M.: Edge detection based on fractional differential. J. Sichuan Univ. (Eng. Sci. Ed.) **40**(1), 152 (2008)

26. Li, B., Ren, W., Fu, D., Tao, D., Feng, D., Zeng, W., et al.: Benchmarking single-image dehazing and beyond. IEEE Trans. Image Process. **28**(1), 492–505 (2018)
27. Wang, Z., Li, Q.: Information content weighting for perceptual image quality assessment. IEEE Trans. Image Process. **20**(5), 1185–1198 (2011)
28. Wang, Z., Bovik, A.C., Sheikh, H.R., Simoncelli, E.P.: Image quality assessment: from error visibility to structural similarity. IEEE Trans. Image Process. **13**(4), 600–612 (2004)
29. Zhang, R., Isola, P., Efros, A.A., Shechtman, E., Wang, O.: The unreasonable effectiveness of deep features as a perceptual metric. In: Proceedings of the IEEE Conference on Computer Vision and Pattern Recognition (CVPR), pp. 586–595. IEEE (2018)
30. Choi, L.K., You, J., Bovik, A.C.: Referenceless prediction of perceptual fog density and perceptual image defogging. IEEE Trans. Image Process. **24**(11), 3888–3901 (2015)
31. Abdi, H.: Z-scores. Encycl. Meas. Stat. **3**, 1055–1058 (2007)
32. Ancuti, C.O., Ancuti, C., Vasluianu, F.A., Timofte, R., Zhou, H., Dong, W., et al.: NTIRE 2023 HR nonhomogeneous dehazing challenge report. In: Proceedings of the IEEE/CVF Conference on Computer Vision and Pattern Recognition Workshops (CVPRW), pp. 1808–1825. IEEE (2023)

Contrastive Learning for Silent Face Liveness Detection Based on A Hybrid Framework

Ying Tang[1], Zhongyue Chen[1], Minchao Ye[1], Zhaojuan Zhang[1], Yaping Qi[1], Huijuan Lu[1,2], and Wanli Huo[1(✉)]

[1] China Jiliang University, Hangzhou 310018, Zhejiang, China
huowl@cjlu.edu.cn
[2] Drore Information and Technology Co., Ltd., Hangzhou 310000, Zhejiang, China

Abstract. Face liveness detection is essential to ensuring the security of face recognition systems. Most current models rely on convolutional neural networks to achieve domain generalization through complete representations on common modules. The limitations of receptive field prevent model getting global context and capturing long-range dependencies, which ignores the global face semantic information and lacks the local focus of the face on more fine-grained features. To tackle these challenges, this paper proposes a silent face liveness detection domain generalization model based on the fusion of convolutional neural network (CNN) and Swin Transformer features, namely, CLCSN. Then, a contrastive learning technique is suggested to highlight liveness-related style aspects, which improves the generalization capacity, in order to generate a generalized representation. Experimental results demonstrate our approach's effectiveness in solving the face liveness detection domain generalization problems.

Keywords: Silent Face Liveness Detection · Domain Generalization · CNN-Swin Transformer · Contrastive Learning

1 Introduction

Recently, computer vision advancements have spurred widespread adoption of face recognition technology across real-world applications. However, presentation attacks (Pas) such as print attacks, video replay attacks, 3D masks, and potential future unknown attack methods are also emerging. To address these concerns, researchers have developed various face liveness detection (FLD) methods, ranging from those based on hand-crafted descriptors [1] to which based on deep representations [2].

Previous domain-specific FLD approaches have demonstrated high accuracy. However, they also exhibit significant degradation in performance when handling cross-domain data or facing novel adversarial attacks. The overfitting due to dataset bias limited by training dataset results in poor generalization to new domains. Domain Adaptation (DA) techniques [4] are employed to reduce distributional differences between source and target domains. However, in many FLD scenarios, collecting large amounts of unlabeled target data, specifically for spoofing attacks, is a challenging and costly task. Additionally, due to privacy concerns, it is typically hardly to access source face data when deploying FLD models in the target domain.

Therefore, the emergence of domain generalization FLD methods [5] solves above problems and ensures the validity of trained model across different domains. In researching domain generalization, it is assumed that the model is trained on datasets from D1 to DK and applied in a zero-shot manner to the unknown target domain dataset DK + 1. The model's insensitivity to domain changes allows it to be successful applicated in unknown domains.

The essence of FLD is to distinguish between real and fake faces, however, many current methods use domain generalization (i.e., CNN-BN-ReLU) on a common module. This approach does not fully consider local and global fine-grained features. Recent studies have utilized the Transformer architecture as the backbone for models employing FLD domain generalization. Since Transformers can provide larger receptive fields than CNN and are adept at capturing remote dependencies [8] and extracting global semantic features. Additionally, the authors [18] discovered reasonably high performance on domain generalization FLD using only a simple concentration loss to centrally embed real faces in space due to powerful entire face feature extraction of Transformer models.

We propose a new framework for FLD domain generalization. Considering that CNN has local relational coding characteristics which is better at extracting local fine-grained features, while Transformer is good at extracting global semantic information and capturing dependencies between long distances. We combine two frameworks, CNN and Swin Transformer, to extract global semantic face features while capturing local key features with differentiation. Therefore, this model can extract key facial features more accurately to classify facial images with unknown attacks. Discriminative information that enhances the distinction between living and spoofing is retained for extracted localized key information. A contrastive learning method is employed to reduce domain-specific style elements and emphasize liveness-related ones, which achieves the purpose of enhancing the generalization ability.

In comparison to previous domain generalization approaches, our contributions can be summarized as follows:

•We propose a novel network architecture that fuses CNN and Swin Transformer for silent face liveness detection.
•The local feature extraction network captures intrinsic detailed patterns by aggregating the intensity and gradient information, which improves the network's ability to discriminate between fine-grained images of faces.
•The proposed method involves comparing different features and placing emphasis on liveness-related style features. This effectively reduces the domain gap between similar samples, thereby enhancing the model's domain generalization capability.

2 Related Work

2.1 RGB Image-Based FLD

FLD methods are broadly classified into two types: traditional methods and methods based on deep learning. In the early stages of research, most traditional approaches heavily relied on manually designed local descriptors like local binary patterns [1] and directed gradient histograms [10]. However, handcrafted features have certain drawbacks such as limited generalization, time-consuming feature extraction, and applicability in specific scenarios only. Since the success of deep learning, CNN approaches have been widely used to solve liveness detection problems. Dual-stage Feature Learning FLD [12] model using generative adversarial training by removing deception traces from images, improving the interpretability of model decisions.

This paper aims to contribute to the field of domain generalization for silent face liveness detection. The aforementioned methods demonstrate satisfactory performance, but only in cases where the difference in distribution between the training and testing domains is relatively minor. As a result, many methods for domain generalization have been proposed. FGHV [13] was proposed with the aim of handling distributional shifts between real faces and known attacks. By utilizing Gaussian inputs to align the generated face features with the assumptions created by the feature generation network, FGHV aims to produce more robust and reliable features that can effectively counter attacks in unknown domains. IADG [14] introduced Asymmetric Instance Adaptive Whitening (AIAW), which improves the feature by adaptively whitening the feature correlations that are sensitive to the domains in question.

2.2 Transformers and FLD

Transformers are gaining popularity in computer vision and natural language processing (NLP). Dosovitskiy et al. [15] proposed the Vision Transformer (ViT) as a method for reducing processing resources and dividing an image into several small portions for projection onto a low-dimensional feature space. MobileViT [17] combines convolution and transformation in a single module to effectively collect local and global data. The model performs well even in shallow scenarios with this module, making visual translator more suitable for edge devices.

The transformer model has only been used in a few previous studies in FLD tasks. To avoid overfitting, Huang et al. [18] proposed a novel Multi-Level Attention Module DropBlock (MAMD) to enrich discriminative features while removing irrelevant spatial features. The enriched convolutional feature sets were combined and fed into the MTSS network for face spoofing. DiVT [9] used converter model to propose domain-invariant concentration loss and attack separation loss to deal with cross-domain FAS problem, which can achieve higher performance than previous methods on domain-generalized FLD problem with better resource consumption efficiency.

3 Method

3.1 Overview

In this section, we introduce our approach shown in Fig. 1. It avoids the interference of external ambient light by using the improved MobileNetV2 as backbone. A Swin Transformer-based network is also employed to facilitate the extraction of global key information. Its sophisticated sliding window module is utilized to effectively accomplish inter-pane interaction and global attention. Contrastive learning is applied to hide style information unique to a domain and highlight liveliness-related ones. In order to optimize the network for consistent and dependable training, the overall loss is finally integrated.

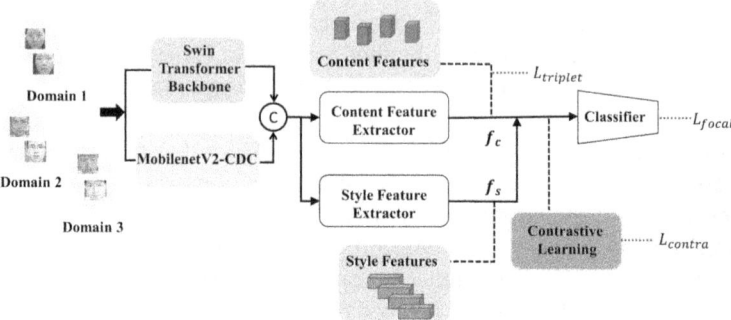

Fig. 1. The overall architecture of our Contrastive Learning based on CNN-Swin Trans-former network (CLCSN).

3.2 Network Architecture

Local Feature Extraction. Current algorithms used for the FLD (fine-grained texture description) task have faced challenges in adequately capturing detailed texture information and often exhibit instability when the environmental conditions, such as lighting levels, change. Our suggested local feature extraction network chooses mobilenetV2 [19] as CNN backbone, which combines Inverted Residuals and Linear Bottlenecks. The model complexity and training time by convolutional substitution while maintaining model performance to make it widely used in real-world scenarios. Specifically, the central difference convolution (CDC) [11] is utilized to replace depthwise separable convolution in mobilenetV2 due to its remarkable ability to represent invariant fine-grained features in different environments, especially its better robustness under ambient light changes. Without introducing any additional parameters, a central differential convolution network is formed with more powerful modeling capabilities as follows:

$$y(p_0) = \theta \sum_{p_n \in R} \omega(p_n) \cdot (x(p_0 + p_n) - x(p_0)) + (1 - \theta) \sum^{\omega}(p_n) \cdot x(p_0 + p_n) \quad (1)$$

where x, y is convolution input and feature map output, p_0 is current input position, p_n is the index of the current position as center neighborhood R, ω is convolution kernel, and θ is hyperparameter. The CDC degenerates into a simple convolution when θ is set to 0, indicating that CDC contains richer information than simple convolution.

Global Feature Extraction. The global feature extractor uses Swin Transformer as backbone in this study [16], which is a network model that includes shifted windows and hierarchical architecture. To achieve global modeling capability, shifted windows operation combines non-overlapping local windows with overlapping cross-windows. It significantly reduces computational load and captures face global features accurately. Patch Partition, Linear Embedding, and four stages make up the Swin Transformer. Multiple Patch Merging and Swim Transformer Block structures are included in each stage. As illustrated in Fig. 2, the output feature maps of Stages 2, 3, and 4 are H/8 × W/8 × 2C, H/16 × W/16 × 4C, and H/32 × W/32 × 8C, respectively. After each Patch Merging, the height and width are cut in half and the depth is doubled.

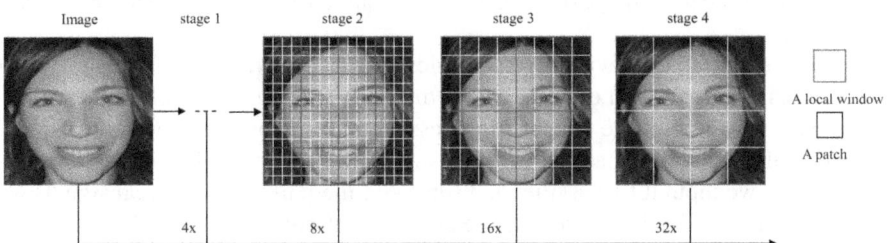

Fig. 2. Hierarchical feature map of Swin Transformer.

In FLD tasks, locating local key discriminatory information is essential. Self-attention or Multi-headed Self-attention (MSA) is used under the assumption that there is a correlation in any portion of the data. Through modeling this correlation, the complete face features can be obtained. Swin Transformer has superior performance in computer vision by using shifted windows instead of conventional Multi-head Self-attention (MSA). Before calculating W-MSA, the second Transformer module uses spatial shuffle, which can prevent the impact of data input order on network training effectively while simultaneously increasing network's randomness and improving its generalization. Shifted Windows Multi-Head Self Attention (SW-MSA) efficiently implements window interaction and global attention with linear computational complexity for image size and a more flexible hierarchical architecture.

Contrastive Learning of Features. One of key challenges when looking at local features is that in cross-domain scenarios, liveness-related style elements could be hidden by domain-specific elements, which could cause mistakes in judgment. We suggest a contrastive learning strategy to suppress domain-specific style elements and highlight liveness-related elements to figure out this problem. We aggregate extracted style and content features. The content features primarily capture physical and global semantic features, such as the size and shape of real or fake faces, which feature space with similar shared semantics. The style features maintain some discriminant information that can be used to improve differentiation between real and fake faces, and also describing certain distinguishing cues.

We hypothesize that, for content feature aggregation, there are only slight differences between attributes based on content information in different domains, but distributional differences between deceptive and real faces are large due to the complexity and variety of deceptive faces as well as various methods used in face database collection. In order to facilitate class boundary optimization for invisible target domains, we employ asymmetric triplet loss [20] to aggregate all real faces to make their distribution in the feature space more compact and to separate deceptive faces from various source domains in order to make their distribution more decentralized. The specific expression is as follows:

$$L_{triplet}(X, Y; G) = \sum_{\forall y_a = y_p, y_a \neq y_n} \left(G(x_a) - G(x_p)_F^2 - G(x_a) - G(x_n)_F^2 + m \right) \quad (2)$$

where $\| \cdot \|_F^2$ represents the square of Frobenius paradigm, m represents the boundary, x_a has the same label as the positive example x_p, but a different label than the negative example x_n.

Because style features with diverse scales, we use a pyramidal [14] strategy for style features aggregation in order to gather multi-layer features as well as hierarchical structures. For example, the scene brightness is mainly concerned with broad-scale features, while a rendered material texture usually focuses on local-scale regions.

For $f_c(x_i)$, we input it to classifier and supervise them using binary real signals with loss function L_{focal}. For $f_s(x_i)$, we use the cosine similarity to measure their difference from $f_c(x_i)$:

$$Sim(a, b) = -a/\|a\|_2 \cdot b/\|b\|_2 \quad (3)$$

where $\| \cdot \|_2$ is l_2-norm, a and b represent two compared features.

As shown in Fig. 3, content features are set as anchors in the style features space. Motivated by [21], a stop-gradient (stop-grad) operation is implemented to fix their position in the feature space. Then, face liveness information extracted from the feature network guides style features away from or close to their corresponding anchors. And this process further aggregates the style information associated with faces. Consequently, the contrastive loss is described as follow:

$$L_{contra} = \sum_{i=1}^{N} Eq(x_i, x_{i*}) \cdot Sim(stopgrad(a), b) \quad (4)$$

where $a = f_c(x_i)$ and $b = f_s(x_i)$. $Eq(x_i, x_{i*})$ measures the consistency of liveness labels between x_i and x_{i*}, which can be formulated as follows:

$$Eq(x_i, x_{i*}) = \begin{cases} +1, & label(x_i) == label(x_{i*}), \\ -1, & otherwise \end{cases} \quad (5)$$

Loss Function. Following the explanation of our network's operation, we gathered the total loss function for stable and reliable training to improve model generalization while addressing positive and negative sample imbalances, which is able to be expressed as follows:

$$L_{overall} = L_{focal} + \lambda_1 \cdot L_{triplet} + \lambda_2 \cdot L_{contra} \quad (6)$$

where λ_1 and λ_2 are hyperparameters used to balance the proportions of different loss functions. We substitute focal loss [22] function for cross-entropy loss function.

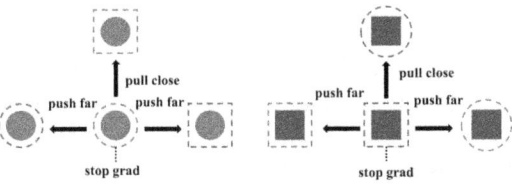

Fig. 3. The illustration of contrastive learning between different features.

4 Experiment

4.1 Datasets and Evaluation Metrics

Within-dataset type protocols, across-dataset intra-type protocols, within-dataset cross-type protocols, and across-dataset cross-type protocols have been developed to assess the efficacy of FLD approaches. In particular, the majority of procedures only include one or two datasets, which can make it more difficult to assess various data distributions. For this reason, the domain generalization performance across different domains is assessed using the OCIM protocol. To assess our method, we used four publicly available worldwide datasets: CASIA-FASD (C) [26], MSU-MFSD (M) [24], Idiap Replay-Attack (I) [27] and OULU-NPU (O) [28]. The quantity of real and fraudulent videos used in our studies is displayed in Table 1. Area Under Curve (AUC) and Half Total Error Rate (HTER) are evaluation metrics used in all of our experiments.

Table 1. Dataset

Dataset	Real videos	Fake videos
CASIA-FASD [26]	150	450
MSU-MFSD [24]	70	210
Replay-Attack [27]	140	700
OULU-NPU [28]	720	2880

4.2 Implementation Details

During the image preprocessing stage, we used all image data directly and employed MTCNN [23] method for face detection on all of the video frames. After that, we cropped facial region and resize it to 256 × 256 as RGB input. We used the same training setup as in [7], that is, randomly sampling one frame as training data from each video because variations between various frames in the videos are not very great. The equal quantity of fake and real data was sampled from all training datasets in every training phase. The proposed models are conducted on Pytorch platform and Ubuntu system, and all the experiments are conducted on a single NVIDIA GTX4090 GPU. The learning rate and weight decay parameters of 1e-4 and 5e-5 were used, respectively, the Adam optimizer was applied after pretraining model on ImageNet1K dataset.

4.3 Domain Generalized Evaluation

Experiment in Leave-One-Out (LOO) Setting. In order to evaluate method performance in Domain Generalization FLD for an overall evaluation, we perform cross-dataset testing using the LOO strategy: three datasets are selected for training and the others remain for testing. We follow this setting principle and show performance comparison between our method and previous competing methods (each dataset is represented using its prefix) in Table 2. The algorithm in this paper is compared with several representative traditional FLD methods in cross-domain FLD performances, including MS-LBP [1], Binary CNN [3], Auxiliary (Depth) [2] and IDA [24]. Performances of recent cross-domain face live detection techniques, including MADDG [6], ANRL [25], and FGHV [13]. Table 2 shows that the algorithm performance proposed in this paper provides more excellent results on four datasets in the cross-dataset scenario, which proves the domain generalization capability of our approach. We provide two figures to better illustrate our results, as shown in the figure of Figs. 4 and 5.

Table 2. The results of cross-dataset testing on OULU-NPU, CASIA-MFSD, Replay-attack, and MSU-MFSD.

Method	O&C&M to I		O&C&I to M		I&C&M to O		O&M&I to C	
	HTER	AUC	HTER	AUC	HTER	AUC	HTER	AUC
MS-LBP [1]	50.30	51.64	29.76	78.50	50.29	49.31	54.28	44.98
Binary CNN [3]	34.47	65.88	29.25	82.87	29.61	77.54	34.88	71.94
IDA [24]	28.35	78.25	66.67	27.86	54.20	44.59	55.17	39.05
Auxiliary [2]	29.14	71.69	22.72	85.88	30.17	77.61	33.52	73.15
MADDG [6]	22.19	84.99	17.69	88.06	27.98	80.02	24.50	84.51
ANRL [25]	16.03	91.04	10.83	96.75	15.67	91.90	17.85	89.26
FGHV [13]	9.17	96.92	12.47	93.47	16.29	90.11	13.59	93.55
Ours	8.16	98.99	7.39	97.66	13.39	93.10	9.46	96.98

Experiment on Limited Source Domains. In this experiment, the algorithms will be evaluated under challenging conditions where the available source domains are extremely limited. Specifically, a smaller training dataset will be used for evaluation purposes, selecting MSU-MFSD and Replay-Attack as the source domains for training. The remaining two domains, CASIA-MFSD and OULU-NPU, will serve as the target domains for testing the algorithms. As shown in Table 3, despite the limited source data, the algorithm proposed in this paper still performs well in more challenging situations. These results strongly verify our network generalization on invisible target domain.

Table 3. Comparison results on limited source domains.

Methods	M&I to C		M&I to O	
	HTER	AUC	HTER	AUC
ANRL [26]	31.06	72.12	30.73	74.10
SSAN-M [5]	30.00	76.20	29.44	76.62
Ours	29.43	79.13	27.35	79.48

4.4 Ablation Study

To demonstrate the superiority of our CLCSN and evaluate the impact of each component, we constructed several incomplete models by varying different variables. All results were measured using the same method, as depicted in Table 4.

Table 4. Evaluations of different components for the method with different architectures.

Method	O&C&M to I		O&C&I to M		I&C&M to O		O&M&I to C	
	HTER	AUC	HTER	AUC	HTER	AUC	HTER	AUC
CLCSN w/o CDC	9.64	94.87	8.24	95.54	14.41	91.94	10.67	94.58
CLCSN w/o Swin Transformer	10.36	93.14	10.37	94.91	15.59	91.39	12.33	93.97
CLCSN w/o L_{contra}	9.49	95.42	9.54	95.24	15.36	91.27	11.67	94.78
Ours (CLCSN)	8.16	98.99	7.39	97.66	13.39	93.10	9.46	96.98

Effectiveness of Different Components. We performed ablation experiments on different backbone branches and components using publicly available datasets to give a thorough and efficient evaluation of our approach. At first, we performed CLCSN w/o CDC experiments. Specifically, the improved CNN network is more conducive to emphasizing local face information through the incorporation of CDC. The CNN is more efficient in capturing fine-grained face features, which is essential for FLD systems deployed in real-world application scenarios. Then, we performed CLCSN w/o Swin Transformer tests to illustrate the significance of the sliding window in the Swin Transformer module and to realize the interaction between panes and the global attention for global feature capture. Quantitative results show that the global feature extraction network using Swin Transformer as backbone is beneficial to improve performance of cross-domain FLD task.

Analysis of Contrastive Learning. The approach in this paper is to perform contrastive learning between global style features and local content features. In previous work, all FLD implemented classical supervised contrastive learning (SCL) on complete representations (CNN-BN-ReLU). To compare them, we conducted w/o L_{contra} experiments. The final experimental results show the effectiveness of the feature space constructed by content features and style features in contrastive learning.

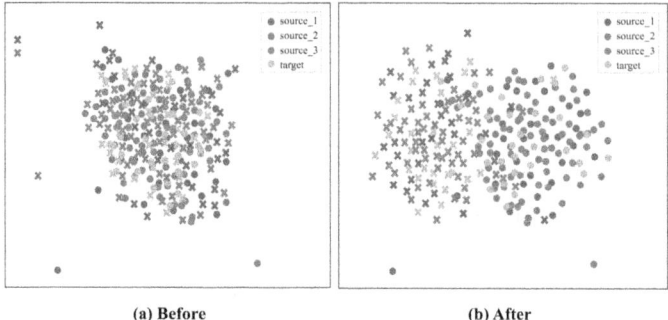

Fig. 4. The various features under protocol O&C&I to M are visualized using t-SNE.

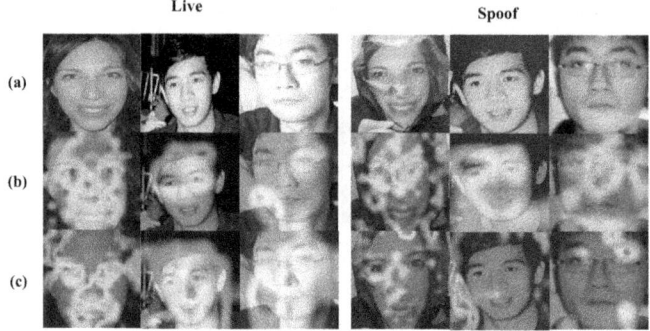

Fig. 5. Feature maps generated at different stages. (a): Original images. (b): Visualizations for content features generation. (c): Visualizations for content and style features generation.

5 Conclusion

In this work, we have proposed a generalizable silent face liveness detection contrastive learning network that combined CNN and Swin Transformer. The enhanced CNN and Swin transformer model were in charge of extracting global semantic features and local fine-grained features, respectively. We used central difference convolution to reduce the impact of ambient light on feature extraction. Considering the attributes of content and style features were distinct, we treated them separately from the prior complete implementation of domain generalization strategy on the common module. For content features, we used asymmetric triplet loss to make them more compact in feature space and promote class boundary optimization in invisible target domain. For style features, to highlight liveliness-related style features, a contrastive learning technique was applied. Experiments conducted using current assessment standards showed our method's superiority.

Acknowledgments. his work was supported by research fundings from National Science Foundation of China (No.82303675, No.61272315 and No.12305404), the National Key R&D Program of China (No.2023YFF0613504), Zhejiang Provincial Major Science and Technology Project (No.2023C01040), Natural Science Foundation of Zhejiang Province (No. LY21F020028, No. LY22F010010 and No. LQ22F020021), Fundamental Research Funds for the Provincial Universities of Zhejiang (No. 2022YW52) and National Platform for basic conditions of science and technology (No.APT2301-7).

Disclosure of Interests. Disclosure of interests. the authors have no competing interests to declare that are relevant to the content of this article.

References

1. Määttä, J., Hadid, A., Pietikäinen, M.: Face spoofing detection from single images using micro-texture analysis. In: 2011 International Joint Conference on Biometrics (IJCB), pp. 1–7. IEEE (2011)
2. Liu, Y., Jourabloo, A., Liu, X.: Learning deep models for face anti-spoofing: Binary or auxiliary supervision. In: Proceedings of the IEEE Conference on Computer Vision and Pattern Recognition, pp. 389–398. IEEE (2018)
3. Yang, J., Lei, Z., Li, S. Z.: Learn convolutional neural network for face anti-spoofing. arxiv preprint arxiv: 1408.5601 (2014)
4. Li, H., Li, W., Cao, H., Wang, S., Huang, F., Kot, A.C.: Unsupervised domain adaptation for face anti-spoofing. IEEE Trans. Inform. Forens. Secur. **13**(7), 1794–1809 (2018)
5. Wang, Z., Wang, Z., Yu, Z., Deng, W., Li, J., Gao, T., Wang, Z.: Domain generalization via shuffled style assembly for face anti-spoofing. In: Proceedings of the IEEE/CVF Conference on Computer Vision and Pattern Recognition, pp. 4123–4133. IEEE (2022)
6. Shao, R., Lan, X., Li, J., Yuen, P.C.: Multi-adversarial discriminative deep domain generalization for face presentation attack detection. In: Proceedings of the IEEE/CVF Conference on Computer Vision and Pattern Recognition, pp. 10023–10031. IEEE (2019)
7. Jia, Y., Zhang, J., Shan, S., Chen, X.: Single-side domain generalization for face anti-spoofing. In: Proceedings of the IEEE/CVF Conference on Computer Vision and Pattern Recognition, pp. 8484–8493. IEEE (2020)
8. Muzammal, N.M.: Intriguing properties of vision transformers. Adv. Neural Info. Process. Syst. **34** (2021)
9. Liao, C. H., Chen, W. C., Liu, H. T., Yeh, Y. R., Hu, M. C., Chen, C. S.: Domain invariant vision transformer learning for face anti-spoofing. In: Proceedings of the IEEE/CVF Winter Conference on Applications of Computer Vision, pp. 6098–6107. IEEE (2023)
10. Komulainen, J., Hadid, A., Pietikäinen, M.: Context based face anti-spoofing. In: 2013 IEEE Sixth International Conference on Biometrics: Theory, Applications and Systems (BTAS), pp. 1–8. IEEE (2013)
11. Yu, Z., Zhao, C., Wang, Z., Qin, Y., Su, Z., Li, X., Zhou, F., Zhao, G.: Searching central difference convolutional networks for face anti-spoofing. In: Proceedings of the IEEE/CVF Conference on Computer Vision and Pattern Recognition, pp. 5295–5305. IEEE (2020)

12. Wang, Y.C., Wang, C.Y., Lai, S.H.: Disentangled representation with dual-stage feature learning for face anti-spoofing. In: Proceedings of the IEEE/CVF Winter Conference on Applications of Computer Vision, pp. 1955–1964. IEEE (2022)
13. Liu, S., Lu, S., Xu, H., Yang, J., Ding, S., Ma, L.: Feature generation and hypothesis verification for reliable face anti-spoofing. Proc. AAAI Conf. Intell. **36**(2), 1782–1791 (2022)
14. Zhou, Q., Zhang, K.Y., Yao, T., Lu, X., Yi, R., Ding, S., Ma, L.: Instance-aware domain generalization for face anti-spoofing. In: Proceedings of the IEEE/CVF Conference on Computer Vision and Pattern Recognition, pp. 20453–20463. IEEE (2023)
15. Dosovitskiy, A., et al.: An image is worth 16 × 16 words: Transformers for image recognition at scale. arxiv preprint arxiv: 2010.11929 (2020)
16. Liu, Z., et al.: Swin transformer: Hierarchical vision transformer using shifted windows. In: Proceedings of the IEEE/CVF International Conference on Computer Vision, pp. 10012–10022. IEEE (2021)
17. Mehta, S., Rastegari, M.: Mobilevit: Light-weight, general-purpose, and mobile-friendly vision transformer. arxiv 2021. arxiv preprint arxiv: 2110.02178. IEEE (2021)
18. Huang, Y.H., Hsieh, J.W., Chang, M.C., Ke, L., Lyu, S., Santra, A.S.: Multi-teacher single-student visual transformer with multi-level attention for face spoofing detection. In: BMVC, p. 125. IEEE (2021)
19. Sandler, M., Howard, A., Zhu, M., Zhmoginov, A., Chen, L.C.: Mobilenetv2: Inverted residuals and linear bottlenecks. In: Proceedings of the IEEE Conference on Computer Vision and Pattern Recognition, pp. 4510–4520. IEEE (2018)
20. Schroff, F., Kalenichenko, D., Philbin, J.: Facenet: A unified embedding for face recognition and clustering. In: Proceedings of the IEEE Conference on Computer Vision and Pattern Recognition, pp. 815–823. IEEE (2015)
21. Chen, X., He, K.: Exploring simple siamese representation learning. In: Proceedings of the IEEE/CVF Conference on Computer Vision and Pattern Recognition, pp. 15750–15758. IEEE (2021)
22. Lin, T. Y., Goyal, P., Girshick, R., He, K., Dollár, P.: Focal loss for dense object detection. In: Proceedings of the IEEE International Conference on Computer Vision, pp. 2980–2988. IEEE (2017)
23. Xiang, J., Zhu, G.: Joint face detection and facial expression recognition with MTCNN. In: 2017 4th International Conference on Information Science and Control Engineering (ICISCE), pp. 424–427. IEEE (2017)
24. Wen, D., Han, H., Jain, A.K.: Face spoof detection with image distortion analysis. IEEE Trans. Inform. Forensic. Secur. **10**(4), 746–761 (2015)
25. Liu, S., et al.: Adaptive normalized representation learning for generalizable face anti-spoofing. In: Proceedings of the 29th ACM International Conference on Multimedia, pp. 1469–1477. IEEE (2021)
26. Zhang, Z., Yan, J., Liu, S., Lei, Z., Yi, D., Li, S.Z.: A face antispoofing database with diverse attacks. In: 2012 5th IAPR International Conference on Biometrics (ICB), pp. 26–31. IEEE (2012)
27. Chingovska, I., Anjos, A., Marcel, S.: On the effectiveness of local binary patterns in face anti-spoofing. In: 2012 BIOSIG-Proceedings of the International Conference of Biometrics Special Interest Group (BIOSIG), pp. 1–7. IEEE (2012)
28. Boulkenafet, Z., Komulainen, J., Li, L., Feng, X., Hadid, A.: Oulu-npu: A mobile face presentation attack database with real-world variations. In: 2017 12th IEEE International Conference on Automatic Face & Gesture Recognition (FG 2017), pp. 612–618. IEEE (2017)

BS2CL: Balanced Self-supervised Contrastive Learning for Thyroid Cytology Whole Slide Image Multi-classification

Wensi Duan[1], Juan Liu[1(✉)] [iD], Lang Wang[1], Yu Jin[1], Peng Jiang[1], Cheng Li[2], Dehua Cao[2], and Baochuan Pang[2]

[1] Institute of Artificial Intelligence, School of Computer Science, Wuhan University, Wuhan, China
liujuan@whu.edu.cn
[2] Landing Artificial Intelligence Center for Pathological Diagnosis, Wuhan, China

Abstract. Thyroid cytology whole slide images (WSIs) hold vital information essential for precise diagnosis. Given the huge size of WSIs, multiple instance learning (MIL) is an effective solution for the WSI classification task when only slide-level labels are accessible. The embedding-based MIL uses a feature extractor pretrained with the self-supervised contrastive learning framework to eliminate the dependence on patch-level labels. However, the distribution of class in thyroid patches is unbalanced, and most existing self-supervised contrastive learning methods take little account of the data imbalance, which makes the features not discriminative enough. To address this problem, we propose a novel balanced self-supervised contrastive learning (BS2CL) framework for pretraining. It first clusters the patches to preserve the class structure of the patches and then assigns the clustering centers to a set of pre-computed uniformly distributed optimal locations. This constraint creates a more uniform distribution of different classes in the feature space which leads to clearer class boundaries between different classes, an unbiased feature space, and more discriminative features. Furthermore, a bag-level data augmentation strategy is introduced to increase bag quantities and improve classification performance. Extensive experiments show that the proposed method outperforms other latest methods on the thyroid cytology WSI dataset.

Keywords: Whole Slide Image · Thyroid Cytology · Self-Supervised Contrastive Learning · Multiple Instance Learning

1 Introduction

Thyroid cancer has seen the fastest growth in incidence of any malignancy worldwide in recent years, and this rising trend continues [1]. Fine-needle aspiration biopsy (FNAB) is the most commonly used preoperative diagnostic technique for thyroid malignancies [2]. Cytopathologists look at the morphology of cells on a liquid-based preparation slide collected by FNAB using a microscope and make a diagnostic classification according to the Thyroid Bethesda System (TBS) [3]. TBS is the universally recognized system for reporting thyroid FNAB, and it is structured into six distinctive categories, from TBS1 to TBS6. TBS 1 is assigned to inadequately prepared slides and is beyond the scope of this work. TBS 2 suggests benign conditions. The next categories, TBS 3 to 5, indicate abnormalities, which escalate from mild to severe as the category number increases. Lastly, TBS 6 is indicative of malignancy. However, the examination process for professional cytopathologists is both time-consuming and strenuous. Additionally, the complex nature of biological specimens results in a certain level of subjectivity and non-repeatability. To improve diagnostic efficiency and accuracy, computer-aided diagnosis is critically important. The development of digital pathology and the widespread adoption of whole slide imaging (WSI) make it possible to employ computerized methods for diagnostic assistance. This can provide more objective and repeatable results and substantially ease the cytopathologists' workload.

Due to the high pixel count of WSIs, reaching up to a trillion, it's hard to analyze a WSI directly limited by computational resources. A common process is to divide a WSI into smaller images called patches. Many studies are based on labeled patches [4–7], and tend to focus on a specific disease like papillary thyroid carcinoma [6, 7]. As for thyroid WSI classification, most approaches follow the multiple instance learning (MIL) setting to the natural structure of WSIs. WSIs serve as labeled bags, while the extracted patches function as the unlabeled instances within these bags. MIL could be modeled in two ways: 1) instance-based approach [8, 9]. Instances are first assigned pseudo-labels or are labeled to train an instance-level classifier in a supervised manner and the instance-level classification aggregates the bag-level classification results. 2) embedding-based approach [10, 11]. Instances are first mapped to feature embeddings through a feature extractor. The instance-level embeddings are then aggregated into a bag-level feature embedding for classification through MIL pooling operators which are typically the mean pooling or max pooling operator, while the latter is mostly used [12–15].

Instance-level labeling is a prerequisite for instance-based MIL, however, the large size of WSI makes the process of detailed annotation both costly and time-consuming. Additionally, the accuracy of diagnosis is heavily dependent on the clinical expertise and medical insight of cytopathologists. For embedding-based MIL, training a feature extractor in an unsupervised way removes the dependency on instance-level labels. Self-supervised contrastive learning has grown rapidly in recent years, even outperforming supervised learning methods. However, most embedding-based MIL methods directly use existing self-supervised contrastive learning frameworks like SimCLR [16], MoCo [17] and DINO [18]. Classical self-supervised contrastive learning explicitly pulls the representations of different transformations or views of the same instance closer and pushes the representations of different instances apart. This may lead to distances of instances belonging to the same class being pulled apart. What's more, these frameworks are pretrained on the class-balanced ImageNet dataset [19] and fail to learn discriminative features when the dataset is imbalanced [20]. Classes with high numbers can dominate the feature space, leading to unclear class boundaries. Figure 1 shows the class distribution of 41077 randomly selected instances annotated by cytopathologists. In a thyroid WSI, the class distribution of follicular cells or clusters is unbalanced but the critical classes for classification tend to be few.

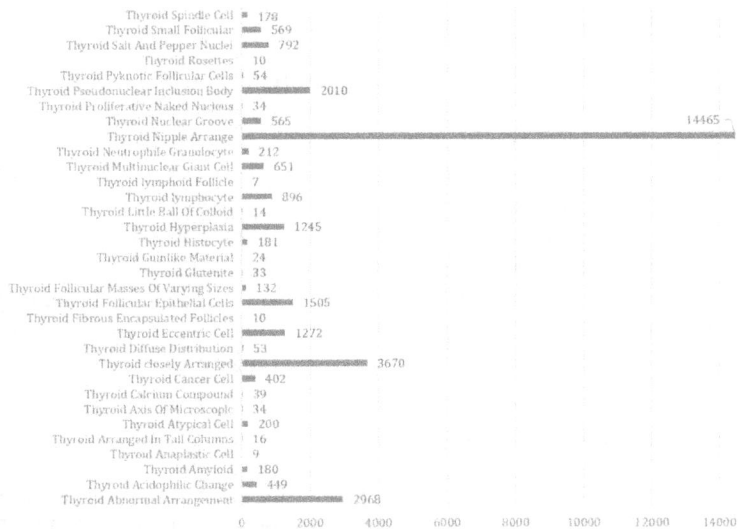

Fig. 1. The class distribution of follicular cells or clusters from 41077 randomly selected instances.

In this paper, we propose a novel **b**alanced **s**elf-**s**upervised **c**ontrastive **l**earning (**BS2CL**) framework based on clustering. When pretraining the feature extractor, we cluster all the instance features and treat each cluster as a class to form the contrastive loss that preserves the semantic structure among instances. Meanwhile, we match the cluster centers to the optimal locations that are generated in advance. These locations are uniformly distributed in the feature space to avoid the feature space being biased and dominated by classes with high numbers. Moreover, deep learning networks are inherently data-intensive, exhibiting enhanced performance metrics when trained on extensive and heterogeneous annotated data which are expensive to collect especially for thyroid cytology WSIs. Therefore, we propose a bag-level data augmentation strategy that amplifies the volume of bags and further improves the utilization of instance features and classification performance. The contributions of this study are as follows:

1) We propose a novel balanced self-supervised contrastive learning framework that captures the implicit semantic structure of instances and avoids the biased feature space.
2) We introduce a bag-level data augmentation strategy to expand the count of thyroid WSIs and improve classification performance further.
3) We further show that our method achieves state-of-the-art thyroid cytology WSI classification performance on the in-house dataset.

2 Related Work

2.1 Self-Supervised Contrastive Learning in MIL

Self-supervised contrastive learning methods have shown promising results in medical imaging [21, 22] and most MIL methods utilize available networks like SimCLR [16], MoCo [17] and DINO [18] For instance, Li et al. [21] applied SimCLR [16] as a feature extractor for WSI classification following the MIL setting. Yet existing self-supervised contrastive learning methods are pretrained on class-balanced datasets such as ImageNet [19] while the instances of the thyroid WSI dataset are unbalanced which may lead to significant drops in performance. To address this problem, we propose a novel BS2CL framework that balances the feature space and makes the class boundaries clearer.

2.2 Thyroid Cytology WSI Classification

Most methods for thyroid WSI classification follow the MIL setting and can be classified into instance-based methods [8, 9] and embedding-based methods [10, 11]. Instance-based methods focus on training an instance-level classifier and studying the instance-level informativeness. For example, Dov et al. propose a maximum likelihood estimation to analyze the instances' contribution beyond the MIL setting [9]. These methods are limited by their dependence on instance-level labels. Using a pretrained feature extractor, embedding-based methods only require WSI labels. However, most works ignore the importance of data augmentation while it's expensive to collect and annotate thyroid WSIs (bags). In this paper, we propose a bag-level data augmentation strategy that increases the quantity of bags.

3 Method

This section introduces our method for thyroid cytology WSI classification including the BS2CL framework and the bag-level data augmentation strategy.

3.1 Preliminary: Problem Description

Given a dataset composed of N thyroid WSIs $W = \{W_1, W_2 \cdots W_N\}$, where each W_i is associated with a corresponding label $Y_i \in \{2, 3, 4, 5, 6\}$ which indicates the TBS category annotated by a cytopathologist. W_i is patched into a bag of small patches (instances) $W_i = \{x_{i,j}, j \in \{1, 2, \ldots n_i\}\}$ without overlapping where n_i is the number of patches in the i-th WSI. Our goal is to predict the label $\widehat{Y}_i$ of W_i, given by:

$$\widehat{Y}_i = c(g(f(x_{i,1}), f(x_{i,2}), \ldots, f(x_{i,j}), \ldots, f(x_{i,n_i}))) \tag{1}$$

where $f(\cdot)$ is the pretrained feature extractor that corresponds to the proposed BS2CL framework. And its output $f(x_{i,j}) \in R^d$ refers to a latent feature vector of d-dimensions. $g(\cdot)$ is an aggregator that integrates instance features. $c(\cdot)$ is a linear classifier that outputs a bag prediction.

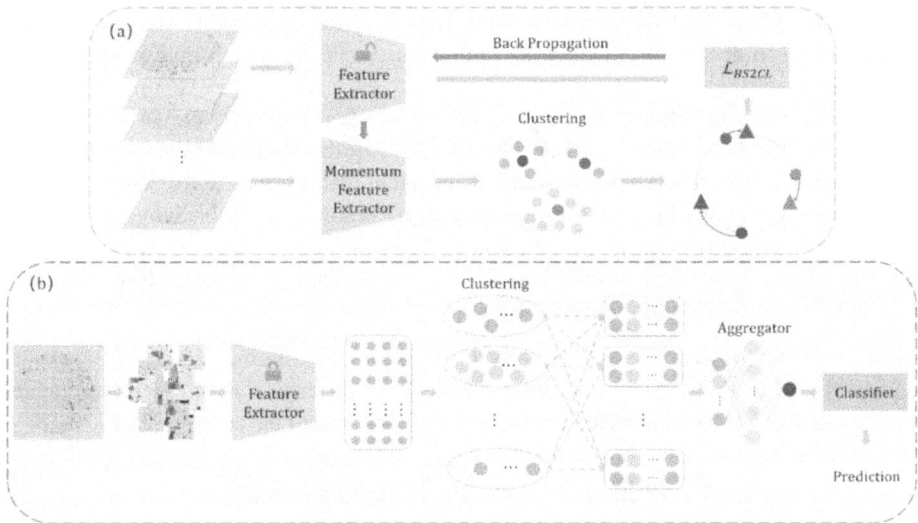

Fig. 2. (a) The overview of the proposed Balanced Self-Supervised Contrastive Learning framework. (b) The pipeline of the thyroid cytology WSI classification based on multiple instance learning.

3.2 Balanced Self-Supervised Contrastive Learning

Within a pertaining set $X = \{x_1, x_2, \ldots, x_n\}$ consisting of n patches extracted from various WSIs, the aim of self-supervised learning is to develop a feature extractor $f_\theta(\cdot)$ that transforms X into a corresponding set of feature vectors $V = \{v_1, v_2, \ldots, v_n\}$, where each $v_i = f_\theta(x_i)$ is generated without utilizing any patch labels. Traditional self-supervised contrastive learning fulfills this goal by minimizing a contrastive loss function such as InfoNCE [23], which is articulated as follows:

$$\mathcal{L}_{InfoNCE} = \sum_{i=1}^{n} -\log \frac{\exp(v_i \cdot v_i'/\tau)}{\exp(v_i \cdot v_i'/\tau) + \sum_{j=1}^{r} \exp(v_i \cdot v_j'/\tau)} \quad (2)$$

where v_i' is extracted from a random augmentation of x_i, and v_j' is extracted from r other patches, and τ is a temperature hyper-parameter [24].

Minimizing the loss function drives the feature of x_i to align more closely with the feature of its randomly augmented counterpart, while simultaneously repelling the feature of x_i from the features of other patches within the training set. But it may lead to pushing apart the features of patches from the same class. What's more, the class distribution of thyroid patches is unbalanced which causes the biased feature space and unclear class boundaries. Uniformity is a fundamental characteristic of contrastive learning. It implies that features from different classes are evenly spread across a hypersphere $\mathcal{S}^{d-1} = \{u \in R^d : ||u|| = 1\}$. However, an imbalanced dataset can undermine uniformity. When certain classes have a significantly larger number compared to others, the majority classes occupy a larger portion of the hypersphere in the feature space, while the minority classes are sparsely distributed. This imbalanced distribution disrupts the clear boundaries between classes in the feature space, making it more challenging for the model to accurately distinguish the minority classes which may be critical for classification.

To solve these problems, we proposed the **BS2CL** framework shown in **Fig. 2(a)**. BS2CL is a framework that improves the uniformity of the feature space. It first extracts features from all patches. Then it clusters all the patch features into K clusters to preserve the class structure avoiding the problem of pulling features from the same class closer together. We define $C = \{c_i\}_{i=1}^{K}$ as the cluster centers and $P = \{p_i^*\}_{i=1}^{K}$ as the points of the optimal positions that are uniformly distributed on the hypersphere. To obtain clear class boundaries, we should assign C to P.

Position Generation and Assignment Computing the optimal positions does not require access to the dataset, and only requires the dimension d of the feature space and the number of classes. We calculate $\{p_i^*\}_{i=1}^{K}$ by gradient descent on

$$\mathcal{L}_u(\{p_i\}_{i=1}^{K}) = \frac{1}{K}\sum_{i=1}^{K} \log \sum_{j=1}^{K} exp(p_i \cdot p_j/\tau) \quad (3)$$

where p_i is restricted to be on the hypersphere and $\{p_i^*\}_{i=1}^{K}$ corresponds to the minimum loss.

Then we should assign each cluster to a corresponding position. Due to the different distances between two optimal positions, random assignment may ruin the semantics of the feature space. The ideal situation is that clusters with semantic proximity close to each other should be assigned to positions that are equally proximate. However, the ground truth of the training set is unknown and it's hard to quantify the semantic proximity. To match a cluster to the corresponding optimal position while keeping semantic similarity between clusters is difficult. To solve this, we compute the assignment during pretraining instead of using a settled assignment. In each epoch, we compute the assignment $\{\sigma_i^*\}_{i=1}^{K}$ with the Hungarian Algorithm [25], defined as:

$$\{\sigma_i^*\}_i = \arg\min_{\{\sigma_i\}_i} \frac{1}{K} \sum_{i=1}^{K} ||p_{\sigma_i} - c_i||. \quad (4)$$

The computed assignment minimizes the distance between cluster centers and the optimal positions.

Balanced Self-Supervised Contrastive Loss. To make the class boundaries clearer and the feature space less biased, we compute the uniformly distributed positions $\{p_i^*\}_{i=1}^{K}$ and the assignment $\{\sigma_i^*\}_{i=1}^{K}$ that matches the clusters to the corresponding positions. Additionally, in order to preserve the property of local smoothness and to facilitate the bootstrap of clustering, we add InfoNCE loss to our balanced self-supervised contrastive Loss $\mathcal{L}_{BS2CL}$, which is defined as:

$$\mathcal{L}_{BS2CL} = \sum_{i=1}^{n} -\left(\log \frac{exp(v_i \cdot v_i'/\tau)}{exp(v_i \cdot v_i'/\tau) + \sum_{j=1}^{r} exp(v_i \cdot v_j'/\tau)} \right.$$
$$\left. + \log \frac{exp(v_i \cdot p_{\sigma_{k_i}}/\tau)}{exp(v_i \cdot p_{\sigma_{k_i}}/\tau) + \sum_{j=1}^{r} exp(v_i \cdot p_{\sigma_{k_j}}/\tau)} \right) \quad (5)$$

where $p_{\sigma_{k_i}}$ is the position corresponding to the centroid c_{k_i} of the cluster to which v_i belongs.

After pertaining the feature extractor $f(\cdot)$ with the BS2CL framework, we freeze its parameters in the stage of classification for thyroid WSIs.

3.3 Bag-Level Data Augmentation Strategy

Considering the cost of collecting and annotating thyroid WSIs, appropriate data augmentation is necessary. We propose a bag-level data augmentation strategy to increase the number of bags.

Figure 2(b) shows the pipeline of thyroid WSI classification. Given a WSI W_i (bag), we split it into small patches $\{x_{i,j}\}_{j=1}^{n_i}$ (instances) which are sent into the pretrained feature extractor. In traditional MIL, the output $\{v_{i,j}\}_{j=1}^{n_i}$ are then aggregated into a bag feature through the aggregator. In this paper, before aggregation, we cluster all instance features $\{v_{i,j}\}_{j=1}^{n_i}$ from W_i and sample random instances from each cluster. After repeating the sampling process M times, we get M pseudo bags $X_i = \{X_i^m | m = 1, 2, \ldots, M\}$ with $n_{i'}$ instances from a bag X_i and each pseudo X_i^m bag is assigned the label of X_i, i.e., $Y_i^m = Y_i$. As instances in the same cluster share similar semantic properties, the $n_{i'}$ instances in a pseudo bag approximate the representation of a bag with n_i instances. Then, we feed these pseudo bags into the aggregator to get the bag features. A bag-level classifier is trained with bag features in a supervised way for thyroid cytology WSI classification.

4 Experiments

Our experiment is conducted on the in-house dataset and demonstrates the superior performance of the proposed method.

4.1 Thyroid Cytology Dataset

We conducted a retrospective analysis and collected 461 thyroid FNAB WSIs from multiple healthcare institutions. Table 1 shows the distribution of the 461 WSIs, wherein each WSI corresponds to a single participant, with liquid-based cytologic preparation. This dataset was labeled by professional cytopathologists and only the TBS category is used for training. 80% of the dataset is used for training and validation and 20% for testing. We divide a WSI into patches with a size of 1024 × 1024 without overlapping.

This study conforms to the ethical standards of the institutional research committee and the tenets of the Helsinki Declaration. As the nature of this study is anonymized and retrospective, the requirement for informed consent has been exempted.

4.2 Experiment Details and Evaluation Metrics

Feature Extractor Pretraining. When pretraining the feature extractor, we build a pretraining dataset consisting of 500629 patches from 56 thyroid WSIs. The self-supervised contrastive methods in this study are all pretrained on this dataset for 200 epochs with four

Table 1. The thyroid cytology WSI dataset description.

	TBS Category	WSI count
1	Nondiagnostic or unsatisfactory	-
2	Benign	33
3	Atypia of undetermined significance or follicular lesion of undetermined significance	18
4	Follicular neoplasm or suspicious for a follicular	6
5	Suspicious for malignancy	67
6	Malignant	337

NVIDIA GeForce GTX 3090Ti GPUs. To ensure an equitable evaluation, our pretraining procedure for the feature extractor mirrors the setting of MoCo [17]. A ResNet-50 [26] is adopted as the feature extractor and its last fully connected layer outputs a 128-dimensional feature that undergoes ℓ_2-normalization. The optimizer is conducted using SGD with a weight decay set at 0.0001, momentum of 0.9, and a batch size of 128. In the initial 20 epochs, we use InfoNCE loss only to warm up the network for better clustering. The learning rate initiates at 0.03 and is scaled down by a factor of 0.1 at epoch 120 and epoch 160. We set the temperature hyper-parameter $\tau = 0.2$ and set $r = 16384$. For each epoch, we utilize the FAISS [27] library for efficient K-means clustering. We set $K = 1000$ and design an ablation experiment to explore the effects of the value of K.

WSI Classification. In this stage, we freeze the parameters of the pretrained feature extractor. We cluster a bag into 100 clusters and randomly sample 5 instances from each cluster to form a pseudo bag. We train the aggregator for 100 epochs and use the Adam [28] optimizer with a cosine decay learning rate scheduler.

Evaluation Metrics. We report the balanced accuracy (ACC) and macro area under the curve (AUC) scores for the task of WSI classification.

Baselines. We utilize 2 classical self-supervised learning frameworks (DINO [18], MoCoV3 [29]) and 6 commonly used aggregators (max poling, mean pooling, ABMIL [15], DSMIL [21], CLAM-SB, CLAM-MB [22]) for experiments. A feature extractor and an aggregator form a combination to perform comparative experiments.

Table 2. Classification results on thyroid cytology dataset

Framework	Max Pooling		Mean Pooling		DSMIL [21]		ABMIL [15]		CLAM-SB [22]		CLAM-MB [22]	
	ACC	AUC	ACC	AUC	ACC	AUC	ACC	AUC	ACC	AUC	ACC	AUC
MoCoV3 [29]	0.258	0.600	0.200	0.500	0.206	0.575	0.200	0.500	0.200	0.500	0.200	0.500
DINO [18]	**0.404**	0.700	0.320	0.675	0.431	0.700	0.341	0.600	0.350	0.600	0.361	0.675
ours	0.356	**0.750**	**0.499**	**0.800**	**0.521**	**0.975**	**0.494**	**0.725**	**0.535**	**0.800**	**0.487**	**0.800**

4.3 Classification Results

The classification results are summarized in Table 2. By examining the quantitative results outlined in Table 2, it is readily apparent that our proposed approach outperformed other existing methods on the task of WSI classification. Surprisingly, we find that certain frameworks utilizing a feature extractor pretrained with MoCoV3 demonstrate performance comparable to random classification. This finding strongly suggests the impact of class imbalance within the instance level on self-supervised learning models. When combined with different aggregators, our proposed approach consistently yields improved performance which validates the robustness of our method as well as its ability to learn discriminative representations suited for the classification task.

Figure 3 (a) and (c) show two example confusion matrices of DINO and our BS2CL combined with the same aggregator CLAM-SB, respectively. For DINO, the off-diagonal values indicate a higher level of misclassification between classes, which suggests that it is not extracting distinguishing features. In contrast, the matrix for BS2CL shows higher diagonal and lower off-diagonal values, demonstrating it can better distinguish different classes attributed to more discriminative features learned through the proposed balanced self-supervised contrastive learning framework.

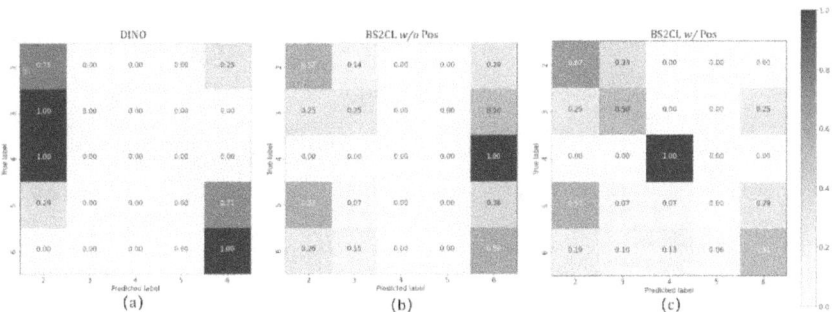

Fig. 3. The example confusion matrices from three compositions: (a) DINO [18] + CLAM-SB [22], (b) BS2CL without positions + CLAM-SB [22], (c) BS2CL(ours) + CLAM-SB [22].

4.4 Ablation Study

We conducted ablation experiments to analyze the impact of the optimal positions in our proposed BS2CL framework. We assign the cluster centers to the optimal positions in our study. This helps alleviate the bias towards majority classes in the learned feature space and yields clearer class boundaries.

As shown in Table 3, classification performance with the optimal positions is better than without applying the positions. This optimization enhances the separability and discrimination of the extracted features. We visualize the features extracted from the pretrained feature extractors in Fig. 4. It can be observed that the boundaries of features from BS2CL with optimal positions are clearer, which further confirms the effectiveness of our approach.

Table 3. Accuracy of BS2CL with/without positions with different values of K

Framework		$K = 500$	$K = 1000$	$K = 5000$
w/o Position Assignment	Max Pooling	0.333	0.238	0.298
	Mean Pooling	0.321	0.340	0.308
	DSMIL [21]	0.374	0.358	0.471
	ABMIL [15]	0.27	0.319	0.39
	CLAM-SB [22]	0.282	0.353	0.363
	CLAM-MB [22]	0.381	0.358	0.466
w Position Assignment	Max Pooling	0.230	**0.356**	0.292
	Mean Pooling	0.277	**0.499**	0.408
	DSMIL [21]	0.444	**0.521**	0.425
	ABMIL [15]	0.452	**0.494**	0.375
	CLAM-SB [22]	0.477	**0.535**	0.411
	CLAM-MB [22]	**0.523**	0.487	0.397

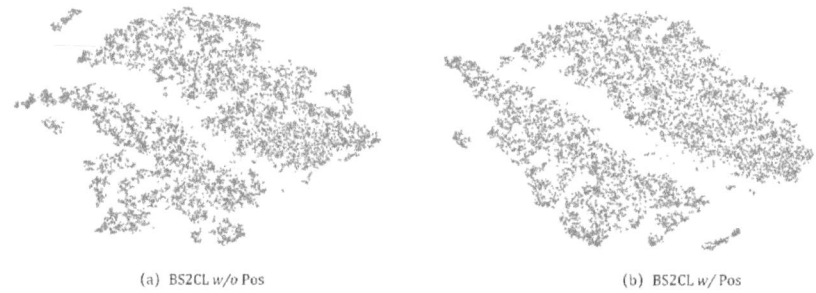

(a) BS2CL w/o Pos   (b) BS2CL w/ Pos

Fig. 4. The t-SNE [30] visualization of instance features from a thyroid WSI: (a) features extracted by BS2CL without positions and (b) features extracted by BS2CL with positions.

We also investigate the impact of the number of clusters K on the classification results. Excessive clustering can have some benefits, but it can also lead to loss of the internal structure of the class when exceeding a certain limit. Therefore, different K values should be adopted for different datasets. For the thyroid dataset used in this study, $K = 1000$ is found to perform best. The confusion matrices shown in Fig. 3 are a further demonstration of our previous experiments.

5 Conclusion

In this study, we propose a balanced self-supervised contrastive learning (BS2CL) framework and a bag-level data augmentation strategy for thyroid cytology WSI multi-classification. The BS2CL framework captures the intrinsic semantic relationships between patches while avoiding biased feature space. The bag-level augmentation strategy is introduced to expand the size of the training dataset effectively. Experimental results on an in-house thyroid cytology WSI dataset demonstrate that the proposed method achieves state-of-the-art classification performance and can be combined with different aggregators. The current work focuses on evaluating the proposed approach at a single-resolution level, future work will explore experiments involving multi-resolution feature learning and classification.

References

1. Cabanillas, M.E., McFadden, D.G., Durante, C.: Thyroid cancer. The Lancet **388**(10061), 2783–2795 (2016)
2. Haugen, B.R., Alexander, E.K., Bible, K.C., et al.: 2015 American Thyroid Association management guidelines for adult patients with thyroid nodules and differentiated thyroid cancer: the American Thyroid Association guidelines task force on thyroid nodules and differentiated thyroid cancer. Thyroid **26**(1), 1–133 (2016)
3. Cibas, E.S., Ali, S.Z.: The 2017 Bethesda system for reporting thyroid cytopathology. Thyroid **27**(11), 1341–1346 (2017)
4. Cochand-Priollet, B., Koutroumbas, K., Megalopoulou, T.M., et al.: Discriminating benign from malignant thyroid lesions using artificial intelligence and statistical selection of morphometric features. Oncol. Rep. **15**(4), 1023–1026 (2006)
5. Gopinath, B., Shanthi, N.: Development of an automated medical diagnosis system for classifying thyroid tumor cells using multiple classifier fusion. Technol. Cancer Res. Treat. **14**(5), 653–662 (2015)
6. Chain, K., Legesse, T., Heath, J.E., et al.: Digital image-assisted quantitative nuclear analysis improves diagnostic accuracy of thyroid fine-needle aspiration cytology. Cancer Cytopathol. **127**(8), 501–513 (2019)
7. Guan, Q., Wang, Y., Ping, B., et al.: Deep convolutional neural network VGG-16 model for differential diagnosing of papillary thyroid carcinomas in cytological images: a pilot study. J. Cancer **10**(20), 4876 (2019)
8. Hirokawa, M., Niioka, H., Suzuki, A., et al.: Application of deep learning as an ancillary diagnostic tool for thyroid FNA cytology. Cancer Cytopathol. **131**(4), 217–225 (2023)
9. Dov, D., Kovalsky, S.Z., Assaad, S., et al.: Weakly supervised instance learning for thyroid malignancy prediction from whole slide cytopathology images. Med. Image Anal. **67**, 101814 (2021)
10. Qiu, S., Guo, Y., Zhu, C., et al.: Attention based multi-instance thyroid cytopathological diagnosis with multi-scale feature fusion. In: 2020 25th International Conference on Pattern Recognition (ICPR), pp. 3536–3541 (2021)
11. Yu, B., Yin, P., Chen, H., et al.: Pyramid multi-loss vision transformer for thyroid cancer classification using cytological smear. Knowl.-Based Syst. **275**, 110721 (2023)
12. Feng, J., Zhou, Z.H.: Deep MIML network. In: Proceedings of the AAAI conference on artificial intelligence, pp. 1884–1890 (2017)
13. Pinheiro, P.O., Collobert, R.: From image-level to pixel-level labeling with convolutional networks. In: Proceedings of the IEEE Conference on Computer Vision and Pattern Recognition, pp. 1713–1721 (2015)
14. Zhu, W., Lou, Q., Vang, Y.S., et al.: Deep multi-instance networks with sparse label assignment for whole mammogram classification. In: Descoteaux, M., Maier-Hein, L., Franz, A., Jannin, P., Collins, D.L., Duchesne, S. (eds.) MICCAI 2017. LNCS, vol. 10435, pp. 603–611. Springer, Cham (2017). https://doi.org/10.1007/978-3-319-66179-7_69

15. Ilse, M., Tomczak, J., Welling, M.: Attention-based deep multiple instance learning. In: International Conference on Machine Learning, pp. 2127–2136 (2018)
16. Chen, T., Kornblith, S., Norouzi, M., et al.: A simple framework for contrastive learning of visual representations. In: International Conference on Machine Learning, pp. 1597–1607 (2020)
17. He, K., Fan, H., Wu, Y., et al.: Momentum contrast for unsupervised visual representation learning. In: Proceedings of the IEEE/CVF Conference on Computer Vision and Pattern Recognition, pp. 9729–9738 (2020)
18. Caron, M., Touvron, H., Misra, I., et al.: Emerging properties in self-supervised vision transformers. In: Proceedings of the IEEE/CVF Conference on Computer Vision and Pattern Recognition, pp. 9650–9660 (2021)
19. Deng, J., Dong, W., Socher, R., et al.: Imagenet: a large-scale hierarchical image database. In: 2009 IEEE Conference on Computer Vision and Pattern Recognition, pp. 248–255 (2009)
20. Assran, M., Balestriero, R., Duval, Q., et al.: The hidden uniform cluster prior in self-supervised learning. arXiv preprint arXiv:2210.07277 (2022)
21. Li, B., Li, Y., Eliceiri, K.W.: Dual-stream multiple instance learning network for whole slide image classification with self-supervised contrastive learning. In: Proceedings of the IEEE/CVF Conference on Computer Vision and Pattern Recognition, pp. 14318–14328 (2021)
22. Lu, M.Y., Williamson, D.F., Chen, T.Y., et al.: Data-efficient and weakly supervised computational pathology on whole-slide images. Nat. Biomed. Eng. **5**(6), 555–570 (2021)
23. Oord, A.v.d., Li, Y., Vinyals, O.: Representation learning with contrastive predictive coding. arXiv preprint arXiv:1807.03748 (2018)
24. Wu, Z., Xiong, Y., Yu, S.X., et al.: Unsupervised feature learning via non-parametric instance discrimination. In: Proceedings of the IEEE Conference on Computer Vision and Pattern Recognition, pp. 3733–3742 (2018)
25. Kuhn, H.W.: The Hungarian method for the assignment problem. Naval Res. Logistics Q **2**(1–2), 83–97 (1955)
26. He, K., Zhang, X., Ren, S., et al.: Deep residual learning for image recognition. arXiv preprint arXiv:1512.03385 (2015)
27. Johnson, J., Douze, M., Jégou, H.: Billion-scale similarity search with GPUs. IEEE Trans. Big Data **7**(3), 535–547 (2019)
28. Kingma, D.P., Ba, J.: Adam: a method for stochastic optimization. arXiv preprint arXiv:1412.6980 (2014)
29. Chen, X., Xie, S., He, K.: An empirical study of training self-supervised vision transformers. arXiv preprint arXiv:2104.02057 (2021)
30. Van der Maaten, L., Hinton, G.: Visualizing data using t-SNE. J. Mach. Learn. Res. **9**(11), 2579–2605 (2008)

Unsupervised Domain Adaptation Method for Medical Image Segmentation Using Fourier Feature Decoupling and Multi-scale Feature Fusion

Wei Hu[1], Qiaozhi Xu[1(✉)], Zhe Lian[1], Yanjun Yin[1], Min Zhi[1], Na Yang[1], Wentao Duan[1], and Lei Yu[2]

[1] School of Computer Science and Technology, Inner Mongolia Normal University, Hohhot 010022, China
ciecxqz@imnu.edu.cn

[2] People's Hospital of Inner Mongolia Autonomous Region, Hohhot 010022, China

Abstract. Unsupervised Domain Adaptation (UDA) is an effective technique for utilizing labeled data from a source domain alongside unlabeled data from a target domain, aiming to mitigate the impact of domain shift on model performance. Feature decoupling-based UDA methods have garnered significant attention due to their ability to address specific challenges, offering superior performance. However, existing methods that employ cycle-consistency and adversarial losses need improvements to better maintain content consistency and preserve the style information of medical images. To address these issues, we propose UDA-F4, an improved UDA method based on the feature decoupling of Fourier transform and multi-scale feature fusion. Experiments on the MICCAI 2017 MM-WHS cardiac dataset demonstrate that our method not only generates higher quality synthetic images and achieves more precise medical segmentation results. Additionally, our method significantly improves both the Dice and ASD metrics compared to traditional methods.

Keywords: Unsupervised Domain Adaptation · Cross-Medical Image Segmentation · Feature Decoupling · Fourier Transform · Multi-Scale Feature Fusion

1 Introduction

In recent years, medical image segmentation models based on deep learning have rapidly evolved [1, 2]. These models typically assume that the training and testing data are independent and identically distributed (i.i.d.) [3]. However, the problem of domain shift challenges this assumption and may lead to a significant decline in model performance upon actual deployment. Consequently, addressing domain shift is crucial for the practical application of these models.

Domain Adaptation (DA) techniques can adapt models to an unseen target domain using knowledge learned from the source domain, offering effective solutions to the domain shift problem. Among these, Unsupervised Domain Adaptation (UDA) technology, which does not require labeled target data, has proven to be an effective approach for addressing cross-domain medical image segmentation tasks where target domain labels are scarce. In recent years, UDA methods based on feature decoupling [4–6] have shown exceptional performance which employed a similar or identical feature decoupling framework to enhance the domain adaptability of models, and we call them Traditional Feature Decoupling Method (TFDM) in this paper. However, these methods had some limitations: firstly, the cycle-consistency loss used by them was less effective in maintaining the content consistency between original and reconstructed images; secondly, the decoupling process, which solely utilizes adversarial loss, might fail to preserve the style information of medical images fully; lastly, the shared content encoder in the feature extraction process may lead to the loss of some crucial semantic information. These limitations led to the inability of traditional methods to effectively preserve the content and style features of original images, which resulted in the poor quality of synthetic images and impacted adaptability in the target domain.

To address these issues, we propose a novel UDA method for medical image segmentation, dubbed UDA-F4. The primary contributions of our work are threefold:

(1) We replace the traditional cycle-consistency loss, which maintains the fidelity between the original and reconstructed images in feature decoupling methods, with a Fourier-based content consistency loss. This approach more effectively preserves content consistency.
(2) We have designed a Fourier-based style transfer loss and incorporated it into the traditional feature decoupling framework. This innovation effectively addresses the challenge of aligning multi-style features in medical images, achieving style consistency.
(3) By introducing a multi-scale feature fusion strategy within a shared content encoder, we merge features across different scales to generate synthesized images that retain more semantic information. This promotes domain adaptation of the model.

2 Related Work

Domain Adaptation (DA) technology can transfer knowledge learned in the source domain to the target domain and enhance adaptation in the target domain by minimizing distribution differences between the source and target domains. Depending on whether the target domain contains labels or not, domain adaptation methods are classified into Supervised Domain Adaptation (SDA), Semi-supervised Domain Adaptation (SSDA), and Unsupervised Domain Adaptation (UDA) [7].

UDA methods, which do not require labels in the target domain, have shown excellence in addressing the scarcity of labels in cross-domain medical image segmentation tasks. Image alignment and feature alignment are the mainstream strategies in this area currently [8–11]. These methods primarily employ Cycle-Consistent Generative Adversarial Networks (CycleGAN) [12] for image alignment strategy. However, CycleGAN can cause content distortion during the image translation process, limiting model adaptability. The feature alignment strategy mainly utilizes adversarial learning, which presents its own challenges, such as training instability, mode collapse, and difficulties in model evaluation [13].

Feature decoupling is an enhanced feature alignment method that can effectively alleviate the aforementioned issues by decomposing input data into multiple meaningful components. Medical images are complex mixtures of anatomical structures and modality factors [14]. Feature decoupling methods separate the medical images of the source and target domains into anatomical structures (content features, which are domain-invariant) and modality factors (style features, which are domain-specific). Then, different features are combined and synthesized into cross-domain medical images that have the content features of the source domain and the style features of the target domain. These synthetic images share labels with their corresponding source domain images, thus improving the adaptability of models in the target domain [15, 16].

3 Method Overview

UDA methods involve two domains with different distributions: the source domain D^s and the target domain D^t. The source domain $D^s = \{(x_i, y_i)\}_{i=1}^{n}$ contains n data samples and their corresponding labels, whereas the target domain $D^t = \{(x_j)\}_{j=1}^{m}$ comprises m data samples and no labels.

The UDA-F4 framework is divided into two stages:

(1) Data alignment: A feature decoupling approach based on the Fourier Transform is designed and integrated with a multi-scale feature fusion strategy. This approach can effectively capture the semantic and style information of the original images and generate high-quality synthetic images.
(2) Network Training: The segmentation model is trained using the high-quality synthetic images mentioned above and learns the knowledge of the target domain to enhance its generalization ability in the target domain.

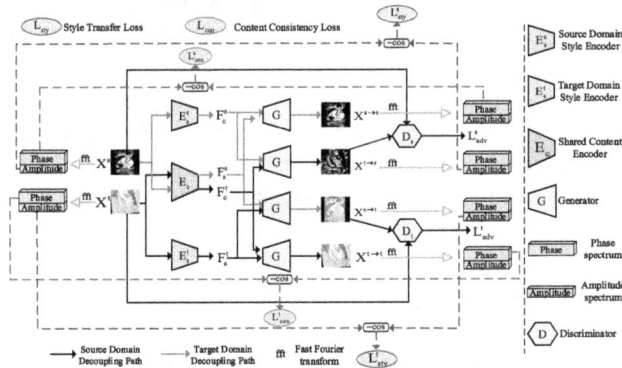

Fig. 1. Structure of the Feature Decoupling based on Fourier Transform.

3.1 Fourier Transform-Based Feature Decoupling Method

In this stage, medical images are decoupled into domain-invariant content features and domain-specific style features using the Feature Decoupling Method based on the Fourier

Transform (FDFF), as shown in Fig. 1. The blue solid line represents the decoupling path for images from the source domain, while the red solid line indicates the decoupling path for images from the target domain. Initially, images from both the source and target domains are input into a shared content encoder E_c and two distinct style encoders (E_s^s, E_s^t) to extract their content features (F_c^s, F_c^t) and style features (F_s^s, F_s^t) respectively. Subsequently, the style and content features are combined and fed into a decoder to generate reconstructed images ($X^{s \to s}, X^{t \to t}$,,) as well as synthetic images ($X^{t \to s}, X^{s \to t}$).

Thereafter, two style discriminators (D_s, D_t) are used to differentiate between real and synthetic images, aiming to make the synthetic images ($X^{t \to s}, X^{s \to t}$) have a similar style to the original images (X^s, X^t). The discrimination loss for the target domain is shown in Eq. (1), where D_t needs to maximize the loss function L_{adv}^t in order to accurately discriminate between the real and synthetic images. Conversely, E_s^t, E_c, and G need to minimize the loss function L_{adv}^t and ensure that the style of the synthetic images $X^{s \to t}$ closely aligns with that of the real target domain images X^t.

$$L_{adv}^t(E_c, E_s^t, G, D_t) = E_{x^t \in D^t}[\log(D_t(x^t))] + E_{x^s \in D^s, x^t \in D^t} \\ [\log(1 - D_t(G(E_c(x^s), E_s^t(x^t))))] \quad (1)$$

Content Consistency Loss and Style Transfer Loss. The amplitude spectrum and phase spectrum of the Fourier Transform can respectively capture the low-level distributional features of images (such as style) and high-level distributional features (such as content) [17]. The phase spectrum contains substantial semantic content. Therefore, by minimizing the phase difference loss between the original image and its corresponding reconstructed image, the strict constraints of pixel-level loss can be relaxed. This encourages the shared content encoder to extract more content features and generate reconstructed images that preserve more semantic content, thereby achieving content consistency. Variations in the amplitude spectrum significantly impact the image style [18]. The style similarity between synthetic and original images is further enhanced by reducing the differences in the amplitude spectrum, which pushes the style encoder to extract more style features.

Based on the analyses above, we propose the Content Consistency Loss (CCL) and Style Transfer Loss (STL) based on the Fourier Transform. Firstly, we apply the Fourier Transform to the original, synthetic, and reconstructed images using Eq. (2) (as shown by the gray solid line in Fig. 1), where H, W, and C represent the height, width, and channels of the ith image, respectively.

$$F(x_i^k)(u, v, c) = \sum_{h=0}^{H-1} \sum_{w=0}^{W-1} x_i^k(h, w, c) e^{-j2\pi(\frac{h}{H}u + \frac{w}{W}v)} \quad (2)$$

Subsequently, the frequency domain signal $F(x_i^k)$ can be further decomposed into its phase spectrum $P_i^k \in \mathbb{R}^{h \times w \times d}$ and amplitude spectrum $A_i^k \in \mathbb{R}^{h \times w \times d}$ [19]. Equation (3) represents the negative cosine of the phase difference between the source domain image and its reconstructed image, where $< \cdot >$ denotes the dot-product, and $|| \cdot ||_2$ represents the L2 norm. Minimizing Eq. (3) can reduce the discrepancies in the phase spectrum, thereby enhancing the consistency of semantic content.

$$L_{con}^s(x^s, x^{s \to s}) = -\frac{1}{N} \sum_{i=1}^{N} \frac{< F(x^s)_i^P, F(x^{s \to s})_i^P >}{||F(x^s)_i^P||_2 \cdot ||F(x^{s \to s})_i^P||_2} \quad (3)$$

The final CCL is shown in Eq. (4), which corresponds to the red dashed line in Fig. 1.

$$\underset{\theta(E_s^s, E_c, G), \theta(E_s^t, E_c, G)}{min} L_{con}((E_s^s, E_c, G), (E_s^t, E_C, G)) = L_{con}^s(x^s, x^{s \to s}) + L_{con}^t(x^t, x^{t \to t}) \quad (4)$$

Finally, a Style Transfer Loss based on the Fourier Transform is added to the base of the adversarial loss, which corresponds to the blue dashed line in Fig. 1. The STL is applied to the amplitude spectrum of the original and synthetic images to further maintain the style similarity.

$$L_{sty}^s(x^s, x^{t \to s}) = -\frac{1}{N} \sum_{i=1}^{N} \frac{<F(x^s)_i^A, F(x^{t \to s})_i^A>}{||F(x^s)_i^A||_2 \cdot ||F(x^{t \to s})_i^A||_2} \quad (5)$$

Equation (5) represents the negative cosine of the amplitude difference between the source domain image and its synthetic image. Minimizing this difference can reduce disparities in the amplitude spectrum and enhance style consistency. The final STL is shown in Eq. (6).

$$\underset{\theta(E_s^s, E_c, G), \theta(E_s^t, E_c, G)}{min} L_{sty}((E_s^s, E_c, G), (E_s^t, E_C, G)) = L_{sty}^s(x^s, x^{t \to s}) + L_{sty}^t(x^t, x^{s \to t}) \quad (6)$$

3.2 Multi-scale Feature Fusion Strategy

Many studies have shown that generating synthetic images that preserve more semantic information is significant for improving the generalization of models [20, 21]. The CCL can help models generate synthetic images with more semantic content, but the fundamental reason for losing important semantic information is the multi-layer convolutional processing during feature extraction. Therefore, we introduce a multi-scale feature fusion strategy (MSFFS) into the shared encoder to preserve and transmit early feature information to subsequent convolutional layers, ultimately reducing the loss of crucial semantic information.

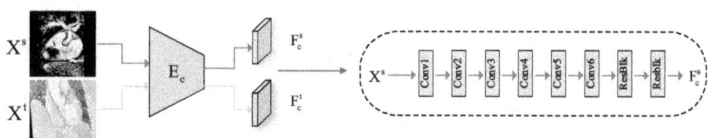

Fig. 2. Detailed Structure of the Content Encoder.

Multi-scale Feature Extraction. The shared content encoder E_c is composed of six two-dimensional convolutional blocks and two residual blocks, as illustrated in Fig. 2.

The kernel size for the first convolutional block is 7×7, whereas the kernel sizes for the subsequent blocks are 4×4. The inclusion of the two residual blocks aims to address the issues of gradient vanishing and slow convergence during the training of the network.

Lower-dimensional features contain more positional and detail information and have a higher resolution but may lack some semantic information because they pass through fewer convolutional layers. Conversely, higher-dimensional features contain stronger semantic information as they pass through more convolutional layers. Therefore, we perform multi-scale feature extraction on the last three layers of the content encoder, as shown in Fig. 3(a).

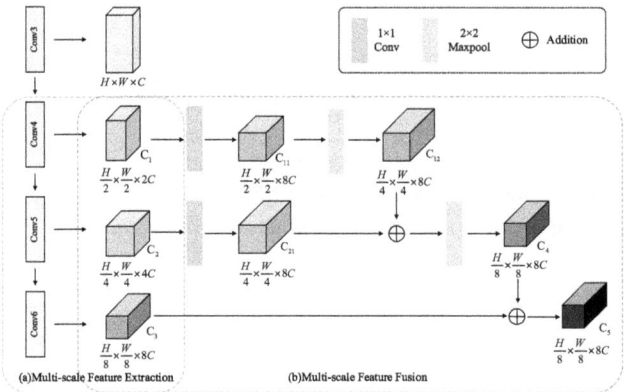

Fig. 3. Multi-scale Feature Fusion Strategy.

Multi-scale Feature Fusion. Multi-scale feature fusion can fully utilize semantic information at various levels to achieve a more comprehensive, richer, and representative feature representation. By integrating features at different scales, it captures more accurate edges and details of the target and synthesizes images that preserve more semantic features, thereby enhancing the precision and robustness of models.

Firstly, a 1×1 convolution is applied to the lower-level features (C_1, C_2) to increase dimensionality, thereby aligning their dimensions with those of the higher-level features, as shown in Eqs. (7) and (8).

$$C_{11} = Reshape\left(c_1, size = \left(\frac{H}{2} \times \frac{W}{2} \times 8C\right)\right), Reshape = conv1 \times 1, c_1 \in \mathbb{R}^{\frac{H}{2} \times \frac{W}{2} \times 2C} \quad (7)$$

$$C_{21} = Reshape\left(c_2, size = \left(\frac{H}{4} \times \frac{W}{4} \times 8C\right)\right), Reshape = conv1 \times 1, c_2 \in \mathbb{R}^{\frac{H}{4} \times \frac{W}{4} \times 4C} \quad (8)$$

Secondly, a 2×2 max pooling layer is employed to reduce the size of the lower-level features ($C_{11}, C_{12} + C_{21}$) by half, as shown in Eqs. (9–10).

$$C_{12} = Reshape\left(c_{11}, size = \left(\frac{H}{4} \times \frac{W}{4} \times 8C\right)\right), Reshape = Maxpool2 \times 2 \quad (9)$$

$$C_4 = Reshape\left(c_{12} + c_{21}, size = \left(\frac{H}{8} \times \frac{W}{8} \times 8C\right)\right), Reshape = Maxpool2 \times 2 \quad (10)$$

Finally, features from different layers are fused to obtain a representation that preserves more semantic information, as shown in Eq. (11). The detailed implementation scheme is illustrated in Fig. 3(b).

$$C_5 = C_3 + C_4, C_3 \in \mathbb{R}^{\frac{H}{8} \times \frac{W}{8} \times 8C} \tag{11}$$

The fused features C_5 are then input into a residual block. Residual blocks only need to learn the differences between inputs and outputs, effectively mitigating the problem of gradient vanishing and obtaining content features that preserve more semantic content.

3.3 Model Training and Testing

After the first phase, UDA-F4 has obtained synthetic images $x^{s \to t}$, and their content features come from the source domain while their style features come from the target domain. Consequently, the labels from the source domain can be shared with the synthetic target domain images [15]. This approach can be used to train the model and enhance its generalization in the target domain, as shown in Fig. 4(a).

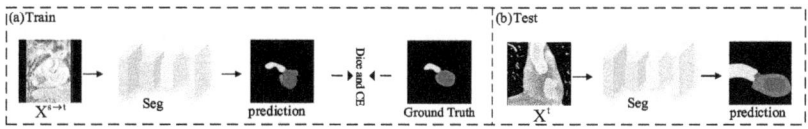

Fig. 4. Training and Testing Process of the Segmentation Network.

The training process uses Dice loss and cross-entropy loss, as shown in Eq. (12). The loss function takes into account both pixel-level and region-level relationships, enabling the model to comprehend the target areas more accurately and produce more precise segmentation results. The total loss is shown in Eq. (13). After training, the real target domain images (x^t) are used for testing, as shown in Fig. 4(b).

$$L_{seg} = Dice(y^s, seg(X^{s \to t})) + CE(y^s + Seg(X^{s \to t})) \tag{12}$$

$$L = L^s_{adv} + L^t_{adv} + L_{con} + L_{style} + L_{seg} \tag{13}$$

4 Experiments

4.1 Dataset and Evaluation Metrics

To validate the effectiveness of the UDA-F4 framework, we utilize the MICCAI 2017 Multi-Modality Whole Heart Segmentation (MM-WHS) dataset [22] for testing, which includes 20 unpaired 3D cardiac MRI images and 20 3D cardiac CT images. For training, sixteen labeled 3D cardiac MRI images are selected, and the remaining four are used for testing segmentation performance. The division of CT images is identical to that of MRI images. Initially, the region of interest (the cardiac area) is cropped from the original 3D images, then the 3D images are sliced into 2D sections, and the cropped images from both datasets are normalized. The slice size during the data augmentation phase is 512 × 512 × 1, and in the segmentation phase, it is 256 × 256 × 1.

The experiment targets four anatomical structures for segmentation, including the Ascending Aorta (AA), Left Atrial Cavity (LAC), Left Ventricular Cavity (LVC), and Myocardium (MYO). We employed the Dice coefficient (Dice) and Average Surface Distance (ASD) as evaluation metrics. The Dice coefficient ranges from 0 to 1, with higher values indicating better segmentation outcomes, while a lower ASD signifies superior model performance at the boundaries.

4.2 Validation of Model Adaptability in the Target Domain

To validate adaptability, experiments were conducted in two directions: CT (source domain) to MRI (target domain) and MRI (source domain) to CT (target domain). To compare the segmentation accuracy of different models, optimal (Supervised) and worst (Without Domain Adaptation, WoDA) performance thresholds were established. The optimal threshold was obtained through supervised training in the target domain, while the worst threshold resulted from testing the target domain data directly on the source domain model without domain adaptation. The WoDA performance is extremely low in both directions due to significant domain shifts between CT and MRI images.

Table 1. Comparison of average Dice & ASD (CT to MRI).

Method name	Dice (%)					ASD (%)				
	AA	LAC	LVC	MYO	Avg	AA	LAC	LVC	MYO	Avg
Supervised	82.8	80.5	92.4	78.8	83.6	3.6	3.9	2.1	1.9	2.9
WoDA	5.4	30.2	24.6	2.7	15.7	15.4	16.8	13.0	10.8	14.0
CyCADA [25]	60.5	44.0	77.6	47.9	57.5	7.7	13.9	4.8	5.2	7.9
CycleGAN [12]	64.3	30.7	65.0	43.0	50.7	5.8	9.8	6.0	5.0	6.6
PnPAdaNe t[23]	43.7	47.0	77.7	48.6	54.3	11.4	14.5	4.5	5.3	8.9
SynSegNet [24]	41.3	57.5	63.6	36.5	49.7	8.6	10.7	5.4	5.9	7.6
SIFA [8]	65.3	62.3	78.9	47.3	63.4	7.3	7.4	3.8	4.4	5.7
TFDM	66.7	63.9	77.4	46.7	**63.7**	5.7	6.5	4.1	4.7	**5.3**
UDA-F4(ours)	**68.8**	**64.7**	**79.0**	**48.1**	**65.2**	**5.2**	**5.9**	**3.8**	**4.5**	**4.9**

We compare UDA-F4 with CycleGAN, PnP-AdaNet [23], SynSegNet [24], SIFA, CyCADA [25], and the TFDM, which utilized cycle-consistency loss and adversarial loss, among others. These methods had performed well on the MM-WHS dataset. Table 1 presents the results from CT (source domain) to MRI (target domain), and Table 2 shows results for MRI (source domain) to CT (target domain). The results indicate that UDA-F4 outperforms other methods, with the average Dice score increasing to 65.2% and 76.6% in both directions, respectively, and the average ASD decreasing to 4.9 and 5.8. This narrows the gap to a 14% difference from supervised training Dice scores. Figure 5 presents the visual results, demonstrating that, apart from the supervised training method, the segmentation results of UDA-F4 are closer to the labels and exhibit better adaptability and effectiveness in the unlabeled target domain.

Table 2. Comparison of average Dice & ASD (MRI to CT).

Method name	Dice(%)					ASD(%)				
	AA	LAC	LVC	MYO	Avg	AA	LAC	LVC	MYO	Avg
Supervised	92.7	91.1	91.9	87.7	90.9	1.5	3.5	1.7	2.1	2.2
WoDA	28.4	27.7	4.0	8.7	17.2	20.6	16.2	N/A	48.4	N/A
CyCADA [25]	72.9	77.0	62.4	45.3	64.4	9.6	8.0	9.6	10.5	9.4
CycleGAN [12]	73.8	75.7	52.3	28.7	57.6	11.5	13.6	9.2	8.8	10.8
PnPAdaNet [23]	74.0	68.9	61.9	50.8	63.9	12.8	6.3	17.4	14.7	12.8
SynSegNet [24]	71.6	69.0	51.6	40.8	58.2	11.7	7.8	7.0	9.2	8.9
SIFA [8]	81.3	79.5	73.8	61.6	74.1	7.9	6.2	5.5	8.5	7.0
TFDM	83.4	81.3	74.2	62.4	**75.3**	6.8	6.0	4.7	7.7	**6.3**
UDA-F4(ours)	**84.1**	**83.4**	**74.7**	**64.1**	**76.6**	**6.3**	**5.5**	**4.6**	**6.8**	**5.8**

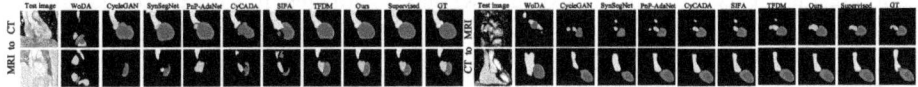

Fig. 5. Visual Results Comparison of Various Methods.

4.3 Ablation Experiment

This experiment incrementally integrates the Fourier Transform-based Content Consistency Loss (CCL), Style Transfer Loss (STL), and Multi-Scale Feature Fusion Strategy (MSFFS) into the TFDM to evaluate the effectiveness of each component.

Table 3. Comparison of average Dice & ASD under different CCL and STL (MRI to CT).

TFDM	CCL	STL	Dice (%)					ASD (%)				
			AA	LAC	LVC	MYO	Avg	AA	LAC	LVC	MYO	Avg
1	✗	✗	83.4	81.3	74.2	62.4	75.3	6.8	6.0	4.7	7.7	6.3
2	✓	✗	84.0	82.6	74.7	62.4	75.9	6.6	5.9	4.7	7.8	6.2
3	✗	✓	83.8	81.5	74.2	62.5	75.5	6.6	6.0	4.8	7.4	6.2
4	✓	✓	**84.0**	**83.2**	**75.1**	**63.1**	**76.4**	**6.4**	**5.7**	**4.6**	**7.3**	**6.0**

Effectiveness of CCL and STL. Firstly, we replace the cycle-consistency loss in the TFDM with the CCL. Figure 6(A) illustrates the visualization results of the reconstruction effects on MRI images (top row) and CT images (bottom row) using two different loss functions. The first column shows the original images, serving as a baseline. The second and third columns display the reconstructed images using cycle-consistency loss and content consistency loss, respectively. Notably, images reconstructed with cycle-consistency loss show discrepancies with the original ones, while those reconstructed using content consistency loss maintain semantic consistency more effectively, as highlighted in the red-boxed areas. These results underscore the effectiveness of content consistency loss in preserving the inherent content features of the images.

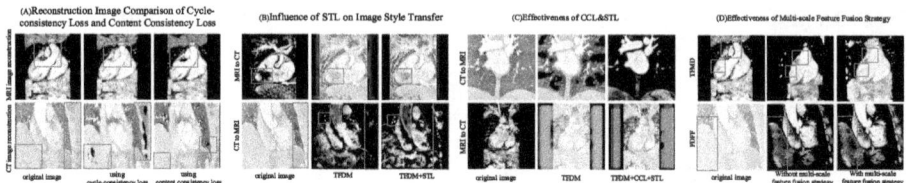

Fig. 6. Visualization of ablation experiment results.

Secondly, the STL is incorporated into the TFDM, and Fig. 6(B) presents the visualization results of style transfer between MRI and CT images. It is observed that images produced with the style transfer loss exhibit enhanced clarity and realism compared to those produced with the TFDM alone.

Finally, the TFDM was enhanced by embedding both the CCL and the STL. Figure 6(C) shows the visual results, which demonstrate that the CCL and STL can successfully accomplish the style shift while preserving more substantial semantic content. The detailed experimental results, shown in Table 3, reveal that, compared to cycle consistency loss, content consistency loss facilitates an improvement of 0.6% in average Dice and a reduction of 0.1 in average ASD. Moreover, the style transfer loss further enhances average Dice and ASD. Their combination results in an increase of 1.1% in the average Dice and a decrease of 0.3 in ASD.

Table 4. Effectiveness of MSFFS on Dice & ASD (MRI to CT)

Method name	Dice(%)					ASD(%)				
	AA	LAC	LVC	MYO	Avg	AA	LAC	LVC	MYO	Avg
TFDM	83.4	81.3	74.2	62.4	75.3	6.8	6.0	4.7	7.7	6.3
TFDM + MSFFS	83.7	82.2	74.3	63.0	75.8	6.6	5.9	4.7	7.4	6.1
FDFF	84.0	83.2	**75.1**	63.1	76.4	6.4	5.7	4.6	7.3	6.0
FDFF + MSFFS	**84.1**	**83.4**	74.7	**64.1**	**76.6**	**6.3**	**5.5**	**4.6**	**6.8**	**5.8**

Validation of the Effectiveness of MSFFS. We add the MSFFS into the TFDM and FDFF respectively, and Fig. 6(D) illustrates the results. It is evident that the MSFFS can preserve more semantic information, thereby significantly enhancing the quality of the generated images. The results in Table 4 also prove the effectiveness of the MSFFS, which enhances the average Dice score of the TFDM by nearly 0.5% and reduces the average ASD by 0.2. When applied to FDFF, there is an increase of 0.2% in the average Dice score and a decrease of 0.3 in ASD.

5 Conclusion

To address the problems of cycle consistency loss in feature decoupling methods, which cannot effectively maintain semantic consistency between the original and reconstructed images, unsatisfactory style preservation between the original and synthesized images, and semantic information loss caused by shared encoders, we propose UDA-F4, a UDA framework based on the feature decoupling of the Fourier transform and multi-scale feature fusion. First, in the feature decoupling process, the content consistency loss based on the Fourier transform is used to replace the cycle consistency loss, enhancing semantic consistency between the original and reconstructed images. Second, a style transfer loss based on the Fourier transform is proposed to effectively address the preservation of diverse styles in medical datasets. Finally, a multi-scale feature fusion strategy is introduced into the shared content encoder to generate synthesized images with richer semantic features. The experimental results based on the MICCAI 2017 MM-WHS cardiac dataset demonstrate the effectiveness and superiority of UDA-F4.

Acknowledgments. This study was funded by Science and Technology Program of Inner Mongolia Autonomous Region (2022YFSH0010) and Natural Science Foundation of Inner Mongolia Autonomous Region (2021MS06031).

References

1. Du, X., Liu, Y.: Constraint-based unsupervised domain adaptation network for multi-modality cardiac image segmentation. IEEE J. Biomed. Health Inform. **26**(1), 67–78 (2021)
2. Yang, F., Liang, F., Lu, L., Yin, M.: Dual attention-guided and learnable spatial transformation data augmentation multi-modal unsupervised medical image segmentation. Biomed. Signal Process. Control **78**, 103849 (2022)
3. Xu, H., Xie, H.T., Zhang, Y.D.: Review of domain generalization in vision. J. Guangzhou Univ. (Nat. Sci. Edn.) **21**(02), 42–59 (2022)
4. Xie, Q., Li, Y., He, N., Ning, M., Ma, K., Wang, G., Zheng, Y.: Unsupervised domain adaptation for medical image segmentation by disentanglement learning and self-training. IEEE Trans. Med. Imag. **43**, 4–14 (2022)
5. Peng, L., Lin, L., Cheng, P., Huang, Z., Tang, X.: Unsupervised domain adaptation for cross-modality retinal vessel segmentation via disentangling representation style transfer and collaborative consistency learning. In: 2022 IEEE 19th International Symposium on Biomedical Imaging (ISBI), pp. 1–5. IEEE (2022)
6. Yao, K., et al.: A novel 3D unsupervised domain adaptation framework for cross-modality medical image segmentation. IEEE J. Biomed. Health Inform. **26**(10), 4976–4986 (2022)
7. Tian, Q., Zhu, Y., Ma, C.: Review on Domain Adaptation Methods Based on Deep Learning Data Collection and Processing **37**(03) (2022)
8. Chen, C., Dou, Q., Chen, H., Qin, J., Heng, P.-A.: Synergistic image and feature adaptation: Towards cross-modality domain adaptation for medical image segmentation. Proc. AAAI Conf. Artif. Intell. **33**(01), 865–872 (2019). https://doi.org/10.1609/aaai.v33i01.3301865

9. Dong, S., et al.: Partial unbalanced feature transport for cross-modality cardiac image segmentation. IEEE Trans. Med. Imaging **42**(6), 1758–1773 (2023)
10. Wang, S., Fu, Z., Wang, B., Hu, Y.: Fusing feature and output space for unsupervised domain adaptation on medical image segmentation. Int. J. Imaging Syst. Technol. **33**(5), 1672–1681 (2023)
11. Cui, H., Yuwen, C., Jiang, L., Xia, Y., Zhang, Y.: Bidirectional cross-modality unsupervised domain adaptation using generative adversarial networks for cardiac image segmentation. Comput. Biol. Med. **136**, 104726 (2021)
12. Zhu, J.Y., Park, T., Isola, P., Efros, A. A.: Unpaired image-to-image translation using cycle-consistent adversarial networks. In: Proceedings of the IEEE international conference on computer vision, pp. 2223–2232 (2017)
13. Hu, W., Xu, Q.Z., Ge, X.W.: A review of unsupervised domain adaptation in medical image segmentation. Comput. Eng. Appl. **60**(06), 10–26 (2024)
14. Chartsias, A., Joyce, T., Papanastasiou, G., Semple, S., Williams, M., Newby, D.E., Tsaftaris, S.A.: Disentangled representation learning in cardiac image analysis. Med. Image Anal. **58**, 101535 (2019)
15. Isola, P., Zhu, J. Y., Zhou, T., Efros, A.A.: Image-to-image translation with conditional adversarial networks. In: Proceedings of the IEEE conference on computer vision and pattern recognition, pp. 1125–1134 (2017)
16. Wang, R., Zhou, Q., Zheng, G.: EDRL: entropy-guided disentangled representation learning for unsupervised domain adaptation in semantic segmentation. Comput. Methods Programs Biomed. **240**, 107729 (2023)
17. Liu, Q., Chen, C., Qin, J., Dou, Q., Heng, P.A.: Feddg: Federated domain generalization on medical image segmentation via episodic learning in continuous frequency space. In: Proceedings of the IEEE/CVF Conference on Computer Vision and Pattern Recognition, pp. 1013–1023 (2021)
18. Zhang, Z., Li, Y., Shin, B.S.: C2-GAN: Content-consistent generative adversarial networks for unsupervised domain adaptation in medical image segmentation. Med. Phys. **49**(10), 6491–6504 (2022)
19. Frigo, M., Johnson, S.G.: FFTW: An adaptive software architecture for the FFT. In: Proceedings of the 1998 IEEE International Conference on Acoustics, Speech and Signal Processing, ICASSP'98 (Cat. No. 98CH36181), vol. 3, pp. 1381–1384. IEEE (1998)
20. Jiang, Z., et al.: O2M-UDA: unsupervised dynamic domain adaptation for one-to-multiple medical image segmentation. Knowl.-Based Syst. **265**, 110378 (2023)
21. Liu, X., et al.: Attentive continuous generative self-training for unsupervised domain adaptive medical image translation. Med. Image Anal. **88**, 102851 (2023)
22. Zhuang, X., Shen, J.: Multi-scale patch and multi-modality atlases for whole heart segmentation of MRI. Med. Image Anal. **31**, 77–87 (2016)
23. Dou, Q., et al.: Pnp-adanet: plug-and-play adversarial domain adaptation network at unpaired cross-modality cardiac segmentation. IEEE Access **7**, 99065–99076 (2019)
24. Huo, Y., et al.: Synseg-net: synthetic segmentation without target modality ground truth. IEEE Trans. Med. Imaging **38**(4), 1016–1025 (2018)
25. Hoffman, J., et al.: Cycada: Cycle-consistent adversarial domain adaptation. In: International Conference on Machine Learning, pp. 1989–1998. Pmlr (2018)

LVMUM: Toward Open-World Object Detection with Large Vision Models and Unsupervised Modeling

Yangyang Huang, Xing Xi, Weiye Wu, and Ronghua Luo[✉]

South China University of Technology, Guangdong 510006, GZ, China
huangyangy@whu.edu.cn

Abstract. Open-world object detection (OWOD), as an emerging and challenging task in object detection, requires the model to have the ability to detect known and unknown objects in dynamic environments. Furthermore, it should have the capability to perform incremental learning based on newly acquired knowledge. However, current OWOD methods focus on labeling regions with high objectness scores as unknown objects. These heuristic annotation methods rely entirely on the supervision of known objects, thus leading to the issue of label bias. To solve this problem, we propose the Object Reconstruction-based Weibull Model (ORWM) method, which uses object-level semantic information for feature reconstruction to perform unsupervised modeling of the foreground and background. In the modeling process, another challenge to detecting unknown objects is the limited annotations for unknown objects. Therefore, we propose an Unsupervised Region Proposal Generation method based on SAM (SAM-URPG) to generate original pseudo labels for unknown objects and use the zero-shot ability of the large visual model to generate pseudo labels for unknown objects. Experimental results show that our proposed method significantly improves the ability to detect unknown objects on the MS-COCO dataset. It increases U-Recall by 14.0, surpassing the previous state-of-the-art (SOTA) method by **34%**, re-aching **50.9** U-Recall, while maintaining competitive performance in detecting known objects. Additionally, in terms of inference speed, our method constructs the model using a pure convolutional neural network, rather than employing a dense attention mechanism. This approach surpasses the SOTA deformable DETR-based method with a speed of **9.95 FPS**, while maintaining an inference speed advantage of the SOTA Faster R-CNN-based methods.

Keywords: Unsupervised · Open World · Incremental Learning · Object Detection

1 Introduction

In the early phase, there has been significant advancement in object detection using deep learning techniques [13, 14, 16, 23]. However, conventional object detection models usually work in a closed set, focusing only on detecting known categories with manual annotations, ignoring other unlabeled objects. However, in specific scenarios, identifying unknown categories is crucial. For example, self-driving cars and robots must be able to identify unexpected obstacles to prevent accidents and maintain safety.

Previous research [2] investigated Open Set Object Detection (OSOD), which involves training detectors with known category labels but requires them to identify unknown categories during testing. Recent research has expanded the OSOD task to a more dynamic situation referred to as OWOD [11], in which the model needs to identify both known and unknown categories and can learn incrementally based on the new knowledge introduced. Prior methods tackled the OWOD challenge [7, 11, 15, 25] through the strategy of assigning pseudo-labels to regions that exhibit high objectness scores and do not intersect with known objects. These methods successfully detected unknown categories with features similar to those of known categories. However, they suffer from a severe label bias issue for known categories, tending to detect all regions as part of the background if they are dissimilar to known categories.

Several prior approaches [3, 15] have investigated the application of unsupervised region proposal generation techniques [1, 17, 18, 24] to enhance the adaptability of OWOD models. These unsupervised region proposals are typically derived from hand engineered low-level attributes such as colour, texture, shape, and contour. These proposals offer preliminary knowledge and physical limitations concerning areas where unknown objects may be located. Nonetheless, these unsupervisedly generated region proposals still necessitate pseudo-labels based on objectness for calibration. Consequently, the issue of label bias, which impedes the detection of unknown objects in OWOD tasks, persists.

To address the label bias problem, we propose a novel method named LVMUM. The primary implementation process is as follows: Firstly, to model unknown objects in an unsupervised manner, we delve into the rapidly emerging Large Vision Models (LVM), such as the Segment Anything Model (SAM) [12]. Leveraging SAM's capability to segment any object, we generate class-agnostic masks for all objects in the image. By identifying the maximum and minimum coordinates x, y, we can obtain the bounding boxes of the objects. Subsequently, we generate pseudo-labels for potential targets, providing the model with supervision for potential unknown objects. However, the generated pseudo-labels contain Ground Truth information and noise. Therefore, we propose an Unsupervised Region Proposal Generation method based on SAM (SAMURPG) to generate original pseudo-labels for unknown objects.

To identify true unknown objects from the original pseudo-labels of unknown objects generated by SAM-URPG, we find that generic background areas (such as walls, sky, and ground) often appear in images, exhibiting repetitive and low-level patterns. On the contrary, foreground areas appear less frequently and have diverse features. Therefore, from the perspective of feature frequency, the background and foreground form two different distributions. Inspired by out-of-distribution (OOD) detection [10, 22] based on data reconstruction, it is observed that the encoder-decoder framework trained on In-Distribution (ID) data exhibits a larger reconstruction error for Out-Of-Distribution (OOD) data. Therefore, during inference, ID and OOD samples can be distinguished based on their reconstruction errors. However, the current reconstruction-based OOD detection methods [4, 5, 10], which compute reconstruction errors at the pixel level, have high training costs and are unable to capture semantic information adequately. We propose the Object Reconstruction-based Weibull Model (ORWM), which utilizes the ability of SAM to segment any object, generating object-level semantic information for feature reconstruction to model foreground and background in an unsupervised manner, thereby improving the model's accuracy in identifying unknown objects, and it significantly reduces the training cost of the model. Compared to previous SOTA methods, the experimental results demonstrate that the proposed method substantially improves over previous leading techniques in identifying unknown objects within the MS-COCO dataset while maintaining competitiveness Performance in detecting known object categories. Furthermore, our model, constructed using a pure convolutional neural network and utilizing fewer parameters, showcases significant advantages in terms of inference speed. We summarize our methods and contributions as follows:

- We propose an Unsupervised Region Proposal Generation method based on SAM (SAM-URPG) to generate original pseudo-labels for unknown objects, providing the model with supervision for potential unknown objects.
- We propose an Object Reconstruction error Weibull Model (ORWM), which utilizes the prior knowledge of object occurrence frequency for unsupervised modeling, enhancing the model's accuracy in identifying unknown objects. Moreover, our modeling method based on object reconstruction error significantly reduces the training cost of the model.
- Through experimental research, it was found that our proposed method, when evaluated on the OWOD task on the MS-COCO dataset, significantly outperforms contemporaneous SOTA methods in terms of recall rate for unknown categories, achieving a U-Recall of **50.9**. At the same time, it maintains competitive performance in detecting known object categories. In terms of inference speed, our method can reach **34.04 FPS**.

2 Methodology

To tackle the previously mentioned issue of label bias for known categories, we propose a method named LVMUM aimed at the unsupervised modeling of unknown objects in the original pseudo-labels generated by the unsupervised region proposal generation method. For this purpose, our method proposes several modules, including the SAM-based Unsupervised Region Proposal Generation method (SAM-URPG) discussed in Sect. 2.2, and the Weibull model based on object reconstruction error (ORWM) discussed in Sect. 2.3. As shown in Fig. 1, SAM-URPG uses SAM to generate original pseudo-labels for unknown objects, providing the model with supervision for potential unknown objects. ORWM uses the prior knowledge of object occurrence frequency for unsupervised modeling, improving the model's accuracy in identifying unknown objects. We use Faster-RCNN [16] as the base detector because Faster-RCNN has a natural advantage [2] in detecting unknown categories, and it has been used as the baseline network for many open vocabulary and open world object detection tasks [6, 11, 21].

2.1 Problem Description

In OWOD defined by ORE [11], the model M_t at time t is tasked not only with detecting the known classes $KN_t = \{1, 2, ..., C\}$, but also with identifying previously unlearned target instances as unknown classes $UN = \{C+1, ...\}$. Subsequently, users can selectively label n new interesting classes and annotate the corresponding unknown instances to train the model, incorporating this new set of classes into the known categories, denoted as $KN_{t+1} = KN_t + \{C + 1, ..., C + n\}$. Finally, the model M_t undergoes incremental learning on KN_{t+1}, avoiding training on the entire dataset to detect all target categories within KN_{t+1}.

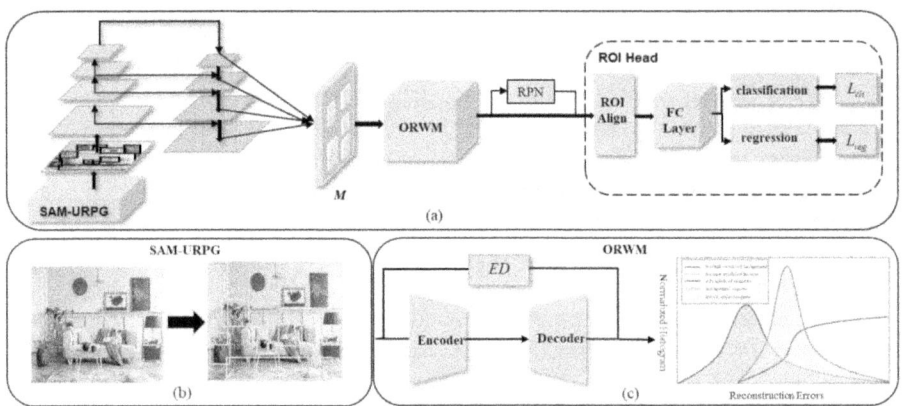

Fig. 1. The overall structure of our model. The proposed method is based on the standard Faster R-CNN [16] with FPN [9]. We first propose SAM-URPG, using the SAM to generate raw pseudo-labels for unknown objects, enhancing the model's recognition of unknown objects. Then, we propose ORWM, which utilizes object-level semantic information generated by SAM for feature reconstruction, improving the model's accuracy in recognizing unknown objects.

2.2 SAM-URPG: SAM Unsupervised Region Proposal Generation

Existing unsupervised region extraction methods can generate a large number of regions, which may contain various types of known and unknown objects. Therefore, region proposals that do not overlap with Ground Truth objects can serve as pseudo-labels for unknown objects. However, these pseudo-labels for unknown objects are coarse and are likely to be non-object bounding boxes of background areas.

To generate accurate initial pseudo-labels for unknown objects in images, we propose an Unsupervised Region Proposal Generation method based on SAM (SAM-URPG). Specifically, as shown in Fig. 2, we first use the SAM model to segment the entire image X to obtain a class-agnostic mask, represented as:

$$M_{sam}(X) = \left\{ i \in [1, nm] | \left(\left(x_1^i, y_1^i\right), ..., \left(x_{np}^i, y_{np}^i\right) \right) \right\} \quad (1)$$

where nm and np represent the number of masks and the pixel count of the current mask, respectively, subsequently, we calculate the maximum x and y coordinates for each mask to obtain the bounding box set for each mask:

$$Bb_i = \left(\min_{j \in [1,np]} \left(x_j^i, y_j^i \right), \max_{j \in [1,np]} \left(x_j^i, y_j^i \right) \right) \tag{2}$$

$$B_{set} = \{Bb_1, Bb_2, ..., Bb_{nm}\} \tag{3}$$

These bounding boxes may contain Ground Truth information and noise. To generate pseudo-labels for unknown objects, we first filter through Non-Maximum Suppression (NMS) and Intersection Over Union (IOU). We use NMS to filter out duplicate bounding boxes, then calculate the IOU of the object bounding boxes generated by SAM with the annotated object bounding boxes. If the IOU is greater than a set threshold IOU_a, it is considered a known object; otherwise, it is an unknown object:

$$B_{rough} = \left(Bb_j \in B_{set} | \left\langle \max_{i \in [1, n_{gt}]} IOU(Bb_j, gt_i) \right\rangle < IOU_a \right) \tag{4}$$

where gt_i is an instance of a known class. Despite SAM's strong zero-shot capability, it still has noise bounding boxes. Upon observation, SAM often predicts new masks for some internal pixels of already segmented objects. If a mask's bounding box has a length-to-width ratio that is too large or too small, then this object may be due to noise or detection errors. Therefore, we can apply appropriate thresholds to effectively filter out noise. If the length-to-width ratio is between thresholds Ba_{min} and Ba_{max}, we consider it as a pseudo-label for an unknown object:

$$B_{uk} = \left\{ Bb_j \in B_{rough} | Ba_{min} < \frac{|x_2^i - x_1^i|}{|y_2^i - y_1^i|} < Ba_{max} \right\} \tag{5}$$

where $x_1^i, x_2^i, y_1^i, y_2^i$ are the bounding box coordinates generated by Eq. (2). Please refer to Sect. 3.3 for the experimental parameter settings.

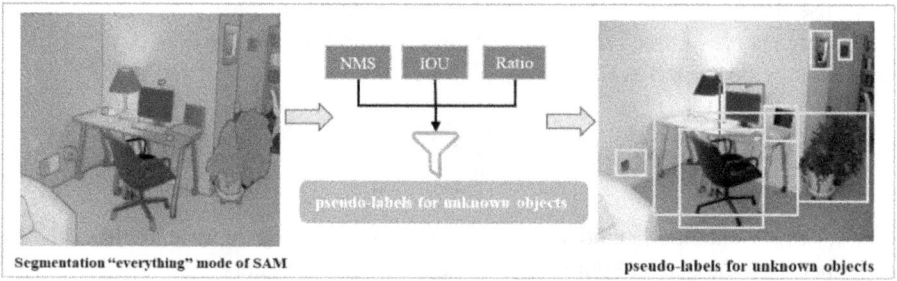

Fig. 2. The process by which SAM generates pseudo-labels, where the yellow box represents an unknown category and the red box represents a known category.

2.3 ORWM: Object Reconstruction Error Weibull Model

Current OOD detection methods based on reconstruction utilize the encoding and decoding process of autoencoders, which present the following issues: Firstly, pixel-level feature reconstruction requires the computation of reconstruction errors for all pixels, leading to high training costs. Secondly, pixel features cannot adequately represent the semantic information of known and unknown objects. To address these issues, we propose an unsupervised modeling method based on object reconstruction.

Specifically, ORWM first uses SAM to segment all objects in the image and generates object bounding boxes based on the mask, as shown in Eq. (3), Bset = {Bb1, Bb2,..., Bbnm}. Then, it extracts the feature map M = [M1, M2, M3, M4] from the input image $X \in R^{H \times W \times C}$ through the backbone network. In order to fully represent the semantic information of objects, the object bounding boxes generated by SAM are mapped to the feature map. That is, referring to the technical details of RoIAlign [8] is used to extract features from the feature map that correspond to the target area in the original image:

$$O_F = R_A(M, B_{set}) = [of_1, of_2, of_3, ..., of_{nm}] \tag{6}$$

Here, R_A represents the features extracted by ROIAlign [18], and of_{nm} represents the feature representation of each object on the feature map. Since the object-level features of_{nm} can fully represent the semantic information of objects (whether foreground or background), we perform feature reconstruction for each object's features generated on the feature map through an autoencoder. The autoencoder consists of an encoder $Ed(.)$ and a decoder $Dd(.)$. The encoder first maps all objects in the feature map to a low-dimensional latent space representation:

$$Ed(of_{nm}) = [of_E^1, of_E^2, ..., of_E^{nm}] \tag{7}$$

Here, of_{nm} represents the original features of each object in the object feature map, and of i represents the features after encoding. Then, the decoder reconstructs all objects in the latent space back to their original dimensions:

$$Dd(of_E^{nm}) = [of_D^1, of_D^2, ..., of_D^{nm}] \tag{8}$$

We use the Euclidean Distance (ED) to calculate the reconstruction error of each object, which serves as the reconstruction loss function for the autoencoder. The above process can be described as follows:

$$L_{ORWM} = \frac{1}{nm} \sum_{i=1}^{nm} \left\| of_E^i - of_D^i \right\|^2 \tag{9}$$

Here, $\|.\|$ represents the Euclidean norm. The formula above represents the square of the ED between the original data of_E^i and the reconstructed data of_D^i.

Each object region feature represents the features of the corresponding bounding box, thus assigning foreground or background labels to each object based on the corresponding bounding box. Since the background region appears more frequently and is easier to reconstruct, its reconstruction error is smaller compared to foreground objects. By arbitrarily extracting object representations from known object regions and background parts in the MS-COCO training dataset, we collected a set of object reconstruction errors, represented as ε_{kn} and ε_{bg}. As shown in part (c) of Fig. 1, we visualized the histogram of object reconstruction errors extracted from known object regions and background parts. The comparison found that the reconstruction error of the background part is smaller than the reconstruction error of the known object region because the frequency of the background region appearing is higher than the frequency of the known object region. Therefore, we can use the reconstruction error extracted from the known object region to estimate the probability distribution of all foreground regions.

Due to the inherent advantage of the Weibull distribution in fitting the shape distribution of many scenarios, it is used as the prior model in ORWM. The forms of the Weibull distributions for known regions and background regions (denoted as ft_{kn} and ft_{bg} respectively) are as follows:

$$ft(L_{ORWM}; k, g) = \frac{g}{k}(\frac{L_{ORWM}}{k})^{g-1} e^{-(L_{ORWM}/k)^g} \qquad (10)$$

Here, L_{ORWM} represents the magnitude of the object's reconstruction error, and ft is the probability distribution function of the Weibull distribution. k and g serve as the scale and shape parameters of ft. The most suitable k and g are calculated using least squares estimation (LS) based on the sampled reconstruction errors from the foreground region (ε_{kn}) and the background part (ε_{bg}).

After establishing the probability distribution models for the background region and foreground objects, we use the probability functions (ft_{kn} and ft_{bg}) to evaluate the likelihood of a pseudo-unknown object being a real unknown object. Equation (5) calculates the pseudo-label B_{uk} of an unknown object in image X. The following equation is used to calculate the soft label, which estimates the likelihood score of the pseudo-object becoming a real unknown object:

$$s(B_{uk}) = \left(\frac{ft_{kn}(L_{ORWM}(B_{uk}))}{ft_{bg}(L_{ORWM}(B_{uk})) + ft_{kn}(L_{ORWM}(B_{uk}))} \right)^\gamma \qquad (11)$$

Here, ftkn and ftbg respectively represent the Weibull functions of the known object area and the background part. γ is a hyperparameter used for score calculation. When $\gamma \to \infty$, the probability of all unknown object pseudo-labels is very low, which can be considered close to 0. However, when $\gamma \to 0$, we consider these pseudo-labels as real unknown objects. Then, the score from Eq. (11) is used as a parameter and added to the loss function of the base detector as a supervisory signal, thereby learning known and unknown objects. The optimized loss function is as follows:

$$L(P_{rpj}) = \frac{1}{N_{cls}} \sum_{rpj} w_{rpj} L_{cls}\left(P_{rpj}, P^*_{rpj}\right) \qquad (12)$$

where w_{rpj} is the loss weight for region proposals rpj. When rpj belongs to a region of pseudo-unknown objects, w_{rpj} equals $s(rpj)$; otherwise, it equals 1. p_{rpj} represents the predicted probability for region proposals rpj, while p^*_{rpj} represents its ground truth, and L_{cls} represents the cross-entropy loss.

3 Experiment

3.1 Dataset

To substantiate our proposed method's efficacy, we evaluated our model on the OWOD benchmark, as proposed by OWOD [11] and OW-DETR [7]. As defined by PROB [25], there exist two benchmarks, namely S-OWODB and M-OWODB. Given that S-OWODB is superclass-separated and the semantics of unknown objects are more challenging to extend, our experiment pertains to the S-OWODB benchmark. We formulated four distinct tasks with 80 categories from the MS-COCO dataset, with the number of training images and instances for each task being: T1 (89490, 421243), T2(55870, 163512), T3(39402, 114452), T4(38903, 160794) respectively. Task one encompasses the categories of PASCAL VOC, and subsequently, each task incorporates 20 new categories based on the preceding task for incremental experiments. The test set comprises all categories with 4952 images and 36781 test instances.

3.2 Metric

We adhere to the standard evaluation metrics for the OWOD task [11]. The widely accepted object detection metric evaluates the model's performance on known categories, Mean Average Precision (mAP). The model's performance on objects without annotations is evaluated using the Unknown Class Recall (U-Recall) for unknown classes. Previously known mAP represents the detection accuracy for classes seen in previous tasks, denoted as mAP_pk. The current known mAP represents the detection accuracy for newly introduced classes in the current task, denoted as mAP_ck. Both indicate the detection accuracy for all categories seen in the current task, denoted as mAP_bo. In the incremental learning tasks (T2 − T4), the performance of known classes is divided into two parts: classes seen before and the classes introduced in the current task.

3.3 Details

Our experiments are built based on Detectron2 [20]. We use ResNet50-FPN [9] as our backbone network, and the base detector adopts Faster-RCNN [16]. The Stochastic Gradient Descent (SGD) is used as the optimizer. Our parameter settings include a learning rate of 0.02, a momentum parameter of 0.9, and a weight decay of e − 4. The model undergoes a standard training schedule for 32 training cycles, with each round consisting of a 6-cycle self-training process. Our experiments utilize 2 NVIDIA RTX3090 GPUs, with a batch size of 16. In this experiment, the hyperparameter $\gamma = 4$ is set by default. In the process of handling pseudo-labels in SAM-URPG, our experiment adopts a data processing strategy to filter Ground Truth information and noise bounding boxes. Firstly, the generated bounding boxes use NMS for deduplication, setting IOUa to 0.8. We calculate the IOU of the object-bounding boxes generated by SAM and the annotated object-bounding boxes. If the IOU is greater than the set threshold IOUa, it is considered a known object. Otherwise, it is an unknown object. Then we proceed to denoise, setting the maximum aspect ratio threshold of the bounding box Bamax to 4 and the minimum threshold Bamin to 0.25. Bounding boxes that do not satisfy the aspect ratio size between 0.25 and 4 are considered noise bounding boxes. Finally, we obtain the pseudo-labels of unknown objects.

3.4 Comparison with State-of-the-Art Models

To provide a clear demonstration of the experimental to provide a clear demonstration of the experimental results of our method, we compared it with several of the latest models in the field of OWOD, including ORE [11], OW-DETR [7], PROB [25], CAT [15] and MEPU [4]. We removed the energy model (EBUI) from ORE, as it could potentially lead to data leakage due to its use of fully annotated categories. All the data used in the papers above originate from the data in the original papers.

Table 1. Compare state-of-the-art of OWOD models

Task IDs (→)	Task 1		Task 2			Task 3			Task 4		
	U-Recall (↑)	mAP (↑) Current known	U-Recall (↑)	mAP (↑)		U-Recall (↑)	mAP(↑)		mAP (↑)		
				Previously known	Current known	Both		Previously known	Current known	Both	Previously known	Current known	Both
ORE-EBUI(CVPR2021)	1.5	71.4	3.9	61.0	30.9	45.6	3.6	43.1	32.2	39.5	33.6	26.3	31.8
OW-DETR(CVPR2022)	5.7	73.1	6.2	65.0	29.0	46.0	6.9	46.7	25.7	39.7	38.2	28.1	33.1
PROB(CVPR2023)	17.6	73.5	22.3	66.3	36.0	50.4	24.8	47.8	30.4	42.0	42.6	31.7	39.9
CAT(CVPR2023)	24.0	74.2	23.0	67.6	35.5	50.7	24.6	51.2	32.6	45.0	45.4	35.1	42.8
MEPU	37.9	74.3	35.8	68.0	1.9	54.3	35.7	50.2	38.3	46.2	43.7	33.7	41.2
Ours(LVMUM)	**50.9**	73.5	**50.7**	**68.2**	37.8	52.3	**43.6**	48.8	36.6	44.1	42.1	32.2	39.8

Identifying Potential Unknown Objects (T_1). As shown in Table 1, our method has achieved a comprehensive lead in the recall rate of unknowns. In terms of the performance of recalling unknown objects, it reached the highest unknown recall rate of 51.9. The closest to this result is MEPU, and our model significantly leads with a recall rate advantage of 34.3% (50.9 vs 37.9). For CAT, the advantage reaches 112.1% (50.9 vs 24.0), and for PROB, the advantage reaches 189.2% (50.9 vs 17.6). In terms of the performance of known categories, the mAP has slightly decreased, lagging behind MEPU's mAP by 0.8 and CAT's mAP by 0.7. This decline in performance is acceptable because the additional unknown supervision makes it more difficult for the model to distinguish known objects.

Incremental Learning ($T_2 - T_4$). As shown in Table 1, our method maintains an advantage in U-Recall (T_2: 141.6% MEPU, T_3: 122.1% MEPU). As the number of known categories increases, the mAP of our model on known categories gradually falls behind that of MEPU. This result is acceptable because the model recalls more unknown targets, which reduces the proportion of seen categories in the top 100 predictions of standard post-processing and faces serious challenges in the classification head (RoI Head).

3.5 Ablation Study

We conducted experiments to compare the model's performance with and without adding these modules to the tasks to validate the effectiveness of the two modules, SAM-URPG and ORWM, in our proposed approach.

Table 2. Different unsupervised region proposal methods generate pseudo labels

Unsupervised Region Propoasl Genenration	U-Recall	mAP_ck
Baseline	33.4	73.2
Selective Search	34.2	73.7
GOP	37.1	73.4
FreeSOLO	37.9	**74.3**
SAM-URGP	**50.9**	73.5

SAM-URGP Effectiveness. We evaluated the effectiveness of unsupervised region proposal generation methods on our model, as shown in Table 2. In Task 1, we compared four unsupervised region proposal generation methods with a baseline method that does not use any proposal generator. These methods are Selective Search [17], DETReg [1], FreeSOLO [18], and SAM-URGP. We found that all proposal generation methods typically produce better results than the baseline method, especially regarding unknown recall (a gain of + 17.5 can be achieved using SAM-URGP), significantly improving the detection results of unknown objects. It is worth noting that although the earliest method, such as Selective Search, generates lower-quality region proposals, it still improves. Our ORWM module can identify true unknown classes from cluttered environments.

ORWM Effectiveness. We conducted a performance analysis of ORWM on the MSCOCO dataset, reporting mAP for known classes and U-Recall for unknown classes in Task 1–4, as shown in Table 3. Without ORWM, the method is equivalent to using proposals generated by the SAM-URGP method directly as pseudo-labels for training Faster-RCNN on unknown objects. Few inaccuracies exist in the pseudo-labels for unknown objects, leading to confusion between foreground and background regions in the detector. The modeling mechanism of ORWM for unknown objects contributes to improving the accuracy of recognizing known and unknown objects. In Task 1, U-Recall improved by 4.6, and mAP_ck improved by 4.1. In Task 2, U-Recall increased by 7.5, and mAPck increased by 2, and there were varying degrees of improvement in other tasks as well.

Table 3. Our complete model with its variants

ORWM	Task 1		Task 2		Task 3		Task 4
	U-Recall	mAP_ck	U-Recall	mAP_ck	U-Recall	mAP_ck	mAP_ck
×	46.3	69.1	43.2	35.8	37.1	**34.7**	31.7
√	**50.9**	**73.5**	**50.7**	**37.8**	**43.6**	34.6	**32.2**

4 Conclusions

In response to the existing label bias problem in OWOD, we propose a novel method to address this problem. Initially, we model unknown objects unsupervised, effectively resolving the label bias problem. Simultaneously, we leverage popular Large Visual.

Models (LVM), such as the SAM model, which can segment any object to extend the effective detection of unknown objects. Experimental findings reveal that our model has significantly improved the detection of unknown objects, substantially surpassing current SOTA methods. At the same time, it maintains competitive performance in detecting known object categories. Our method can inspire insights into OWOD, especially in detecting unknown objects.

Acknowledgements. This work was also partially supported by Guangdong Artificial Intelligence and Digital Economy Laboratory (Guangzhou).

References

1. Bar, A., et al.: Detreg: unsupervised pretraining with region priors for object detection. In: Proceedings of the IEEE/CVF Conference on Computer Vision and Pattern Recognition, pp. 14605–14615 (2022)
2. Dhamija, A., Gunther, M., Ventura, J., Boult, T.: The overlooked elephant of object detection: Open set. In: Proceedings of the IEEE/CVF Winter Conference on Applications of Computer Vision, pp. 1021–1030 (2020)
3. Dong, N., Zhang, Y., Ding, M., Lee, G.H.: Open world detr: transformer based open world object detection. arXiv preprint arXiv:2212.02969 (2022)
4. Fang, R., Pang, G., Zhou, L., Bai, X., Zheng, J.: Unsupervised recognition of unknown objects for open-world object detection. arXiv preprint arXiv:2308.16527 (2023)
5. Graham, M.S., et al.: Denoising diffusion models for out-of-distribution detection. In: Proceedings of the IEEE/CVF Conference on Computer Vision and Pattern Recognition, pp. 2947–2956 (2023)
6. Gu, X., Lin, T.Y., Kuo, W., Cui, Y.: Open-vocabulary object detection via vision and language knowledge distillation. arXiv preprint arXiv:2104.13921 (2021)
7. Gupta, A., et al.: Ow-detr: Open-world detection transformer. In: Proceedings of the IEEE/CVF Conference on Computer Vision and Pattern Recognition, pp. 9235–9244 (2022)
8. He, K., Gkioxari, G., Dollár, P., Girshick, R.: Mask r-cnn. In: Proceedings of the IEEE international conference on computer vision, pp. 2961–2969 (2017)

9. He, K., Zhang, X., Ren, S., Sun, J.: Deep residual learning for image recognition. In: Proceedings of the IEEE conference on computer vision and pattern recognition, pp. 770–778 (2016)
10. Jiang, W., et al.: Read: Aggregating reconstruction error into out-of-distribution detection. In: Proceedings of the AAAI Conference on Artificial Intelligence, vol. 37, pp. 14910–14918 (2023)
11. Joseph, K., Khan, S., Khan, F.S., Balasubramanian, V.N.: Towards open world object detection. In: Proceedings of the IEEE/CVF conference on computer vision and pattern recognition, pp. 5830–5840 (2021)
12. Kirillov, A., et al.: Segment anything. arXiv preprint arXiv:2304.02643 (2023)
13. Lin, T.Y., Goyal, P., Girshick, R., He, K., Dollár, P.: Focal loss for dense object detection. In: Proceedings of the IEEE international conference on computer vision, pp. 2980–2988 (2017)
14. Lu, Y., Chen, X., Wu, Z., Yu, J.: Decoupled metric network for single-stage few-shot object detection. IEEE Transactions on Cybernetics **53**(1), 514–525 (2022)
15. Ma, S., et al.: Cat: Localization and identification cascade detection transformer for open-world object detection. In: Proceedings of the IEEE/CVF Conference on Computer Vision and Pattern Recognition, pp. 19681–19690 (2023)
16. Ren, S., He, K., Girshick, R., Sun, J.: Faster r-cnn: Towards real-time object detection with region proposal networks. Advances in neural information processing systems 28 (2015)
17. Uijlings, J.R., Van De Sande, K.E., Gevers, T., Smeulders, A.W.: Selective search for object recognition. Int. J. Comput. Vision **104**, 154–171 (2013)
18. Wang, X., et al.: Freesolo: Learning to segment objects without annotations. In: Proceedings of the IEEE/CVF Conference on Computer Vision and Pattern Recognition, pp. 14176–14186 (2022)
19. Wei, F., Gao, Y., Wu, Z., Hu, H., Lin, S.: Aligning pretraining for detection via object-level contrastive learning. Adv. Neural. Inf. Process. Syst. **34**, 22682–22694 (2021)
20. Wu, Y., Kirillov, A., Massa, F., Lo, W., Girshick, R.: Detectron2 [www document] (2019). URL https://github.com/facebookresearch/detectron2. Accessed 3 March 2021
21. Zhao, X., et al.: Revisiting open world object detection. IEEE Transactions on Circuits and Systems for Video Technology (2023)
22. Zhou, Y.: Rethinking reconstruction autoencoder-based out-of-distribution detection. In: Proceedings of the IEEE/CVF Conference on Computer Vision and Pattern Recognition, pp. 7379–7387 (2022)
23. Zhu, X., et al.: Deformable detr: Deformable transformers for end-to-end object detection. arXiv preprint arXiv:2010.04159 (2020)
24. Zitnick, C.L., Dollár, P.: Edge boxes: Locating object proposals from edges. In: Computer Vision–ECCV 2014: 13th European Conference, Zurich, Switzerland, September 6–12, 2014, Proceedings, Part V 13, pp. 391–405. Springer (2014)
25. Zohar, O., Wang, K.C., Yeung, S.: Prob: probabilistic objectness for open world object detection. In: Proceedings of the IEEE/CVF Conference on Computer Vision and Pattern Recognition, pp. 11444–11453 (2023)

Implementation and Application of Violence Detection System Based on Multi-head Attention and LSTM

Fengping Cao(✉), Yi Miao, and Wangyi Zhang

Southeast University Chengxian College, Nanjing 210000, JS, China
cfp423@126.com

Abstract. The extensive expansion of surveillance has enabled the identification of numerous threats in advance. By examining surveillance footage, violent activities can be identified in time to prevent disastrous repercussions. In this paper, a method for detecting violence is proposed. Initially, GoogLeNet is chosen for feature extraction in time and space based on the loss of pre-trained CNN feature extraction results and the running efficiency of each model. Some convolutional layers of GoogLeNet are frozen in accordance with the concept of migration learning to meet the demand for accurate feature extraction on tiny data sets. Multi-head Attention (MHA) was used in order to increase the model's precision and operating efficiency by focusing on key features. The results are then input into the long short-term memory (LSTM) violence detection model. In addition, an ablation study on the input characteristics was carried out, comparing the outcomes with and without the MHA. It revealed that including the MHA enhanced the outcomes by 7.31%. Finally, the model obtains 100% accuracy on the Daily Violence and Movies Fight datasets and 94.36% accuracy on the RWF-2000 dataset, which is commendable. As can be seen, our model on daily violence and Movies Fight has produced the best results, and it is 4% more accurate than the best method currently available for RWF-2000. To put the model in this paper to use in practice, we also created an Android application (APP). Violence in hospitals is common, but not all hospitals can deal with it promptly. Our APP can detect violent behavior in hospital surveillance videos in real time and promptly alert security officers. The usefulness is excellent.

Keywords: Violence Detection · Application · Multi-head Attention · LSTM

1 Introduction

Identification of human behavior is a topic of intense interest in computer vision. The detection of anomalies in contemporary intelligent video surveillance systems has a significant research value [1]. Violence detection, a key component of anomaly detection, has become an active study subject in computer vision, drawing a large number of researchers [2].

Research [3, 4] has shown that action recognition and behavior detection of videos using deep learning techniques are more efficient and accurate than manual monitoring.

With the progress of artificial intelligence, it is now possible to detect violence by convolutional neural networks (CNN) to extract and classify data at temporal and spatial levels [5]. To predict violent acts, Ullah FUM [6] et al. utilized lightweight CNN and an improved 3D-CNN model. CNN was employed as a spatial feature extractor and Long Short Term Memory Network (LSTM) [7] as a temporal feature extractor for a real-time violence detector by Abdali et al. [8]. For violence detection, Pang et al. [9] utilized an audiovisual dependency attention (AVD-attention) module. Nevertheless, the currently available approaches for violence detection cannot combine efficiency and precision.

In this paper, we use a pre-trained GoogLeNet to extract spatiotemporal video features. Then classify using LSTM. Subsequently, MHA is added to improve the model's precision and efficiency. Finally, we obtain a violence detection model. Using this model, a violence detection software application was designed for use in hospitals.

The rest of the paper is laid out as follows: Sect. 2 provides an overview of related works on abnormal behavior and violence detection. Section 3 demonstrates the proposed method in detail. Section 4 explains experiments, results, and application. Finally, Sect. 5 concludes our work.

2 Related Work

2.1 Abnormal Behavior Detection

Analysis and monitoring, recognition, and detection of abnormal human behavior have become one of the hot spots in the field of computer vision, which plays a crucial role in freeing up labor and boosting productivity. Researchers usually define aberrant behavior as unusual, unexpected, and unpredictable behavior that deviates from existing patterns [10]. Currently, approaches to abnormal behavior recognition are divided into two groups, one based on manual feature extraction and the other on deep network learning features.

The method based on manual feature extraction frequently employs traditional machine learning techniques. Its advantages lie in need-based orientation, strong pertinence, and simple implementation. However, as the necessity for recognizing aberrant activity develops, manual feature extraction can become increasingly time-consuming and ineffective.

Nowadays, deep feature-based models have achieved tremendous success in a variety of nonlinear high-dimensional data applications [11], including activity recognition and video summarization, etc. In the study of abnormal behavior detection, Deng et al. [12] presented a model of a "spatiotemporal auto-encoder". Deep neural networks were used to extract the movie's temporal and spatial data and learn the film's motion characteristics. Ma et al. [13] used YOLO for real-time detection and feature extraction of specified surveillance targets and then LSTM to make the final behavioral discrimination of behavioral action sequences. Zhou et al. [14] present a behavior recognition model based on spatiotemporal convolution (ST-CNN) and attention-based LSTM (ATT-LSTM). Integrating spatial information at a granular level into each network segment increases network recognition performance.

2.2 Violence Detection

As part of deviant behavior, violent acts, such as fights, assaults, and knife wounds, are included. Traditional methods for violence identification have largely centered on manually generated characteristics that indicate motion trajectory, limb orientation, local appearance, inter-frame variations, etc. Deniz et al. [15] proposed a hybrid "handcrafted/learned" feature framework, which used the Hough Forests classifier and 2DCNN.

Li et al. [16] suggested a 3D CNN based on the DenseNet architecture that requires fewer parameters and is more efficient. Halder et al. [17] used a Convolutional Neural Network-based Bidirectional LSTM for violence detection. This demonstrates that LSTM is a more prevalent classification method for violent behaviors. Mumtaz et al. [18] propose a deep representation-based violence scene detection model that uses the concept of transfer learning to identify human aggressive behavior. Results show the highest accuracies of 99.28% and 99.97% on Hockey Fight [19] and Movies Fight [20] datasets respectively. This demonstrates that migration learning and LSTM can yield superior results in the detection of violence.

3 Method

Each frame of the video is transformed into a 240 × 240 RGB picture with three channels. For temporal space feature extraction, the processed video frames are fed into a CNN model with partially frozen convolutional layers. The results are entered into a Long short-term memory (LSTM) model for the classification of violent and non-violent behaviors. To improve the accuracy of the model, we identify many significant video frame elements utilizing multi-headed attention (MHA) [21]. The outputs are fused with spatiotemporal information for feature fusion and then fed into an LSTM classifier. The overall model structure of this paper is shown in Fig. 1 In addition, the procedure is discussed in detail below.

3.1 Feature Extraction

Feature extraction is the main core in classification, clustering, recognition, and detection. Using useful feature variables can result in high performance, even if the machine learner is simple. In contrast, using unhelpful feature variables with an advanced complex machine learner might lead to decreased performance [22]. Therefore, it is important to choose a suitable feature extraction method to obtain features for each frame. There are numerous approaches to extracting features. Common methodologies in deep learning include Recurrent Neural Networks (RNNs), Autoencoders (AE), Convolutional Neural Networks (CNNs), Generative Adversarial Networks (GANs), and others.

Research [8, 22]indicates that CNNs perform better at behavior recognition. Meanwhile, the CNN models that performed well on ImageNet for glomerulus classification, mineral prospectivity prediction, object detection, etc. can also perform better. Transfer learning [23] is the process of transferring knowledge from one domain to another, in order to improve learning outcomes in the target domain. This paper utilizes a pre-trained CNN model for temporal and spatial information extraction from violent video clips.

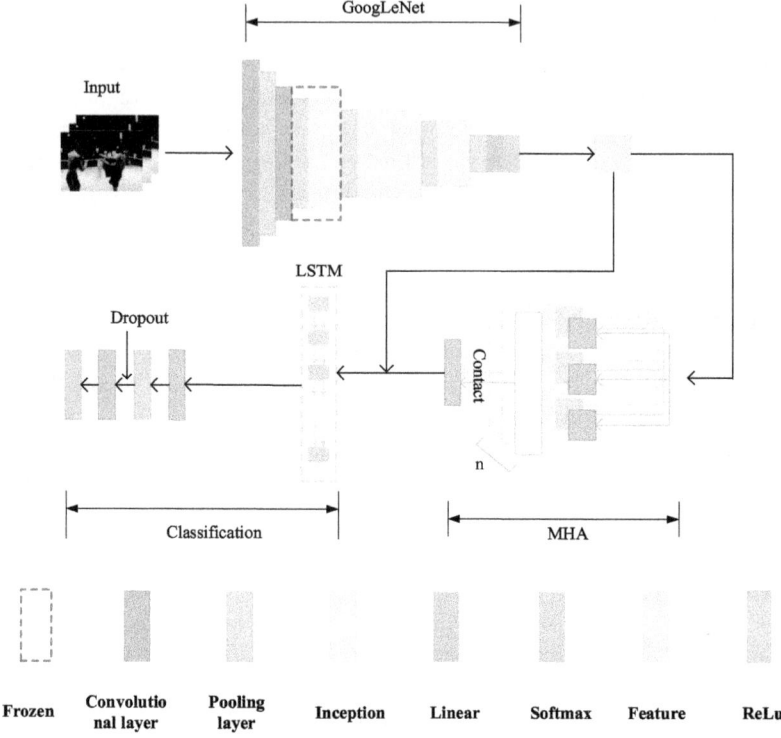

Fig. 1. Overall model structure

According to the requirement of real-time surveillance video monitoring, consideration is given to which pre-trained CNNs will be utilized for migration learning. In this study, VGG, which has more parameters and higher computational demand, was not selected as the pre-trained CNN model. Initially, ResNet, GoogLeNet, and DenseNet were chosen for training. They have excellent performance and consume less memory than VGG computation. ResNet is capable of avoiding gradient disappearance and preserving the original characteristics. GoogLeNet's global average pooling layer reduces parameters, while inception raises recognition accuracy and decreases overfitting. DenseNet uses dense connectivity to enhance feature reuse and mitigate gradient disappearance.

However, in some tiny datasets, it is inappropriate to employ large and deep models. In addition to causing arithmetic overload, it may also overfit the network and fail to produce a widely applicable model. Thus, in this paper, we consider frozen convolutional layers when employing a pre-trained CNN model. For smaller datasets, more convolutional layers are frozen to minimize the model depth, whereas, on larger datasets, fewer or no convolutional layers are frozen to place greater emphasis on precise feature extraction.

3.2 Optimization Using Attention Mechanism

The attention mechanism [24] is capable of focusing on the most important aspects of a huge amount of information while paying less attention to irrelevant details. After Vaswani et al. [21] proposed the Transformer structure in 2017, the attention mechanism is frequently implemented in models of neural network architectures. Attention mechanisms are present in domains such as picture caption creation, text categorization, action recognition, image-based analysis, etc. In this study, after employing CNN for feature extraction, we use an attention mechanism to zero out the most salient elements of violent actions.

Each frame offers a variety of information regarding the recognition of violence, such as knives, swinging fists, firearms, etc. It is not scientific to recognize only the smallest amount of information in a frame, as this will drastically lower the accuracy and applicability of the model. MHA enables the model to simultaneously attend to multiple sections of the input sequence, which can enhance the model's capacity to grasp complex dependencies and interactions within the data. Additionally, using MHA can provide greater flexibility in modeling different types of relationships within the data, like capturing both local and global dependencies. This can increase the efficiency of model detection while maintaining the model's precision. So, we employ MHA to concentrate on the most important information in each frame. Hence, the model's retrieved features are more representative.

The subsequent part will provide a concise overview of the concept of MHA. The specific steps are shown in the Fig. 2.

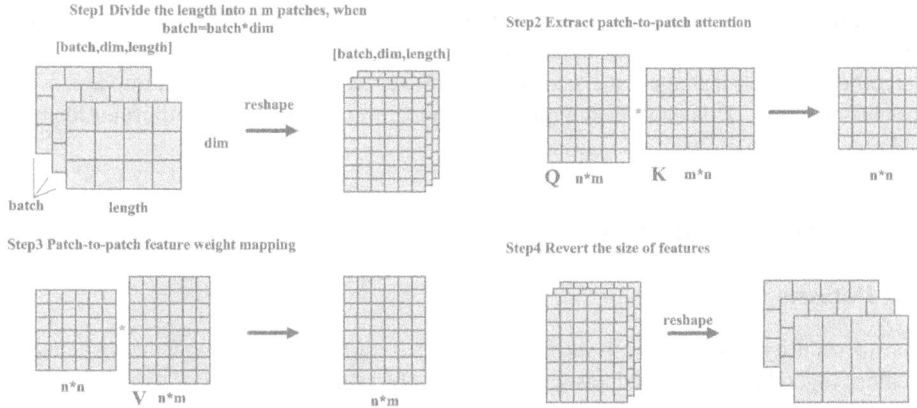

Fig. 2. Step in MHA

In The first step, the feature matrix that GoogleNet has extracted is entered into MHA. Its length is divided into n patches of length m. At this time, the batch becomes batch*dim. The input is divided into matrices that can be computed with MHA in this step. Additionally, a preliminary depiction of the violent behavior's characterization QVK is obtained. In the second step, the features between patches are extracted. Each layer comprises n blocks and each patch is of length m. To create a n*n feature matrix, multiply the Q matrix by its transposed K matrix. The inter-patch features are represented by this matrix. In the third step, doing the mapping of features to weights between patches. The V matrix is used to multiply the second step's outcome. In the second and third steps, the original features are split to get more detailed features. The relevance of the features is "ranked" by weighting them, emphasizing the primary features while ignoring the supporting ones. For instance, if swinging a fist is the primary characteristic of violent conduct, the higher weight is multiplied by its matrix. More focus is placed on it in the future detection process so that it is simpler to identify the occurrence of violent conduct using the many traits of human behavior.

After getting the extracted features, their dimensions are finally lifted to the input dimensions. The model can better focus on the key characteristics of a violent act thanks to feature extraction by MHA, which improves violence detection.

3.3 Classification

LSTM is a temporal recurrent neural network that processes time-dependent information well.

These are the specific phases of the original categorization presented in this research. First, the extracted features from the pre-trained CNN are used as the prediction input for the LSTM. The results of the prediction are input into the fully connected layer. With the Relu activation function, increase each neuron's expressiveness. Using the gradient descent process, the loss function's lowest point is identified. The results are then projected in two dimensions to the fully linked layer. Finally, the prediction is generated using the softmax function.

In this paper, the model is once again optimized to improve its precision. Using the MHA technique, the crucial information in the retrieved characteristics is extracted. The outcomes are then reshaped, merged with the retrieved features, and sent into an LSTM for classification. This enables the model to concentrate on the most important features and enhances the model's precision.

4 Experiment and Analysis

4.1 Datasets

Due to security and privacy issues, access to surveillance footage of the violence is challenging. The following datasets are frequently used in the field of violence detection: Crowd Violence [25], Hockey Fight [19], Movies Fight [20], and RWF-2000 [26]. Specific information for each dataset is shown in Table 1.

Crowd Violence Dataset is comprised of 246 segments of violent and non-violent activities in crowded, low-resolution situations. With the advancement of modern surveillance technologies, the resolution of surveillance video is now greater than that of Violent Flow, making its use for training models impractical. Hockey Fight Dataset is video captured from National Hockey League games, which contains some of the moves that might be involved in the fight. The Movies Fight Dataset contains footage of double fights from movies. RWF-2000 is a collection of 2,000 videos collected by surveillance

Table 1. The dataset used in this paper

Dataset	Data Scale	Resolution	Scenario
Movies Fight [20]	200 Clips	720*480	Movie
RWF-2000 [26]	2000 Clips	Variable	Surveillance
Hockey Fight [19]	1000 Clips	Variable	Hockey
Daily Violence	42 Clips	Variable	Natural

cameras in real-world circumstances, containing a variety of violent actions that are consistent with real-world scenarios. A model generated from it as a training dataset is capable of detecting a variety of violent behaviors in daily life.

To improve the detection of violent behavior, this study collects behavioral patterns from the web to produce a Dataset titled Daily Violence, which spans numerous scenarios. It contains both violent and non-violent behaviors in a crowded area and activities involving two combatants. Videos are captured from real-life security footage or from movies that show daily life. For example, in the same scene, we artificially distinguish its violent and non-violent actions.

The successful identification of these behaviors has positive implications for the application of the model in this paper.

4.2 Experiment

The hardware environment used for the experiment is as follows:

- CPU: i7-10710U 1.10 GHz
- GPU: NVIDIA Geforce MX350; P100 on Kaggle

We utilized Restnet34, DenseNet121, and GoogLeNet for feature extraction on the Movies Fight dataset, respectively, to determine a suitable CNN model. Since there are only 200 clips in Movies Fight, we freeze the same proportion of convolutional layers for each training model. Given that freezing different convolutional layers could result in different feature extraction outcomes, we evaluated each model multiple times and then calculated the mean. The final cross-entropy loss was used to judge which model had superior results for feature extraction.

Figure 3 displays the results, with the loss of GoogLeNet being the lowest at 0.36. GoogLeNet is therefore selected for feature extraction in this work.

In the process of behavioral classification, various activation functions and hidden layers provide various outcomes. Numerous experiments have shown that, in short-batch datasets, a mere 40 hidden layers are needed for accurate video classification. Stated differently, detecting violence in tiny areas can yield greater results with fewer resources. Whereas in RWF-2000, more hidden layers are used for classification. However, adding more hidden layers all at once does not provide desirable outcomes. 200 hidden layers were employed in one experiment, which not only wasted a lot of resources but also produced subpar results.

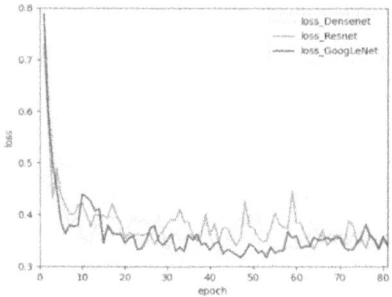 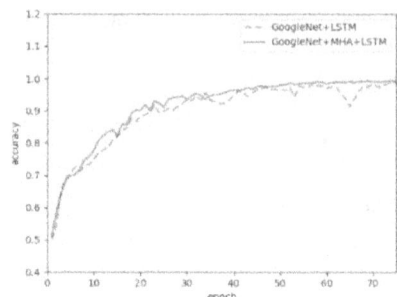

Fig. 3. Losses with different CNNs   **Fig. 4.** Model accuracy before and after enhancement in RWF-2000

To assess the performance of our model, it was implemented on three datasets. After dividing the dataset into training (80%) and testing (20%), the model was used for detection. Finally, the accuracy of the tests for Daily Violence and Movies Fight both reached 100 percent. Nonetheless, the outcomes of RWF-2000 were disappointing. So, we added the MHA module and retested it. Figure 4 shows a line graph depicting the change in accuracy before and after the improvement.

As seen in Fig. 4, the addition of attention somewhat improves the model's convergence speed. What's more, the mean recall rate before improvement was 0.951 after improvement was 0.967. In the meantime, the accuracy rate rises from 87.05 percent to 94.36 percent. As seen in Table 2, our model outperforms others.

Table 2. Comparison of accuracy on datasets

Model/Dataset	RWF-2000	Movie Fights	Hockey Fight	Daily Violence
ConvLSTM [3]	77%	100%	97.10%	-
I3D (Optical-flow only) [27]	75.50%	100%	-	-
Cheng et al. (P3D) [26]	87.20%	100%	98%	-
SSHA model (RGB only) [28]	90.40%	99%	98%	-
SSHA model (Optical-flow only) [28]	76%	98.50%	86.20%	-
Ours	94.30%	100%	98%	100%

The above accuracy rates are explained in this study. Movies Fight is easier to categorize because it only consists of one scene, has a small amount of high-definition clips overall, and primarily features two people performing violent activities in a single scene. Therefore, most approaches produce superior outcomes. The above accuracy rates are examined in this study.

Movie Fights is easier to categorize because it only consists of one scene, has a small amount of high-definition clips overall, and primarily features two people performing violent activities in a single scene. Therefore, most approaches produce superior outcomes. The accuracy percentage is greater in Hockey Fight because the majority of the videos feature two-person incidents of violence in lesser resolution.

Nonetheless, the majority of the movies in RWF-2000 have diverse settings, colors, and definitions. The span is very large, which is a good reproduction of the diversity of video sources in daily life. Owing to the wide range of movies, it is required to convert the videos to the same size and color. The information currently has a certain loss, which affects the outcome as well. Despite having a tiny sample size, Daily Violence offers a wide variety of video formats. High-resolution films of individuals acting violently or peacefully in pairs, multiples, and masses were gathered. It is also clearly detectable by our model. We will also gather more information for the dataset in the future so that we can finish this job more effectively.

4.3 Application

The purpose of violence detection is to reduce damage. When violence happens, if the relevant staff notices it in a timely manner and takes the necessary steps to prevent it from continuing, or if the victim is treated in a timely way. Then, violence would not divide so many families from one another.

Thus, we design an app for hospitals that detects violence based on the model presented in this research. Use this model to detect surveillance video. When an odd incident is identified, the app will notify hospital security officers in time for them to respond. With the app, security staff can view the location details of the violent occurrence and

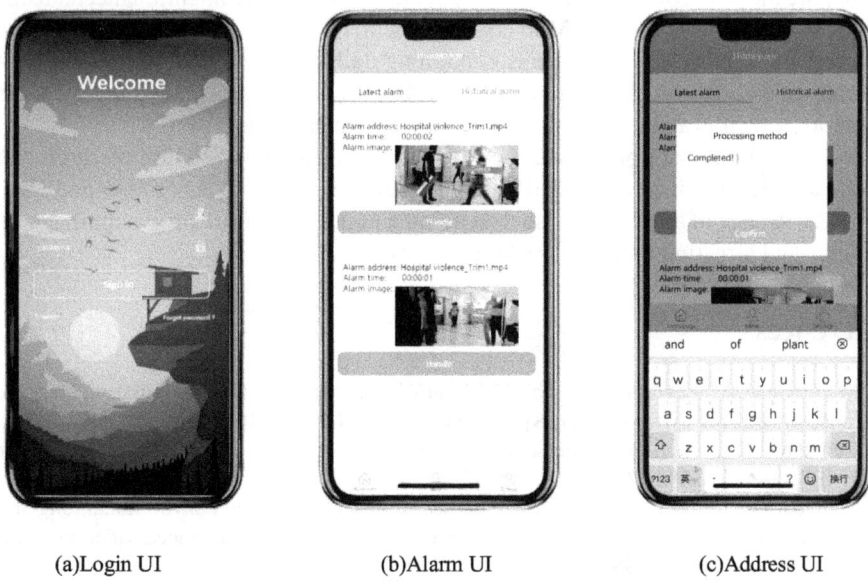

(a)Login UI   (b)Alarm UI   (c)Address UI

Fig. 5. The main UI of the application

the live scenario map, allowing them to make more informed decisions about how to respond.

The Android application is built using the GSON framework and Android Jetpack. Focusing on the user experience, it satisfies use criteria while being simple and straightforward. The main UI of the APP is shown in Fig. 5. The web-facing management information of the backend is developed using Spring Boot. Within the application, the administrator can manage the content of notifications, user information, alarm information, etc.

The database connects the detection model and APP to create a three-tier design. When the model identifies violence, the location and site information are saved to the database, and the APP is refreshed every 0.1s to receive the database information. This enables the detection of violence in surveillance footage in real-time and the notification of the appropriate staff for processing.

5 Conclusion

In this paper, a methodology for detecting violence is laid out and applied practically. The model's processing phases are as follows. In terms of picture recognition, models like GoogLeNet, DenseNet, ResNet, and others perform well. Based on the concept of transfer learning, we apply it to the detection of violent behavior in surveillance videos. We perform feature extraction separately using them and conclude that GoogLeNet is the most effective in this regard based on the loss. To improve model accuracy on smaller datasets such as Movies Fight, we freeze part of the convolutional layer of GoogLeNet for feature extraction. The extracted features are then subjected to ablation experiments to compare the effect of including or excluding the multi-headed attention mechanism on the results. Finally, we use LSTM to classify whether an act is violent or not. Our model achieved 100% accuracy on datasets containing daily violence and Movies Fight. An accuracy of 94.36% was achieved on RWF-2000, which contains many types of violent behaviors, which is about 4% higher than that of Mohammadi et al. [28].

Our model does not process facial recognition for tracking. Future research could include a face recognition module to better reduce the impact of violent events and expand our model's range of applications, such as helping police officers identify ongoing violent incidents and targeting them for tracking.

References

1. Mabrouk, A.B., Zagrouba, E.: Abnormal behavior recognition for intelligent video surveillance systems: A review. Expert Syst. Appl. **91**, 480–491 (2018)
2. Ramzan, M., et al.: A review on state-of-the-art violence detection techniques. IEEE Access **7**, 107560–107575 (2019)
3. Sudhakaran, S., Lanz, O.: Learning to detect violent videos using convolutional long short-term memory. In: 2017 14th IEEE international conference on advanced video and signal based surveillance (AVSS), pp. 1–6. IEEE (2017)
4. Tran, D., Bourdev, L., Fergus, R., Torresani, L., Paluri, M.: Learning spatiotemporal features with 3d convolutional networks. In: Proceedings of the IEEE international conference on computer vision, pp. 4489–4497 (2015)

5. Traor´e, A., Akhloufi, M.A.: Violence detection in videos using deep recurrent and convolutional neural networks. In: 2020 IEEE International Conference on Systems, Man, and Cybernetics (SMC), pp. 154–159. IEEE (2020)
6. Ullah, F.U.M., Ullah, A., Muhammad, K., Haq, I.U., Baik, S.W.: Violence detection using spatiotemporal features with 3d convolutional neural network. Sensors **19**(11), 2472 (2019)
7. Hochreiter, S., Schmidhuber, J.: Long short-term memory. Neural Comput. **9**(8), 1735–1780 (1997)
8. Abdali, A.M.R., Al-Tuma, R.F.: Robust real-time violence detection in video using cnn and lstm. In: 2019 2nd Scientific Conference of Computer Sciences (SCCS), pp. 104–108. IEEE (2019)
9. Pang, W., Xie, W., He, Q., Li, Y., Yang, J.: Audiovisual dependency attention for violence detection in videos. IEEE Transactions on Multimedia, pp. 1–12 (2022)
10. Khaleghi, A., Moin, M.S.: Improved anomaly detection in surveillance videos based on a deep learning method. In: 2018 8th Conference of AI and Robotics and 10th RoboCup Iranopen International Symposium (IRANOPEN), pp. 73–81. IEEE (2018)
11. Ullah, W., Ullah, A., Hussain, T., Khan, Z.A., Baik, S.W.: An efficient anomaly recognition framework using an attention residual lstm in surveillance videos. Sensors **21**(8), 2811 (2021)
12. Zhao, Y., et al.: Spatio-temporal autoencoder for video anomaly detection. In: Proceedings of the 25th ACM international conference on Multimedia, pp. 1933–1941 (2017)
13. Ma, Y., Tan Li, D.X., Chong, Y.C.: Behavior recognition for intelligent surveillance, pp. 282–290 (2019)
14. Zhou, K., Hui, B., Wang, J., Wang, C., Wu, T.: A study on attention-based lstm for abnormal behavior recognition with variable pooling. Image Vis. Comput. **108**, 104120 (2021)
15. Serrano, I., Deniz, O., Espinosa-Aranda, J.L., Bueno, G.: Fight recognition in video using hough forests and 2d convolutional neural network. IEEE Trans. Image Process. **27**(10), 4787–4797 (2018)
16. Li, J., Jiang, X., Sun, T., Xu, K.: Efficient violence detection using 3d convolutional neural networks. In: 2019 16th IEEE International Conference on Advanced Video and Signal Based Surveillance (AVSS), pp. 1–8 (2019)
17. Halder, R., Chatterjee, R.: CNN-BiLSTM model for violence detection in smart surveillance. SN Computer Science **1**(4), 201 (2020)
18. Mumtaz, A., Sargano, A.B., Habib, Z.: Violence detection in surveillance videos with deep network using transfer learning. In: 2018 2nd European Conference on Electrical Engineering and Computer Science (EECS), pp. 558–563 (2018)
19. Bermejo Nievas, E., Deniz Suarez, O., Bueno Garc´ıa, G., Sukthankar, R.: Violence detection in video using computer vision techniques. In: Computer Analysis of Images and Patterns: 14th International Conference, CAIP 2011, Seville, Spain, August 29–31, 2011, Proceedings, Part II 14, pp. 332–339. Springer (2011)
20. Nievas, E.B., Suarez, O.D., Garcia, G.B., Sukthankar, R.: Movies fight detection dataset. In: Computer Analysis of Images and Patterns, pp. 332–339. Springer (2011)
21. Vaswani, A., et al.: Attention is all you need. Adv. Neural Info. Proc. Sys. **30** (2017)
22. Ko, K.E., Sim, K.B.: Deep convolutional framework for abnormal behavior detection in a smart surveillance system. Eng. Appl. Artif. Intell. **67**, 226–234 (2018)
23. Pan, S.J., Yang, Q.: A survey on transfer learning. IEEE Trans. Knowl. Data Eng. **22**(10), 1345–1359 (2010)
24. Mnih, V., Heess, N., Graves, A., et al.: Recurrent models of visual attention. Adv. Neural Info. Proce. Sys. **27** (2014)
25. Hassner, T., Itcher, Y., Kliper-Gross, O.: Violent flows: Real-time detection of violent crowd behavior. In: 2012 IEEE Computer Society Conference on Computer Vision and Pattern Recognition Workshops, pp. 1–6. IEEE, Providence, RI, USA (2012)

26. Cheng, M., Cai, K., Li, M.: Rwf-2000: an open large scale video database for violence detection. In: 2020 25th International Conference on Pattern Recognition (ICPR), pp. 4183–4190. IEEE (2021)
27. Carreira, J., Zisserman, A.: Quo vadis, action recognition? a new model and the kinetics dataset. In: proceedings of the IEEE Conference on Computer Vision and Pattern Recognition, pp. 6299–6308 (2017)
28. Mohammadi, H., Nazerfard, E.: Video violence recognition and localization using a semi-supervised hard attention model. Expert Syst. Appl. **212**, 118791 (2023)

GFFNet: An Efficient Image Denoising Network with Group Feature Fusion

Lijun Gao[1], Youzhi Zhang[1(✉)], Xiao Jin[1], Qin Xin[2], Zeyang Sun[1], and Suran Wang[1]

[1] College of Computer Science, Shenyang Aerospace University, Shenyang 110136, China
zhangyouzhi@stu.sau.edu.cn
[2] Faculty of Science and Technology, University of the Faroe Islands, Faroe Islands, Denmark

Abstract. Image denoising is a critical pre-processing step for a wide range of image processing and computer vision applications, where the primary goal is to remove noise interference from corrupted images while preserving the essential features of the image. Although recent research has made significant progress in images denoising using deep learning methods, problems such as loss of detail, difficulty in recovering edge textures, and low image processing performance still persist. To tackle these issues, we develop an effective network architecture. This study introduces a Group Feature Fusion (GFF) module, which leverages image feature grouping and fusion techniques to enhance the representation capacity and computational efficiency of features in our network. Additionally, this artical introduce a Cross-Information Integration (CII) Module to enhance the network's ability to utilize input data features by integrating low-level and high-level channel information. Finally, the network was enhanced in its effectiveness for edge texture restoration by optimizing it with the PSNR loss function in conjunction with a novel edge loss function. This architecture achieves significant performance improvements on nine benchmark test datasets for image denoising tasks. Extensive experiments have demonstrated the efficiency and superior performance of this architecture.

Keywords: Image Denoising · Computer Vision · Deep Learning

1 Introduction

Recent advancements in deep learning techniques have greatly enhanced image denoising. Utilizing Convolutional Neural Networks (CNNs) [1–3] and Transformers [23, 33], these models effectively capture complex image features and noise distribution patterns, resulting in more accurate noise removal. Several image denoising methods based on deep learning have yielded remarkable results, including Auto-encoder [2, 4], Generative Adversarial Networks (GAN) [28], and Transformer-based encoder-decoder networks [6, 7, 29], offering innovative solutions for the task.

Preserving image details and texture while removing noise is crucial in image denoising. Although deep learning boosts denoising effectiveness via abundant data and high representation, challenges persist in detail preservation and computational efficiency.

Hence, current research focuses on improving denoising efficiency while retaining image details. This entails exploring efficient network architectures, optimization algorithms, and acceleration techniques to reduce computational load and parameters, thus improving real-time performance and scalability.

In this paper, we propose an enhanced denoising network by incorporating the GFF module and CII module into U-Net architecture and optimizing them with a novel loss function. Major contributions include:

- We introduce the Group Feature Fusion (GFF) module, dividing channels into two subprocesses for joint processing across different channels, leveraging inter-channel correlations to enhance denoising accuracy and computational efficiency.
- We developed a Cross-Information Integration (CII) module to enhance feature transfer across layers and introduce additional pathways for information flow. This module effectively merges low-level features from the encoder with high-level features from the upsampling module, transmitting them to the decoder for enhanced processing. The goal is to enrich captured details and minimize information loss across the network architecture.
- By combining the edge loss function with the PSNR loss function, we've optimized the network to markedly improve its ability to restore intricate edge textures in images.

2 Related Work

2.1 Convolutional Neural Network

Recent advancements in image denoising leveraging deep learning, particularly Convolutional Neural Networks (CNNs), have shown remarkable progress. These models can learn intricate features and noise distributions, leading to more precise and resilient denoising outcomes. For example, Zhang et al. [2] achieved efficient denoising through multi-layer convolution and residual connections, while Guo et al. [3] introduced a CNN-based blind denoising method for real photograph noise, demonstrating strong performance on real-world datasets. However, CNNs employed in denoising may inadvertently blur image edges and details due to the local receptive field of convolution operations and information loss from pooling. Additionally, some complex CNN architectures demand substantial computational resources and memory, limiting real-time application in resource-constrained environments.

2.2 U-Net Network

The U-Net network excels in image denoising due to its robust feature extraction, skip connections for information propagation, and effective contextual information usage. Ronneberger et al.'s U-Net architecture [5] is widely adopted and achieves remarkable denoising results. Researchers have adapted U-Net's structure and concept for denoising tasks, yielding significant improvements. For example, Fan et al. [6] proposed SUNet, integrating Swin Transformer layers into U-Net for enhanced performance. Wang et al. [8] introduced Uformer, replacing convolutional layers with Transformers in a U-Net structure, achieving exceptional results in image restoration. U-Net's flexibility allows customization for various denoising tasks, adjusting model complexity and capacity by adding or removing layers [7, 8, 22, 23, 29].

3 Method

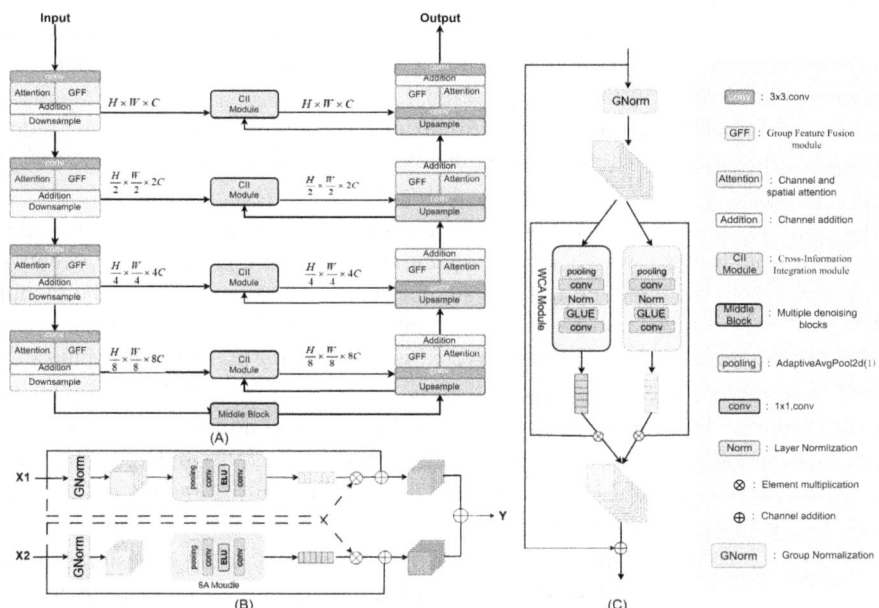

Fig. 1. GFFNet framework diagram. (A) shows the overall framework diagram, (B) shows the CII module and (C) displays the GFF module.

3.1 Network Architecture

In this section, we provide a comprehensive description of our meticulously designed denoising network model for efficient image restoration. As depicted in Fig. 1(A), our model adopts a U-Net-based architecture, consisting of four well-balanced encoder-decoder levels. When presented with a noisy image $I \in \mathbb{R}^{H \times W \times 3}$, we employ convolutions to extract low-level features $F_0 \in \mathbb{R}^{H \times W \times C}$. Subsequently, these features F_0 undergo denoising operations through the integration of Group Feature Fusion (GFF) modules and Attention modules within the encoder. The resulting denoised features from both modules are then fused together. Moreover, the image features F_0 are further processed through downsampling operations to obtain $F_1 \in \mathbb{R}^{\frac{H}{2} \times \frac{W}{2} \times 2C}$. This multi-scale processing is iteratively performed, yielding $F_3 \in \mathbb{R}^{\frac{H}{8} \times \frac{W}{8} \times 8C}$, and so forth. The intermediate layers further refine the features F_3, which are subsequently fed into the decoder for the corresponding operations. Ultimately, the processed features F_3 generate the denoised image $\tilde{I} \in \mathbb{R}^{H \times W \times 3}$.

3.2 Group Feature Fusion (GFF) Module

The Group Feature Fusion (GFF) module is designed for image denoising, aiming to reduce noise and preserve intricate image details through orchestrated operations like normalization, channel segmentation, convolution, weight calculation, and fusion. Shown in Fig. 1(C), this module effectively manipulates feature maps to alleviate noise effects and enhance overall image quality. By intelligently segmenting and combining channel information, along with weight calculation and fusion, the GFF module selectively processes distinct features from different channels, resulting in precise denoising outcomes and preserved intricate image details.

This module initially applies group normalization to the input image to remove redundant information across channels. Subsequently, the normalized image $X \in \mathbb{R}^{H \times W \times C}$ is segmented into $X_1 \in \mathbb{R}^{H \times W \times \frac{C}{2}}$ and $X_2 \in \mathbb{R}^{H \times W \times \frac{C}{2}}$ based on channels.

To determine the importance weights for each group of channels, the WCA module is used to compute these weights. The module extracts and computes the weights of each channel from the input tensor for weighted fusion operations. Firstly, the module performs adaptive average pooling on each channel group by reducing its dimensionality to $X^* \in \mathbb{R}^{1 \times 1 \times C}$. Next, a convolutional layer is used to map the pooled feature map $X^* \in \mathbb{R}^{1 \times 1 \times C}$ to a lower dimensional channel space becoming $X^{**} \in \mathbb{R}^{1 \times 1 \times \frac{C}{2}}$. Following this, the output of the convolutional layer undergoes channel normalization to enhance model stability and generalization. Finally, the normalized features undergo a nonlinear transformation using the GELU activation function. Additionally, the number of channels of the feature map is restored to be consistent with the number of channels of the input tensor by another convolutional layer, i.e., $X^{**} \in \mathbb{R}^{1 \times 1 \times \frac{C}{2}}$ is restored to the form $X^* \in \mathbb{R}^{1 \times 1 \times C}$. The channel weights are computed and then mapped to their corresponding channel groups, resulting in a weighted fusion operation.

$$\overline{X_1} = X_1 \cdot WCA(X_1), \overline{X_2} = X_2 \cdot WCA(X_2) \tag{1}$$

where $\overline{X_1}$ and $\overline{X_2}$ represent the weighted outputs of each group of channels, and $WCA(\cdot)$ represents the module in which the channel weights are calculated.

Finally, the weighted fused channel sets are spliced by channel dimension and added to the original input image through residual linking.

3.3 Cross-Information Integration (CII) Module

The Cross-Information Integration (CII) module begins with normalizing the input to ensure consistent statistical properties. Next, features are extracted via a convolutional layer with a "groups" parameter for feature localization. To enhance information flow and fusion between encoder and decoder, this module normalizes the feature maps of both inputs, reducing redundancy and enhancing stability. It employs the Simple Attention (SA) module to calculate channel weights, reducing dimensionality to 1×1 using average pooling and convolution to halve channel numbers, reducing complexity. ELU activation introduces nonlinearity, handling negative noise and preventing mapping to zero values, aiding detail preservation and mitigating the vanishing gradient problem. A subsequent convolution operation restores the original channel count for precise feature scaling and fusion.

$$ELU(x) = \begin{cases} e^x - 1 & x < 0 \\ x & x \geq 0 \end{cases} \tag{2}$$

$$W_1 = SA(LN(X_1)), W_2 = SA(LN(X_2)) \tag{3}$$

In this network, X_1 and X_2 represent the encoder output and the upsampling module output, respectively. $SA(\cdot)$ calculates the weights of the feature map channels, and $LN(\cdot)$ performs the normalization operation.

Element-wise multiplication is employed to multiply the features from the encoder and upsampling modules by their respective weights following feature scaling and fusion weight acquisition. This process realizes the weighted fusion of encoder and upsampling features. The ultimate output features result from adding the weighted fused features to the original input.

3.4 Network Optimization

To guide the model in the right learning direction, accelerate convergence, and improve generalization ability, we first optimize it using the L_1 loss function, which measures the difference between the reconstructed image and the original clean image. By minimizing this loss, the network is compelled to learn to generate denoised images that closely resemble the clean original images. This encourages the network to learn the details and structure required for denoising tasks, thereby improving the denoising performance.

Our experiments have shown that using L_1 loss as the loss function results in the loss of details and high frequency texture information in the denoised image. To prevent this, we use PSNR loss as the reconstruction loss function and edge loss to preserve edge texture information between X and Y. The overall loss function is designed as follows:

$$Loss = \lambda_1 \cdot L_{PSNR} + \lambda_2 \cdot L_{Edge} \tag{4}$$

By adjusting λ_1 and λ_2, we control the importance of the two loss functions in the composite loss, balancing low-level pixel reconstruction quality (PSNR loss) with high-level structural similarity (edge loss) during network optimization. PSNR loss focuses on pixel-level details, while edge loss emphasizes structural preservation, ensuring clear pixel details and good structural sense. Setting λ_1 to 0.9 and λ_2 to 0.1 in experiments, we tailor the significance of the loss functions, enhancing training effectiveness and generation results.

$$L_{PSNR} = 10 \cdot log_{10}(\frac{MAX_I^2}{MSE}) \tag{5}$$

where, m, n is the spatial dimension of the image, MSE is the mean square error, and PSNR is derived based on MSE, and MAX_I is the maximum value that indicates the color of an image point(If each sampling point is represented by 8 bits, its value is 255.). The edge loss function L_{Edge} is denoted as:

$$L_{Edge} = SmoothL_1(\nabla X, \nabla Y) \tag{6}$$

where, L_{Edge} is mainly derived using $SmoothL_1$ loss and $\nabla X, \nabla Y$ are the edge gradients of the noisy and real images respectively. The L_{Edge} loss adds the consideration of image structure information. By extracting and comparing the blurred edges of the image gradient, the quality of image reconstruction can be effectively measured.

4 Experiment

4.1 Experimental Details

The following is a description of our experimental setup, unless otherwise noted. In the image denoising task, the number of blocks for each stage of the encoder and decoder in this network is set to {2, 2, 4, 8} and {2, 2, 2, 2}. For the Group Feature Fusion (GFF) Module, the number of groups is set to 2 by default. We used the Adam optimizer and the PyTorch framework for training (where $\beta_1 = 0.9$, $\beta_2 = 0.9$, and weight decay is 0). The total number of iterations was 500 K, and the initial learning rate was set to 1e-3 and gradually decreased to 1e-7. We used 256 × 256 training patches and set the batch size to 8. Finally, in our experiments, we used peak signal-to-noise ratio (PSNR) and structural similarity (SSIM) as evaluation metrics. Among them, the best results are marked in bold.

4.2 Gaussian Noise Cancellation

This study utilized the DIV2K dataset for training Gaussian denoising, consisting of 1000 high-resolution images. From these, 256 × 256 sized patches were randomly cropped and Gaussian noise (15–50 range) added for training. The network was trained on 700, validated on 150, and tested on 150 images. Evaluation during testing covered various image types using standard test sets.

Table 1 presents denoising results for grayscale images. We tested on standard sets (Set12, BSD68, Urban100) at noise levels of 15, 25, and 50, evaluating using PSNR and visual inspection, comparing with classical methods. Our approach achieved state-of-the-art performance, particularly outperforming others at high noise levels. Visual comparisons at noise level 25 (Fig. 2) show our network's ability to recover richer details and produce more realistic images than classical methods.

In the context of color image denoising, our experiment evaluated performance on established benchmark datasets: CBSD68, Kodak24, and McMaster. Applying the same

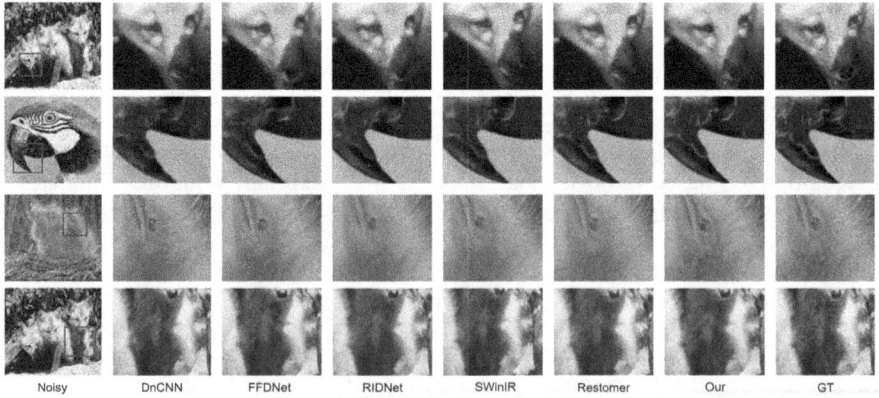

Fig. 2. Gaussian noise removal(where Noisy is the noisy image and GT is the real image)

testing conditions as for grayscale images, we consistently observed commendable denoising performance. Visual results in Fig. 2 vividly illustrate the network's effectiveness in recovering texture information, demonstrating its proficiency in color image denoising.

Table 1. Gaussian gray scale image denoising.

Method	Set12			BSD68			Urban100		
	$\sigma=15$	$\sigma=25$	$\sigma=50$	$\sigma=15$	$\sigma=25$	$\sigma=50$	$\sigma=15$	$\sigma=25$	$\sigma=50$
DnCNN [2]	32.67	30.35	27.18	31.62	29.16	26.23	32.28	29.80	26.35
FFDNet [4]	32.75	30.43	27.32	31.63	29.19	26.29	32.40	29.90	26.50
IRCNN [11]	32.76	30.37	27.12	31.63	29.15	26.19	32.46	29.80	26.22
RIDNet [12]	–	–	–	31.81	29.34	26.40	–	–	–
DRUNet [13]	33.25	30.94	27.90	31.91	29.48	26.59	32.44	31.11	27.96
DRANet [18]	–	–	–	31.79	29.36	26.47	–	–	–
SwinIR [24]	33.36	31.01	27.91	31.97	29.50	26.58	33.70	31.30	27.98
Restormer [29]	**33.42**	31.08	28.00	31.96	29.52	26.62	**33.79**	31.46	28.29
Our	33.41	**31.13**	**28.06**	**32.00**	**29.58**	**26.65**	**33.79**	**31.52**	**28.32**

Table 2. Gaussian color image denoising.

Method	CBSD68			Kodak24			McMaster		
	$\sigma=15$	$\sigma=25$	$\sigma=50$	$\sigma=15$	$\sigma=25$	$\sigma=50$	$\sigma=15$	$\sigma=25$	$\sigma=50$
DnCNN [2]	33.90	31.24	27.95	34.60	32.14	28.95	33.45	31.52	28.62
FFDNet [4]	33.87	31.21	27.96	34.63	32.13	28.98	34.66	32.35	29.18
IRCNN [11]	33.86	31.16	27.86	34.69	32.18	28.93	34.58	32.18	28.91
DRANet [18]	34.18	31.56	28.37	35.02	32.59	29.50	35.09	32.84	29.77
BRDNet [20]	34.10	31.43	28.16	34.88	32.41	29.22	35.08	32.75	29.52
SwinIR [24]	**34.42**	31.78	28.56	35.34	32.89	29.79	35.61	33.20	30.22
Restormer [29]	34.39	31.78	**28.59**	35.44	33.02	30.00	35.55	**33.31**	30.29
AirNet [30]	33.92	31.26	28.01	34.68	32.21	29.06	34.70	32.44	29.26
ADNet [31]	33.99	31.31	28.04	34.76	32.26	29.10	34.93	32.56	29.36
Our	34.41	**31.80**	28.58	**35.48**	**33.05**	**30.03**	**35.65**	**33.31**	**30.33**

4.3 Real Image Denoising

This study trained the network using the SIDD dataset to denoise real images, enabling the model to learn to remove complex real-world noise. Evaluation involved multiple standard test datasets like SIDD, DND, and SenseNoise, covering diverse real-world scenarios and shooting conditions, comprehensively assessing the method's generalization performance.

SIDD. Using the SIDD benchmark with 1280 color images for validation, we assess our method's performance in real-world denoising tasks. Table 3 demonstrates our network's superior results compared to 10 denoising algorithms, particularly outperforming other CNN-based methods. Visual comparisons reveal our network's ability to restore richer colors and texture details, with sharper image edges compared to alternative methods (Table 2 and Fig. 3).

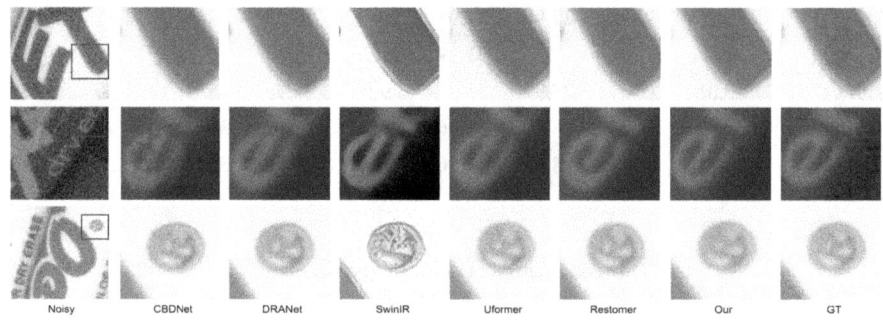

Fig. 3. Visualization and comparison of denoising results on SIDD dataset.

DND. Our method was evaluated on the DND dataset consisting of 50 pairs of real noisy images and corresponding clean references. Since no training data was available in the DND dataset, we trained our model using the SIDD dataset. We employed the same model that performed best on the SIDD benchmark and submitted the results to the DND benchmark. Table 3 shows that our method outperformed other networks on the DND dataset.

SenseNoise. The SenseNoise dataset comprises training and test sets. Training set: 39,345 pairs of real noisy and clean images. Test set: real noisy and clean images from 120 scenes, diverse in types, scenes, and lighting conditions. Our experiments compare denoising techniques' effectiveness in recovering image clarity and detail. Evaluation based on denoised images and quantitative metrics like PSNR and SSIM, alongside visual perception assessment. Results presented in Table 3 and Fig. 4.

Table 3. Denoising results demonstrated on three standard real noisy image test sets.

Method	SIDD		DND		SenseNoise	
	PSNR	SSIM	PSNR	SSIM	PSNR	SSIM
DnCNN [2]	23.66	0.583	32.43	0.790	34.06	0.904
CBDNet [3]	30.78	0.801	38.06	0.942	–	–
NBNet [7]	39.75	0.973	39.89	0.955	–	–
Uformer [8]	39.77	0.956	39.80	0.954	35.43	0.920
RIDNet [12]	38.71	0.951	39.26	0.953	34.88	0.915
BM3D [14]	25.65	0.685	34.51	0.851	–	–
MPRNet [22]	39.71	0.958	39.88	0.956	35.43	0.922
Restomer [29]	40.02	0.960	40.03	0.956	35.52	0.924
MIRNet [32]	39.72	0.956	39.80	0.954	35.30	0.919
SADNet [33]	39.46	0.957	39.59	0.952	–	–
Our	**40.28**	**0.967**	**40.26**	**0.961**	**35.58**	**0.927**

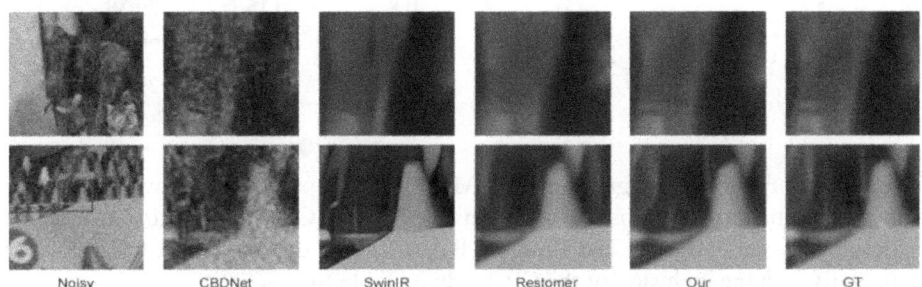

Fig. 4. Comparison of denoising results visualization in SenseNoise dataset.

4.4 Ablation Experiment

We conducted extensive ablation studies to validate the effectiveness of our method. All ablation studies were conducted based on Gaussian denoising. We trained the model for 150,000 iterations. The other training settings were kept consistent with the main experiments of Gaussian denoising on color images.

Group Feature Fusion (GFF) Module. In this experiment, the network architecture incorporating the Group Feature Fusion (GFF) Module was compared with the baseline model for gaussian denoising tasks. As shown in Table 4(a), the peak signal-to-noise ratio(PSNR) significantly increased by 0.11 dB when introducing the Group Feature Fusion (GFF) Module compared to the baseline model.

Table 4. Comparison of each module

Network	PSNR
Baseline	29.36
(a)Baseline + GFF	29.47
(b)Baseline + CII	29.45
(c)Baseline + GFF + CII	29.55
(d)Baseline + GFF + Loss	29.52
(e)Baseline + GFF + CII + Loss	**29.64**

Table 5. Loss function selection

Loss Function	PSNR
PSNR Loss	29.36
L1 Loss	29.19
Edge Loss	29.15
L1 + Edge Loss	29.30
PSNR + Edge Loss	**29.41**

Table 6. The selection of λ_1 and λ_2 in the loss

λ_1	λ_2	PSNR
0.95	0.05	29.39
0.9	0.1	**29.41**
0.85	0.15	29.38
0.8	0.2	29.37
0.5	0.5	29.34

Cross – Information Integration(CII) Module. Comparing the network structure with the addition of the cross-information Integration (CII) Module to the baseline model in gaussian denoising task (Table 4(B)), it's noted that the PSNR has increased by 0.09 dB with the inclusion of the CII Module (Table 6).

Network Optimization. In this experiment, different loss functions were added to the same baseline model for comparing denoising results. As shown in Table 5, it can be observed from the data that the denoising performance of the network significantly improved after incorporating the edge loss function.

The Selection of λ_1 and λ_2 in the Network Optimization. As shown in the table above, we conducted experiments to find optimal values for hyperparameters λ_1 and λ_2. results show $\lambda_1 = 0.9$ and $\lambda_2 = 0.1$ produced the best outcomes. Deviating from these values resulted in reduced PSNR. When λ_2 exceeded 0.1, fine edge details were overly emphasized, diminishing optimization efficiency for non-edge details. Conversely, excessive focus on non-edge details led to significant loss of critical edge details.

5 Conclusion

Our study presents the Group Feature Fusion (GFF) module to enhance computational efficiency and accuracy in image denoising. This module divides image processing into two subprocesses, reducing complexity via channel grouping. Additionally, we introduce the Cross-Information Integration (CII) module, facilitating direct low- to high-level feature connections, enhancing detail retention and quality. After optimizing with an improved loss function, a high-performance image denoiser is developed. Experimental results demonstrate the method's outstanding performance across nine benchmark datasets for image denoising.

References

1. Luo, E., Chan, S.H., Nguyen, T.Q.: Adaptive image denoising by mixture adaptation. IEEE Trans. Image Process. **25**(10), 4489–4503 (2016)
2. Zhang, K., Zuo, W., Chen, Y., Meng, D., Zhang, L.: Beyond a gaussian denoiser: Residual learning of deep cnn for image denoising. IEEE Trans. Image Process. **26**(7), 3142–3155 (2016)
3. Guo, S., Yan, Z., Zhang, K., Zuo, W., Zhang, L.: Toward convolutional blind denoising of real photographs (2018)
4. Zhang, K., Zuo, W., Zhang, L.: Ffdnet: Toward a fast and flexible solution for cnn-based image denoising. IEEE (9) (2018)
5. Ronneberger, O., Fischer, P., Brox, T.: U-net: Convolutional networks for biomedical image segmentation (2015)
6. Fan, C.M., Liu, T.J., Liu, K.H.: Sunet: Swin transformer unet for image denoising (2022)
7. Cheng, S., et al.: Nbnet: Noise basis learning for image denoising with subspace projection. In: Computer Vision and Pattern Recognition (2021)
8. Wang, Z., Cun, X., Bao, J., Liu, J.: Uformer: A general u-shaped transformer for image restoration (2021)
9. Hu, J., Shen, L., Sun, G.: Squeeze-and-excitation networks. In: 2018 IEEE/CVF Conference on Computer Vision and Pattern Recognition (CVPR) (2018)
10. Woo, S., Park, J., Lee, J.Y., Kweon, I.S.: Cbam: Convolutional block attention module (2018)
11. Zhang, K., Zuo, W., Gu, S., Zhang, L.: Learning deep cnn denoiser prior for image restoration. IEEE (2017)
12. Anwar, S.: Real image denoising with feature attention. IEEE (2019)
13. Zhang, K., et al.: Plug-and-play image restoration with deep denoiser prior. IEEE Transactions on Pattern Analysis and Machine Intelligence (01) (2021)
14. Dabov, K., Foi, A., Katkovnik, V., Egiazarian, K.: Image denoising by sparse 3-d transform-domain collaborative filtering. IEEE Trans. Image Process. **16**(8), 2080–2095 (2007)
15. Gu, S., Zhang, L., Zuo, W., Feng, X.: Weighted nuclear norm minimization with application to image denoising. In: 2014 IEEE Conference on Computer Vision and Pattern Recognition (CVPR) (2014)
16. Portilla, J., Strela, V., Wainwright, M.J., Simoncelli, E.P.: Image denoising using scale mixtures of gaussians in the wavelet domain. IEEE (11) (2003)
17. Rudin, L.I., Osher, S., Fatemi, E.: Nonlinear total variation based noise removal algorithms. Physica D **60**(1–4), 259–268 (1992)
18. Wu, W., Liu, S., Xia, Y., Zhang, Y.: Dual residual attention network for image denoising. Pattern Recognition 110291 (2024)

19. Peng, Y., Zhang, L., Liu, S., Wu, X., Zhang, Y., Wang, X.: Dilated residual networks with symmetric skip connection for image denoising. Neurocomputing **345**, 67–76 (2019)
20. Tian, C., Xu, Y., Zuo, W.: Image denoising using deep cnn with batch renormalization. Neural Netw. **121**, 461–473 (2020)
21. Plötz, T., Roth, S.: Neural nearest neighbors networks. Advances in Neural Information Processing Systems 31 (2018)
22. Zamir, S.W., et al.: Multi-stage progressive image restoration. In: Proceedings of the IEEE/CVF conference on computer vision and pattern recognition. pp. 14821–14831 (2021)
23. Chen, L., Chu, X., Zhang, X., Sun, J.: Simple baselines for image restoration. In: European Conference on Computer Vision, pp. 17–33. Springer (2022)
24. Liang, J., et al.: Swinir: Image restoration using swin transformer. In: Proceedings of the IEEE/CVF international conference on computer vision, pp. 1833–1844 (2021)
25. Li, D., et al.: No attention is needed: Grouped spatial-temporal shift for simple and efficient video restorers. arXiv preprint arXiv:2206.10810 (2022)
26. Nah, S., Son, S., Lee, S., Timofte, R., Lee, K.M.: Ntire 2021 challenge on image deblurring. In: Proceedings of the IEEE/CVF Conference on Computer Vision and Pattern Recognition, pp. 149–165 (2021)
27. Zamir, S.W., et al.: Learning enriched features for real image restoration and enhancement. In: Computer Vision--ECCV 2020: 16th European Conference, Glasgow, UK, August 23--28, 2020, Proceedings, Part XXV 16, pp. 492–511. Springer (2020)
28. Cai, Y., et al.: Learning to generate realistic noisy images via pixel-level noise-aware adversarial training (2022)
29. Zamir, S.W., et al.: Restormer: Efficient transformer for high-resolution image restoration. In: Proceedings of the IEEE/CVF conference on computer vision and pattern recognition, pp. 5728–5739 (2022)
30. Tian, C., Xu, Y., Li, Z., Zuo, W., Liu, H.: Attention-guided cnn for image denoising. Neural Netw. **124**, 117–129 (2020)
31. Li, B., et al.: All-in-one image restoration for unknown corruption. In: 2022 IEEE/CVF Conference on Computer Vision and Pattern Recognition (CVPR), pp. 17431–17441 (2022). https://doi.org/10.1109/CVPR52688.2022.01693
32. Zamir, S.W., et al.: Learning enriched features for fast image restoration and enhancement. IEEE Trans. Pattern Anal. Mach. Intell. **45**(2), 1934–1948 (2022)
33. Menteş, S., Kınlı, F., Özcan, B., Kıraç,, F.: [re] spatial-adaptive network for single image denoising. In: ML Reproducibility Challenge 2020 (2021)

End-to-End Object Detection with YOLOF

Xing Xi, Yangyang Huang, Weiye Wu, and Ronghua Luo(✉)

South China University of Technology, Guangzhou, China
xxyzll@yeah.net

Abstract. Within the field of computer vision, object detection is a core issue. A technique extensively utilized in convolution-oriented detectors is Non-Maximum Suppression (NMS), designed to suppress redundant predictions. However, the sequential nature intrinsic to NMS inhibits its capacity for parallel execution, consequently restricting the inference speed. Furthermore, the recall rate of detectors with NMS is also affected in scenes with high object density and overlap. In this paper, we propose a real-time and end-to-end detector with YOLOF (You Only Look One-level Feature). The proposed methods do not introduce additional parameters or attention mechanisms, making them practical for real-time applications. Specifically, we propose the stop-gradient strategy to train only a portion of parameters to address the problem of weak supervision in one-to-one label assignment. We also present auxiliary losses to strengthen the supervision of negative samples during training and use semantic anchor optimization to suppress other anchors in the same location. These techniques allow the improved YOLOF to discard NMS within a 1 mAP gap and achieve faster inference speed. Our YOLOF-CSP-D53-DC5 achieves 42.7 mAP, only 0.5 mAP lower than the original version. Additionally, our YOLOF-R50 achieves a 37.1 mAP at 38 FPS and exceeds state-of-the-art networks by more than 1.5 times in inference speed.

Keywords: YOLOF · End-to-end Detector · Non-Maximum Suppression · Object Detection

1 Introduction

Object detection, a fundamental component of computer vision, is instrumental in a range of real-world applications, including but not limited to autonomous vehicles, security monitoring, and robotic systems. A common obstacle encountered in object detection is the problem of Non-Maximum Suppression (NMS), which is used to discard the reduplicative bounding boxes by the detection algorithm (left in Fig. 1).

Despite the widespread adoption of NMS in standard post-processing workflows, it presents two potential issues: computational burden and recall rate. NMS is a ranking-based algorithm that iteratively suppresses duplicate predictions within the same category. However, the entire computation process is not parallelizable. As a result, it significantly impacts the inference speed of the model, especially on edge devices.

Subsequent work [15, 18, 19] has proposed modifications to its process to achieve higher execution speeds, but the computational burden it brings is still considerable.

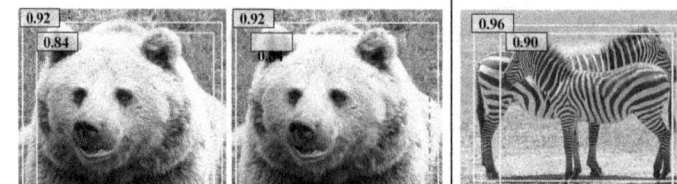
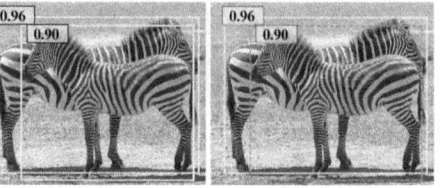

Fig. 1. The purpose and shortcomings of the NMS. The aim of NMS is to suppress redundant predictions with lower scores (left). However, the algorithm exhibits recall issues when two objects are in close proximity (right).

In addition, NMS has the problem of reducing the recall rate (right in Fig. 1). The principle of NMS in suppressing duplicate predictions is to calculate the Intersection over Union (IOU) of two targets of the same class. If this value exceeds a predefined threshold, the one with the lower confidence among them will be suppressed. This flaw is particularly prominent in dense tasks, such as the CrowdHuman [7] task, where the theoretical upper bound of the recall rate using NMS is 95%. Therefore, in this paper, we focus on how to discard NMS in detectors with dense predictions. We adopt YOLOF (You Only Look One-level Feature [3]) as our baseline model because it only uses single-layer features and has an advantage in inference speed.

We noted a substantial reduction in the mean average precision (mAP) by 27.7 when NMS was excluded from YOLOF, suggesting that its NMS-dependent version generated reduplicative predictions. Although PSS [14] and DATE [4] have effectively solved this issue, they have yet to produce satisfactory outcomes in YOLOF, a single-feature-map detector. We attribute the subpar performance of the end-to-end model to the insufficient supervision signal provided by π_{oto}.[1] Consequently, we introduce the stop-gradient strategy, which utilizes only a subset of the model's parameters to fit the results of π_{oto}.

To further narrow the performance gap between YOLOF$_{nms}$ and YOLOF$_{end}$, we conducted an analysis using TIDE [1]. Our investigation disclosed that YOLOF$_{end}$ classifies numerous background regions as positive samples. To diminish the error and enhance model performance, we propose the negative loss and introduce the ranking loss [14] for training. The proposed negative loss function has only one hyperparameter and provides supervision effectively for the background error.

Lastly, given that YOLOF$_{nms}$ is an anchor-based detector, we conducted a visual analysis and discovered that predictions generated by anchors of varying sizes at the same position are similar. π_{oto} allocates only one prediction to each instance in the image, resulting in one anchor being matched as a positive sample while another scale anchors as the negative sample. However, those anchors share similar feature regions; the only difference is their receptive fields. Thus, treating one as positive and the other as negative samples causes an optimized conflict. Therefore, we propose an innovative solution to

---

[1] For simplicity, we use π_{oto} and π_{otm} to denote one-to-one and one-to-many label assignments, respectively. YOLOF$_{nms}$ and YOLOF$_{end}$ represent the NMS-dependent and NMS-independent YOLOF, respectively.

the problem. Specifically, we select an optimal anchor for each position in the feature map to serve as its prediction. The remaining predictions are disregarded and do not participate in model supervision. This approach reduces the number of predictions and prevents optimization conflicts.

Compared to $\text{YOLOF}_{\text{nms}}$, our proposed method achieves end-to-end object detection with slight sacrifice within one mAP. For instance, the YOLOF-CSP-D53-DC5 implementation yields 43.2 mAP, while its NMS-free counterpart yields 42.7 mAP, just 0.5 mAP gap. Furthermore, the improved YOLOF is NMS-independent and runs approximately 1 FPS faster than the original implementation. Compared with other NMS-free detectors, our proposed YOLOF NMS-free version can attain similar performance with over 1.5 + times the inference speed. It's worth noting that the speed evaluation is based on RTX TAITAN (24). Therefore, on edge devices, the impact of NMS is greater, and our improvements will be more significant. We summarize the contributions of this article as follows:

- In our quest to eliminate the necessity for NMS, we proposed three novel approaches: the Stop-Gradient Strategy, the Auxiliary Loss, and the Semantic Anchor Optimization.
- Notably, these proposed techniques, devoid of any additional parameters or attention mechanisms, successfully achieve $\text{YOLOF}_{\text{end}}$ while maintaining a marginal 1 mAP disparity and demonstrating superior inference speed.
- By conducting experiments on COCO, the improved model achieves 37.1 mAP at 38 FPS and exceeds other SOTA methods by more than 1.5 times in inferencespeed.

2 Our Approach

2.1 Overall Architecture

Figure 2 illustrates the outline of the proposed model. Firstly, we observed that π_{oto} provided insufficient supervision, greatly compromising the performance. Thus, we propose the Stop-Gradient strategy (Sect. 2.2). Secondly, we noticed that $\text{YOLOF}_{\text{end}}$ classifies numerous background regions as positive samples. Therefore, we propose the Auxiliary Loss to mitigate this (Sect. 2.3). Finally, we observed that anchors corresponding to different scales share feature regions, and treating one as positive and the other as negative samples causes the optimized conflict. To tackle this, we propose Semantic Anchor Optimization (Sect. 2.4).

2.2 Stop Gradient

The dataset is denoted as $D = \{X, Y\}$, where X and Y represent the input image and corresponding label, respectively. The label of the i-th instance in the k-th image, denoted as y_i^k, is defined as $\{l^k, c_x^k, c_y^k, w^k, h^k\}$, where l^k, c_x^k, c_y^k, w^k and h^k correspond to the category, bounding box center coordinates, width, and height, respectively. Traditional object models often employ π_{otm} to optimize the model:

$$L = \sum_{\pi_{otm}} f_{cls}(p_j^k, y_i^k | \pi_{i,j}) + f_{loc}(p_j^k, y_i^k | \pi_{i,j}). \tag{1}$$

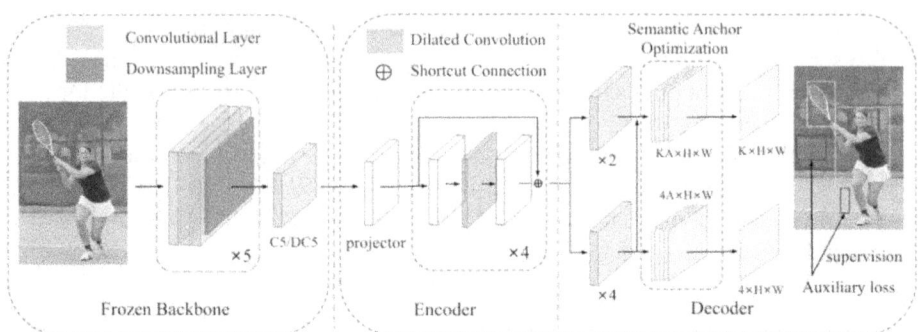

Fig. 2. The overall architecture of the proposed method. Consistent with YOLOF, the model comprises three key components: the Backbone, Encoder, and Decoder. The Backbone serves as the feature extractor for image classification tasks, employing architectures such as ResNet50 [10]. The Encoder incorporates dilated convolutions and residual connections, with the aim of enlarging the receptive field to cover objects of all scales. The Decoder follows a RetinaNet-style [5] prediction head. C5/DC5 represents the output of the Backbone network, while the Project layer is designed to adjust the channel count of feature maps.

Here, $p_j^k \in P^k$ means the j-th prediction in the k-th image, and $\pi_{i,j}$ indicates that the i-th ground truth is assigned to the j-th prediction. The loss functions f_{cls} and f_{loc} correspond to classification and location, respectively. π_{otm} forces the detector to adopt additional post-processing to suppress these redundant predictions. To alleviate the need for NMS, an alternative is π_{otm}. However, YOLOF-ono achieves only 31.6 mAP, indicating a significant performance gap compared to YOLOF$_{nms}$ (Table 1). Furthermore, YOLOF-woNMS attains a mere 10.0 mAP, suggesting a strong reliance on NMS.

In addition, several existing methods have achieved successful end-to-end object detection. DATE [4] introduces an additional π_{otm} branch for training. PSS [14] improves performance by incorporating a sample selector into the regression branch. These methods exhibit competitive performance on FPN-based detectors like FCOS [11] and oneNet [8]. However, these methods do not translate effectively to YOLOF. DATE[4] and PSS [14] achieve mAP values of 31.0 and 23.3, respectively, indicating declines of 6.7 and 14.4 mAP compared to the NMS version of YOLOF.

The question arises: Why do detectors heavily depend on π_{otm}? We deem that this isdue to the adequate supervisory signal it provides to train the entire model. However, the signal supplied by π_{oto} is insufficient for the training model with numerous parameters.

Thus, we propose the stop-gradient strategy to reduce the number of trainable parameters in the backbone. During training, we employ the encoder and decoder to fit π_{oto} while transferring the knowledge from YOLOF to the backbone (Table 1 YOLOF-detach). YOLOF-detach achieves 35.1 mAP, marking a 3.5 mAP improvement over YOLOF-ono, demonstrating that parameter reduction significantly alleviates the supervisory signal issues.

Table 1. Comparison of various end-to-end methods in object detection. All experiments were conducted using the mmdetection [2].

Method	AP	AP50	AP75	AP$_S$	AP$_M$	AP$_L$
YOLOF	37.7	56.9	40.6	19.1	42.5	53.2
YOLOF-woNMS	10.0	13.3	11.0	12.1	18.9	14.3
YOLOF-ono	31.6	52.6	33.0	16.1	35.6	42.3
YOLOF-PSS	23.3	32.8	25.4	10.2	24.7	37.7
YOLOF-DATE	31.0	51.8	32.0	13.6	34.9	44.5
YOLOF-datach	35.1	55.0	37.3	18.7	39.5	48.2

2.3 Auxiliary Loss

Furthermore, we investigate the impact of π_{oto} and π_{otm} on model prediction. To prevent the Stop-Gradient strategy from introducing noise into the results, we conduct an error analysis using YOLOF-ono and YOLOF, with the results displayed in Fig. 3. The result reveals that YOLOF-ono exhibits a notably higher background prediction error rate, suggesting that YOLOF-ono erroneously categorizes many background samples as positive instances. Thus, we propose an additional loss function to supervise those background predictions to address this.

The post-processing procedure entails three steps: (1) For model predictions P^2, retain predictions P_t that exceed the threshold hyperparameter t, and discard the rest. (2)Sort P_t based on their confidence. (3) Select the top-k samples from P_t as the model's output, denoted as $P_{t,k}$. To reduce the Bkg error, we propose a negative loss to attenuate the confidence of background samples, leading to their filter in step (1):

$$f_{negative}(P, Y | \pi_{oto}) = \frac{1}{n_-} \sum_{i=1}^{n_-} max(e^{t-p_{i_-}+m} - 1, 0). \qquad (2)$$

where, n_- is the number of negative samples, and $p_{i_-} \in P$ denotes the negative sample. The hyperparameter $m \in [0, t]$ controls the desired margin between negative samples and t. The parameter t is utilized in step (1) to filter out samples with low scores. It is set in YOLOF$_{nms}$ (0.05). Thus, the proposed loss function contains only a single hyperparameter m.

To further decrease the Bkg error, we introduce the Rank loss [14], which aims to widen the gap between positive and negative samples:

$$f_{rank}\left(P, Y | \pi_{oto}\right) = \frac{1}{n_- n_+} \sum_{i_-}^{n_-} \sum_{j_+}^{n_+} max\left(0, \alpha - p_{j_+} + p_{i_-}\right) \qquad (3)$$

where n_+ denote the number of positive samples. α is a hyperparameter used to control the gap between positive and negative samples.

---
[2] For clarity, we omit image indices k.

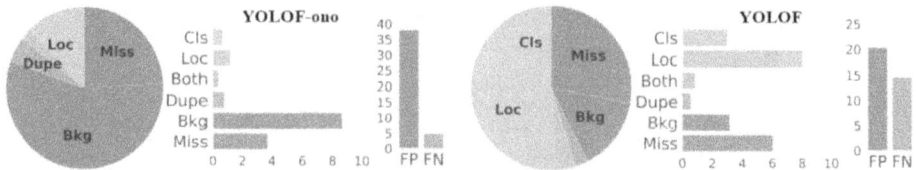

Fig. 3. Error Analysis of TIDE [81]. The image displays six types of errors: Cls (classification error), Loc (location error), Both (both classification and location error), Dupe (duplication error), Bkg (background error), and Miss (missing error).

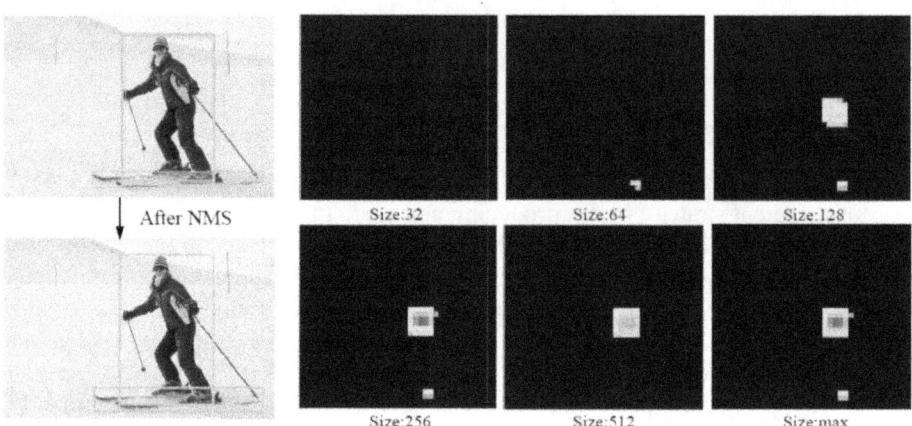

Fig. 4. Visualization of predicted classification scores from different anchors. The input image contains two instances. Size denotes the corresponding anchor scale, while max indicates the maximum value of the proposed channel.

The total loss function is defined as follows:

$$L = f_{cls}(P_{t,k}, Y | \pi_{ono}) + f_{loc}(P_{t,k}, Y | \pi_{ono}) + f_{negative}(P_{t,k}, Y | \pi_{ono}) + f_{rank}(P_{t,k}, Y | \pi_{ono}), \quad (4)$$

where f_{cls} is classification loss, and we use the Focal loss [5] with default setting. The term f_{loc} corresponds to the GIOU [6]. Notably, it is important to emphasize that, in alignment with the conventional post-processing procedure, all loss computations are performed based on $P_{t,k}$ rather than the complete prediction set P.

2.4 Semantic Anchor Optimization

YOLOF operates as an anchor-based detector, employing five preset anchors at each position. The Uniform Match strategy [3] assigns multiple predictions to the same instance based on the bounding box L1 distance. However, replacing it with the one-to-one label assignment introduces optimization conflicts. As illustrated in Fig. 4, anchors of sizes 64, 128, and 256 produce duplicate predictions for the same instance, and similar scenarios also occur with anchors of sizes 54, 128, and 256. However, those anchors share

Table 2. Effect of Different Anchor Sizes on Model Performance. Anchor size denotes the side length of the anchor. ALL indicates the use of pre-set anchors.

Anchor size	AP	AP50	AP75	AP_S	AP_M
32	35.4	53.9	38.0	18.5	40.8
64	36.1	54.5	39.1	18.5	41.2
128	35.7	53.7	39.0	18.3	40.5
256	34.9	52.5	37.9	17.3	39.7
512	36.0	54.1	39.0	18.3	40.7
ALL	35.1	55.0	37.3	18.7	39.5

similar feature regions; the only difference is their receptive field. Consequently, optimization conflicts arise when one anchor is assigned as a positive sample and other anchors are treated as negative samples. To illustrate this, we experimented to assess their impact. Table 2 reveals that using all preset anchors achieved only 35.1 mAP. However, a model with an anchor size of 64 attained 36.1 mAP, marking a 1.0 mAP improvement. Remarkably, all experimental configurations, except for anchor size 256, outperformed the baseline.

To address the optimization conflict, we propose the Semantic Anchor Optimization strategy. As depicted in Fig. 4, we select the most suitable anchor for each position by suppressing non-maximum predictions at the same position:

$$p_i = p_i \cdot I\{\max_{1 \leq j \leq n}(p_i, p_{i+j}) = p_i\}. \tag{5}$$

Here, n denotes the number of preset anchors, and $I()$ denotes the Kronecker delta function, equal to 1 when the input condition holds and 0 otherwise. The confidence of these non-maximum predictions is set to 0, leading to their exclusion in step (1).

3 Experiments

3.1 Baseline Settings

Details. All experiments were conducted on the COCO [15]. We utilized the official train2017 split, which contains approximately 118,000 images for training, and the eval2017 split, which includes 5,000 images for evaluation. We adhered to the standard COCO evaluation metric mAP 0.5–0.95 as our evaluation metric, and instances were divided into large (AP_L), medium (AP_M), and small (AP_S) objects to evaluate their performance separately. For clarity, in the table, we only display the current average indicator (AP) for 0.5–0.95 and the mAP at 0.5 (AP50) and 0.75 (AP75). All experiments standard conduct 1x schedule, which total contain 12 epoch.

Table 3. Main Experimental Results.

Model	NMS	FPS	GFLOPs	#par	AP	Gap	AP50	AP75	AP_S	AP_M	AP_L
YOLOF-R50*our*	N	38	88	44.1 M	37.1	0.6	55.2	40.2	18.8	41.9	52.4
YOLOF-R50	Y	37	88	44.1 M	37.3	0.4	57.1	39.6	18.7	42.0	52.9
YOLOF-R50*	Y	37	86	44.1 M	37.7	-	56.9	40.6	19.1	42.5	53.2
YOLOF-R101*our*	N	26	154	63.1 M	39.0	0.8	57.6	42.5	20.5	44.2	53.8
YOLOF-R101	Y	25	154	63.1 M	39.2	0.6	59.4	42.0	20.6	44.3	54.6
YOLOF-R101*	Y	25	151	63.1 M	39.8	-	59.4	42.9	20.5	44.5	54.9
YOLOF-CSP-D53-DC5*our*	N	-	211	48.3 M	42.7	0.5	60.4	46.5	23.0	47.2	59.4
YOLOF-CSP-D53-DC5	Y	-	211	48.3 M	42.8	0.4	62.1	45.9	23.2	47.2	59.4
YOLOF-CSP-D53-DC5*	Y	-	209	48.3 M	43.2	-	62.2	46.6	22.8	47.2	59.8

* denotes the official version, while R50 and R101 denote ResNet50 and ResNet101, respectively. CSP-D53-DC5 indicates the use of DarkNet53 as the backbone with no downsampling performed in the final stage. The FPS for R101 was calculated with a batch size of 1 on TAITAN, based on the total pure inference time reported in Detectron2 [13]. For R50, FPS was calculated using mmdetection [2]. GFLOPs were measured with a shorter edge size of 800 and a longer edge below 1333 using the first 100 images of COCO val2017. #par denotes the number of parameters in the model.

3.2 Main Experimental Results

We conducted experiments to evaluate our proposed method (Table 3). Our approach successfully implements the NMS-free version of YOLOF with an absolute gap of only 1 mAP. In the first section, YOLOF-R50 achieves a mAP of 37.1, which is only 0.6 mAP lower than its NMS-based counterpart. In the last section, YOLOF-CSP-D53-DC5 achieves a mAP of 42.7, which is only 0.5 mAP lower than the NMS-based version.

The original YOLOF relies on traditional NMS to suppress duplicate predictions, and the sorting nature of NMS slows down its detection speed. Our method does not rely on NMS, and the Semantic Anchor Optimization only retains 1/5 of the detection results, which further speeds up the processing speed. Therefore, our method surpasses the original YOLOF in terms of detection speed. In addition, our method realizes end-to-end detection without any additional parameters, adding only 2 GFlops of computational burden during inference. Notably, all inference speed evaluations were conducted on a TAITAN (24 G). When deployed on specific edge devices, the proposed method can achieve significant improvements, as our model does not rely on the non-parallelizable NMS.

3.3 Ablation Experiments

Auxiliary Loss. Due to the limitations of π_{ono}, which provides less supervision, the YOLOF$_{end}$ predicts a large number of background samples as positive samples. To solve the issue, we propose the $f_{negative}$, and introduce the f_{rank}. We analyze their impact on performance. The results are presented in Table 4a, where $f_{negative}$ achieves a 0.7 mAP improvement, achieving 35.8 mAP, while f_{rank} leads to a 0.5 mAP improvement,

Table 4. Ablation Study. We conduct an ablation comparison for all potential choices of the method proposed in this paper.

f_n	f_r	AP	APs	APM	APL
N	N	35.1	18.7	39.5	48.2
Y	N	35.8(+0.7)	18.4	40.5	49.8
N	Y	35.6(+0.5)	18.8	40.1	49.4
Y	Y	36.1(+1.0)	19.4	41.1	50.3

(b) The impact of auxiliary loss functions on model performance. f_n denotes that we proposed $f_{negative}$. f_r means f_{rank}.

k	AP	AP50	AP75	APs	APM	APL
100	36.7	54.7	39.8	18.9	41.7	51.5
150	36.7	54.7	39.9	19.0	41.7	51.1
200	**36.8**	55.0	39.7	18.8	41.6	51.3
ALL	36.5	54.6	40.1	18.5	41.3	50.5

(a) Effect of different number of top on model performance. ALL indicates that all predictions are used to calculate lo

m	AP	AP50	AP75	APs	APM	APL
0.01	**36.2**	53.8	39.5	19.2	41.3	49.9
0.02	36.0	53.6	39.4	19.4	41.0	50.0
0.03	36.1	53.8	39.5	18.8	41.1	50.5

(d) Effect of different number of top on model performance. ALL indicates that all predictions are used to calculate loss

Loc	AP	AP50	AP75	APs	APM	APL
1	36.8	54.8	39.8	19.0	41.7	51.0
2	**37.1**	55.2	40.2	18.8	41.9	52.4
N	35.7	53.6	38.6	17.9	40.5	50.0

(c) Efficiency of different locations. Location: 1 decoder, 2 encoder. N presents no stop gard.

resulting in 35.6 mAP. Additionally, the model attains its peak performance, an mAP of 36.1, upon applying both $f_{negative}$ and f_{rank}, marking a 1.0 mAP enhancement.

Top-k Strategy. In step (3), only the top-k samples are utilized for the ultimate prediction. Consequently, the classification loss calculation takes into account merely the top-k samples. This section delves into the influence of varying k values on the model's performance. The findings are depicted in Table 4b. YOLOF, devoid of the top-k strategy, attains a mere 36.5 mAP. The model's performance is further improved by treating all predictions as binary classification problems and training only on the top-k examples. When the k value is set to 200, YOLOF achieves a 0.3 mAP improvement over the model without the top-k strategy, reaching 36.8 mAP.

Hyperparameter m. The parameters m and t play crucial roles in our model. Precisely, m adjusts the score gap, whereas t is employed in the first step to eliminate low-score samples. In most detection models, including YOLOF, a small value is typically assigned to ensure a high recall rate. To minimize the number of hyperparameters, we maintain the value of t constant (0.05). We perform experiments in this section to explore the influence of varying m values on the model's performance. As depicted in Table 4c, the model delivers optimal performance when m is set to 0.01, yielding a mAP of 36.2.

Table 5. Comparison with different state-of-the-art NMS-free decectors. All FPS are evaluated on a single TAITAN. To be fair, all networks are evaluated on input images with 800 short edges and 1333 long edges. Sparse R-CNN, DATE-F, DATE-R and OneNet are all evaluated on mmdetection [2]. For DeFCN, we evaluate the obtained on cvpods [15].

Model	FPS	AP	AP50	AP75	AP$_S$	AP$_M$	AP$_L$
Sparse R-CNN [10]	21(+17)	37.9(-0.8)	56.0	40.5	20.7	40.0	53.5
OneNet [9]	22(+16)	35.4(+1.7)	53.3	38.1	19.3	38.6	45.4
DATE-F [4]	22(+16)	37.3(-0.2)	55.3	40.7	21.2	40.3	48.8
DATE-R [4]	23(+15)	37.0(+0.1)	54.9	40.4	20.5	39.8	49.0
DeFCN [13]	20(+18)	37.8(-0.7)	55.6	41.8	22.1	41.3	48.7
YOLOF$_{our}$	38	37.1	55.2	40.2	18.8	41.9	52.4

Stop-Gradient Location. The YOLOF-ono yielded only 31.6 mAP, which is 5.9 mAP lower than the NMS version of YOLOF. As shown in Table 1, using the stop-gradient strategy significantly improves the model's performance, increasing it from 31.6 mAP to 35.1 mAP, resulting in a gain of 4.1 mAP. This section delves into the effects of varying stop-gradient locations on the model's performance. The results are presented in Table 4d. Stopping the gradients at the classification and regression subnetworks yields the poorest model performance, with only 30.1 mAP. Stopping the gradient at the prediction head leads to a model with 36.8 mAP, while stopping the gradient at the encoder achieves the highest model performance of 37.1 mAP.

3.4 Comparison with Other NMS-Free Detectors

Our implementation of the NMS-free version achieves the fastest inference speed within the absolute gap of 1 mAP (Table 5). Sparse R-CNN [9] reaches 37.9 mAP at 21 FPS. Compared to it, our model falls in precision 0.8 mAP, but we achieve a significant advantage in inference speed, up to 17 FPS. Compared to OneNet [8], our model outperforms it by 1.7 mAP and is 16 FPS faster. When compared to DATE [4], our model is 15 FPS faster than DATE-F and 16 FPS faster than DATE-R. DeFCN [12] is an end-to-end detector based on FCOS [12]. DeFCN uses one-to-one matching, auxiliary loss, and 3DMF to eliminate NMS successfully. Compared to DeFCN, our method has a slightly lower model performance by less than 0.7 mAP, but our detector is nearly twice as fast.

4 Conclusion

This article illustrates the limitations of NMS in practical application and proposes a real-time end-to-end model based on YOLOF. To discard NMS, this paper presents three methods, including the gradient termination strategy that trains only a subset of the model parameters and an auxiliary loss function to supervise background samples during training, as well as the semantic anchor optimization strategy to eliminate the prediction of other scales of Anchor at the same position. The NMS-free version of YOLOF implemented in this paper achieves a performance difference of within 1 mAP compared to the original version. In addition, improved YOLOF without NMS increases the detection speed by 1 FPS and can correctly detect objects with high overlap. We hope that the approach presented in this paper can facilitate the practical application of real-time and end-to-end object detection models.

Acknowledgements. This work was also partially supported by Guangdong Artificial Intelligence and Digital Economy Laboratory (Guangzhou).

References

1. Bolya, D., Foley, S., Hays, J., Hoffman, J.: Tide: a general toolbox for identifying object detection errors. In: Computer Vision–ECCV 2020: 16th European Conference, Glasgow, UK, August 23–28, 2020, Proceedings, Part III 16, pp. 558–573. Springer (2020)
2. Chen, K., et al.: MMDetection: Open mmlab detection toolbox and benchmark. arXiv preprint arXiv:1906.07155 (2019)
3. Chen, Q., Wang, Y., Yang, T., Zhang, X., Cheng, J., Sun, J.: You only look one-level feature. In: Proceedings of the IEEE/CVF conference on computer vision and pattern recognition, pp. 13039–13048 (2021)
4. Chen, Y., Chen, Q., Hu, Q., Cheng, J.: Date: dual assignment for end-to-end fully convolutional object detection. arXiv preprint arXiv:2211.13859 (2022)
5. Lin, T.Y., Goyal, P., Girshick, R., He, K., Dollár, P.: Focal loss for dense object detection. In: Proceedings of the IEEE international conference on computer vision, pp. 2980–2988 (2017)
6. Lin, T.Y., et al.: Microsoft coco: Common objects in context. In: Computer Vision– ECCV 2014: 13th European Conference, Zurich, Switzerland, September 6–12, 2014, Proceedings, Part V 13, pp. 740–755. Springer (2014)
7. Rezatofighi, H., et al.: Generalized intersection over union: a metric and a loss for bounding box regression. In: Proceedings of the IEEE/CVF conference on computer vision and pattern recognition, pp. 658–666 (2019)
8. Shao, S., et al.: Crowdhuman: A benchmark for detecting human in a crowd. arXiv preprint arXiv:1805.00123 (2018)
9. Sun, P., et al.: What makes for end-to-end object detection? In: Proceedings of the 38th International Conference on Machine Learning. Proceedings of Machine Learning Research, vol. 139, pp. 9934–9944. PMLR (2021)
10. Sun, P., et al.: Sparse r-cnn: End-to-end object detection with learnable proposals. In: Proceedings of the IEEE/CVF conference on computer vision and pattern recognition, pp. 14454–14463 (2021)
11. Targ, S., Almeida, D., Lyman, K.: Resnet in resnet: Generalizing residual architectures. arXiv preprint arXiv:1603.08029 (2016)
12. 12Tian, Z., Shen, C., Chen, H., He, T.: Fcos: Fully convolutional one-stage object detection. In: Proceedings of the IEEE/CVF international conference on computer vision, pp. 9627–9636 (2019)
13. Wang, J., et al.: End-to-end object detection with fully convolutional network. In: Proceedings of the IEEE/CVF conference on computer vision and pattern recognition, pp. 15849–15858 (2021)

14. Wu, Y., Kirillov, A., Massa, F., Lo, W.Y., Girshick, R.: Detectron2 (2019). https://github.com/facebookresearch/detectron2
15. Zheng, Z., et al.: Enhancing geometric factors in model learning and inference for object detection and instance segmentation (2021)
16. 16Zhou, Q., Yu, C., Shen, C., Wang, Z., Li, H.: Object detection made simpler by eliminating heuristic nms (2021)
17. Zhu*, B., et al.: cvpods: All-in-one toolbox for computer vision research (2020)
18. Bolya, D., Zhou, C., Xiao, F., Lee, Y.J.: Yolact: Real-time instance segmentation. In: Proceedings of the IEEE/CVF international conference on computer vision, pp. 9157–9166 (2019)
19. Zheng, Z., et al.: Distance-iou loss: Faster and better learning for bounding box regression. In: The AAAI Conference on Artificial Intelligence (AAAI) (2020)

BiRGAN: Bi-directional Deep Image Retargeting

Di Sun[1], Yunxiang Wang[1], Tingting Yang[1], Yijing Mei[2], and Gang Pan[2]($^{\boxtimes}$)

[1] College of Artificial Intelligence, Tianjin University of Science and Technology, Tianjin 300222, China
[2] College of Intelligence and Computing, Tianjin University, Tianjin 300350, China
pangang@tju.edu.cn

Abstract. Current single retargeting operators perform poorly on diverse images and varying target sizes, rendering them unsuitable for both image reduction and expansion simultaneously. In this paper, we present a deep bi-directional image retargeting network, BiRGAN. The network performs two opposite processes: one training a generator to learn the process of downsizing images, and another learning the upsizing process. The output from the first process is fed into the second, creating a comprehensive closed loop. This network is designed to comprehend the deformation process of retargeted images by employing multiple methodologies and executing retargeting operations within the feature space. Experimental results demonstrate that BiRGAN outperforms previous methods in terms of overall image retargeting results.

Keywords: Image Retargeting · GAN · Bi-directional · IRQA

1 Introduction

Multimedia devices with various screen sizes are becoming increasingly prevalent. Normally, these devices possess diverse aspect ratios and image resolutions, necessitating the adaptation of images to fit the specific target devices. We define the task of adapting an image to best suit a target display device as image retargeting or resizing.

Early content-aware methods [1–8] initially estimate the salient regions of the image and then resize the image while preserving the content of such regions. Since the salient regions are obtained from low-level semantic features, it is common for these methods to result in structural distortion and the creation of artificial artifacts.

In recent years, there are some deep learning measures that implement a complete end-to-end training process [9–16]. However, these approaches rely heavily on calculating importance maps, once the calculation of importance map fails, it usually leads to poor quality of the retargeting results, which significantly limits the generality of these methods.

Moreover, current single retargeting operators may not perform well on multifarious images and various target sizes. Therefore, synthesizing multiple operators is an effective solution. Unlike Multi-operator [3] and Photo Squarization [10], which combine different

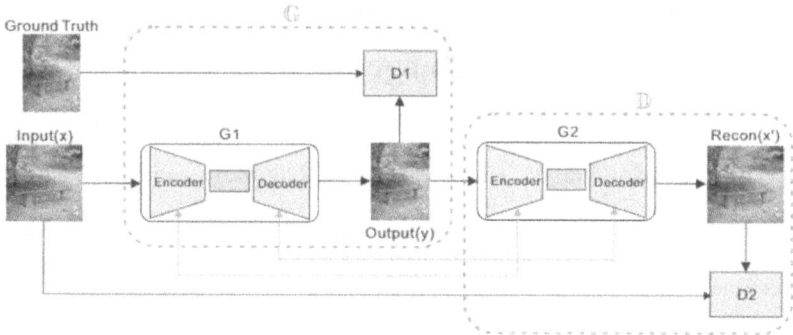

Fig. 1. Overview of the BiRGAN: The model implements a bi-directional retargeting process. It feeds the input image Input(x) into the generator G_1 to generate a width-reduced image Output(y), and then sends y and the corresponding ground truth to the discriminator D_1 for distinguishing. At the same time, y is fed into generator G_1 as input to generate an image Recon(x′) with expanded width, after which x′ and x are input to the discriminator D_2 together.

operators in an optimal way and then operate directly on the pixel space, we try to start from the retargeting process of different operators. The key idea is put the best performance of retargeting results of different images together, and then learn how to deform the original image into the best through a complete end-to-end training. Finally, retargeting operation is carried out in the feature space, so that the result can be better expressed.

In this paper, we propose a generative adversarial network (GAN) based bi-directional retargeting network (BiRGAN) in this paper. The network needs to complete two reciprocal retargeting processes respectively. One is training a generator to learn the process of resizing images to smaller sizes, and the other is a discriminator that learns the process of resizing images to larger sizes. The output of the first process is fed into the second process as the input over here, causing the network to form a complete closed loop, and the two processes compete with each other in the hope that both can produce preferable results. Our main contributions can be summarized as:

- We offer a new perspective into supervised image retargeting that utilizes data from multiple operators within the feature space. The proposed strategy can circumvent the constraints associated with relying solely on a single calculation method for determining the importance map.
- We propose the BiRGAN network, a bi-directional image retargeting framework. It can achieve visually pleasing results for both image reduction and expansion. Furthermore, it offers a comprehensive framework that accommodates a diverse range of tasks involving reciprocal processes.

2 Related Work

Most of conventional image retargeting approaches are based on content perception. Discrete methods [1–3] usually extract the saliency information of pixels in an image, and then define an operation method to insert or delete pixels to obtain the retargeted image. Continuous methods [5, 6] typically cover a uniform grid on an original image, and assign a different zoom factor to each grid unit. The zoom factor of important areas is larger than other areas. Nevertheless, these traditional content-aware methods normally extract and utilize low-level features, ignoring high-level semantics, so their effects are limited.

Existing image retargeting quality assessment algorithms can be roughly classified into subjective methods and objective methods. Subjective approaches require many participants to vote repeatedly on a large number of retargeted images and then evaluate the retargeted images according to the votes. For example, Castillo et al. use eye tracking to compare image retargeted images by examining gaze fixations and viewing patterns. Objective methods are evaluated based on the analysis of the salient region and structure of image.

Many deep learning based image retargeting approaches have been invented. However, these approaches mainly perform retargeting operation by means of the depth feature maps extracted from the pre-training network, which are not an end-to-end training process. Subsequently, Song et al. [10] present a CNN-based framework to introduce user preference into a multi-operator retargeting algorithm. Cho et al. [11] propose a weakly and self-supervised deep network to learn a shift map from the original image to the retargeting map. Although these methods are end-to-end training, they are essentially dependent on the importance map obtained by calculation, so their results are also limited by the calculation measure of the importance map. After that, Tan et al. [12] develop an unsupervised deep cyclic image retargeting method (CycleIR) that improves the quality of retargeted images by introducing cyclic perception consistency loss. However, all of these methods [9–13, 15–17] directly perform retargeting in the image space but not in the feature space, which can lead to unnatural distortions in results.

Recently, GAN has been applied to image retargeting. For example, Shocher et al. [14] suggest a fully unsupervised image-specific GAN(InGAN) that trains on a single input image and learns its internal distribution of patches. However, InGAN [14] learns a local block in the original image as ground truth. In other words, InGAN [14] mainly considers the texture information of the image, and does not take into account the semantics or scene information of the image. Mei et al. [18] introduce a deep supervised technique into the image retargeting task. This deep model learns a shift map to implement pixel-wise mapping from the source image to the target image in the feature space. But MRGAN only considers retargeting images to smaller sizes.

2.1 Retargeting Dataset

Three public datasets exist for image retargeting, namely MIT RetargetMe, CUHK, and NIRD. Each of these datasets comprises retargeted images generated through various methods, accompanied by corresponding subjective evaluation scores.

MIT RetargetMe Dataset. This dataset contains 37 original images and 296 retargeted results. The retargeted results are generated by eight retargeting algorithms, incluing CR, SCL, SC, MULTIOP, SM, SNS, SV, and WARP. The retargeting is set to either 50% or 25% of the original image's height or width respectively. Each original image is labeled with six attributes.

CUHK Dataset. The CUHK dataset comprises 57 original images and 171 retargeted results. For each original image, three retargeting operators are randomly selected from ten representative retargeting algorithms, resulting in the generation of corresponding retargeted images.

NRID Dataset. The NRID dataset comprises 35 original images, with five distinct retargeting algorithms applied to generate retargeted images: MO, SCL, SC, SM, and WARP. The original image in NRID dataset also has the same six attributes as MIT RetargetMe dataset.

However, the above three public datasets are currently insufficiently populated to adequately support the training process of the network. Furthermore, most of these datasets are utilized for comparing IRQA methods, which implies that we cannot identify the optimal retargeted image (ground truth). Consequently, a significant impediment to research in image retargeting based on GAN is the absence of benchmark datasets.

TIReD Dataset. Mei et al. introduce a new dataset named TIReD, which consists of 6,576 pairs generated by multiple operators using Image Retargeting Quality Assessment (IRQA) algorithm. Each pair consists of an original image and its corresponding retargeted image, which is selected from results of seven retargeting algorithms using the IRQA algorithm. The retargeted image that corresponds to the original image serves as the ground truth.

3 Retargeting TIReD ++ Dataset

Our goal is to achieve retargeting by learning the target retargeted images using the GAN network. The focal point and challenge in this process, however, lies in the selection of the target image. In the realm of image retargeting, numerous methods have been proposed, however, there exists no stringent standard to assess which type of retargeted image is superior. To solve this problem, we contribute a comprehensive dataset named TIReD ++ for image retargeting. The overview of data generation is shown in Fig. 2. We implement certain representative prior retargeting algorithms, including: uniform scaling (USL), seam-carving (SC) [1], improved seam-carving (ISC) [2], scale-and-stretch (SNS) [22], shift map (SM) [4], Cycle-IR [13], WSSDCNN [12], SAMIR [11]. We employ the eight retargeting operators implemented to perform the identical retargeting on the same original input image. We divide the retargeted image with the same input and this input image (9 images in total) into the same group.

We then adopt the IRQA algorithm, TRASIM [19] as the evaluation criteria, to score the retargeted image based on original input image in each group. We finally consider the retargeted image with the highest score within the group as the best performance (ground truth) and pair it with the original image for training purposes. We consider the ground truth as a reference, and create a pair of input images that correspond with the original image for training purposes. There are 7,074 image pairs in total. They are with different width scaling ratios, one for the ratio of 0.5 and the other for 0.75. Specifically, each has 3,537 retargeting-image pairs, including the original images and retargeted images (ground truth). The training dataset has 2,800 pairs, and the test dataset has 737

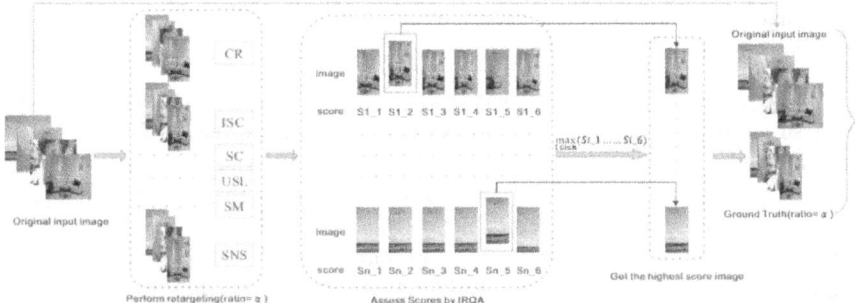

Fig. 2. Overview of Data Collection. We use the collected original image as input. Then we use the IRQA algorithm in [19] to generate the retargeted image as the ground truth.

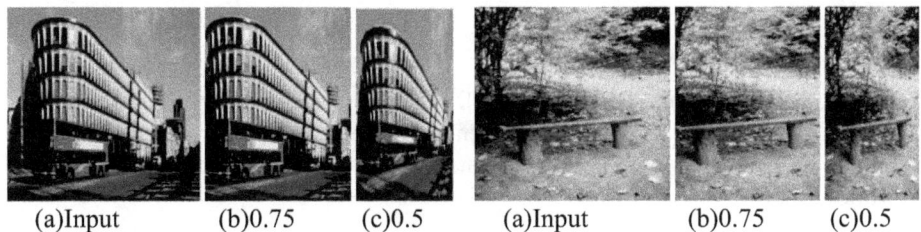

(a)Input   (b)0.75   (c)0.5   (a)Input   (b)0.75   (c)0.5

Fig. 3. Some example images in the constructed dataset. (a) is the original image; (b) is the ground truth at a width scaling ratio of 0.75; and (c) is the ground truth at a width scaling ratio of 0.50.

pairs. Figure 3 shows some images in our dataset. In each group, we display the selection of the corresponding ground truth for different styles of images.

4 Approach

4.1 BiRGAN Model

In this section, only the width adjustment of the image is described as an example. The overall architecture of BiRGAN is shown in Fig. 1. BiRGAN has two subnetworks, Retargeting Generation (G) and Retargeting Verification (D). G is based on GAN to generate images with reduced width. D uses a structure similar to G to expand the image width. In general, G first generates a width-reduced retargeted image, and then D takes this retargeted image and the original image as input. D reconstructs the original image, and evaluates the similarity of the reconstructed image and the original image, so as to verify whether the result of G completely retains the important features of the original image. That is, G and D form a GAN-like structure. G is similar to the generator of the GAN network, and D is equivalent to the discriminator analogously.

Retargeting Generation (Generator). Retargeting Generation (G), similar to the generator in GAN network, which realizes the retargeting operation of reducing the image width. As shown in Fig. 1. It includes a complete GAN structure with a generator G_1 and a discriminator D_1. It feeds the input image into G_1 to generates a width-reduced image Y. Then it sends y together with the corresponding ground truth to D_1 for discrimination.

For the G_1, we adopt a "U-Net" network as the generator which follows an encoder-decoder structure similar to the one used in [18]. Based on the U-Net structure, we add the Dilated Convolutions and the 1 x 1 Convolution. The encoder part splices a common layer of convolution and the output feature map of the convolution layer into the next layer of convolution to encode, in this way, the features extracted from different receptive fields can be fused to obtain more complete features, which is also beneficial to the redirection at different resolutions, and 1 x 1 convolution can increase the interaction between channels, increase online learning capabilities. For discriminator D_1, it uses the full convolution patch discriminator [20]. Since that the difference between the retargeted image and the original image is relatively small. Patches in patch discriminator has better local characteristics. During the training, the resulting image is fed into D with ground truth, and a matrix of N × N is output, where N is the size of patch, and the value of the matrix is the result of the patch.

Retargeting Verification (Discriminator). The structure of Retargeting Verification module (D) is the same as Retargeting Generation module (G), including a generator G_2 and a discriminator D_2. Therefore, it may be regarded as a discriminator in GAN network formally.

The structure of Retargeting Verification module (D) is the same as Retargeting Generation module (G), including a generator G_2 and a discriminator D_2. Its generator takes the retargeted image from Retargeting Generation module as input, and mainly implements the retargeting of expanding the image width. It then seeds the generated expanded image and original input image into the D_2 for distinguishing. In general, D verifies or discriminates whether the generated image of G completely preserves the important features in the original input image by reconstructing the input image and evaluating the similarity of the reconstructed image and the input image. Therefore, it may be regarded as a discriminator in GAN network formally.

Since that Retargeting Generation and Retargeting Verification are equivalent to a GAN structure, when the G starting point is high, if D' is trained from the beginning, the generator and discriminator function in GAN structure will be out of balance. Affect the effectiveness of the network. Therefore, in order to avoid this effect, the D module is also pre-trained in this paper. Considering that G and D are an interactive and reciprocal process, and when the original image is input into G, this module is based on the ground truth in the retargeting dataset established in the paper.

Therefore, if ground truth is used as input for D, the module should be trained with the original image as the standard. The G_1 and D_1 of Retargeting Generation G are the same as G_2 and D_2 of Retargeting Verification D. However, in the process of pre-training, the generator G_2 takes the ground truth in G as the input, and then generates the generated image with expanded width. Then the retargeted image of G_2 and the original input image in G are fed into the discriminant D_2 for line discrimination.

When both G and D are pre-trained, the G_1 and D_1 of G remain unchanged, while the G_2 and D_2 of D turn to an approximate discriminator during the actual combined training. That is to say, when a retargeted image with a reduced width is generated in the process of G, it needs to be input to the generator G_2 in D to generate the retargeted result with a wider width. At the same time, the ground truth in G needs to be input to G_2 to generate the retargeted image. Not only that, in the pre-training process, the ground truth in G has been used as input, and the original image in G has been used as the standard to adjust the network parameters. In this way, the global training of bi-directional retargeting can be performed with D as the discriminator of G in the form.

4.2 Loss Design

Adversarial Loss. The network of GANs require simultaneous training both the generator and the discriminator. We design the adversarial losses for the two GANs. The equations are as follows:

$$Ł_{GAN_1}(G_1, D_1) = \mathbb{E}_{x_{gt} \sim p_{ddta}(x_{gt})}[\log D_1(x_{gt})] \\ + \mathbb{E}_{x \sim p_{data}(x)}[\log(1 - D_1(G_1(x)))], \quad (1)$$

$$Ł_{GAN_2}(G_1, G_2, D_2) = \mathbb{E}_{x_{gt} \sim p_{data}(x_{gt})}\left[\log D_2\left(G_2(x_{gt})\right)\right] \\ + \mathbb{E}_{x \sim p_{data}(x)}\left[\log\left(1 - D_2(G_2(G_1(x)))\right)\right], \quad (2)$$

where L_{GAN1} is the adversarial loss for the G, and xgt is the corresponding width reduced image in the dataset of ground truth. L_{GAN2} is the adversarial loss for the D, x is the original input image.

Since that D is used as the discriminator of G, the adversarial loss of BiRGAN is as follows:

$$Ł_{BiRHGAN}(G_1, G_2, D_2) = \mathbb{E}_{x_{gt} \sim p_{data}(x_{gt})}\left[\log D_2\left(G_2(x_{gt})\right)\right] \\ + \mathbb{E}_{x \sim p_{data}(x)}\left[\log\left(1 - D_2(G_2(G_1(x)))\right)\right], \quad (3)$$

Other Loss. For training stability, we use L_1 loss [20] to emphasize the matching of each corresponding pixel between the generated image and the real image, encouraging robustness and less fuzziness. They are defined as follows:

$$Ł_{G_1L_1}(G_1) = \|x_{gt} - G_1(x)\|_1, \quad (4)$$

$$Ł_{G_2L_1}(G_1, G_2) = \|x - G_2(x_{gl})\|_1, \quad (5)$$

where $L_{G1!L1}$ is the L_1 loss designed for the network represented by G_1, and $L_{G2!l1}$ is designed for G_2. $\|\cdot\|_1$ is the L_1 norm.

In addition, the ideal retargeting model should generate a retargeted image that is highly consistent with the input image in terms of visual perception, without obvious distortion and artificial artifacts, and can completely preserve important image information. Therefore, we use the reconstruction loss to keep the uniformity of the image before redirection and the mapping after redirection through a reciprocal redirection.

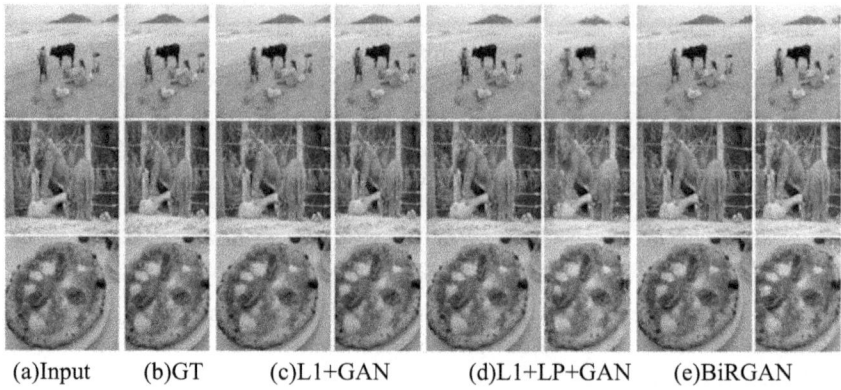

(a)Input (b)GT (c)L1+GAN (d)L1+LP+GAN (e)BiRGAN

Fig. 4. Ablation Study. (a) and (b) are the original image and ground truth, ((c)-(e)) are results trained with a different loss. For each group, the left shows the image generated by expanding the width in the bi-directional process, and the right side is the result of the width reduced, and the image on the right side is the input for generation process of the left.

This loss is to perform the consistency constraint between pixels between the original reconstructed image and the original input image in G_1 generator after the retargeted image generated by G_1 is passed through G_2 the reconstruction loss not only keeps the structure and content of the two independent redirection processes, but also promotes and restrains each other between the two processes. Lres Loss as Eq. 6:

$$L_{\text{res}}(G_1, G_2) = x - G_2(G_1(x))_1, \tag{6}$$

Total Loss. After we have defined different losses to evaluate the network, we get the target equation for BiRGAN. Here λ are the set parameters of contribution weight to the total loss, which are obtained according to the experiment. The expression is as follows:

$$\begin{aligned} G^* = \underset{G_1}{\text{argmin}}\underset{D_1}{\text{max}} L_{GAN_1}(G_1, D_1) + \underset{G_1}{\text{argmin}}\underset{\mathbb{D}}{\text{max}} L_{GAN_2}(G_1, G_2, D_2) \\ + \lambda_{G_1L_1} L_{G_1L_1}(G_1) + \lambda_{G_2L_2} L_{G_2L_2}(G_1, G_2) + \lambda_{\text{res}} L_{\text{res}}(G_1, G_2), \end{aligned} \tag{7}$$

5 Experiment

BiRGAN is implemented based on python and tensorflow. In the training, we set the value of λ_{G1L1}, λ_{G2L2} and λ_{res} to 1000. We also employ batch normalization [21] in most convolutional blocks to encourage stability of the proposed model. In the experiment, our model performed a complete end-to-end training using the Adam optimizer [22].

The batch size is set to 4. We trained it on NVIDIA Tesla V100 GPU with 32GB GPU memory.

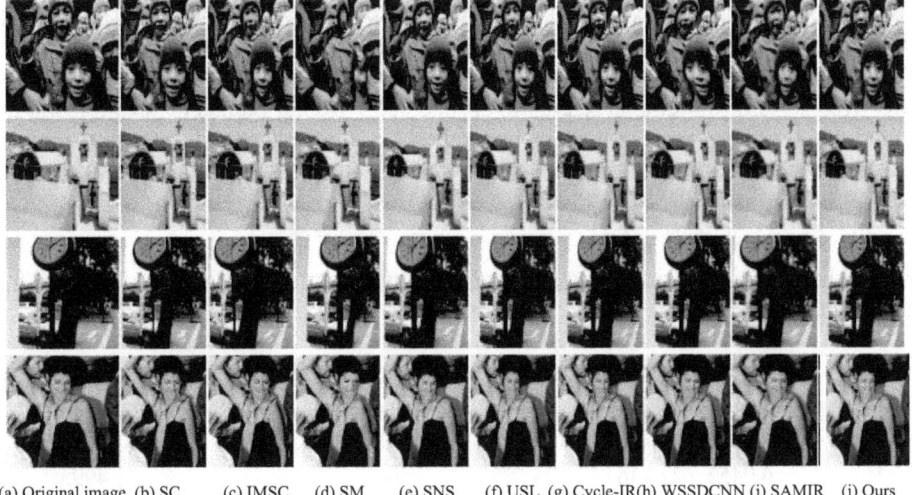

(a) Original image (b) SC   (c) IMSC   (d) SM   (e) SNS   (f) USL (g) Cycle-IR(h) WSSDCNN (i) SAMIR   (j) Ours

Fig. 5. Visual comparison of our method with representative retargeting approaches. (a) is the original image, (b)-(i) are retargeting images by prevous methods, (j) is our results.

5.1 Ablation Study

In order to train two GANs in our model and improve their stability, in addition to Adversarial Loss, we also use L1 Loss and Reconstruction Loss to assist in it. Here, we conducted an ablation study to verify the importance of these losses.

Figure 4 illustrates their differences in optimizing the BiRGAN with several examples of retargeted images. It can be seen that L_1 loss pays more attention to matching at pixel-level and lacks high-frequency information, so its introduction can improve the visual effect of generated images. Conversely, Reconstruction loss is more concerned with content perception and structural similarity. Therefore, only BiRGAN (which use Adversarial loss, L_1 loss and Reconstruction loss simultaneously) achieves the best results, producing rationally meaningful images and reducing artifacts dramatically.

5.2 Comparison with Previous Methods

Figure 5 shows a visual comparison between BiRGAN and several previous retargeting methods by adjusting the width of the input image to 0.75 of its original width on both TIRED ++ dataset and RetargetMe dataset. Among them, (a) is the original image, and (b)-(k) are the retargeted images by SC [1], IMSC [2], SM [4], SNS [22], USL, Cycle-IR [13], WSSDCNN [12], SAMIR [11] and our method. It can be seen that SC and IMSC may deform important objects when the seam passes through them. SNS pays too much attention to the retention of all information and neglects the retention of important information. When the shift map in SM fails to calculate, the original image will lose or seriously distort important information. USL simply merges adjacent pixels together, resulting in an excessive reduction of significant objects. In addition, Cycle-IR has the same problem as SNS. The retargeted results of the WSSDCNN are often distorted.

InGAN does not consider semantic information because it is not a traditional retargeting algorithm, so it works well on texture images, but not on semantic images such as people. Thanks to the large retargeting dataset TIRED + +, powerful supervised learning, and the effectiveness of bi-directional retargeting processes, BiRGAN can generate high quality target images. Compared with previous methods, it can be seen that our approach can not only avoid image distortion during retargeting, but also keep the lines in the image well without causing the color distortion of the image.

Table 1. Retargeting results in terms of NIQE, BRISQU and NBIQA on the new dataset and RetargetMe(RM).

Method	NIQE	BRISQUE	NBIQA	NIQE(RM)	BRISQUE(RM)	NBIQA(RM)
SC	6.2021	25.306	24.2240	7.2791	29.540	24.9689
IMSC	6.2237	23.5643	23.6607	7.4080	28.668	24.5436
USL	6.0452	22.146	23.7220	7.4080	23.827	23.4995
SM	6.1605	23.398	24.6454	6.8286	25.925	25.9928
SNS	5.7373	20.302	24.7172	5.9054	17.364	20.9607
Cycle-IR	5.8676	22.562	23.2554	6.1286	21.008	20.9531
WSSDCNN	5.9394	22.014	23.4985	6.4185	23.161	23.2155
SAMIR	6.8352	39.7886	42.1039	6.6493	38.7707	41.9513
Ours	5.6302	21.1829	22.9749	5.6985	17.5583	18.1242

5.3 Quantitative Assessment

Table 1 presents the quantitative assessment results using objective evaluation methods on the proposed dataset TIRED ++ and RetargetMe(RM). It can be seen that the BIRGAN model has the best performance in NIQE and NBIQA, although it is not perfect in BRISQUE compared with other advanced methods.

6 Conclusion

In this paper, we have proposed a bi-directional retargeting network based on GAN. It conducts two completely opposite retargeting processes independently, and competes to achieve preferable results. Simultaneously, the retargeting operation is performed in feature space of the image which allows for a reduction in artifacts and distortions through reconstruction of the retargeted image, enhancing its naturalness and authenticity. The proposed network implements two operations that are inverse to each other, so it also provides a unified framework for a variety of different tasks involving reciprocal processes.

Acknowledgments. This work was funded by the Natural Science Foundation of Tianjin Municipality (No. 21JCYBJC00640), 2023 CCF-Baidu Songguo Foundation (Research on Scene Text Recognition Based on PaddlePaddle).

References

1. Avidan, S., Shamir, A.: Seam carving for content-aware image resizing. In: ACM Transactions on Graphics (TOG), vol. 26, p. 10. ACM (2007)
2. Rubinstein, M., Shamir, A., Avidan, S.: Improved seam carving for video retargeting. In: ACM Transactions on Graphics (TOG), vol. 27, p. 16. ACM (2008)
3. Rubinstein, M., Shamir, A., Avidan, S.: Multi-operator media retargeting. ACM Transactions on graphics (TOG) **28**(3), 23 (2009)
4. Pritch, Y., Kav-Venaki, E., Peleg, S.: Shift-map image editing. In: 2009 IEEE 12th International Conference on Computer Vision, pp. 151–158. IEEE (2009)
5. Panozzo, D., Weber, O., Sorkine, O.: Robust image retargeting via axis-aligned deformation. In: Computer Graphics Forum, vol. 31, pp. 229–236. Wiley Online Library (2012)
6. Lin, S.-S., Yeh, I.-C., Lin, C.-H., Lee, T.-Y.: Patch-based image warping for content-aware retargeting. IEEE Trans. Multimedia **15**(2), 359–368 (2012)
7. Chen, R., Freedman, D., Karni, Z., Gotsman, C., Liu, L.: Content-aware image resizing by quadratic programming. In: 2010 IEEE Computer Society Conference on Computer Vision and Pattern Recognition-Workshops, pp. 1–8. IEEE (2010)
8. Shi, M., Yang, L., Peng, G., Xu, D.: A content-aware image resizing method with prominent object size adjusted. In: Proceedings of the 17th ACM Symposium on Virtual Reality Software and Technology, pp. 175–176. ACM (2010)
9. Song, E., Lee, M., Lee, S.: Carvingnet: Content-guided seam carving using deep convolution neural network. IEEE Access **7**, 284–292 (2018)
10. Song, Y., et al.: Photo squarization by deep multi-operator retargeting. In: ACM Multimedia, pp. 1047–1055 (2018)
11. Cho, D., Park, J., Oh, T.-H., Tai, Y.-W., So Kweon, I.: Weakly-and self-supervised learning for content-aware deep image retargeting. In: Proceedings of the IEEE International Conference on Computer Vision, pp. 4558–4567 (2017)
12. Tan, W., Yan, B., Lin, C., Niu, X.: Cycle-ir: Deep cyclic image retargeting. IEEE Trans. Multimedia **22**(7), 1730–1743 (2019)
13. Shocher, A., Bagon, S., Isola, P., Irani, M.: Internal distribution matching for natural image retargeting. arXiv preprint arXiv:1812.00231 (2018)
14. Zhou, Y., Chen, Z., Li, W.: Weakly supervised reinforced multi-operator image retargeting. IEEE Trans. Circuits Syst. Video Technol. **31**(1), 126–139 (2020)
15. Kajiura, N., Kosugi, S., Wang, X., Yamasaki, T.: Self-play reinforcement learning for fast image retargeting. In: Proceedings of the 28th ACM International Conference on Multimedia, pp. 1755–1763 (2020)
16. Tang, Z., Yao, J., Zhang, Q.: Multi-operator image retargeting in compressed domain by preserving aspect ratio of important contents. Multimedia Tools and Applications, 1–22 (2022)
17. Mei, Y., Guo, X., Sun, D., Pan, G., Zhang, J.: Deep supervised image retargeting. In: 2021 IEEE International Conference on Multimedia and Expo (ICME), pp. 1–6. IEEE (2021)
18. Liang, Y., Liu, Y.-J., Gutierrez, D.: Objective quality prediction of image retargeting algorithms. IEEE Trans. Visual Comput. Graphics **23**(2), 1099–1110 (2016)
19. Isola, P., Zhu, J.-Y., Zhou, T., Efros, A.A.: Image-to-image translation with conditional adversarial networks. In: Proceedings of the IEEE Conference on Computer Vision and Pattern Recognition, pp. 1125–1134 (2017)
20. Ioffe, S., Szegedy, C.: Batch normalization: Accelerating deep network training by reducing internal covariate shift. arXiv preprint arXiv:1502.03167 (2015)
21. Kingma, D.P., Ba, J.: Adam: A method for stochastic optimization. arXiv preprint arXiv:1412.6980 (2014)
22. Wang, Y.-S., Tai, C.-L., Sorkine, O., Lee, T.-Y.: Optimized scale-and-stretch for image resizing. In: ACM Transactions on Graphics (TOG), vol. 27, p. 118. ACM (2008)

MulTIR: Deep Multi-Target Image Retargeting

Di Sun[1], Yitong Guo[1], Chaojie Yao[1], Yijing Mei[2], Dufeng Chen[3], and Gang Pan[2(✉)]

[1] College of Artificial Intelligence, Tianjin University of Science and Technology,
Tianjin 300222, China
[2] College of Intelligence and Computing, Tianjin University, Tianjin 300350, China
pangang@tju.edu.cn
[3] Beijing Geotechnical and Investigation Engineering Insititute, Beijing 100080, China

Abstract. Image retargeting aims to resize images to fit various devices while maintaining good viewing experiences. Normally, multi-operator image retargeting shows better performance than single operator strategy, however, there is still no single method that performs well on all cases. This inspires us to provide a general image retargeting framework that can adaptively learns from multiple methods. We present a multi-target image retargeting model named MulTIR, which learns the deformation process from multiple diverse outputs and automatically pick the optimal target in feature space. We also introduce a Mean-GAN-Min-Task loss to adapt the additional targets in each training example. Experimental results indicate the superiority of MulTIR against representative methods.

Keywords: Image retargeting · Multi-target · GAN · 1-to-M mapping

1 Introduction

The rise of media devices necessitates adjusting images and videos for full-screen display with appropriate aspect ratios and resolutions. Traditional scaling techniques often result in distortions like shrinking, clipping, or stretching. Image retargeting technology addresses this by adjusting aspect ratios while preserving essential information. Recent content-aware methods have seen success by utilizing saliency maps and various importance measures like pixel gradient and color contrast [1–8]. However, these methods are constrained by fixed designs, and a single retargeting operator may not perform well for all scenarios.

In recent years, deep learning has shown its excellent performance in various applications. Recently, some learning based retargeting technologies have been presented [9–15]. Most methods use pre-trained network or improved network to extract deep features to calculate the corresponding importance map, and then directly perform retargeting operation in image space. The first end-to-end learning-based method is WSSDCNN ([13]), which utilizes an encoder-decoder to learn an attention map. Although the great progress has been made, this method has a limit on the sizes of the input images. Tan et al. ([14]) develop Cycle-IR, an unsupervised method that improves the quality of retargeted images by introducing cyclic perception consistency loss, however, it can not handle the situations when the important areas cover high proportion of the whole images. In general, there are little studies that attempt to address image retargeting problem by using supervised methods. This is because the evaluation of retargeted images from the perspective of vision is highly subjective, so it's difficult to construct a dedicated dataset to train the deep retargeting models.

Different from the task with clear objective or evaluation criteria, the image retargeting task is an uncertain problem, that is, the method to produce the desired retargeted result is unfixed, and the way to evaluate retargeted results is subjective. In some work, multiple operator-mixed measures are presented to accommodate the variation on various images and target sizes [2, 12, 16–20]. In general, multi-operator approaches perform better than single operator strategy, but they essentially arrange the order of operators to find the best combination, which is easy to fall into local optimum.

In this paper, we present a multiple target image retargeting method that deals with the aforementioned challenges. Rather than 1-to-1 training with an unavailable ground truth, we provide more than one target for each input image to automatically learn the optimal target in feature space. To our knowledge, this is the first attempt to address image retargeting in a deep multi-target learning manner. To accommodate the research, we construct a 1-to-M image retargeting dataset that consists of multiple diverse target images.

How to model for guiding 1-to-M mapping learning? We design MulTIR, a deep multi-target model based on Generative Adversarial Network(GAN) [21]. MulTIR performs retargeting operations in feature space, this makes it possible to pay attention to the generation of image details while learning the overall deformation of target images, so as to improve the naturalness and authenticity of the image. The last challenge for training such a retargeting generator is to solve the diversity among the target images obtained from multiple retargeting operators for the same input. We design a MeanGAN-Min-Task loss that carefully employs two different aggregate functions to guide the generation from multiple diverse targets encountered during training. Moreover, we provide in-depth experiments and demonstrate that MulTIR achieves superior performance compared with the state-of-the-art algorithms. The major contributions are as below:

- We provide a new solution into deep image retargeting that exploits information from multiple operators within the feature space. To our knowledge, this is the first attempt to address image retargeting in a deep multi-target learning manner.
- We present a deep learning-based image retargeting network that resolves uncertain target images by exploring 1-to-M mapping learning in feature space.

2 Related Work

Image retargeting requires adjusting input images into arbitrary size on the premise of preserving regions of importance. Early attempts usually employ some content-aware approaches to transform image to the target size. They can be generally divided into discrete and continuous methods. A typical discrete method is seam carving(SC) ([1]) which iteratively deletes or inserts pixels that produce the least loss of energy to preserve the visual saliency. Rubinstein et al. ([7]) modify seam carving by removing a seam from the minimum energy change to determine the energy of a pixel. Pritch et al. ([3]) present a Shift-Map (SM) technique to remove or add band regions. Normally, these methods [1–3, 7] resize the image by removing discrete regions, which easily bring visual distortions. In contrast, continuous measures [5, 8] utilize non-uniform grid deformation to preserve important areas. For example, Wang et al. ([8]) iteratively calculate the optimal scaling factor of each local area, and update the image with the help of saliency map. Guo et al. ([5]) construct a saliency-based mesh representation which is consistent with the underlying image structures. In general, these traditional approaches require computing a salience map based on hand-drafted features. The quality of salience map directly affects the performance of these approaches.

More recently, many learning-based retargeting methods have been developed, such as CarvingNet [9], DeepIR [10]. However, above approaches require separate steps to perform retargeting operation, rather than an end-to-end training process. Whereafter, Cho et al. [13] pose a weakly and selfsupervised end-to-end model to learn a shift map from the original image to the retargeting map. Although the methods are end-to-end training, they are essentially dependent on the importance map obtained by calculation, so their results are also limited by the calculation measure of the importance map. Besides, Tan et al. [14] develop an unsupervised deep cyclic image retargeting method (Cycle-IR) that improves the quality with cyclic perception consistency loss, however, it cannot handle images with large areas of visual importance. Shocher et al. [22] pose a fully unsupervised image specific GAN(InGAN). It uses a single input image to learn its internal patch distribution to synthesize a different size output. Therefore, the time cost is intolerable for abundant synthesis task. it does not take into account the semantics or scenes of the image.

As for multi-operator image retargeting, Rubinstein et al. [2] are the earliest to propose multi-operator retargeting by combining several representative operators in an optimal manner. Song et al. [12] present a CNN-based framework that introduces user preference for researching the photo squarization problem in the image retargeting field. Zhou et al. [19] utilize reinforcement learning to perform global optimization. These methods generally arrange the order of operators to find the best combination, and then perform the retargeting operation in image space. They are essentially searching for the optimal operator according to different strategies.

3 Approach

Our aim is to design a deep model which can produce visually pleasing ratargeted images. A key aspect is that each original input corresponds to multiple target images obtained by different methods, as shown in Fig. 1.

3.1 Formulation

We use the power of Generative Adversarial Network (GAN) [21]. It contains a generator G and a discriminator D. The generator takes the input image x, and together with a transformation T (which determines the target size), it maps to a target y. The generator G is designed to produce "real" images, while the discriminator D undergoes adversarial

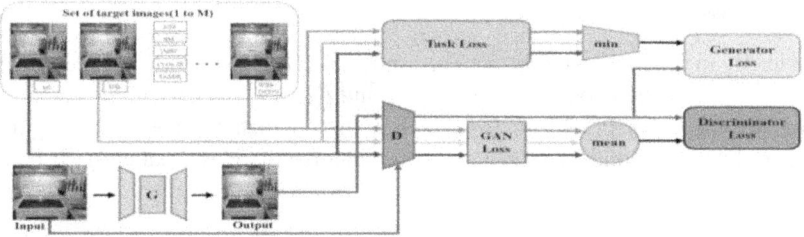

Fig. 1. MulTIR architecture. A generative adversarial network for image retargeting that illustrates multiple different outputs encountered during training.

training to determine whether an image is real or fake. Mathematically, this optimization problem can be written as:

$$G^* = \min_G \max_D L_{gan}(x, y) \tag{1}$$

$$L_{gan}(x, y) = \mathbb{E}_{(y)} \log D(y) + \mathbb{E}_{(x,T)} \log(1 - D(G(x; T))) \tag{2}$$

The L_{gan} encourages the distribution of $G(x; T)$ is matched to that of x. In fact, applying only L_{gan} may cause mode collapse, so the GAN loss is normally combined with a task loss. We follow the common way to include a task loss which aims to avoid mode collapse. The total loss function is summarized as:

$$L_{total}(x, y) = \lambda L_{gan}(x, y) + L_{task}(x, y), \tag{3}$$

However, we have multiple targets $y_i^{(1)}, y_i^{(2)}, ..., y_i^{(M_i)}$ for the same input x_i. It's w-orth emphasizing that the number of M_i may vary for different inputs, so this 1-to-M mapping can be viewed as a regular 1-to-1 mapping problem: $\left(x_1, y_1^{(1)}\right), ..., (x_1, y_1^{(M_1)}), ..., \left(x_N, y_N^{(1)}\right), ..., \left(x_N, y_N^{(M_i)}\right)$. Motivated by [23], our method treats $(x_i^{(1)}, y_i^{(1)}, y_i^{(2)}, ..., y_i^{(M_i)})$ as a single training example, and these pairs are randomly fetched to train the network. To fit the additional targets in each training case, we introduce a Mean-GAN-Min-Task loss. The generator G and the discriminator D employ two different aggregate functions, respectively. The final loss is formulated as:

$$L(x_i, y_i^{(1)}, ..., y_i^{(M_i)}) = \frac{\lambda}{M_i} \sum_{j=1}^{M_i} L_{gan}(x_i, y_i^{(j)}) + \min_{j \in (1,...,M_i)} L_{task}(x_i, y_i^{(j)}) \tag{4}$$

Here we average over the target images to aggregate the GAN loss. The generator adaptively pick the most suitable target to generate on-the-fly by means of the min aggregate function. The discriminator learns to distinguish the generated ratargeted image from all target images with equal importance by using the mean aggregate function. Hence, the issue of conflicting gradients caused by diverse modalities is effectively alleviated.

3.2 Task Loss

As previously mentioned, we follow the common in GAN to include a task loss. For our retargeting task, the task loss includes L_1, L_{tv} and L_p.

First, we use a per-pixel loss L_1, which is the L1 distance between the generated image and the corresponding target image to enhance the pixel matching. It is defined as below:

$$L_1 = \|y - G(x)\|_1, \tag{5}$$

In order to maintain the object shape and enhance the smoothness in generated images, we also adopt a total variation loss L_{tv} as shown in equation:

$$L_{tv} = \frac{1}{CWH} \|\nabla G(x) - \nabla y\|_1, \tag{6}$$

where C denotes the channel number, ∇ represents the image gradient, and W and H are width and height, respectively.

In addition, we employ a perceptual loss L_P to constrain the feature similarity between the generated image and the corresponding target.

$$L_p = \sum_{l=L-2}^{L-1} \beta_l \cdot \|\Phi_l(y) - \Phi_l(G(x))\|_2, \tag{7}$$

where L represents the number of convolution blocks in the pre-trained *VGG*19. β contributes the weight of each item to the total perceptual loss. Φ_l is used to extract the feature map of the l-th convolution block in *VGG*19. $\|\cdot\|_2$ is the Euclidean norm.

Finally, the combined task loss function is as follows:

$$L_{task}(x, y) = \lambda_1 L_1(x, y) + \lambda_2 L_{tv}(x, y) + \lambda_3 L_p(x, y), \tag{8}$$

here λ_i is the set parameter of contribution weight to the task loss, which is obtained according to the experiment.

3.3 Network Details

The generator G follows the hourglass architecture [24]. Dilated convolutionsare utilized to expand the receptive field of the convolutions, so as to preserve global characteristics of the image and enhance the network applicability for different scale images. At the same time, the 1×1 convolution can increase the interaction among 6 channels and increase the network learning ability. The bottleneck uses ResNet module that consists of six residual-blocks. The decoder of G is completely symmetrical with the encoder part. Resize-convolution layer is used as an alternative instead of regular deconvolution, and skip connections are also employed between the mirrored layers of the encoder and decoder part. The network architecture of the generator is shown in Fig. 2.

For discriminator D, we use the patch discriminatorwith full convolution. Normally, PatchGAN helps to generate nice texture and shape. Because the generator part has taken overall information into account, we focus on local features in the discriminator.

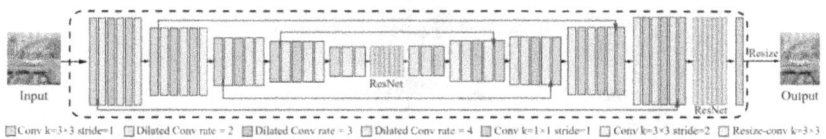

Fig. 2. The architecture of generator G. The red lines demonstrate skip-connections, and k is the kernel size. (Color figure online)

4 Experiments

4.1 Experimental Settings

TIReD Dataset ([25]). TIReD is a deep paired dataset in image retargeting. It composed of 6,576 pair images. Instead of directly using these pair images, we focus on retargeted images obtained by different methods, so we use the original input and its corresponding retargeted results.

Experimental Settings. The experiments are carried out under the configuration of NVIDIA TITAN V GPU with 12GB memory and Intel i7-10700K processor. The proposed network is implemented in PyTorch. We train and update the network parameters by the ADAM optimizer with an initial leaning rate 2×10^{-4}. We train the model on the TIReD which includes 5,000 groups with multiple target images. In training, we set the value of β_{L-1} in L_P to 2 and β_{L-2} to 1. The values of λ is set to 10. And in formula 8, the values of $\lambda 1$, $\lambda 2$ and $\lambda 3$ are 1000, 10 and 0.01, respectively. The activation functions of the encoder and decoder use LReLU and ReLU respectively. We also employ batch normalization in most convolutional blocks to encourage stability of the proposed model. Here the batch size is set to 4.

4.2 Ablation Study

Figure 3 shows the results in ablation study, where column (a) shows the original input, column (b) indicates the result of MulTIR model, and column (c)–(e) are the results without using L_1, L_{tv} and L_p respectively. It can be found that the design of L_1 makes the network more stable and has a more positive effect on the truthiness of the generated image (the first line in Fig. 3). L_{tv} has a great effect on maintaining straight lines and object shapes(see the first and second rows in Fig. 3), the circle of wheels and the boundary of people and animals are maintained better. It makes the model more sensitive to pure edge lines and generate results with more correct contours. L_p makes the semantic information of the retargeted image more correct. It can be observed that the semantic information is better preserved in the two cases in Fig. 3. In addition, as we can see from Table 1, the evaluation achieves the best performance when all the loss functions are included. It is thus proved that each loss function has a definite effect.

4.3 Performance Comparison

We compare MulTIR with the following state-of-the-art image retargeting algorithms, which include SC [1], ISC [7], SM [3], SNS [8], USL, Cycle-IR [14], WSSDCNN [13] and SAMIR [19] on TIReD and RetargetMe.

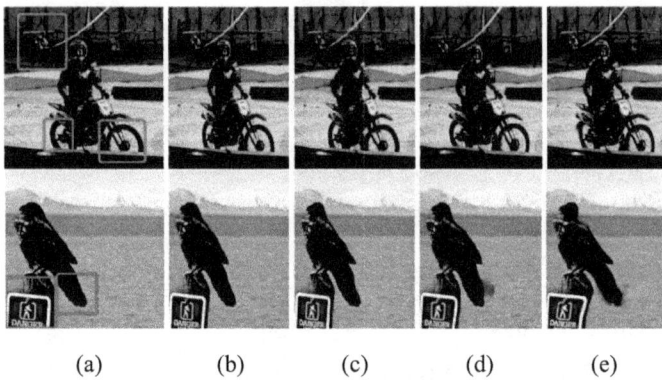

Fig. 3. Ablation study. (a) Original images. (b) Our results. (c)-(e) Results without $\mathcal{L}_1$, $\mathcal{L}_{tv}$ and $\mathcal{L}_P$, respectively.

Table 1. Retargeting results for ablation study. The values in bold indicate the best performances.

Metric	No-$\mathcal{L}_P$	No-$\mathcal{L}_{tv}$	No-$\mathcal{L}_1$	Ours
NIQE	6.3466	5.9318	6.0561	**5.7364**
BRISQU	24.4563	22.3521	23.2343	**20.2025**
NBIQA	25.3482	20.7672	22.8723	**20.3855**

Qualitative Evaluation. Figure 4 provides visual comparisons of our results with other methods. The first three rows depict results on TIReD. While most methods preserve contents with semantic importance, there are deformations of lines and edges. SC and ISC tend to generate shape inconsistencies, SM creates discontinuous artifacts, and SCL excessively reduces important objects by merging adjacent pixels. WSSDCNN exhibits shape deformations on the tower and pencil (Fig. 4(i)). Some semantic content loss is observed in Fig. 4(g), while Cycle-IR experiences similar issues with missing details affecting visual experience (Fig. 4(h)). In contrast, MulTIR performs better, preserving both human and shadow parts well (Fig. 4(j)). The last three rows showcase cases on RetargetMe, where most methods cause varying degrees of shape distortions as highlighted in the red box. In contrast, MulTIR better preserves content and avoids distortions, benefiting from deep supervised learning and semantic information effectiveness. MulTIR's ability to learn from multiple methods enables high-quality retargeted images across various inputs.

Quantitative Evaluation. We numerically compare our algorithm with three image quality evaluation metrics NIQE [26], BRISQU [27] and NBIQA [28]. Among them, NIQE algorithm is closer to the human vision system, which is effective enough to evaluate image quality. BRISQU algorithm needs to calculate the feature vectors based on extracted natural scene statistics, so as to evaluate image quality from the perspective of spatial domain. The NBIQA algorithm mainly considers the feature information from both transform and spatial domain and trains the regression model to predict the image

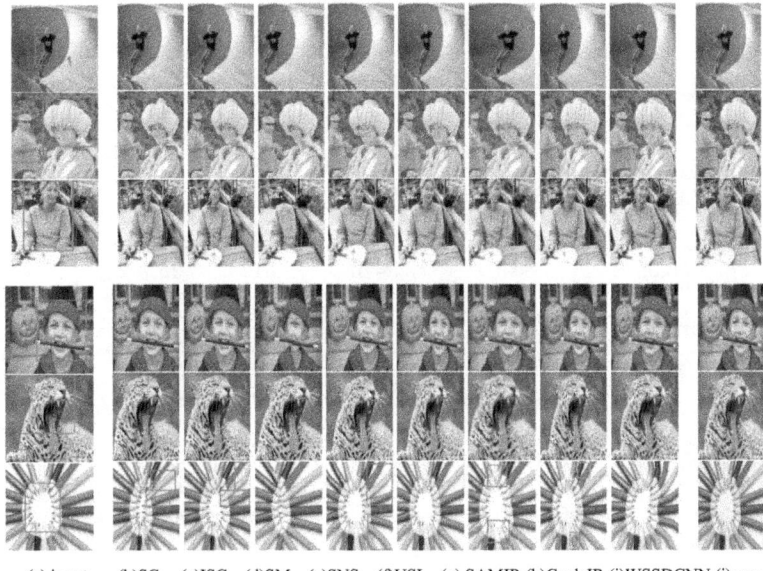

(a) input　(b)SC　(c)ISC　(d)SM　(e)SNS　(f)USL　(g) SAMIR (h)CycleIR (i)WSSDCNN (j)ours

Fig. 4. Visual comparison of our method with representative retargeting approaches on TIReD and RetargetMe dataset.

quality score. Table 2 presents the objective evaluation of the proposed algorithm with 8 representative methods, our model achieves the best or the second best performance.

User Study. We further conduct a user study to evaluate the subjective quality of the proposed method. 20 participants from different backgrounds are recruited (age from 25 to 50, 10 males and 10 females). 30 groups of images are displayed randomly for each participant in turn. The leftmost side of each group is the original image, followed by 9 randomly arranged retargeted images. Each switch from one group to another would rearrange the 9 choices randomly. Each participant chooses two images he likes from the nine image options, without time limit. As shown in Table 3, our work receives the highest number of votes. In addition, considering that the uniform scaling method is a moderate baseline, it is qualitatively meaningful that our method records the most votes.

Table 2. Comparison with recent works on TIReD and RetargetMe. The values in bold and underlined demonstrate the best and the second best performance respectively.

Method	NIQE	BRISQUE	NBIQA	NIQE (RM)	BRISQUE (RM)	NBIQA (RM)
SC	6.1959	25.306	24.085	7.2971	29.540	24.950
ISC	6.2171	23.564	23.508	7.4080	28.668	24.525

(*continued*)

Table 2. (*continued*)

Method	NIQE	BRISQUE	NBIQA	NIQE (RM)	BRISQUE (RM)	NBIQA (RM)
SM	6.1496	23.398	24.441	6.8255	25.925	25.951
SNS	5.7299	**20.302**	24.393	5.9060	**17.364**	20.899
USL	6.0372	22.146	24.007	6.6481	23.827	23.478
SAMIR	6.0672	22.841	24.470	7.0125	25.172	24.346
Cycle-IR	5.8608	22.562	23.211	6.1486	21.008	20.953
WSSDCNN	5.9312	22.214	23.300	6.4185	23.161	23.216
Ours	**5.6912**	22.135	**23.181**	5.9157	18.327	**19.851**

Table 3. The voting results of user study for comparing with representative methods. There are 20 participants with 2 votes each, and 1200 votes in the total. Our results have received more votes and more user preferences.

Method	USL	SC	ISC	SM	SNS	SAMIR	Cycle-IR	WSSDCNN	Ours
Votes	125	116	114	116	151	106	143	150	179
Proportion	10.4%	9.5%	9.7%	9.5%	12.6%	8.8%	11.9%	12.5%	14.9%

5 Conclusion

This study provide new insights into supervised image retargeting. For the first time, multiple ground truths learning is exploited to address the uncertain target image problem in image retargeting task. We employ a comprehensive dataset with groups of target images generated by different retargeting methods to ensure data diversity. We then present an effective deep model to implement the proposed MulTIR. Extensive experiments indicate the superior performance of the proposed method.

Acknowledgments. This work was funded by the Natural Science Foundation of Tianjin (No. 21JCYBJC00640), 2023 CCF-Baidu Songguo Foundation Research on Scene Text Recognition Based on PaddlePaddle).

References

1. Avidan, S., Shamir, A.: Seam carving for content-aware image resizing. ToG (2007)
2. Rubinstein, M., Shamir, A., Avidan, S.: Multi-operator media retargeting. ToG **23** (2009)
3. Pritch, Y., Kav-Venaki, E., Peleg, S.: Shift-map image editing. In: ICCV, pp. 151–158. IEEE (2009)
4. Lin, S.-S., Yeh, I.-C., Lin, C.-H., Lee, T.-Y.: Patch-based image warping for content-aware retargeting. TMM **15**(2), 359–368 (2012)

5. Guo, Y., Feng, L., Jian, S., Zhou, Z.H., Gleicher, M.: Image retargeting using mesh parametrization. TMM **11**(5), 856–867 (2009)
6. Asheghi, B., Salehpour, P., Khiavi, A.M., Hashemzadeh, M.: A comprehensive review on content-aware image retargeting: from classical to state-of-the-art methods. Signal Process. **195**, 108496 (2022). https://doi.org/10.1016/j.sigpro.2022.108496
7. Rubinstein, M., Shamir, A., Avidan, S.: Improved seam carving for video retargeting. ToG **27**, 16–1169 (2008)
8. Wang, Y.-S., Tai, C.-L., Sorkine, O., Lee, T.-Y.: Optimized scale-and-stretch for image resizing. In: ToG, p. 118. ACM (2008)
9. Song, E., Lee, M., Lee, S.: CarvingNet: content-guided seam carving using deep convolution neural network. Access, 284–292 (2018)
10. Lin, J., Zhou, T., Chen, Z.: DeepIR: a deep semantics driven framework for image retargeting. arXiv preprint arXiv:1811.07793 (2018)
11. Arar, M., Danon, D., Cohen-Or, D., Shamir, A.: Image resizing by reconstruction from deep features. arXiv preprint arXiv:1904.08475 (2019)
12. Song, Y., Tang, F., Dong, W., Zhang, X., Deussen, O., Lee, T.-Y., et al.: Photo squarization by deep multi-operator retargeting. In: MM, pp. 1047–1055. ACM (2018)
13. Cho, D., Park, J., Oh, T.-H., Tai, Y.-W., So Kweon, I.: Weakly-and self-supervised learning for content-aware deep image retargeting. In: ICCV, pp. 4558–4567. IEEE (2017)
14. Tan, W., Yan, B., Lin, C., Niu, X.: Cycle-IR: deep cyclic image retargeting. TMM **22**(7), 1730–1743 (2020)
15. Imani, H., Islam, M.B., Wong, L.-K.: Saliency-aware stereoscopic video retargeting. In: Proceedings of the IEEE/CVF Conference on Computer Vision and Pattern Recognition (CVPR) Workshops, pp. 1230–1239 (2023)
16. Qiu, Z., Ren, T., Liu, Y., Bei, J., Yang, Y.: Multi-operator image retargeting based on automatic quality assessment. In: ICIG, pp. 428–433 (2013)
17. Qian, Z., Tang, Z., Jiang, H., Kan, C.: Multi-operator image retargeting with preserving aspect ratio of important contents, pp. 306–315 (2017)
18. Wu, L., Yan, C., Jian, M., Liu, S., Dong, W., Chen, C.W.: A fast hybrid retargeting scheme with seam context and content aware strip partition. Neurocomputing **286**, 198–213 (2018)
19. Zhou, Y., Chen, Z., Li, W.: Weakly supervised reinforced multi-operator image retargeting. TCSVT **PP**(99), 1 (2020)
20. Tang, Z., Yao, J., Zhang, Q.: Multi-operator image retargeting in compressed domain by preserving aspect ratio of important contents. Multimedia Tools Appl. **81**, 1–22 (2022)
21. Goodfellow, I., et al.: Generative adversarial nets. In: NeurIPS, pp. 2672–2680 (2014)
22. Shocher, A., Bagon, S., Isola, P., Irani, M.: Internal distribution matching for natural image retargeting. arXiv preprint arXiv:1812.00231 (2018)
23. Li, M., Lin, Z., Mech, R., Yumer, E., Ramanan, D.: Photo-sketching: inferring contour drawings from images. In: WACV, pp. 1403–1412. IEEE (2019)
24. Ronneberger, O., Fischer, P., Brox, T.: U-net: Convolutional networks for biomedical image segmentation. In: Navab, N., Hornegger, J., Wells, W.M., Frangi, A.F. (eds.) MICCAI 2015. LNCS, vol. 9351, pp. 234–241. Springer, Cham (2015). https://doi.org/10.1007/978-3-319-24574-4_28
25. Mei, Y., Guo, X., Sun, D., Pan, G., Zhang, J.: Deep supervised image retargeting. In: ICME, pp. 1–6. IEEE (2021)
26. Mittal, A., Soundararajan, R., Bovik, A.C.: Making a "completely blind" image quality analyzer. SPL **20**, 209–212 (2012)
27. Mittal, A., Moorthy, A.K., Bovik, A.C.: No-reference image quality assessment in the spatial domain. TIP **21**(12), 4695–4708 (2012)
28. Ou, F.-Z., Wang, Y.-G., Zhu, G.: A novel blind image quality assessment method based on refined natural scene statistics. In: ICIP, pp. 1004–1008 (2019)

PAAM (Parameter-free Attentional Aggregation Model)

Xuan-Hao Qi, Min Zhi(✉), Zeng Mi, Wei Hu, Yan-Jun Yin, Yue-Ning Zhang, Wen-Tao Duan, and Zhe Lian

College of Computer Science and Technology, Inner Mongolia Normal University, Hohhot 010022, China
cieczm@imnu.edu.cn

Abstract. The channel attention mechanism and spatial attention mechanism are crucial in enhancing the performance of convolutional neural networks. However, most existing methods focus on developing more intricate attention modules to improve performance, which inevitably increases the number of model parameters. To address the trade-off between performance and parameter count, this paper introduces an efficient Parameter-free Attention Aggregation Model (PAAM) plug-and-play module. The module first creates a Local Feature Enhancement Module (LFEM) using adaptive pooling. Firstly, the local feature enhancement module (LFEM) is constructed through adaptive pooling to enhance the expression of local features; secondly, the local-global feature interaction module (L-GFIM) is used to realize the mutual compensation between local and global features, which effectively extends the coverage of local-global interaction. The experimental results indicate that PAAM outperforms the SOTA model in ImageNet-1K, Cifar-10, and Cifar-100 image classification datasets.

Keywords: Attention Mechanism · Parameter-free · Local-global Feature Mutual Compensation · Computer Vision

1 Introduction

The field of deep learning has led to a significant focus on image recognition using convolutional neural networks [1] (CNNs). In 2012, AlexNet [2] gained recognition for its ability to learn representations, generalize, and maintain translation invariance, leading to its success in the ILSVRC ImageNet competition. Following this, VGGNet [3] achieved second place in 2014 and has since been used as the foundation for further research. In 2014, Ian Goodfellow's team proposed the generative adversarial network [4] (GAN), which achieved great success in image generation and natural language processing (NLP). In 2015, Microsoft Labs proposed the residual network [5] (ResNet), which successfully mitigated the problem of gradient vanishing in deep neural networks by using jump connections. In the same year, Ronneberger's team [6] proposed U-Net, initially for biomedical image segmentation, and later widely used for image semantic segmentation. In 2017, two lightweight network architectures were proposed: MobileNet

[7] and ShuffleNet [8]. DenseNet [9] improved performance through dense connectivity and feature reuse. Currently, the mainstream research trend aims to enhance the feature extraction capability of CNNs and improve their performance by improving the network structure. This is achieved through the design of stacked convolution, residual connectivity, and dense connectivity. This is an important research direction in the current field of computer vision [10].

Another area of research has concentrated on constructing plug-and-play attention modules. The plug-and-play attention modules are designed to be flexible and versatile, allowing for easy integration into various network architectures without significant modifications to the overall structure. They refine the output features within the convolutional layer, enabling the entire network to learn more feature information. Additionally, the attention mechanism assigns different weights to the features, highlighting important ones and suppressing minor ones, ultimately improving network performance. Using SE-Net [11] as an example, the SE module, which is an independent network architecture, can be directly inserted into various networks, such as VGG, ResNet, and ResNeXts [12], to significantly enhance the performance of the baseline model.

Currently, plug-and-play attention modules have limitations. (1) Most attention modules focus on extracting local features independently along the channel or spatial dimension. However, this approach often ignores the correlation between spatial and channel information, resulting in the model losing key information about local features across channels and spaces, which affects its overall performance. (2) Many existing attention modules are connected in series, acquiring only local or global feature information, which limits the model's expressive ability and scope of application by failing to realize the mutual compensation of local-global features. To address these issues, this paper proposes a plug-and-play, lightweight, parameterless attention mechanism.

The main contribution of this paper is specifically 3 points:

1. The LFEM module is inspired by the human attention mechanism. It uses adaptive pooling to dynamically select feature regions of interest, filter out redundant information, and focus on critical local information in the image. This enhances the ability to capture key local features and ultimately improves pixel-level feature extraction.
2. The L-GFIM module utilizes a new local-global feature interaction strategy to combine channel attention, spatial attention, cross-channel, and spatial attention, achieving mutual compensation between local and global features. Additionally, the residual structure is employed to preserve the original image information, preventing information loss caused by network deepening and ensuring the model accurately captures the image's detail information.
3. PAAM has zero parameters and is highly flexible, making it easy to integrate into various deep learning architectures. In comparison to other popular attention models, this algorithm demonstrates significant advantages in terms of accuracy, parameter count, and speed.

2 Related Work

Attention mechanism is an effective method to improve the accuracy of image processing tasks, and its core idea is to mimic the selective perception mechanism of the human visual system, dynamically adjusting the feature weights of the input image, focusing the attention on the most important regions in the image and suppressing the irrelevant parts, so as to improve the performance and accuracy of the computer vision system. In the process of machine learning, the attention mechanism can enhance its ability to discriminate between useful and redundant data information to improve model performance. This technique has been widely used in various fields of deep learning, such as target detection, image super-resolution, and human pose estimation. Currently existing attention mechanisms are mainly categorized into channel attention mechanisms and hybrid channel and spatial attention.

1. Almost all current models of channel attention are based on the composition of the compression and expansion module of SE-Net. This module enhances and suppresses feature information in the channels to obtain the correlation between them, resulting in high-quality feature maps.
2. ECA-Net [13] uses one-dimensional convolution to obtain neighboring channel information, resulting in more accurate channel attention information. This allows high-dimensional channels to interact over a longer range while introducing fewer parameters and minimal computation.
3. GCT [14] combines gating mechanisms and normalization methods to selectively use different channel feature information for modeling.
4. SK-Net [15] uses Selective Kernel convolution instead of ordinary convolution to obtain receptive fields of different sizes by dynamically selecting convolution kernels. This allows for better adaptation to different object shapes and sizes.
5. CG [16] starts with the overall semantics and information of the image and uses a lightweight global context module to capture the image's overall structure and semantic relations. The four types of channel attention can be combined into the form shown in Fig. 1. Channel attention and Channel and spatial mixed attention methods.
6. CBAM [17] extracts refined feature map information sequentially from two dimensions using channel attention and spatial attention to comprehensively capture the long-term dependency relationship between features.
7. BAM [18] uses parallel channel and spatial attention mechanisms to achieve the complementarity of channel and spatial information without losing any information.
8. PSA [19] introduces nonlinear transformations while maintaining high resolution in space and channels by polarizing the self-attention module to output more detailed feature maps.
9. A2-Net [20] collects key features from the entire space into a compact set. The first level of attention selectively collects key features from the entire space, while the second level of attention adaptively distributes the collected key features. (6) to (9) These four types of attention for channel and spatial mixing can be combined in the form of Fig. 1. Channel attention and Channel and spatial mixed attention methods.

Figure 1. Channel attention and Channel and spatial mixed attention methods. Presents methods of channel attention and hybrid channel-spatial attention. While these approaches have achieved excellent performance, each attention model still has limitations, specifically in that they can only capture either channel or spatial feature information separately, failing to establish an information flow between channels and spaces.

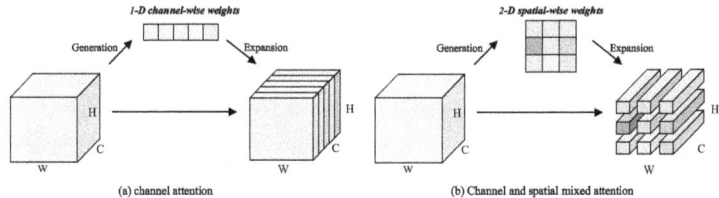

Fig. 1. Channel attention and Channel and spatial mixed attention methods.

This results in insufficient capability of the models to capture contextual semantic information. To address these issues, this paper effectively establishes contextual dependencies through the LFEM and L-GFEM modules. Experiments conducted on the public datasets ImageNet-1K, Cifar-10, and Cifar-100 demonstrate that, without requiring any additional parameters, PAAM outperforms other SOTA models in image classification tasks.

3 Method

This paper proposes a novel attention mechanism that utilizes mutual compensation between local and global features to capture both global context information and local detail features of an image. This approach addresses the issue of relying on single information and eliminates incomplete overall structure of the target, resulting in refined target contours compared to other attention mechanisms. The proposed model effectively integrates rich global and local feature information. The importance of image classification and target detection cannot be overstated.

Figure 2. Overall framework diagram of the network. Illustrates the PAAM network structure, which comprises three main components: the local feature enhancement module (LFEM), the global feature enhancement module (GFEM), and the local-global feature interaction module (L-GFIM). LFEM utilizes adaptive pooling to extract local enhancement features across channels and spaces in adjacent local regions. GFEM adopts the energy function to obtain global features across channels and spaces simultaneously. L-GFIM fuses the parallel extracted global features and local features. The fusion of global and local features compensates for local-global features, allowing the model to better understand and utilize feature information at different scales. The residual structure is used to obtain the original image information, avoiding network deepening that leads to information loss and ensuring that the model accurately captures detail information in the image. Where C, H, and W represent the channel size, height, and width of the image.

3.1 Local Feature Enhancement Module

To address the challenge of obtaining local information on subtle differences in the feature map, we designed a Local Feature Enhancement Module (LFEM) inspired by the BAM model. The LFEM enhances local feature expression by applying it to adjacent local regions. It consists of a parallel attention mechanism, which effectively suppresses

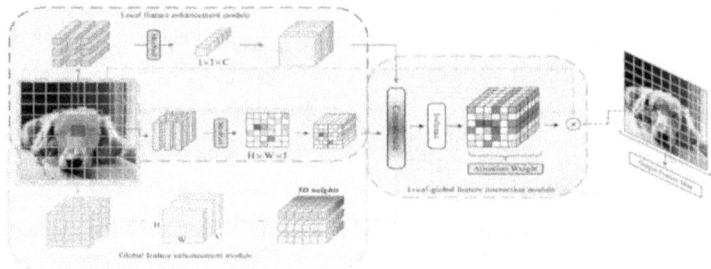

Fig. 2. Overall framework diagram of the network.

various interferences. Please refer to Fig. 1. Channel attention and Channel and spatial mixed attention methods. For a visual representation of the LFEM. Please refer to Fig. 1. Channel attention and Channel and spatial mixed attention methods. For a visual representation of the LFEM. Part 1 is channel attention, which redistributes the channel weights in the feature map through the maximum pooling operation to increase the weights of the relevant channels and reduce the weights of the remaining channels; part 2 is spatial attention, which re-gives the spatial weights more reasonably through the maximum pooling approach to give the potential spatial information in the feature map a higher weight, and reduces the remaining region weights; By adjusting the feature weights of the input image dynamically, attention is focused on the most critical local regions in the image while suppressing irrelevant parts. This effectively improves the performance and accuracy of the model.

Channel Attention. A global maximum pooling operation is performed along the spatial dimensions (i.e., height and width) of the input feature maps to compress the feature maps from $H \times W \times C$ to $1 \times 1 \times C$, thus obtaining a one-dimensional vector as the channel attention map, which is essentially a local representation of the most salient features of each channel in the entire spatial extent, and $y_C \in \mathbb{R}^{H \times W}$ is used as the weight coefficients of each channel, which is computed as shown in Eq. (1):

$$A_{ch}(y_C) = max\left(\frac{1}{H \times W}\sum_{i=1}^{H}\sum_{j=1}^{W} y_C(i,j)\right) \quad (1)$$

The channel attention mechanism selects the most representative feature values in each channel through maximum pooling and calculates channel weights accordingly to emphasize key channels and suppress non-key channels.

Spatial Attention. To achieve focused attention on the most important feature part of the spatial feature map, a global maximum pooling operation is performed along the channel dimensions of the input feature map to compress the feature map from $H \times W \times C$ to $H \times W \times 1$, generating a spatial attention weight map. The weight coefficient $x_{H \times W} \in \mathbb{R}^C$ for each space is calculated as shown in Eq. (2):

$$A_{sp}(x_{H \times W}) = max\left(\frac{1}{C}\sum_{i=1}^{C} x_{H \times W}(i)\right) \quad (2)$$

Spatial attention captures local spatial information across the feature map by calculating the maximum value of each spatial element on each channel and using it as the generated spatial attention weights.

3.2 Global Feature Enhancement Module

The GFEM module addresses the limitation of traditional methods in feature extraction, which only have a single method and struggle to obtain cross-channel and spatial attention information simultaneously. By calculating the linear divisibility between neurons, the module obtains cross-channel and spatial attention information at once. This approach not only overcomes the limitations of traditional methods but also comprehensively understands the feature structure of the data, enabling the refinement of global feature processing. The module defines an energy function for each neuron, as shown in Eq. (3):

$$e_t(\omega_t, b_t, y, x_i) = (y_t - \hat{t})^2 + \frac{1}{M-1} \sum_{i=1}^{M-1} (y_o - \hat{x}_i)^2 \tag{3}$$

where y_t and y_o represent the outputs of the target neuron and other neurons, respectively. $\hat{t}$ and x_i represent the true values of the target neuron and other neurons, respectively. M is the number of neurons per channel, and i represents the neuron index. Additionally, ω_t and b_t are the neuron weights and biases, respectively.

Secondly, this paper calculates the linear separability between the target neuron and other neurons in the same channel by minimizing the energy function. To simplify the calculation, binary labels of $y_t = 1$ and $y_o = -1$ are used, and a regular term is added to obtain the final energy function, as shown in Eq. (4):

$$e_t(\omega_t, b_t, y, x_i) = \frac{1}{M-1} \sum_{i=1}^{M-1} (-1 - (\omega_t x_i + b_t))^2 + (-1 - (\omega_t x_i + b_t))^2 + \lambda \omega_t^2 \tag{4}$$

Then, the mean $\mu_t = \frac{1}{M-1} \sum_{i=1}^{M-1} x_i$ and variance $\sigma_t^2 = \frac{1}{M-1} \sum_{i=1}^{M-1} (x_i - \mu_t)^2$ of all neurons on a single channel were used in order to calculate the reduction of the number of model parameters to obtain the minimum energy for each position as shown in Eq. (5):

$$e_t^* = \frac{4(\hat{\sigma}^2 + 2\lambda)}{(t - \mu_t)^2 + 2\sigma_t^2 + 2\lambda} \tag{5}$$

where the smaller the value of e_t^*, the more separable the target neuron and other neurons of the current feature map are, and the more significant the contribution is, proving that the neuron is more important.

Finally, each neuron weight on the feature map is evaluated using $1/e_t^*$ to obtain the final output feature map $\tilde{X}$ as shown in Eq. (6):

$$\tilde{X} = sigmoid\left(\frac{1}{E}\right) \tag{6}$$

where E is the set of all neuron e_t^* values for the feature map, and the addition of a sigmoid function limits the values in E from being too large.

The GFEM module demonstrates its unique advantage in the process of feature extraction by fully considering the interaction of information across different channels and spatial locations in the feature map. This allows for simultaneous attention to information across different channels (such as color and texture) and spatial locations in the image. The GFEM module is able to improve target recognition accuracy by considering multiple features in the image, thus avoiding the recognition bias caused by the traditional method that relies on single information acquisition.

3.3 Local-Global Feature Interaction Module (L-GFIM)

The Local-Global Feature Interaction Module (L-GFIM) integrates the features generated by the parallel local feature enhancement module and the global feature enhancement module to realize mutual compensation between the local and global features without losing any important information. The Local-Global Feature Interaction Module (L-GFIM) integrates the features generated by the parallel local feature enhancement module and the global feature enhancement module to realize mutual compensation between the local and global features without losing any important information. L-GFIM comprises the channel attention module $A_{ch} \in \mathbb{R}^{1 \times 1 \times C}$, the spatial attention module $A_{sp} \in \mathbb{R}^{H \times W \times 1}$, and the 3D attention module $A_{3D} \in \mathbb{R}^{H \times W \times C}$.

First, the maximum pooling operation is used to convert channel features and spatial features into local features, which are then used as feature weights. Next, 3D attention constructs an optimized energy function to compute uniform global weights in the feature maps and calculates the linear divisibility between neurons to determine the importance of each neuron. Finally, the channel and spatial attention maps are expanded along the reduced dimension, recombined with the 3D attention map, and the representation of the reorganized attention map is enhanced using the sigmoid gating mechanism. The enhanced attention map is then multiplied with the original input feature map to form the final output feature map. The entire process is shown in Eq. (7):

$$F' = \sigma \left(A_{sp} \otimes A_{ch} \otimes A_{3D} \right) \otimes F \qquad (7)$$

where $\otimes$ denotes the element-by-element multiplication operation, σ is the sigmoid function $\sigma(x) = \frac{1}{1+e^{-x}}$, and F' is used as the output of the PAAM module.

The L-GFIM module has a significant advantage in capturing channel and spatial correlations, which enhances the diversity and expressiveness of features. This is achieved by skillfully fusing the weight distributions of the channel and spatial dimensions, and integrating local and global information to capture complementary features. This design allows the model to concentrate on the most crucial parts of the input feature map, emphasize the most significant feature regions, and effectively suppress various interfering factors. This improves recognition accuracy and provides robust support for complex tasks.

4 Experimental Results

To test the model's effectiveness and generalization ability, this paper conducts numerous experiments on standard public datasets, including ImageNet-1K, CIFAR-10, CIFAR-100, in the field of image classification. The results are compared with those of other similar attention models with representative parametric quantities.

4.1 Experimental Details

This paper utilizes CUDA 11.6 as the computing platform for the deep learning framework, PyTorch 2.0.1, and Python 3.8 to develop the model. The NVIDIA GeForce RTX 3090 high-performance graphics card is used to train the model. Figure 3. Top-1 and Top-5 accuracy curves. Displays the curves of Top-1 and Top-5 accuracy during model training and testing, where the PAAM module is utilized to enhance the ResNet-50 baseline network. The Fig. 3. Top-1 and Top-5 accuracy curves. Shows that the introduction of the PAAM module significantly improves the performance of the baseline model in both the training and testing phases. The PAAM module enhances the recognition accuracy of the model by strengthening the relationship between the channels and spaces of the features. This validates the effectiveness of the parameter-free attention model proposed in this paper for image recognition tasks.

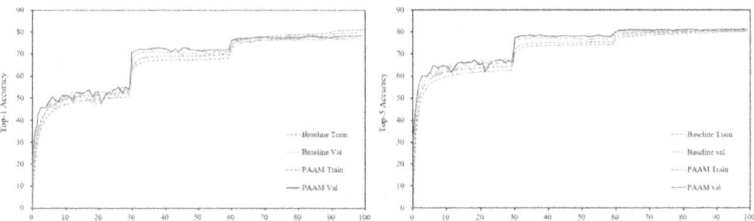

Fig. 3. Top-1 and Top-5 accuracy curves.

4.2 Experiment Comparing Parameter Count

Attention models currently in use employ additional sub-networks to generate attention weights, which increases model complexity compared to PAAM. PAAM, on the other hand, extracts 1D, 2D, and 3D information from input feature maps simultaneously by performing only element-by-element operations. Table 1. Comparison of structural design and parameters of different attention modules.lists the operations and parametric quantities of mainstream attention modules.

Operators are: k and r are the number of filters and the reduction ratio, respectively, and C stands for the number of channels; GAP, CAP, GMP, and CMP refer to spatially averaged pooling, channel averaged pooling, spatially maximal pooling, and channel maximal pooling, respectively; and C2D, C1D, FC, and BN refer to the standard convolution, the channel convolution, the standard fully-connected layer, and the bulk normalisation, respectively.

Table 1. Comparison of structural design and parameters of different attention modules.

Attention Modules	Operators	Parameters	Value
CBAM	GAP, GMP, FC, ReLU, CAP, CMP, BN, C2D, /, +, ⊙	$2C^2/r + 2k^2$	0.09M
SE	GAP, FC, ReLU, /, +, ⊙	$2C^2/r$	0.09M
ECA	GAP, C1D, /, +, ⊙	k	0M
PAAM	GAP, /, +, ⊙	0	0M

4.3 Image Classification Experiments

The ImageNet dataset comprises over 1.2 million color images, each of a specific size, and divided into 1000 categories. The dataset is further divided into a training set of 1.2 million images and a test set of 50,000 images. In this paper, the model is trained on the training set and the Top-1 accuracy of the output is tested on the test set. Top-1 accuracy refers to the accuracy of the first-ranked category that matches the actual results. The training process consists of 100 epochs, with an initial learning rate of 0.1. The learning rate is reduced by a factor of 10 at rounds 30, 60, and 90. For the MobileNet model, the initial learning rate is set to 0.5, and the weight decay rate is 4e-5. The training process for this model consists of 150 epochs. Table 2. ImageNet-1K dataset classification performance comparison. Presents the experimental results of the compared models on the ImageNet dataset. The PAAM model designed in this paper outperforms other existing attention-based models with zero parameters. Specifically, in ResNet-18, the Top1 accuracy is improved by 0.17% compared to CBAM, and better results are also achieved in ResNet-101. Furthermore, PAAM outperforms all other attention-based modules when using ResNet-34, ResNet-50, ResNeXt-50, and MobileNet as baseline models. It can also be added to existing networks without any additional parameters. Table 2. ImageNet-1K dataset classification performance comparison. Shows that SE and ECA have faster inference speeds than CBAM and SRM, and PAAM has even further speed improvements compared to other attention modules.

Table 3. Comparison of results with other methods on the CIFAR-10 and CIFAR-100 datasets. Presents the relevant data. The method proposed in this paper demonstrates significant advantages over several baseline models. When ResNet-20 and PreResNet-20 are used as the baseline models, the method in this paper outperforms other attention models in terms of accuracy and achieves the highest accuracy rate. In the PreResNet-101 network, SimAM achieved the best accuracy on CIFAR-10 (94.90) and CIFAR-100 (76.24), respectively. However, PAAM outperforms SimAM with a Top-1 accuracy of 94.91 compared to 76.57, respectively. Additionally, PAAM is capable of enhancing the performance of the WideResNet-20x10 large-scale network while maintaining its flexibility and versatility as a parameter-free attention module.

Table 2. ImageNet-1K dataset classification performance comparison.

Model	Top-1 Acc.	Top-5 Acc.	Baseline	+ Parameters	# FLOPs	Speed
ResNet-18	70.33%	89.58%	**11.69 M**	0	**1.82 G**	215 FPS
+SE	71.19%	**90.21%**	11.78 M	0.087 M	1.82 G	144 FPS
+CBAM	71.24%	90.04%	11.78 M	0.090 M	1.82 G	78 FPS
+ECA	70.71%	89.85%	11.69 M	36	1.82 G	148 FPS
+SRM	71.09%	89.98%	11.69 M	0.004 M	1.82 G	115 FPS
+PAAM	**71.41%**	89.88%	**11.69 M**	0	1.82 G	147 FPS
ResNet-34	73.75%	91.60%	**21.80 M**	0	**3.67 G**	119 FPS
+SE	74.32%	91.99%	21.95 M	0.157 M	3.67 G	81 FPS
+CBAM	74.41%	91.85%	21.96 M	0.163 M	3.67 G	38 FPS
+ECA	74.03%	91.73%	21.80 M	74	3.67 G	82 FPS
+SRM	**74.49%**	92.01%	21.81 M	0.008 M	3.67 G	59 FPS
+PAAM	74.47%	**92.04%**	21.80 M	0	3.67 G	78 FPS
ResNet-50	76.34%	93.12%	**25.56 M**	0	**4.11 G**	89 FPS
+SE	77.51%	93.74%	28.07 M	2.515 M	4.12 G	64 FPS
+CBAM	**77.63%**	**93.88%**	28.09 M	2.533 M	4.12 G	33 FPS
+ECA	77.17%	93.52%	25.56 M	88	4.12 G	64 FPS
+SRM	77.51%	93.06%	25.59 M	0.030 M	4.11 G	56 FPS
+PAAM	77.47%	93.69%	**25.56 M**	0	4.11 G	64 FPS
ResNet-101	77.82%	93.85%	**44.55 M**	0	**7.83 G**	47 FPS
+SE	78.39%	94.13%	49.29 M	4.743 M	7.85 G	33 FPS
+CBAM	78.57%	**94.18%**	49.33 M	4.781 M	7.85 G	14 FPS
+ECA	78.46%	94.12%	44.55 M	171	7.84 G	33 FPS
+SRM	78.58%	94.15%	44.68 M	0.065 M	7.83 G	25 FPS
+PAAM	**78.70%**	94.12%	**44.55 M**	0	7.83 G	32 FPS
ResNeXt-50	77.47%	93.52%	**25.03 M**	0	4.26 G	70 FPS
+SE	77.96%	93.93%	27.54 M	2.51 M	4.27 G	53 FPS
+CBAM	**78.06%**	**94.07%**	27.56 M	2.53 M	4.27 G	32 FPS
+ECA	77.74%	93.87%	25.03 M	86	4.27 G	54 FPS
+SRM	78.04%	93.91%	25.06 M	0.030 M	4.26 G	46 FPS
+PAAM	78.02%	93.96%	**25.03 M**	0	4.26 G	53 FPS
MobileNet	71.90%	90.51%	**3.50 M**	0	**0.31 G**	99 FPS
+SE	72.46%	**90.85%**	3.53 M	0.028 M	0.31 G	65 FPS

(*continued*)

Table 2. (*continued*)

Model	Top-1 Acc.	Top-5 Acc.	Baseline	+ Parameters	# FLOPs	Speed
+CBAM	**72.49%**	90.78%	3.54 M	0.032 M	0.32 G	35 FPS
+ECA	72.01%	90.46%	3.50 M	59	0.31 G	66 FPS
+SRM	72.32%	90.70%	3.51 M	0.003 M	0.31 G	53 FPS
+PAAM	72.40%	90.72%	**3.50 M**	0	**0.31 G**	66 FPS

Table 3. Comparison of results with other methods on the CIFAR-10 and CIFAR-100 datasets.

Attention Method	ResNet-20		ResNet-56		ResNet-101		MobileNetV2	
	C10	C100	C10	C100	C10	C100	C10	C100
Baseline	92.33	68.88	93.58	72.24	94.51	75.54	91.86	71.32
+SE	92.42	69.45	93.69	**72.84**	94.68	**76.56**	91.79	71.54
+CBAM	92.60	69.47	93.82	72.47	**94.83**	76.45	91.88	71.79
+ECA	92.35	68.89	93.68	72.45	94.72	76.33	92.34	71.24
+GC	92.47	69.16	93.58	72.50	94.78	76.21	91.73	71.78
+SimAM	92.73	69.57	93.76	72.82	94.72	76.42	**92.36**	**72.08**
+PAAM	**92.83**	**69.67**	**93.82**	72.73	94.77	76.45	92.35	71.98
Attention Method	PreResNet-20		PreResNet-56		PreResNet-101		WideResNet-20x10	
	C10	C100	C10	C100	C10	C100	C10	C100
Baseline	92.14	68.70	93.71	71.83	94.22	75.95	95.78	81.31
+SE	92.24	68.70	93.57	72.57	94.40	76.57	96.24	81.30
+CBAM	92.19	68.76	93.67	72.16	94.37	76.01	95.98	80.54
+ECA	92.16	68.31	93.78	72.43	94.70	76.11	**96.12**	80.35
+GC	92.19	68.96	93.77	72.44	94.85	75.48	96.12	79.98
+SimAM	92.47	69.13	93.80	72.36	94.90	76.24	96.09	81.51
+PAAM	**93.33**	**71.42**	**93.80**	**74.12**	**94.91**	**76.57**	96.03	**81.46**

5 Conclusion

This paper proposes a LFEM local feature enhancement module and a L-GFIM local-global feature interaction module to address the issue of existing attention mechanism models not fully realizing the complementarity of local and global information, resulting in information flow failure. The combination of the features of two different local attention mechanisms in LFEM effectively promotes information interaction between local windows. The experimental results indicate that the algorithm proposed in this paper outperforms the SOTA model when the number of parameters is zero. This demonstrates that the L-GFIM proposed in this paper achieves information flow between local and global windows through the local-global feature compensation strategy, capturing more semantic information of the feature maps and having a more powerful contextual modeling capability.

Acknowledgments. This work was supported by Natural Science Foundation Program of Inner Mongolia (No. 2023MS06009).

References

1. Chen, Y.: Convolutional neural network for sentence classification. Master's thesis, University of Waterloo (2015)
2. Krizhevsky, A., Sutskever, I., Hinton, G.E.: ImageNet classification with deep convolutional neural networks. Commun. ACM **60**(6), 84–90 (2017)
3. Simonyan, K., Zisserman, A.: Very deep convolutional networks for large-scale image recognition. arXiv preprint arXiv:1409.1556 (2014)
4. Goodfellow, I., et al.: Generative adversarial nets. Adv. Neural Inf. Process. Syst. **27** (2014)
5. He, K., Zhang, X., Ren, S., Sun, J.: Deep residual learning for image recognition. In: Proceedings of the IEEE Conference on Computer Vision and Pattern Recognition, pp. 770–778 (2016)
6. Ronneberger, O., Fischer, P., Brox, T.: U-net: Convolutional networks for biomedical image segmentation. In: Navab, N., Hornegger, J., Wells, W.M., Frangi, A.F. (eds.) MICCAI 2015. LNCS, vol. 9351, pp. 234–241. Springer, Cham (2015). https://doi.org/10.1007/978-3-319-24574-4_28
7. Howard, A.G., et al.: MobileNets: Efficient convolutional neural networks for mobile vision applications. arXiv preprint arXiv:1704.04861 (2017)
8. Zhang, X., Zhou, X., Lin, M., Sun, J.: ShuffleNet: an extremely efficient convolutional neural network for mobile devices. In: Proceedings of the IEEE Conference on Computer Vision and Pattern Recognition, pp. 6848–6856 (2018)
9. Huang, G., Liu, Z., Van Der Maaten, L., Weinberger, K.Q.: Densely connected convolutional networks. In: Proceedings of the IEEE Conference on Computer Vision and Pattern Recognition, pp. 4700–4708 (2017)
10. Yin, Y., et al.: Artificial neural networks for finger vein recognition: a survey. arXiv preprint arXiv:2208.13341 (2022)
11. Hu, J., Shen, L., Sun, G.: Squeeze-and-excitation networks. In: Proceedings of the IEEE Conference on Computer Vision and Pattern Recognition, pp. 7132–7141 (2018)
12. Xie, S., Girshick, R., Doll´ar, P., Tu, Z., He, K.: Aggregated residual transformations for deep neural networks. In: Proceedings of the IEEE Conference on Computer Vision and Pattern Recognition, pp. 1492–1500 (2017)
13. Wang, Q., Wu, B., Zhu, P., Li, P., Zuo, W., Hu, Q.: ECA-Net: efficient channel attention for deep convolutional neural networks. In: Proceedings of the IEEE/CVF Conference on Computer Vision and Pattern Recognition, pp. 11534–11542 (2020)
14. Yang, Z., Zhu, L., Wu, Y., Yang, Y.: Gated channel transformation for visual recognition. In: Proceedings of the IEEE/CVF Conference on Computer Vision and Pattern Recognition, pp. 11794–11803 (2020)
15. Li, X., Wang, W., Hu, X., Yang, J.: Selective kernel networks. In: Proceedings of the IEEE/CVF Conference on Computer Vision and Pattern Recognition, pp. 510–519 (2019)
16. Wu, T., Tang, S., Zhang, R., Cao, J., Zhang, Y.: CGNet: a light-weight context guided network for semantic segmentation. IEEE Trans. Image Process. **30**, 1169–1179 (2020)

17. Woo, S., Park, J., Lee, J.Y., Kweon, I.S.: CBAM: convolutional block attention module. In: Proceedings of the European Conference on Computer Vision (ECCV), pp. 3–19 (2018)
18. Park, J., Woo, S., Lee, J.Y., Kweon, I.S.: BAM: Bottleneck attention module. arXiv preprint arXiv:1807.06514 (2018)
19. Zhao, H., et al.: PSANet: Pointwise spatial attention network for scene parsing. In: Proceedings of the European Conference on Computer Vision (ECCV), pp. 267–283 (2018)
20. Xu, K., Wang, Z., Shi, J., Li, H., Zhang, Q.C.: A2-net: Molecular structure estimation from cryo-EM density volumes. In: Proceedings of the AAAI Conference on Artificial Intelligence, vol. 33, pp. 1230–1237 (2019)

FRFT Domain Watermarking Algorithm Based on GA Adaptive Optimization

Qiaoqiao Du, Yanchen Zhao, Weijie Hao, and Wenyin Zhang(✉)

Linyi University, Lanshan District, Linyi City 276000, China
zhangwenyin@lyu.edu.cn

Abstract. In the field of digital communication and copyright protection, digital watermark technology is extremely critical to ensure the security of secret communications and copyrighted information. This paper proposes an improved hybrid watermark optimization scheme. This scheme takes advantage of the multilevel wavelet transform (MDWT) to embed watermark information in the fractional Fourier transform domain by modifying the singular values of the image. At the same time, a genetic algorithm (GA) is designed to optimize system parameters. Ensure adaptive and efficient embedding of watermarks. To further enhance the security of the watermark, the Arnold transform (AT) is used to process the watermark, adding an extra layer of security to it. In addition, this solution conducts a comprehensive evaluation of watermarks of different sizes, and the experimental results confirm the efficiency of the system: the peak signal-to-noise ratio (PSNR) values are all above 48dB, and the structural similarity (SSIM) and normalized correlation coefficient (NC) are all close to 1. Compared with some existing algorithms, this scheme performs well in resisting common image processing attacks and has strong robustness while maintaining good invisibility and security.

Keywords: MDWT · GA · singular value decomposition (SVD) · fractional Fourier transform (FRFT) · watermark

1 Introduction

The rapid development of the Internet and signal processing technology makes it easier to copy and process data, which undoubtedly increases the demand for copyright data protection. As a cutting-edge copyright protection technology, digital watermarking [1] uses specific algorithms to cleverly embed identification information into the original multimedia content without affecting its value and use. Early digital watermarking algorithms were mainly based on spatial domain methods. Among them, the least significant bit (LSB) [2] method is popular for its simple pixel replacement strategy, but its security and robustness are relatively low. Transform domain algorithms are widely used due to their strong robustness. Liu X L et al. [3] used DWT to embed robust watermarks in YCbCr color space to achieve blind extraction. Ko et al. [4] proposed a robust and transparent watermarking method by modifying the discrete cosine transform (DCT) coefficient difference. Srivastava et al. [5] combined DWT and pixel modification methods to improve system performance. In addition, SVD has also attracted much attention. Zhou et al. [6] combined DWT, All-Phase Discrete Cosine Biorthogonal Transform (APDCBT), and SVD to achieve watermark embedding and recovery. Zhu T et al. [7] proposed an optimized watermarking algorithm based on SVD and integer wavelet transform (IWT), which provides a valuable direction for further improvement and application of watermarking technology. In addition, the integration of multiple technologies is becoming a trend. Nazir H et al. [8] integrated DWT, Heisenberg decomposition (HbD), SVD, and 4D hyperchaotic system, and used an improved fruit fly optimization algorithm to optimize the watermark embedding process, and the experimental results were satisfactory. Gao H et al. [9] combined various technologies such as the Random Sample Consistency (RANSAC) algorithm and improved artificial bee colony to solve the geometric distortion correction and false positive problem (FPP), etc., and made contributions to the development of the watermarking field. To enhance the security of watermarks, Loan N A et al. [10] proposed a method of blind digital image watermarking technology based on chaotic encryption. Garg P et al. [11] combined DWT, SVD, entropy, and pixel position shuffling methods. In addition, Wu J Y et al. [12] used SVD ghost imaging for watermark encryption, which further enhanced the security of the watermark system. Makbol N M et al. [13] designed an image watermarking scheme based on SVD. Su et al. [14] proposed a blind color image watermarking algorithm based on LU decomposition and applied the AT and MD5-based Hash pseudo-random number algorithm to enhance the security and robustness of the watermark. To find a balance between robustness and imperceptibility, researchers have conducted a lot of exploration. Ansari et al. [15] used IWT and SVD combined with the artificial bee colony (ABC) algorithm to optimize watermark performance. Liu J et al. [16] combined DWT, Heisenberg decomposition (HD), and SVD, and used the fruit fly optimization algorithm to optimize and achieve watermark embedding. In addition, some research also focuses on adaptive watermarking methods. Wang B et al. [17] combined SVD and Wang-Landau sampling methods to propose an adaptive image watermarking method by selecting the principal component as the embedding position. In addition, Ernawan F et al. [18] designed an adaptive scaling factor method based on DWT and DCT coefficients. Wang X et al. [19] proposed a parallel multiple watermarking method with adaptive inter-block correlation to improve watermarking capacity. The proposal of these methods provides new ideas and methods for improving the performance and security of watermarking systems. In terms of the computational efficiency of watermark processing, Cao Y et al. [20] optimized the DCT algorithm and data accuracy and used the FPGA cloud platform to accelerate watermark processing, achieving a highly scalable, widely shareable, and more secure digital watermark application. The above research shows that watermark technology has made significant progress in terms of security, robustness, embedding capacity, and computational efficiency, providing a more comprehensive and efficient solution for copyright protection and security of digital media. To better balance the robustness and imperceptibility of the digital watermarking system, this paper proposes an FRFT domain watermarking algorithm based on GA adaptive optimization. This method aims to design a digital watermarking system with better performance to achieve better performance in copyright.

2 Main Related Technologies

2.1 Discrete Wavelet Transform (DWT)

DWT is a mathematical transformation method used in science and engineering. It provides a compact representation of image energy and shows good results in resisting image processing attacks. By applying DWT, four sub-band representations of the original image are obtained, namely LH, HL, HH, and LL sub-bands. Among them, the LL subband contains most of the information of the image and has strong attack resistance, which makes the LL subband the preferred subband for embedding robust watermarks.

2.2 Singular Value Decomposition (SVD)

SVD is a linear algebra tool that is applied to orthogonal matrices and plays an important role in the field of image processing. It has good stability. Even if a slight perturbation is applied to the image, the change of its matrix singular value will not exceed the maximum singular value of the perturbation matrix. In addition, since singular values mainly reflect the brightness characteristics of the image and are not directly related to its visual details, this makes SVD an effective watermark embedding method.

2.3 Fractional Fourier Transform (FRFT)

FRFT is a transform that takes into account both time domain and frequency domain characteristics. Its rotation characteristics and angular continuity make it have broad application prospects in the field of digital watermarking, providing great flexibility for watermarking solutions. When the fractional order transforms from 0 to 1, the time domain information of the image gradually decreases and the frequency domain information gradually increases. In watermark embedding, the flexibility and adaptability of information embedding can be enhanced by selecting an appropriate fractional order.

2.4 Genetic Algorithm (GA)

GA simulates the natural selection and genetic evolution process in nature, allowing individuals in the population to experience natural reproduction, crossover, and mutation. Following the evolutionary principle of "survival of the fittest, survival of the fittest", the algorithm eliminates individuals with poor performance from generation to generation, while retaining and replicating individuals with excellent performance. After successive generations of selection and genetic mechanisms, the best individuals can eventually be gradually cultivated. When mapped into the problem solution space, it is equivalent to finding the best solution through N generations of iterative optimization. This process is not only efficient but also highly adaptable, making GA a powerful tool for solving complex optimization problems.

3 Watermark Scheme

This paper proposes an FRFT domain watermarking algorithm based on GA adaptive optimization to achieve more covert and robust watermark embedding. First, AT is performed on the watermark to disperse the information in the entire frequency domain and reduce the local characteristics of the watermark, thereby encrypting the image. Secondly, by adjusting the order of FRFT, the spatial frequency domain representation of the image is obtained, and information can be selectively embedded into different frequency components according to the characteristics of different images. Use FRFT and GA adaptive optimization to improve the watermarking algorithm to make it more flexible and adaptable. It can adaptively adjust according to different characteristics of the image to obtain optimal parameters. Then certain rules are used to embed the singular values of the watermark into the singular values of the host image to improve the robustness of the watermark system and make it more difficult to detect and delete. Therefore, better embedding and extraction effects can be achieved, allowing the watermarking system to achieve a better balance between invisibility and robustness.

In addition, the design of GA and the watermark embedding process have been optimized to minimize time complexity. GA uses appropriate crossover and mutation operations to increase the convergence speed and reduce the number of iterations. During the watermark embedding process, we select mathematical transformations and parameter settings while considering computational efficiency and time overhead. This paper also conducts experiments on watermarks of different sizes to verify the performance of the proposed watermark scheme. The proposed watermark scheme will be comprehensively discussed below, including watermark embedding and extraction methods and GA-based watermark optimization algorithm.

3.1 Watermark Embedding and Extraction Methods

The watermark embedding algorithm takes the carrier image and grayscale watermark as input and takes the watermarked image as output. The extraction algorithm takes watermarked images as input and uses the extracted watermark as output. The pseudocode representation of embedding and extraction is given below (Algorithm 1, 2).

3.2 GA-Based Digital Watermark Algorithm

This paper uses GA to optimize system parameters to find the optimal watermark embedding strength α and FRFT transformation order a. In the population initialization stage, the optimal value range determined by the experience of PSNR and NC in previous papers is used as the individual value range to solve the problem of gradually slowing down the convergence speed when processing a large amount of data. To avoid falling into local optimality, the elite retention strategy is first adopted. This method can prevent the loss of effective solutions, help improve the convergence speed of the algorithm, and obtain better samples under the guidance of excellent fitness modes. Furthermore, appropriate crossover and mutation operations are introduced to maintain the diversity of the population. The crossover operation should ensure that the search space can be effectively explored when operating on the PSNR and NC of two crossed individuals.

The mutation operation needs to have sufficient randomness, such as random addition and subtraction of PSNR and NC values, to avoid the algorithm falling into the local optimal solution prematurely. In this article, GA is run individually 30 times while maintaining a large population size each time, and when the optimal fitness stagnates, iteration end measures are taken. Finally, through a comprehensive comparison of these running results, the risk of falling into the local optimal solution can be better avoided, thereby improving the global search effect.

Algorithm 1: Watermark Embedding

Input: Original image C, Watermark W   **Output**: Watermarked image C_W
1: C_YUV ← RGB_to_YUV(C)
2: U ← Extract_U(C_YUV)
3: W_arnold ← Arnold(W)
4: a ← Optimize_FRFT_GA(U, W_arnold)
5: α ← Optimize_Embedding_Strength_GA(U, W_arnold)
6: Cf ← FRFT(U, a)
7: Wf ← FRFT(W_arnold, a)
8: R ← Size_Ratio(U, W)
9: Cf_LL ← Multi_Level_DWT(Cf, R)
10: S_c, U_c, V_c ← SVD(Cf_LL)
11: S_w, U_w, V_w ← SVD(Wf)
12: S_cw ← S_c + α * S_w
13: Cu_watermarked ← Reconstruct_U(S_cw, U_c, V_c)
14: Cu_IDWT ← IDWT(Cu_watermarked)
15: Cu_final ← IFRFT(Cu_IDWT, a)
16: C_W_YUV ← Merge_Y_U_V(C_YUV.Y, Cu_final, C_YUV.V)
17: C_W ← YUV_to_RGB(C_W_YUV)
18: Return C_W

Algorithm 2: Watermark Extraction

Input: Watermarked image C_W   **Output**: Extracted watermark W
1: C_YUV ← RGB_to_YUV(C_W)
2: U ← Extract_U(C_YUV)
3: a ← Optimize_FRFT_GA(U)
4: Ef ← FRFT(U, a)
5: R ← Determine_Size_Ratio(U)
6: Ef_LL ← Multi_Level_DWT(Ef, R)
7: S_Cw ← Extract_Singular_Value_Matrix(Ef_LL)
8: α ← Optimal_Embedding_Strength_GA(U)
9: E_Sw ← Extracted_Singular_Value_Matrix(S_Cw, S_c, α)
10: E_W ← Reconstruct_Watermark(E_Sw)
11: E_W ← IFRFT(E_W, a)
12: W ← Arnold(E_W)
13: Return W

$$\text{fitness} = \frac{PSNR}{100} + 1.1 \frac{\sum_{i=1}^{n} NCarr[i]}{NCnum} \qquad (1)$$

In terms of evaluating the performance of the watermark algorithm, this paper designs a fitness function based on PSNR and NC. The weighted sum of PSNR and NC is shown in Eq. (1). Where $\sum_{i=1}^{n} NCarr[i]$ represents the sum of all elements in the normalized correlation coefficient array, and PSNR is normalized to the range [0,1]. In order to balance transparency and robustness, we need to multiply by a weighting factor to adjust the importance of the normalized correlation coefficient to fully evaluate the performance of the watermarking algorithm. The following is the pseudo code representation of GA (Algorithm 3).

Algorithm 3: Genetic Algorithm for Watermarking Parameters Optimization

Input: popSize, individualSize; **Output**: bestIndividual(optimized watermark parameters);
1: a = rand(); alpha = rand();
2: for each individual in population do
3:   psnr, nc = EmbedWatermark(a, aplha); fitness = CalculateFitness(psnr, nc);
4:   individual = [a, alpha, psnr, nc, fitness]; insertPop(individual);
5: end for
6: While iteration <= maxIterations && stagnationCount < stagnationThreshold do
7:   newPopulation = zeros(populationSize, individualSize);
8:   newPopSize = 0;
9:   While newPopSize < populationSize do
10:    eliteIndividuals = sortedPop(1:eliteSize, :);
11:    for each selected pair of individual do
12:      if rand () <= crossoverProb then
13:        crossOverMethod(eliteIndividuals);
14:      end if
15:      if rand () <= mutationProb then
16:        mutationMethod(eliteIndividuals);
17:      end if
18:      updatePsnrAndNc(individual);
19:      updateFitness(individual);
20:      insertNewPop(individuals);
21:    end for
22: end while
23: if improvement is found then
24:    updateFitness(bestIndividual);
25: end if
26: bestIndividual = population(bestIndividualIndex,:);
27: stagnationCount += 1
28: end while
29: finalBestIndividual = newBestIndividual < bestIndividual ? newBestIndividual:bestIndividual

4 Experimental Results and Performance Analysis

To conduct a fair performance comparison and verify the effectiveness and stability of the proposed scheme, this scheme was tested on 128*128, 64*64, and 32*32 watermarks, and the experimental programming environment was Matlab2023b. Six 512*512 color images are selected as carrier images (shown in Fig. 1, namely Barbara, Monarch, Airplane, Boat, Wall, and Flower), and Pepper grayscale image watermark is used as the watermark image. In addition, the GA-related operating parameter settings are shown in Table 1.

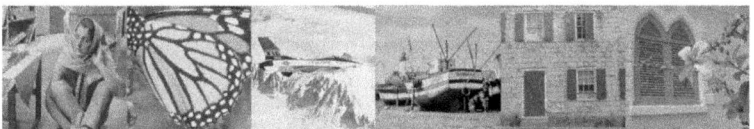

Fig. 1. Carrier picture.

Table 1. GA operating parameters.

Operating parameters	Experience	Experimental parameters
Population size M	20–100	50
Number of iterations T	50–500	50
Crossover probability P1	0.4–1.0	0.8
Mutation probability P2	0.0001–0.1	0.5

4.1 Evaluation Indicators

PSNR and SSIM are used to evaluate the imperceptibility of the algorithm, and their definitions are shown in formulas (2) and (3) respectively. In formula (2), MAX represents the maximum possible value of the signal, and MSE is the mean square error between the original signal and the distorted signal. Generally speaking, when the PSNR is greater than or equal to 30dB, the human eye cannot perceive the embedded watermark information; when it is greater than 40dB, the image quality is considered to be high and very close to the original image. In formula (3), x and y represent the original image and the distorted image respectively, σ_{xy} represents the mean of the image, σ represents the standard deviation of the image, μ represents the covariance between the images x and y, and C_1 and C_2 are constants. Generally, the closer the SSIM is to 1, the stronger the structural similarity between the two images and the better the quality of the image. Compared with PSNR, SSIM pays more attention to the structural information of the image and can better reflect the human eye's perception of image quality.

$$PSNR(dB) = 10\lg\left[\frac{MAX^2}{MSE}\right] = 10\lg\left[\frac{255^2}{MSE}\right] \qquad (2)$$

$$SSIM(x, y) = \frac{(2\mu_x\mu_y + C_1)(2\sigma_{xy} + C_2)}{(\mu_x^2\mu_y^2 + C_1)(\sigma_x^2 + \sigma_y^2 + C_2)} \quad (3)$$

$$NC = \frac{\sum_{i=0}^{M-1}\sum_{j=0}^{N-1} w(i,j)v(i,j)}{\sum_{i=0}^{M-1}\sum_{j=0}^{N-1} [w(i,j)]^2} \quad (4)$$

NC is used to evaluate the similarity between the extracted watermark and the original watermark. Its definition is as shown in formula (4), where w is the original watermark, v is the extracted watermark, and the watermark size is recorded as $M * N$.

4.2 Solution Performance Analysis and Comparison

To verify the effectiveness of the proposed scheme, this section conducts two sets of experiments: one uses random embedding parameters, and the other uses GA to find the best parameters. The experimental results of using random embedding parameters when embedding a 128*128 watermark on some carrier images are given below (Table 2). Experimental results optimized by GA (Table 3). Through analysis, it can be found that for different carrier images, embedding larger-sized watermarks will reduce the PSNR of the image, because more information will lead to greater distortion. Therefore, when embedding a 128*128 watermark, the PSNR is relatively low; while when embedding a 32*32 watermark, the PSNR is relatively high. This is due to the smaller amount of watermark information and relatively less distortion. However, no matter what size of the watermark is embedded, the solution optimized by GA shows significant performance improvement. In all experiments, the PSNR of the GA-optimized scheme is higher than 48dB, and both SSIM and NC are close to 1. In contrast, the scheme using random parameters is far inferior to the optimized scheme. Experimental results show that the scheme optimized by GA performs well in terms of PSNR, SSIM, and NC. This shows that this solution has achieved remarkable results in improving the stability and effectiveness of the watermarking system, and has good invisibility and image quality maintenance capabilities.

Table 2. Watermark model performance test (without GA).

Host Image	Parameter 1 = 0.1				Parameter 2 = 0.01			
	Parameter 2	PSNR	SSIM	NC	Parameter 1	PSNR	SSIM	NC
Barbara	0.01	15.2212	0.5857	0.0319	0.1	15.2212	0.5857	0.0319
	0.02	15.2267	0.5862	0.0422	0.2	14.8594	0.5557	0.0080
	0.03	15.2322	0.5866	0.0458	0.3	14.5509	0.5501	0.0369
Monarch	0.01	17.2443	0.7900	0.0250	0.1	17.2443	0.7900	0.0250
	0.02	17.2507	0.7904	0.0294	0.2	16.7130	0.7656	0.0067
	0.03	17.2568	0.7907	0.0317	0.3	16.3748	0.7556	0.0492

(continued)

Table 2. (continued)

Host Image	Parameter 1 = 0.1				Parameter 2 = 0.01			
	Parameter 2	PSNR	SSIM	NC	Parameter 1	PSNR	SSIM	NC
Airplane	0.01	11.3131	0.2068	0.0076	0.1	11.3131	0.2068	0.0076
	0.02	11.3177	0.2076	0.0157	0.2	10.8672	0.1722	0.0038
	0.03	11.3220	0.2083	0.0189	0.3	10.4234	0.1824	0.0012

To further verify the superiority of this algorithm in terms of imperceptibility, this scheme is compared with [3, 8, 9, 11–14, 17, 18] and [20] were compared. According to the data in Table 4, it can be seen that the PSNR of the proposed method is better than that of the comparison scheme, indicating that the scheme can effectively embed watermark information while maintaining image quality, and has good imperceptibility, further proving the effectiveness of this method.

Table 3. Watermark model performance test (with GA).

Host Image		Parameter 1.2(Optimized)		PSNR	SSIM	NC
Barbara	128*128	0.5055	0.0200	48.8587	0.9994	0.9991
Monarch		0.5049	0.0200	48.9544	0.9998	0.9989
Airplane		0.5026	0.0255	48.8129	0.9986	0.9996
Barbara	64*64	0.5186	0.0343	49.6097	0.9991	0.9993
Monarch		0.5206	0.0324	49.8866	0.9999	0.9987
Airplane		0.5051	0.0400	49.8389	0.9998	0.9988
Barbara	32*32	0.5526	0.0400	50.7233	0.9996	0.9991
Monarch		0.5347	0.0400	50.9853	0.9999	0.9974
Airplane		0.5677	0.0400	50.4023	0.9987	0.9995

Table 4. Comparison of imperceptibility with some jobs (PSNR).

128*128			64*64				
[8]	[17]	Propose	[9]	[8]	[20]	[3]	Propose
35.2342	40.4600	**48.8221**	32.5550	41.1389	35.9700	40.8500	**49.6707**
32*32							
-	[18]	[11]	[12]	[14]	[13]	Propose	-
-	47.1120	42.6029	46.2504	39.4164	42.9449	**50.7790**	-

4.3 Attack Experiment

To test the robustness of the scheme, eight different image processing attacks were performed on watermarked images, namely Wiener Filter (WF), Median Filter (MF), Gaussian Low-pass Filter (GLF), and Average Filter (AF), Speckle Noise (SN 0.001), Crop (Cr 2%), JPEG 2000 Compression (J2 CR = 8) and Sharpening (SH 0.8). Taking Barbara and Monarch as carrier images and embedding watermarks of different sizes as examples, the NC values are calculated respectively, as shown in Table 5. Through analysis, it can be seen that after common attack processing, the average value of NC of this watermark system is above 0.96 and close to 1, indicating that the watermark information can still maintain its integrity and stability well after being attacked.

In addition, the changing trends of NC values in watermark images of different sizes are generally similar. For example, filtering attacks such as MF and GLF have little impact on watermarks, and the NC value remains at a high level; while attacks such as J2 and Cr will have a certain impact on watermark extraction, but the watermark still has a relatively high degree of rashness. Great sex. After the watermark image size is reduced, the watermark's robustness decreases, and the NC value under some attack methods decreases, but overall it still maintains a high stability. It shows that this scheme can still maintain a good watermark extraction effect after some attacks and has good robustness.

Finally, we compare the proposed watermarking scheme with some existing methods to evaluate its robustness. The specific comparison results are shown in Table 6–7. For Table 6, we observe that for the 128*28 watermark, most of the NC values after the attack are above 0.96, indicating that the watermark can be extracted relatively completely. After AF and SH attacks, the NC values are 0.9961 and 0.9966 respectively, indicating that the extracted watermark has high quality. For the 64*64 watermark, the NC value after most attacks is above 0.97. Among them, GLF and Cr attacks have less impact on watermarks, and their NC values are 0.9981 and 0.9947 respectively. For the 32*32 watermark, the NC value after most attacks also remains above 0.96. Among them, after AF and Cr attacks, the extracted watermark performs better in terms of integrity, and its NC values are 0.9918 and 0.9917 respectively.

Overall, the NC value of our watermarking scheme under most attacks is higher than that of the contrasting scheme. For Table 7, it can be known that: except for MF attacks, the average NC value of our watermark scheme is significantly higher than other schemes, indicating that this method has high robustness and stability against common image processing attacks. This provides strong support for its reliability in practical applications.

In general, this watermarking scheme can still extract nearly complete watermark information after some common attacks. It shows that the algorithm has good robustness against attacks such as filtering, shearing, sharpening, and noise, which further verifies the effectiveness of the method.

Table 5. Extract watermark from the attacked image and find NC.

Attacks	128*128		64*64		32*32	
	Barbara	Monarch	Barbara	Monarch	Monarch	Monarch
WF	0.9604	0.9645	0.9811	0.9813	0.9629	0.9569
MF	0.9762	0.9805	0.9891	0.9914	0.9760	0.9676
GLF	0.9882	0.9903	0.9958	0.9984	0.9880	0.9838
AF	0.9972	0.9969	0.9910	0.9944	0.9889	0.9890
SN	0.9741	0.9709	0.9927	0.9802	0.9895	0.9922
Cr	0.9797	0.9836	0.9976	0.9941	0.9885	0.9895
J2	0.9753	0.9803	0.9700	0.9867	0.9606	0.9642
SH	0.9977	0.9966	0.9907	0.9942	0.9888	0.9888

Table 6. Comparison of NC-based robustness under some attacks.

Attacks	OurNC128 (ref NC)	Our NC64 (ref NC)	Our NC32 (ref NC)
WF	**0.9641** (0.9880 [16])	**0.9792**	**0.9626**
MF	**0.9754**	**0.9874** (0.9258 [4])	**0.9608** (0.9338 [14], 0.9793 [6])
GLF	**0.9877**	**0.9981** (0.9992[16])	**0.9878** (0.9905 [7])
AF	**0.9960** (0.9539[16])	**0.9943**	**0.9918** (0.9561 [11], 0.9741 [6])
Cr	**0.9846** (0.9785 [16])	**0.9947** (0.9760 [16])	**0.9917**
SH	**0.9967** (0.9842 [17])	**0.9940** (0.9591 [10], 0.9855 [5], 0.9807 [4])	**0.9915**

Table 7. Robustness comparison of the scheme based on average NC under certain attacks.

Attacks	Scheme [8]	Scheme [10]	Scheme [15]	Our NC
MF	0.8474	0.9235	0.9894	**0.9745**
GLF	0.8272	0.9173	-	**0.9912**
AF	0.8269	-	0.9747	**0.9940**
SN	0.9518	-	-	**0.9792**
SH	0.8565	0.9591	0.9485	**0.9941**

5 Conclusion

In this study, we design and verify an innovative hybrid watermark optimization scheme. The watermarking algorithm is improved by integrating MDWT, SVD, and FRFT technology to effectively embed watermark information in the FRFT domain. The GA is designed to adaptively optimize the key parameters of the watermark, which significantly improves the performance of the watermark system. The results show that the proposed scheme is satisfactory in terms of concealment, robustness, and security. In the future, it is planned to combine the current method with neural networks to explore and solve large-capacity and adaptive location embedding problems. At the same time, we will continue to strengthen the security protection of watermarking algorithms, especially against attacks such as encryption analysis and reverse engineering, and continuously improve and strengthen the watermarking scheme to ensure its robustness in the face of various attacks.

Acknowledgments. This study was funded by Natural Science Foundation of Shandong Province (ZR2020MF058).

Disclosure of Interests. The authors have no competing interests to declare that are relevant to the content of this article.

References

1. Cox, I.J., Miller, M.L., Bloom, J.A., et al.: Digital Watermarking. Morgan Kaufmann, San Francisco (2002)
2. Chan, C.K., Cheng, L.M.: Hiding data in images by simple LSB substitution. Pattern Recogn. **37**(3), 469–474 (2004)
3. Liu, X.L., Lin, C.C., Yuan, S.M.: Blind dual watermarking for color images' authentication and copyright protection. IEEE Trans. Circuits Syst. Video Technol. **28**(5), 1047–1055 (2016)
4. Ko, H.-J., et al.: Robust and blind image watermarking in DCT domain using inter-block coefficient correlation. Inf. Sci. **517**, 128–147 (2020)
5. Srivastava, R., et al.: Image watermarking approach using a hybrid domain based on performance parameter analysis. Information **12**(8), 310 (2021)
6. Zhou, X., Zhang, H., Wang, C.: A robust image watermarking technique based on DWT, APDCBT, and SVD. Symmetry **10**(3), 77 (2018)
7. Zhu, T., Qu, W., Cao, W.: An optimized image watermarking algorithm based on SVD and IWT. J. Supercomput. **78**(1), 222–237 (2022)
8. Nazir, H., Bajwa, I.S., Samiullah, M., et al.: Robust secure color image watermarking using 4D hyperchaotic system, DWT, HbD, and SVD based on improved FOA algorithm. Secur. Commun. Netw. **2021**, 1–17 (2021)
9. Gao, H., Chen, Q.: A robust and secure image watermarking scheme using SURF and improved artificial bee colony algorithm in DWT domain. Optik **242**, 166954 (2021)
10. Loan, N.A., Hurrah, N.N., Parah, S.A., et al.: Secure and robust digital image watermarking using coefficient differencing and chaotic encryption. IEEE Access **6**, 19876–19897 (2018)

11. Garg, P., Rama, K.R.: Secured and multi optimized image watermarking using SVD and entropy and prearranged embedding locations in transform domain. J. Discrete Math. Sci. Crypt. **23**(1), 73–82 (2020)
12. Wu, J.Y., Huang, W.L., Wen, R.H., et al.: Hybrid watermarking scheme based on singular value decomposition ghost imaging. Optica Appl. **50**(4) (2020)
13. Makbol, N.M., Khoo, B.E., Rassem, T.H., et al.: A new reliable optimized image watermarking scheme based on the integer wavelet transform and singular value decomposition for copyright protection. Inf. Sci. **417**, 381–400 (2017)
14. Su, Q., et al.: A new algorithm of blind color image watermarking based on LU decomposition. Multidimension. Syst. Signal Process. **29**, 1055–1074 (2018)
15. Ansari, I.A., Pant, M., Ahn, C.W.: Robust and false positive free watermarking in IWT domain using SVD and ABC. Eng. Appl. Artif. Intell. **49**, 114–125 (2016)
16. Liu, J., Huang, J., Luo, Y., et al.: An optimized image watermarking method based on HD and SVD in DWT domain. IEEE Access **7**, 80849–80860 (2019)
17. Wang, B., Zhao, P.: An adaptive image watermarking method combining SVD and Wang-Landau sampling in DWT domain. Mathematics **8**(5), 691 (2020)
18. Ernawan, F., Ariatmanto, D., Firdaus, A.: An improved image watermarking by modifying selected DWT-DCT coefficients. IEEE Access **9**, 45474–45485 (2021)
19. Wang, X., Yuan, X., Li, M., et al.: Parallel multiple watermarking using adaptive Inter-Block correlation. Expert Syst. Appl. **213**, 119011 (2023)
20. Cao, Y., Yu, F., Tang, Y.: A digital watermarking encryption technique based on FPGA cloud accelerator. IEEE Access **8**, 11800–11814 (2020)

Joint Semantic Feature and Optical Flow Learning for Automatic Echocardiography Segmentation

Juan Lyu[1], Jinpeng Meng[2], Yu Zhang[1(✉)], Sai Ho Ling[3], and Lin Sun[1]

[1] College of Artificial Intelligence, Tianjin University of Science and Technology, Tianjin 300457, China
{Lvjuan,Zhangyuai,Sunlin}@tust.edu.cn
[2] College of Light Industry Science and Engineering, Tianjin University of Science and Technology, Tianjin 300457, China
22062212@mail.tust.edu.cn
[3] School of Electrical and Data Engineering, Faculty of Engineering and Information Technology, University of Technology Sydney, Sydney, NSW 2007, Australia
Steve.Ling@uts.edu.au

Abstract. The left ventricle ejection fraction is an important index for assessing cardiac function and diagnosing cardiac diseases. At present, EchoNet-Dynamic dataset is the unique large-scale resource for studying ejection fraction estimation by echocardiography. Through segmentation of the end-systolic and end-diastolic frames, the ejection fraction can be calculated based on the volumes at these phases. However, existing segmentation methods either mostly focus on single-frame segmentation and rarely consider information across consecutive frames, or they fail to effectively exploit temporal information between consecutive frames, resulting in suboptimal segmentation performance. In our study, we constructed a dual-branch spatial-temporal feature extraction model for achieving echocardiogram video segmentation. One branch was dedicated to extracting semantic features of frames under supervision, while the other branch learned the optical flows between frames in an unsupervised manner. Subsequently, we jointly trained these two branches using a temporal consistency mechanism to acquire spatial-temporal features of the frames. This approach enhances both video segmentation performance and the consistency of transition frame segmentation. Experimental results demonstrate that our proposed model achieves promising segmentation performance compared to existing methods.

Keywords: Echocardiography Segmentation · Optical Flow · Joint Learning

1 Introduction

Cardiovascular diseases are the leading cause of death worldwide, accounting for 32% of the total global deaths, of which heart attack and stroke represent 85% of these deaths. It is recommended by World Health Organization (WHO) that early diagnosing is crucial for cardiovascular diseases. For evaluating heart function and structure, echocardiography is a commonly utilized tool in any stage of clinical practice [1]. At present, deep learning has been the most popular way of echocardiography segmentation task and achieved much better performance. Paper [2, 3] utilized U-Net-based networks to segment the ES and ED frames. Li et al. proposed a multi-level and multi-scale dense pyramid and deep supervision network (DPSN) for segmentation of key frames in multi-chamber views [4]. Other approaches [5, 6] integrated convolutional neural network (CNN) models with transformer modules to utilize image patches for segmentation. Some researchers have also incorporated attention techniques such as pyramid local attention [7], bridge attention [6], and attention refinement modules [8] to enhance feature fusion effectiveness for segmentation. However, the above single-image segmentation methods typically overlook the temporal information and inter-frame correlations between video frames, resulting in challenges in accurately delineating the left ventricular region, particularly in intermediate transition frames.

Recently, more studies started to focus on the echocardiographic video segmentation, which located the ES and ED frames based on the volumes obtained by the segmentation of all frames. To introduce temporal information, some of the methods adopted 3D structures to extract the semantic and temporal features at the same time. For example, Wei et al. proposed a co-learning network that trains both at the appearance level and the shape level based on 3D U-Net [9, 10]. Chen et al. proposed a 3D U-Net for echocardiography video segmentation by learning the ED and ES segmentation and motion tracking between the frames at the same time [10]. However, the 3D-based networks cannot be used in single image cases, which has limitations in clinical practice. Other approaches employed the 2D plus time (2D + t) architecture to discover spatial-temporal information, which take videos or image sequences as inputs. Li et al. proposed a multi-view echocardiographic video segmentation network based on long-short term memory (LSTM), named MV-RAN [11]. Although the MV-RAN can model the temporal consistency, the LSTM structure is time-consuming and causes the end frames of the video to perform worse than the beginnings due to the errors accumulated. Sirhani et al. proposed a EchoRCNN model based on the mask region-based CNN (Mask RCNN) [12]. However, the ground truth mask of the first frame of the video should be delineated, which increases the cost of clinical application. Moreover, the proposed EchoRCNN was validated on a small dataset with only 750 videos. Painchaud et al. proposed an enforced temporal consistency post-processing approach to achieve echocardiographic video segmentation [13]. However, its performance improvement is limited. Wu et al. proposed an adaptive spatiotemporal semantic calibration (ASSC) module to utilize the spatio-temporal information between consecutive frames and to overcome the drawback that the optical-flow-based models are sensitive to speckle noise [14]. However, the ASSC module used a series of transformations and imported several learnable transformation metrics for both coordinate warping calibration and channel-wise feature weighting calibration, which made the model more complex and difficult to learn these metrics.

In this research, we introduced a novel dual-branch spatial-temporal joint learning network for echocardiographic video segmentation. The network consists of a 2D image segmentation branch to learn the spatial features of the inputs and to achieve the frames segmentation, and an optical flow learning branch to extract the optical flow between every two frames. Based on the optical flow learned from two consecutive frames, we jointly learned spatial and temporal information using a temporal consistency module between the warped segmentation prediction and the real segmentation prediction at t time. The contributions of this paper are as follows.

- We developed a dual-branch network which consists of a supervised semantic segmentation branch, and an unsupervised optical flow learning branch to learn the consistency between the consecutive frames.
- We jointly trained the two branches using the temporal consistency technique to learn the spatial-temporal features of the videos.
- The proposed model achieved a promising segmentation performance on the EchoNet-Dynamic dataset and demonstrated higher consistency in transition frames than other approaches.

The rest of the paper is organized as follows: Sect. 2 presents the details of the proposed method, the framework workflow, the segmentation learning and optical flow learning processes, and the joint learning mechanism. Section 3 introduces the materials of this paper, including the dataset we used and implementation details. Section 4 shows the experimental results of our proposed algorithm and demonstrates the comparison results with existing approaches. Finally, we conclude the paper in Sect. 5.

2 Methods

In this work, we presented a dual-branch echocardiographic video segmentation approach that uses video clips as inputs. As illustrated in Fig. 1, the proposed network consists of two branches. The segmentation branch was employed to segment the left ventricle area in each frame. The optical flow branch was used to learn the optical flow changes and temporal information between frame pairs. Finally, we jointly trained two branches by the proposed temporal consistency mechanism.

2.1 Overview of Framework Workflow

The architecture of the proposed model is a spatial and temporal combination structure, composed of two branches: the segmentation branch and the optical flow branch. The videos in the EchoNet-Dynamic dataset are typically large, with an average duration of more than 176 frames, while only two frames in each video are labeled. When training the frames in pairs, only two frames can be used to update the segmentation branch, while all frame pairs are used to update the optical flow branch.. In this paper, in the training stage, we set two clips for each video, the ES frame and its former and later two frames as clip one, the ED frame and its former and later two frames as clip two. They are defined as $c1$: $\{I_{ES-1}, I_{ES}, I_{ES+1}\}$ and $c2$: $\{I_{ED-1}, I_{ED}, I_{ED+1}\}$. All clips were used in the training in pairs to learn the semantic segmentation and optical flow parallelly according to the model shown in Fig. 1. In the testing stage, we tested all the frames of each video and output their predicted left ventricle masks only using the segmentation branch.

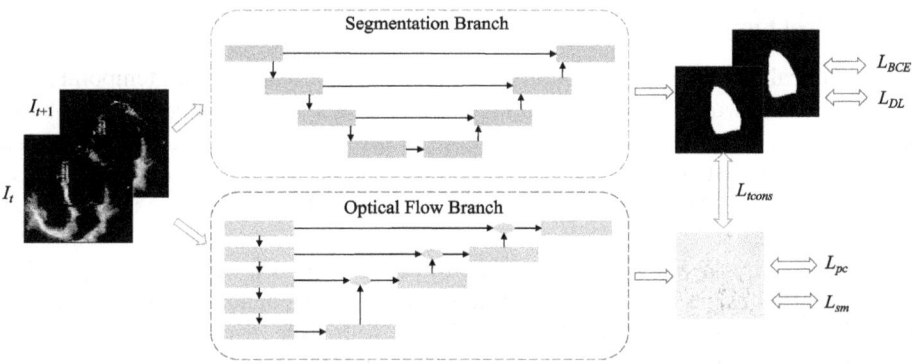

Fig. 1. The architecture of the proposed echocardiography segmentation network. The structure of each branch is presented in corresponding box roughly.

2.2 Segmentation Learning

For the segmentation branch, we adopted a 2D image segmentation network to learn the spatial semantic features of the input echocardiography. The main target of this branch is to distinguish between the region of interest (left ventricle) and the background. Therefore, in this branch, we adopted the baseline model U-Net to focus on spatial semantic feature extraction, more details can be found in paper [15].

As shown in Fig. 2, the input images are trained in pairs between two consecutive frames, denoted as I_t and I_{t+1}. We represented the segmentation branch as $S_g(x)$, where g is its corresponding parameter, and simply referred to it as the S branch for convenience. The corresponding outputs of two input pairs are $S_g(I_t)$ and $S_g(I_{t+1})$, respectively. The S branch was trained using two common semantic segmen-tation loss functions: binary cross−entropy (BCE) loss and dice loss (DL), which are defined as

$$L_{BCE} = -y \log \hat{y} - (1-y)\log(1-\hat{y}), \tag{1}$$

where y and $\hat{y}$ denote semantic region label and the predicted result, respectively.

$$L_{Dice} = 1 - \frac{2|Y \cap G|}{|Y| + |G|}, \tag{2}$$

where we set the predicted segmentation results as Y and its corresponding label as G; the numerator denotes the twice of the overlap area of two sets Y and G, the denominator is the sum of elements in the two sets.

The total loss function of the S branch is defined as

$$L_S = L_{BCE} + L_{Dice}. \tag{3}$$

Notably, the segmentation learning was supervised, with human experts annotating the masks. That is, the segmentation branch can only output their predicted masks for frames without mask labels; they cannot be used to update the weights of the network.

2.3 Optical Flow Learning

For the optical flow branch, we employed a specialized network to learn temporal information between two adjacent frames through the optical flow. Compared to region-based networks, it is more suitable to use a pixel-level algorithm to discover the pixel-scale movement between two consecutive frames. In particular, most of the brightness changes occur at the edge of the heart chambers, which can also help to distinguish the edge from the background.

In this section, we designed a modified FlowNet based on FlowNetSimple [16]. Figure 2 illustrates the architecture of the modified FlowNet, denoted as mFlowNet. The blue component is derived from the original FlowNetSimple, which we customized by importing part of layers. The green section represents our modifications, in which we added more up-sampled layers to ensure that the outputs are of the same size as the inputs. The reason is that we hope to use deconvolutions to learn the up-sampling process, instead of the interpolation during the warping computation. The corresponding hyperparameters for each operation are provided below them in Fig. 2, where f denotes the number of features, k denotes the kernel size of the convolution, s denotes the step size, p denotes the padding size. The number of features of the deconvolution in refine operation is specified below the Refine block. "Up flow" represents the up-sampled operation to predict flow. In mFlowNet, we also adopted the encoder and decoder structures to learn the optical flow between every two frames. In detail, it contains five normal convolution and down-sampling blocks in the encoder. For the decoder, we introduced two additional up-sampling layers and one more feature fusion layer to ensure that the output size matches that of the input.

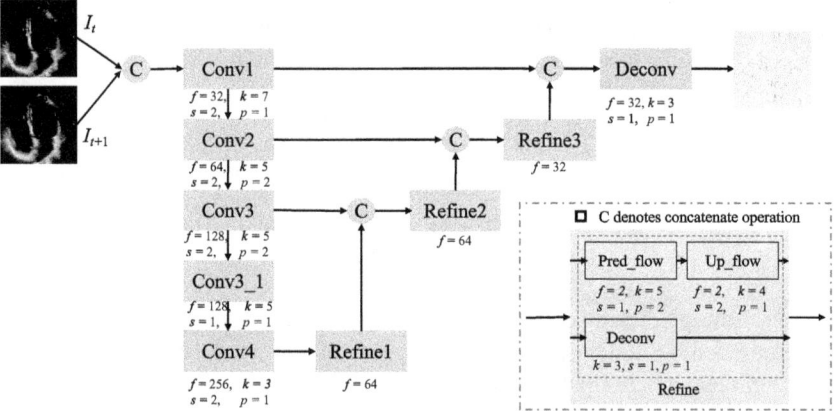

Fig. 2. The architecture of the mFlowNet. The blue rectangles represent the original FlowNet blocks, while the green rectangles represent the modified parts by this work. (Color figure online)

We represented the optical flow branch as $O_p(x)$, where p is its corresponding parameter, and simply named it as O branch. The inputs of the O branch are still in pairs, I_t and I_{t+1}, which are the same as the inputs of the S branch. Two frames of inputs were concatenated in pairs at the channel level, forming a 6−channel input. The output of the mFlowNet is the optical flow between the two input frames, presented as $M_{t \to t+1}$. The mFlowNet was trained in an unsupervised manner and its update was depended on the basic characteristics of optical flow, photometric consistency and motion smoothness.

Photometric consistency loss [16, 18] is to constrain a frame and the warped image from its adjacent frame, which is defined as

$$L_{pc} = \alpha \frac{1 - SSIM(I - I_w)}{2} + (1 - \alpha)\|I - I_w\|_1, \tag{4}$$

where I_w is the warped image, $SSIM$ is the structural similarity index and α is set to 0.85 accordingly [18]. The purpose of motion smoothness is intended to eliminate erroneous predictions while preserving crisp details, which is defined as

$$L_{sm} = \sum_{x,y} |\nabla M(x, y)| \cdot (e^{-|\nabla I(x,y)|}), \tag{5}$$

where ∇ is the vector differential operator, $|\cdot|$ denotes element-wise absolute value. The total loss function for O branch is presented as

$$L_O = \lambda_1 L_{pc} + \lambda_2 L_{sm}, \tag{6}$$

where λ_1 and λ_2 is the corresponding weights of two losses, respectively.

2.4 Cooperation Mechanism and Joint Learning

For the above two branches, the S branch is to learn the spatial semantic features, and the O branch is to discover the temporal features between the frames. We utilized temporal consistency constraints to fuse the learned features to further improve the segmentation performance. We adopted the temporal consistency module in [19]. They defined the temporal consistency constraint as the function of the encoder output features at time t and the warped features from time $t + 1$. However, in this paper, the temporal consistency constraint is defined as a function of the segmentation output at time t and the warped output from time $t + 1$ using the learnt optical flow from the O branch. The rationale behind this choice is that the edges between the left ventricle and the background tend to be blurred in ultrasound imaging. Therefore, the temporal consistency module that only works on the segmentation output can help filter out the background and noise from non-left ventricle regions. Since the segmentation output is binary, that is, the pixel values of the segmented background are all zero, only the segmented left ventricle region is used for the optical flow warping computation.

Given a pair of input frames I_t and I_{t+1}, we got their semantic segmentation results from branch S, Y_t and Y_{t+1}, respectively, and obtained their predicted optical flow from branch O, $M_{t \to t+1}$. Then we warped Y_{t+1} to Y_t' by optical flow $M_{t \to t+1}$, which is calculated by

$$Y_t' = \text{Warp}(Y_{t+1}, M_{t \to t+1}), \tag{7}$$

where we also used differentiable bilinear interpolation for warping. Since our dataset does not have the occluded issue, the temporal consistency loss is defined as

$$L_{tcons} = \sum_{x,y} \|Y'^{xy} - Y^{xy}\|. \tag{8}$$

In this way, we introduced temporal features into spatial space through optical flow and warping. Consequently, we are able to use the temporal O branch to extract features from the unlabeled frames and then enhance the semantic segmentation result through warping. Two branches work together in an end-to-end manner to achieve the video segmentation and improve the performance of the model.

The total loss function of the proposed model is

$$L = L_S + L_O + \lambda_3 L_{tcons} = L_{BCE} + L_{Dice} + \lambda_1 L_{pc} + \lambda_2 L_{sm} + \lambda_3 L_{tcons}, \quad (9)$$

where the weights of L_S and L_O are set to 1, the weights of L_{tcons} is λ_3

3 Materials

3.1 Data

EchoNet-Dynamic is a large-scale, publicly available echocardiography video dataset for cardiac function assessment that we employed in this paper. The EchoNet-Dynamic dataset contains 10,030 echocardiographic videos recorded independently by 10,030 people. For each video, the video length, the positions (time points), masks and volumes of ES and ED frames, and the correspondingly calculated EF are provided. The size of all the frames in the dataset is 112×112. All the annotations are supplied by experienced experts.

3.2 Implementation Details

The experiments were implemented using the Pytorch library version 1.6.0. The training and testing were done on a machine with an Intel Core i7-9700K CPU processor, 31.2 GB of memory, and a GeForce 2080 Ti 11GB GPU, under the Ubuntu 18.04 operating system.

The dataset was divided into training, validation, and testing sets in the ratios of 75%, 12.5%, and 12.5%, respectively, which is the same as the setting of EchoNet–Dynamic [20]. For fair comparison with parts of other models, we also evaluate the proposed method following their training and testing ratio of 80%:20%. During the training stage, as mentioned previously, we utilized video clips to train the proposed model. Each clip generates four pairs of inputs for every video. In the testing stage, we tested all the frames in each video. We trained the model for 100 epochs with a batch size of one. We used the Adam optimizer to update the model weights with an initial learning rate of 1.6 $\times$ 10−5. For the loss function, we experimentally set the λ_1, λ_2, and λ_3 to be 5, 0.2, and 0.4, respectively. In this work, we utilized Dice coefficient score and Hausdorff distance (HD) to evaluate the segmentation performance of the proposed model. Dice score is related to the dice loss and defined as

$$Dice(Y, G) = 1 - L_{Dice}. \quad (10)$$

HD is used to valuate the maximum distance between the prediction Y and ground truth G, HD is defined as

$$H(Y, G) = \max(h(Y, G), h(G, Y)), \quad (11)$$

we take direct Hausdorff distance from Y to G as an example, it is presented as

$$h(Y, G) = \max_{y \in Y}(\max_{g \in G}(d(y, g))), \qquad (12)$$

where $d(y, g)$ denotes the Euclidean distance between y and g.

4 Experiment

First, we investigated the effectiveness of introducing temporal features into the spatial feature extraction network for left ventricle segmentation of echocardiogram video. Second, we evaluated relations between the performance of the proposed method with the number of samples in the training clips. Third, we validated the advancement of the proposed method by comparing it with the existing networks on the EchoNet-Dynamic dataset.

4.1 Evaluation of Introducing Optical Flow Branch

We evaluated the effectiveness of importing the optical flow branch by comparing it with the spatial semantic network, U-Net. The comparison results are shown in Table 1. It turns out that extracting both spatial and temporal features at the same time is better for video segmentation than extracting only spatial features. The temporal features contain the information between the adjacent frames, thereby the network can provide spatial-temporal information for neighboring frames in the videos.

Table 1. Evaluation of Introducing Optical Flow Branch

Structure	Dice score (%)
U-Net	88.76
U-Net + FlowNetSimple	92.50
U-Net + mFlowNet (this work)	**92.64**

4.2 Affection of Training Sample Numbers

In Table 2, we compared the results of training with different amounts of samples, including 6 (this work), 10, 18, and ES to ED frames.

It can be seen that the segmentation performance decreases as the number of samples increases. This suggests that when more unlabeled data is introduced, the segmentation heavily relies on accurate optical flow estimation. However, since the learning process of the optical flow is unsupervised, it may lead to an accumulation of errors during the warping phase if the training samples are too numerous, resulting in decreased segmentation accuracy. Therefore, the optimal training length for this project is 6 samples.

Table 2. Comparison Results of Using Different Samples for Training

Num of Samples per Video	Dice score (%)
6 (this work)	**92.64**
10	92.44
18	92.12
ES to ED frames	89.44

4.3 Comparison with Existing Methods

We compared the proposed model with existing approaches on the EchoNet-Dynamic dataset to validate its segmentation performance, as shown in Table 3. For the 2D ES and ED frames segmentation methods, we compared several algorithms, including the primary algorithm by Ouyang et al., the **EchoNet-Dynamic** method [20] and three recent models: TransBridge [5] (offering **TransBridge-B** and **TransBridge-L** variants), **PLANet** [7], and **Bi-DCNet** [8]. They were evaluated on the training, testing, and validation sets provided by the EchoNet-Dynamic dataset, with a ratio of 75:12.5:12.5, referred to as ratio-1 for convenience. For echocardiographic video segmentation algorithms, we compared two approaches: **Joint-Net** [21] and a recent network [14] named **BSSF-Net**. Training and testing sets were randomly selected from the EchoNet-Dynamic dataset in an 80:20 ratio, denoted as ratio-2. These methods employed 5-fold cross-validation for evaluation and did not include a separate validation set. For comparison, we evaluated our proposed model and the baseline EchoNet-Dynamic algorithm using both ratios.

Table 3. Comparison Result with Existing Methods

Methods	Year	Train/Val/Test: 75/12.5/12.5		Train/Val/Test:80/-/20	
		Dice Score(%)	HD(mm)	Dice Score (mean ± STD)(%)	HD (mean ± STD)(mm)
EchoNet-Dynamic	2020	91.97	2.32	93.79 ± 0.22	2.27 ± 0.47
Joint-net	2020	-	-	90.91 ± 0.36	3.85 ± 0.92
TransBridge-B	2021	91.39	4.41	-	-
TransBridge-L	2021	91.64	4.19	-	-
PLANet	2021	-	-	91.92 ± 0.34	3.42 ± 0.67
BSSF-Net	2022	-	-	92.87 ± 0.16	2.93 ± 0.72
Bi-DCNet	2023	92.25	-	-	-
Ours	2024	**92.64**	**2.23**	**96.99 ± 0.12**	**1.76 ± 0.47**

In Table 3, our proposed method achieves the best segmentation results in both data ratios. For ratio-1, we achieved a Dice score of 92.64%, which is 0.39% higher than Bi-DCNet. In ratio-2, the proposed model demonstrates outstanding performance with a mean Dice score of 96.99%, surpassing ESSF-Net by 4.12% and EchoNet-Dynamic algorithm by 3.2%. This suggests that our spatial-temporal joint learning model excels in identifying the blurred edges of the left ventricle. Additionally, it indicates that the joint learning of semantic features and optical flows better exploits spatial-temporal information compared to 2D image segmentation methods and strategies proposed by Joint-net and BSSF-Net.

The comparison results were then represented in two different ways. Firstly, we compared the segmentation results of expert-labeled ES and ED frames. As depicted in Fig. 3, it is evident from the orange boxes that the contours segmented by our proposed technique are closer to the labels than those segmented by the EchoNet-Dynamic algorithm, indicating that our method can more accurately segment the left ventricle borders.

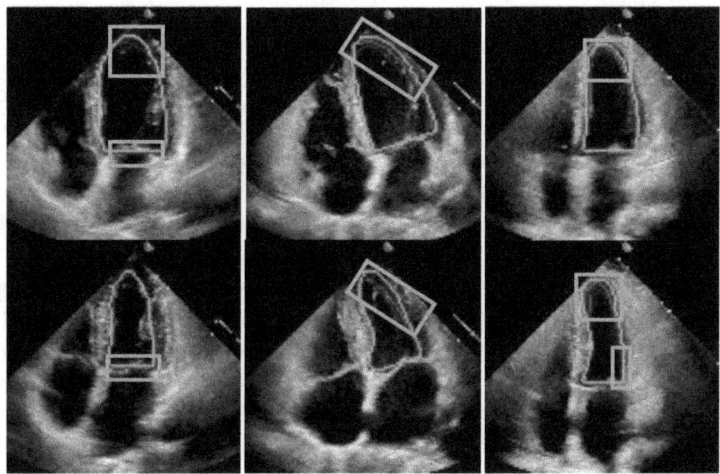

Fig. 3. Comparison results of ES and ED frames. Every column is an example of ES and ED frames in a video. The red circles are the results of this work, the blues are the results of the EchoNet-Dynamic algorithm, and the greens are the labels. (Color figure online)

Second, we exhibited the comparison results of unlabeled transition frames between this work and the EchoNet-Dynamic algorithm in Fig. 4. It can be seen that the EchoNet-Dynamic method was able to roughly segment the targets of ES and ED frames in the orange boxes. However, it is not able to distinguish targets in transition frames correctly, which is supposed to be affected by the imaging quality and noise. It indicates that the proposed method can not only more properly segment the ES and ED frames, but also more stably and reliably segment the transition frames in each video by learning the information between the key frames as well as the transition frames.

To summarize, the proposed method attained superior performance in echocardiography video segmentation by extracting the spatial-temporal properties of the frames. Compared to existing approaches, our method not only surpasses them in segmenting ES and ED frames but also demonstrates more consistent segmentation ability across other transition frames.

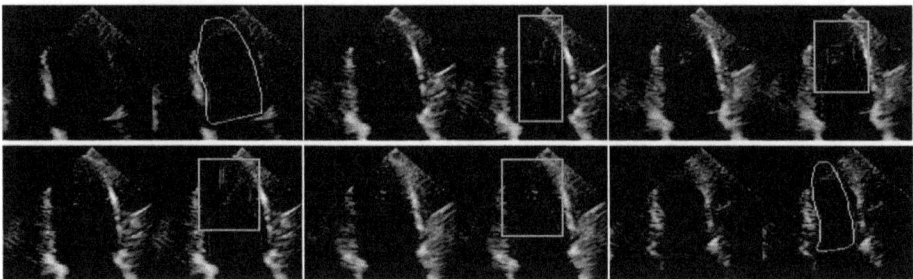

Fig. 4. Comparison results of unlabeled transition frames are depicted in pictures (a) and (b) for two separate videos, respectively. Each picture displays the original image on the left and the corresponding comparison visualization on the right.

5 Conclusion

In this paper, we developed a novel echocardiography video segmentation network on the EchoNet-Dynamic dataset, which consists of a semantic features extraction branch and an optical flow learning branch. The two branches work together to combine the spatial and temporal information of the videos using a temporal consistency module to improve the performance of the left ventricle segmentation. The experimental results reveal that the proposed model achieves a promising performance compared with 2D ES and ED frames segmentation and echocardiographic video segmentation approaches, with a dice score of 92.46%. In the future, we will investigate more advanced temporal feature extraction strategies and the fuse mechanism to improve model segmentation performance.

References

1. Spencer, K.T., Kimura, B.J., Korcarz, C.E., Pellikka, P.A., Rahko, P.S., Siegel, R.J.: Focused cardiac ultrasound: recommendations from the american society of echocardiography. J. Am. Soc. Echocardiogr. **26**(6), 567–581 (2013)
2. Ali, Y., Janabi-Sharifi, F., Beheshti, S.: Echocardiographic image segmentation using deep res-u network. Biomed. Signal Process. Control **64**, 102248 (2021)
3. Puyol-Antón, E., et al.: Ai-enabled assessment of cardiac systolic and diastolic function from echocardiography. arXiv preprint arXiv:2203.11726 (2022)
4. Li, M., et al.: Unified model for interpreting multi-view echocardiographic sequences without temporal information. Appl. Soft Comput. **88**, 106049 (2020)
5. Deng, K., Meng, Y., Gao, D., Bridge, J., Shen, Y., Lip, G., Zhao, Y., Zheng, Y.: TransBridge: a lightweight transformer for left ventricle segmentation in echocardiography. In: Noble, J.A., Aylward, S., Grimwood, A., Min, Z., Lee, S.-L., Hu, Y. (eds.) ASMUS 2021. LNCS, vol. 12967, pp. 63–72. Springer, Cham (2021). https://doi.org/10.1007/978-3-030-87583-1_7
6. Shi, S., Alimu, P., Mahemuti, P., Chen, Q., Wu, H.: The study of echocardiography of left-ventricle segmentation combining transformer and CNN. SSRN 4184447 (2022)
7. Liu, F., Wang, K., Liu, D., Yang, X., Tian, J.: Deep pyramid local attention neural network for cardiac structure segmentation in two-dimensional echocardiography. Med. Image Anal. **67**, 101873 (2021)

8. Ye, Z., Kumar, Y.J., Song, F., Li, G., Zhang, S.: Bi-DCNet: bilateral network with dilated convolutions for left ventricle segmentation. Life **13**(4), 1040 (2023)
9. Wei, H., Cao, H., Cao, Y., Zhou, Y., Xue, W., Ni, D., Li, S.: Temporal-consistent segmentation of echocardiography with co-learning from appearance and shape. In: Martel, A.L., Abolmaesumi, P., Stoyanov, D., Mateus, D., Zuluaga, M.A., Zhou, S.K., Racoceanu, D., Joskowicz, L. (eds.) MICCAI 2020. LNCS, vol. 12262, pp. 623–632. Springer, Cham (2020). https://doi.org/10.1007/978-3-030-59713-9_60
10. Chen, Y., Zhang, X., Haggerty, C.M., Stough, J.V.: Assessing the generalizability of temporally coherent echocardiography video segmentation. In: Medical Imaging 2021: Image Processing, vol. 11596, pp. 463–469. International Society for Optics and Photonics (2021)
11. Li, M., Wang, C., Zhang, H., Yang, G.: MV-RAN: multiview recurrent aggregation network for echocardiographic sequences segmentation and full cardiac cycle analysis. Comput. Biol. Med. **120**, 103728 (2020)
12. Sirjani, N., et al.: Automatic cardiac evaluations using a deep video object segmentation network. Insights Imaging **13**(1), 1–14 (2022)
13. Painchaud, N., Duchateau, N., Bernard, O., Jodoin, P.-M.: Echocardiography segmentation with enforced temporal consistency. IEEE Trans. Med. Imaging **41**(10), 2867–2878 (2022)
14. Wu, H., Liu, J., Xiao, F., Wen, Z., Cheng, L., Qin, J.: Semi-supervised segmentation of echocardiography videos via noise-resilient spatiotemporal semantic calibration and fusion. Med. Image Anal. **78**, 102397 (2022)
15. Ronneberger, O., Fischer, P., Brox, T.: U-net: Convolutional networks for biomedical image segmentation. In: Navab, N., Hornegger, J., Wells, W.M., Frangi, A.F. (eds.) MICCAI 2015. LNCS, vol. 9351, pp. 234–241. Springer, Cham (2015). https://doi.org/10.1007/978-3-319-24574-4_28
16. Dosovitskiy, A., et al.: FlowNet: learning optical flow with convolutional networks. In: Proceedings of the IEEE International Conference on Computer Vision, pp. 2758–2766 (2015)
17. Godard, C., Mac Aodha, O., Brostow, G.J.: Unsupervised monocular depth estimation with left-right consistency. In: Proceedings of the IEEE Conference on Computer Vision and Pattern Recognition, pp. 270–279 (2017)
18. Yin, Z., Shi, J.: GeoNet: unsupervised learning of dense depth, optical flow and camera pose. In: Proceedings of the IEEE Conference on Computer Vision and Pattern Recognition, pp. 1983–1992 (2018)
19. Ding, M., Wang, Z., Zhou, B., Shi, J., Lu, Z., Luo, P.: Every frame counts: joint learning of video segmentation and optical flow. In: Proceedings of the AAAI Conference on Artificial Intelligence, vol. 34, pp. 10713–10720 (2020)
20. Ouyang, D., et al.: Video-based AI for beat-to-beat assessment of cardiac function. Nature **580**(7802), 252–256 (2020)
21. Ta, K., Ahn, S.S., Stendahl, J.C., Sinusas, A.J., Duncan, J.S.: A semi-supervised joint network for simultaneous left ventricular motion tracking and segmentation in 4D echocardiography. In: Martel, A.L., Abolmaesumi, P., Stoyanov, D., Mateus, D., Zuluaga, M.A., Zhou, S.K., Racoceanu, D., Joskowicz, L. (eds.) MICCAI 2020. LNCS, vol. 12266, pp. 468–477. Springer, Cham (2020). https://doi.org/10.1007/978-3-030-59725-2_45

FMUnet: Frequency Feature Enhancement Multi-level U-Net for Low-Dose CT Denoising with a Real Collected LDCT Image Dataset

Yu Zhang[1], Xinqi Yang[1], Guoliang Gong[1](✉), Xianghong Meng[2], Xiaoliang Wang[2], and Zhongwei Zhang[1]

[1] College of Artificial Intelligence, Tianjin University of Science and Technology, No. 9 Dishisan Dajie, Tianjin 300457, China
gongguoliang@tust.edu.cn
[2] Radiology Department, Tianjin Hospital, No.406 Jiefang South Road, Tianjin 300211, China

Abstract. Accompanying the widespread use of CT systems in medical diagnostics has highlighted concerns about the health risks associated with X-ray radiation exposure. Despite reducing the use of X-rays, low-dose computed tomography (LDCT) as a method to mitigate radiation risk is often plagued by quantum noise due to the scarcity of X-ray photons in low-dose scenarios. This results in image edge discontinuities, smoothing of small target structures, and the emergence of low-contrast visual effects. These manifestations of visual degradation primarily occur within the high-frequency band of the image, this study focuses on enhancing the quality of LDCT images by optimizing the utilization of frequency domain features. Specifically, we adopt a multi-level supervised U-shaped neural network and introduce a novel Frequency Feature Attention (FFA) mechanism. FFA utilizes convolution to diversify frequency features, then modulates them using channel weights to enhance learning of beneficial frequencies. We also introduce frequency domain loss based on fast Fourier transform to supervise the model's learning in the frequency domain. Furthermore, considering that synthetic data might introduce biases or distribution mismatches absent in real data, we established a real LDCT dataset. For each volunteer, one regular-dose CT scan and one low-dose CT scan are conducted respectively, resulting in a total of 4310 pairs of NDCT-LDCT images. Through experiments on the contributed dataset, our method produces superior results and outperforms other methods, significantly improving the quality of low-dose CT images, and providing strong technical support for reducing X-ray radiation risks while ensuring the accuracy of image diagnosis.

Keywords: Low-dose CT · CT denoising · LDCT image dataset · U-net · Frequency Feature Attention

1 Introduction

Computerized Tomography (CT) is a reliable and non-invasive medical imaging modality that aids in detecting pathological abnormalities in the human body, such as tumors, vascular diseases, pulmonary nodules, internal injuries, and fractures, and it has found extensive use in clinical treatment and diagnosis [1, 2] Concerns regarding the heightened exposure to X-ray radiation have emerged as an inevitable challenge for both CT manufacturers and healthcare institutions [3], thus drawing considerable social attention to the problem of low-dose computed tomography (LDCT) due to its potential for reducing X-ray radiation. However, due to the principles of X-ray imaging [4], CT images typically suffer from quantum noise and various artifacts during LDCT acquisition. Among these, quantum noise is embedded in LDCT due to the scarcity of X-ray photons during image acquisition. The scarcity of X-ray photons leads to visual degradation manifestations such as edge discontinuities, smoothing of fine structures, and the formation of low-contrast visual effects, which are visual manifestations of quantum noise. Therefore, enhancing the quality of CT images under low X-ray radiation doses is a highly meaningful research endeavor.

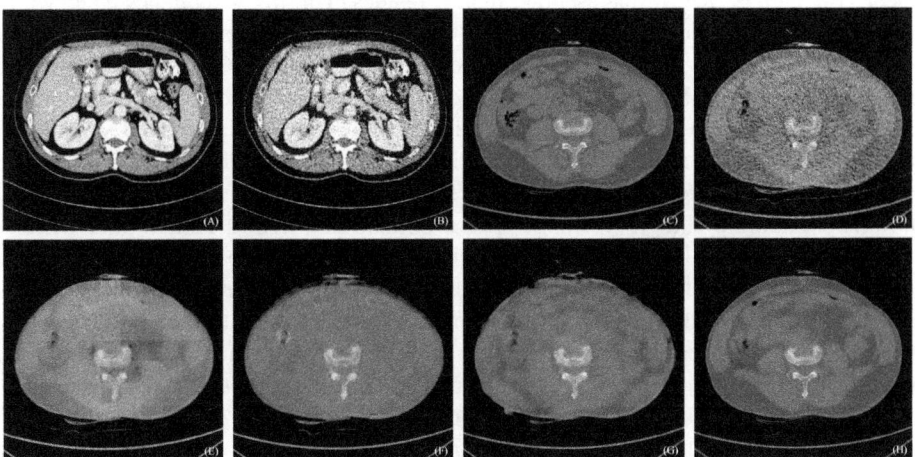

Fig. 1. Comparison between the public dataset and our contributed dataset, as well as comparison between our highlighted model and other LDCT models. (A) Mayo LDCT Challenge's NDCT (B) Mayo LDCT Challenge's LDCT (C) our dataset's NDCT (D) our dataset's LDCT (E) CTformer (F) EDCNN (G) RED-CNN (H) FMUnet

With the emergence of deep learning, it have become the mainstream method for denoising LDCT images [5], but it also has many problems.

Firstly, deep learning, as a data-driven approach, relies heavily on large volumes of supervised data to achieve optimal performance, where the quality of the dataset directly impacts the accuracy and generalization capabilities of the model. However, in existing methods for constructing public datasets, taking AAPM-Mayo Dataset as an example, low-dose computed tomography (LDCT) images are simulated only by adding mixed Poisson-Gaussian distribution (MPGD) noise to normal-dose computed tomography (NDCT) images [6, 7]. As shown in Fig. 1(A) (B), despite the addition of noise, organ boundaries remain clear. However, this approach may not accurately reflect the distribution characteristics of real LDCT images. For instance, in LDCT images, factors such as the shortage of X-ray photons and patient motion can contribute to image blurring [8–10] and streak artifacts [11–14] typically manifest along the long axis of highly absorbing objects. Existing datasets may not simulate these degradation characteristics of LDCT images, making the noise distribution learned by models trained on these public datasets unable to accurately reflect the characteristics of real LDCT images, affecting their generalization ability. Therefore, we organized volunteers and collected complete real LDCT-NDCT image pairs to fill the gap in the lack of real datasets in this field. As shown in Fig. 1(A) (B), our real LDCT images show more blurred organ boundaries and lower contrast, and unlike MPGD noise, real noise has a distribution similar to scattering from the center. This also confirms a clear difference between the distribution of artificial and real noise. The details of collecting the dataset will be covered later.

Secondly, the existing LDCT image deep learning models only consider the features of the image domain, but ignore the more obvious characteristics of CT images in the frequency domain. In LDCT images, noise mainly resides in the high-frequency band, while the low-frequency band of the image primarily contains essential texture information and other useful information. For example, in the field of sparse view CT reconstruction and image reduction or enhancement, many models combine frequency domain and spatial domain information to improve image quality. Arabi et al. [15] combined spatial and transform domain filtering to reduce quantization uncertainty while enhancing image texture. Lee et al. [16] proposed a deep learning model using a fully convolutional network combining sinogram, image spatial domain and hybrid domain and wavelet transform. Lal et al. [17] applied the original image domain based super-resolution reconstruction method to the frequency domain to achieve higher performance. Uetani et al.[18] processed the high frequency and low frequency in the image separately, and performed deep learning reconstruction specifically for the high frequency domain, which effectively reduced the noise in the image. In the above methods, dual-domain or multi-domain is used to improve the image quality in the process of model inference or reconstruction. In recent studies, many advanced results have been achieved by working with convolutional advance frequency features. The study by Park et al. [19] found that the convolution operator has the property of a high-pass filter, which can amplify the high-frequency components in the feature map. Wang et al. [20] also revealed that CNN has the ability to capture high-frequency components of images that are imperceptible to humans and that high-frequency components help explain the generalization of convolutional neural networks. This is also confirmed by Cui's research [21], where his network using convolution to extract frequency features achieves the best performance in several degraded image reduction fields such as image motion blur. Inspired by this observation, we propose a multi-level supervised U-shaped network, called FMUnet, and introduce a Frequency Feature Attention (FFA). This attention mechanism can enhance beneficial frequencies, strengthening the model's learning of LDCT frequency domain features. To address the issue of excessive smoothing in pixel-based loss functions and enhance supervision of frequency domain learning, we introduce a frequency domain loss based on the Fast Fourier Transform, combining it with pixel-based loss functions to supervise model training using dual-domain loss functions. Subsequently, we will retrain and test the proposed model and current well-performing models on our proposed dataset. Objective experiments demonstrate that method produces superior results and outperforms other methods on our contributed dataset. As seen in Fig. 1(E–H), our model exhibits stronger noise suppression capability and boundary texture inpainting capabilities.

In summary, our work makes the following key contributions:

- We first build a real LDCT image dataset. Twice CT scans are executed for each volunteer, once with low-dose and once with high-dose, resulting in 4310 pairs of 0.625mm slice images.
- We proposed a multi-level supervised U-shaped network (FMUnet) tailored to the characteristics of LDCT. Additionally, we designed a Frequency Feature Attention (FFA) mechanism to enhance the model's learning of beneficial frequencies based on the frequency domain characteristics of LDCT. To address the issue of excessive smoothing in pixel-based loss functions and to strengthen frequency domain learning, we introduced a frequency domain loss based on the Fast Fourier Transform.
- We retrained and tested our proposed model on the introduced dataset and compared it with mainstream models. The objective experimental results demonstrate the superior performance of our method on the dataset compared to others. Our approach exhibits stronger noise suppression capabilities and clearer texture restoration effects, resulting in significant improvements both visually and metrically.

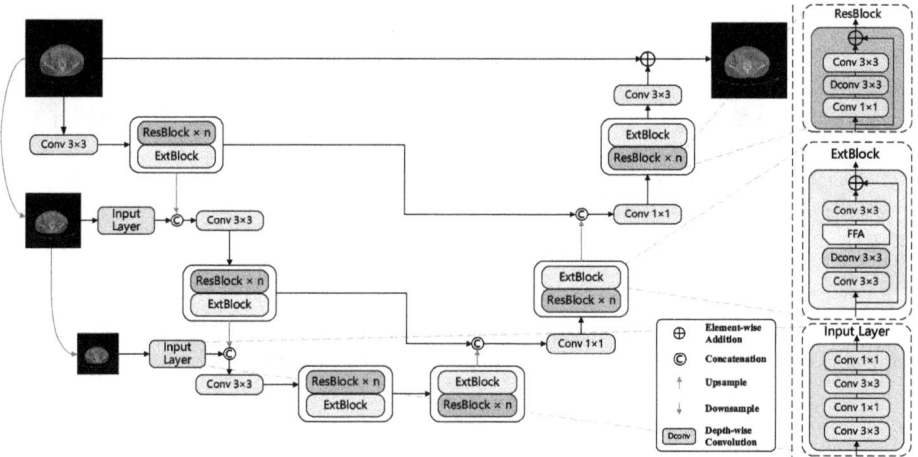

Fig. 2. The structure of the proposed network consists of multiple encoder and decoder architectures for hierarchical feature learning. Both the encoder and decoder are composed of ExtBlock layers and several ResBlock layers, albeit in different sequences.

2 Methods

In this section, we firstly introduce the overall architecture of our prominent network. Subsequently, we provide a detailed description of our highlighted FFA attention module. Finally, we present the design of the loss function.

2.1 FMUnet

Figure 2 illustrates the overall architecture of our proposed framework. Our convolutional neural network adopts an encoder-decoder architecture, where each encoder consists of 12 residual blocks followed by an attention module, and the decoder mirrors this structure but in reverse order. Between the two 3 × 3 convolutional layers within each residual block, we insert a 3 × 3 depth-wise convolutional layer (transposed convolution) to enhance feature learning during the encoding and decoding processes.

Initially, starting from the input LDCT image, a 3 × 3 convolutional layer is used to extract shallow features. Subsequently, the image undergoes three encoding stages. After the first and second encoding layers, the downsampled image is merged into the feature map, followed by a 3 × 3 convolutional layer to fuse features and adjust channel numbers. Upon completion of the final encoder, the network has performed deep and global feature extraction. Subsequently, the image resolution is gradually increased through three decoders. In the decoding process, 1 × 1 convolutional layers are used to reduce channel numbers. Finally, the decoding results are adjusted by a 3 × 3 convolutional layer, and two skip connections are added during the encoding-decoding process, connecting the input image and the predicted image.

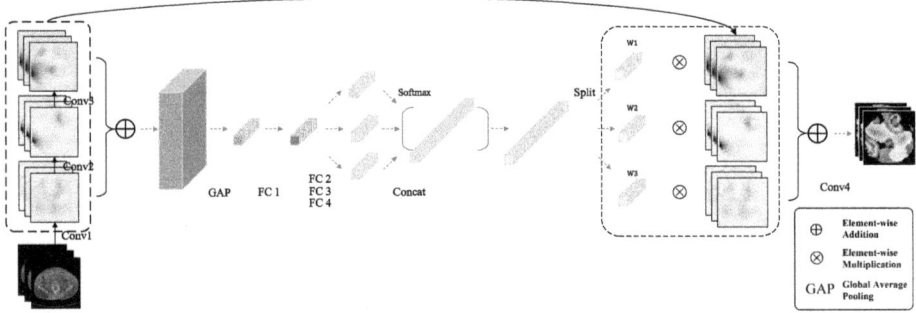

Fig. 3. The FFA (Frequency Feature Attention) extracts and enhances beneficial features in the frequency domain. For clarity, the figure contains only three frequency extraction branches.

2.2 Frequency Feature Attention (FFA)

In addition to the U-shaped backbone network, we propose a frequency-domain channel attention module to enhance the model's learning of LDCT image frequencies (see Fig. 3). Typically, noise primarily resides in the high-frequency bands of LDCT images, and furthermore, the remaining low-frequency bands not only contain the main content of the image but also include weakened image textures, which are noise-free [22]. Under this premise, inspired by [19, 20], we recognize that the convolution operator has the property of a high-pass filter and that high-frequency components help explain the generalization of convolutional neural networks, that is, it is able to amplify the high-frequency components in the feature map. Therefore, we first exploit this property to enhance and amplify the high-frequency feature signal layer-by-layer. Subsequently, we calculate the weights of different frequency channels and modulate them to ultimately improve the model's ability to recover beneficial signals in the frequency domain.

Firstly, for the input feature map $I \in R^{C \times H \times W}$ I, multiple parallel 3×3 convolutional layers are utilized to separate and extract different frequency segment features F_1, F_2 and F_i as follows:

$$F_1 = f_{3\times 3}^1(I) \tag{1}$$

$$F_2 = f_{3\times 3}^2\left(f_{3\times 3}^1(I)\right) \tag{2}$$

$$F_i = f_{3\times 3}^i\left(\ldots\left(f_{3\times 3}^2\left(f_{3\times 3}^1(I)\right)\right)\right) \tag{3}$$

where $f_{3\times 3}$ represents a 3×3 convolutional layer. (For simplicity, we only show the case of using three convolutional layers in Fig. 3) After extracting three frequency bands, the weights of the three frequency channels are calculated through global pooling and fully connected layers, as follows:

$$\left| W_i = FC_i(FC_0(GAP(\sum_i F_i))), i \in \{1, \ldots, i\} \right| \tag{4}$$

where FC represents a fully connected layer, $W \in R^C$ denotes the initial weights, and GAP represents global average pooling. We process the preliminary weights obtained from the two fully connected layers of the second layer through a Softmax function to obtain the final frequency attention weights:

$$W_i' = \frac{e^{W_i}}{\sum_{j=1}^{i \times C} e^{W_j}} \tag{5}$$

where W_i' represents the final weight of the corresponding channel, i.e., the channel attention weight. After applying the weights, the overall output of FFA is as follows:

$$\hat{I} = f_{1\times 1}\left(\sum_i W_i' \cdot F_i\right) \tag{6}$$

2.3 Loss Function

Since previous methods typically used only pixel-level loss (such as mean squared error), this may lead to over-smoothing issues. However, the imaging principle of CT images involves the frequency domain, and the features in our proposed network also utilize the frequency domain. Therefore, in the loss function, in addition to using the spatial domain L_1 loss function, we also add the loss $L_\mathcal{F}$ after the fast Fourier transform. This makes the loss function pay more attention to the differences in the frequency content of the image, including the overall structure and texture of the image, rather than just comparing at the pixel level. The formula is as follows:

$$L_1 = \frac{1}{N}\sum_{i=1}^{W}\sum_{j=1}^{H}\left|I(i,j) - \hat{I}(i,j)\right| \tag{7}$$

$$L_{\mathcal{F}} = \frac{1}{N} \sum_{i=1}^{W} \sum_{j=1}^{H} \left| \mathcal{F}(I(i,j)) - \mathcal{F}(\hat{I}(i,j)) \right| \tag{8}$$

where $\mathcal{F}$ is the Fast Fourier Transform, N is the total number of pixels in the image, W and H represent the width and height of the image, respectively. The final loss function is as follows, where λ is empirically set to 0.1:

$$L = L_1 + \lambda L_{\mathcal{F}} \tag{9}$$

3 Experiments

3.1 Datasets

Existing publicly available datasets simulate quarter-dose images by artificially adding noise to NDCT images, but there may be significant differences between the distribution of this artificial noise and the distribution of real noise. Models trained on datasets with artificially added noise may not generalize well in real-world applications. With this in mind, we propose a real LDCT dataset. In our dataset, we obtained NDCT and LDCT images with a slice thickness of 0.625 mm from lung and abdominal CT scans of six anonymous volunteers, totaling 4310 pairs of 512 × 512 images. The tube current settings for the X-ray tube were distributed as 120 kV and 80 kV, with tube currents of 250 ms and 10 ms, respectively. Our dataset is more challenging, with fewer boundary and texture information in the CT images and higher noise levels. Although this setup makes the task more challenging, it can increase the robustness of the trained models and ensure that the models learn the real noise distribution of LDCT images.

3.2 Implementation Details

We divided the proposed dataset into two parts randomly at a ratio of 2:8, with 3448 pairs of 512 × 512 images used for training and the remaining 862 pairs used as the test set. Our network was trained using the Adam optimizer($\beta_1 = 0.9$, $\beta_2 = 0.999$) with an initial learning rate of $1e^{-4}$, which was decreased to $1e^{-6}$ using cosine annealing. The batch size was set to 4. For data augmentation, we employed horizontal flipping of images with a probability of 0.5. The model was trained on patches of size 256 × 256 and tested on full resolution. Training was conducted for 300 epochs on an NVIDIA GeForce RTX 4090.

3.3 Performance Comparisons

In this session, we compared FMUnet with three advanced methods, and the comparative algorithms are trained for 300 epochs on our real LDCT dataset. A brief introduction of the three algorithms is as follows:

1. CTformer[23]: A Transformer-based model that achieves superior denoising effects by using convolution-free operations and the Token2Token mechanism, thereby improving the model's interpretability.
2. EDCNN[24]: Designed an edge-enhancement module based on trainable Sobel convolutions to enhance edge information extraction, and achieved better denoising effects by introducing the edge-enhancement module and composite loss functions.
3. RED-CNN[25]: Adopted a residual autoencoder structure, combining the advantages of autoencoders and convolutional neural networks, using symmetric convolutional and deconvolutional layers to enhance denoising and structure preservation for low-dose CT images.

Table 1. On the proposed dataset, quantitative evaluations of different models are conducted using PSNR, SSIM, and RMSE.

Method	PSNR↑	SSIM↑	RMSE↓
LDCT	22.27	0.4890	22.01
RED-CNN	29.98	0.8788	8.869
EDCNN	27.57	0.8486	11.58
CTformer	26.66	0.7765	12.67
ours	**36.60**	**0.9325**	**4.2370**

Specific training methods and dataset information are introduced below (Table 1).

Quantitative Analysis. We compared high-performance LDCT methods such as CTformer, EDCNN, and RED-CNN, and retrained these models on our dataset. We employed peak signal-to-noise ratio (PSNR), Structural Similarity Index (SSIM), and Root Mean Square Error (RMSE) evaluation metrics. For image quality evaluation. From the results table, we observe an enhancement in image quality across all three metrics for all the methods evaluated. Specifically, our proposed model achieved a gain of 14.33 dB PSNR relative to LDCT, outperforming previous prominent models. This also indicates that models designed for previous datasets lack sufficient recovery and reconstruction capabilities when faced with strong noise, strong blurring, weak boundaries, and weak contour features in real datasets. Our model not only considers noise suppression but also addresses the reconstruction of various details in LDCT images. This sets a precedent for future models.

Qualitative Analysis. As depicted in Fig. 4, these results were randomly selected from the test set. Compared to Low-Dose CT (LDCT), all methods show effectiveness in denoising, but our proposed FMUnet method approaches the quality of conventional Dose CT (NDCT) more closely. Upon comprehensive analysis of the complete volumetric CT images, we observed that our model outperforms others in edge sharpness and noise suppression, with relatively less noise present in the images. Upon careful examination of the region highlighted by the red box in the first image, we observed that

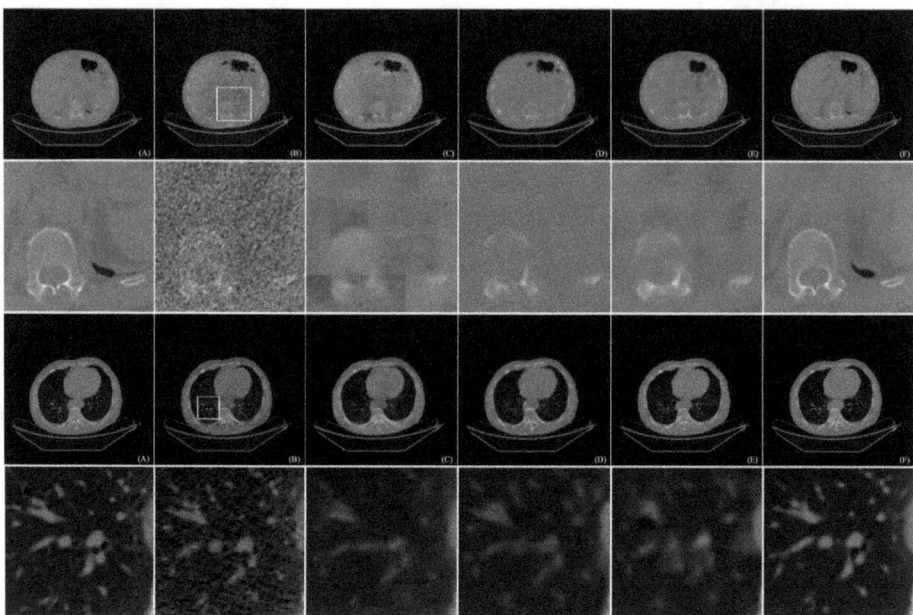

Fig. 4. Visual comparison of various models, the second and fourth rows are the zoomed areas marked by red boxes (A) NDCT, (B)LDCT, (C) CTformer, (D) EDCNN, (E) RED-CNN, (F) FMUnet

our model almost perfectly restored the shape and boundaries of the spine, with contours of dark and light tissues closer to NDCT. While other models achieved some noise suppression, they struggled to restore the contours and shapes of the spine and tissues. In the second image, the white shadow area in the lung region of our model exhibits higher contrast and clearer edges. The over-smoothing issue caused by pixel-wise loss, mentioned in the article, is particularly evident in the comparative models, as they tend to blur the edges of the white shadow in the lungs while reducing noise to some extent. Through comparison, we found that our proposed model demonstrates stronger capabilities in noise suppression, image restoration, and edge preservation. This is attributed to our introduced frequency-domain loss function, which mitigates the over-smoothing issue caused by pixel-wise loss, and our proposed FFA attention model, which strengthens the low-frequency domain's organizational texture information (such as spine edges and lung white shadows) while attenuating noise in the high-frequency domain.

Table 2. Conducting ablation experiments on FMUnet using the proposed dataset.

Method	PSNR	Params(M)
Baseline	35.72	6.89
Baseline + FFA	36.51	8.61
Baseline + FFA + Dconv(Full)	**36.60**	**8.65**

3.4 Ablation Study

We conducted ablation experiments to validate our modules. The dataset used in the ablation experiments remained the one proposed by us. We created a baseline network by eliminating the FFA attention module and deformable convolution (Dconv). The model's parameter variations are on the right side of the table. The results of the channel experiments indicate that our prominent attention mechanism enhances the performance of the model compared to the baseline network. The training method is consistent with the above. The baseline network achieved a PSNR of 35.72 dB on the dataset. By enhancing the frequency signal, our FFA attention yielded a progress gain of 0.79 dB PSNR on the baseline model (see Table 2). Using Dconv can improve by 0.09 dB. The complete network structure integrating FFA and Dconv achieved the highest score. Our results clearly demonstrate the effectiveness of our design (Fig. 5).

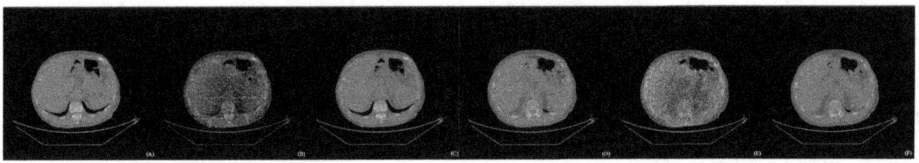

Fig. 5. Robustness of FMUnet for organ migration (A) NDCT-1, (B) LDCT-1, (C) output-1, (D) NDCT-2, (E) LDCT-2, (F) output-2

4 Discussion

In the real LDCT dataset we propose, despite the presence of more realistic noise distribution, image blur, and streak artifacts, these significant degradation characteristics actually enhance the generalization capability and accuracy of deep learning models. However, upon careful analysis of the dataset, we noted an average displacement of 2 to 3 pixels in organ positions between the same set of LDCT and Normal Dose CT (NDCT) images. This displacement is primarily due to minor organ movements caused by the subject's breathing during the two different dose scanning processes, which is unavoidable. Observing the predictions of our model, we found that it not only effectively denoises and reconstructs LDCT images but also demonstrates robustness to organ position displacement caused by breathing. For example, As shown in Fig. 4(A–C), a randomly selected pair of images demonstrates that despite shape changes in the black low-density areas marked by red boxes in the input LDCT images due to breathing, our model can still correct this displacement, making its shape more akin to that of the NDCT images. In Fig. 4(D–F), this corrective effect is more pronounced, with the predicted black contours closely matching those of the NDCT images. To assess the clinical value of this finding, we invited several doctors to review the test results of the model. They generally agreed that the model's predictions are within an acceptable range and can assist doctors in making diagnostic judgments to a certain extent.

5 Conclusion

We established a real LDCT image dataset by recruiting volunteers for image acquisition, addressing the shortcomings of existing publicly available datasets in artificially introducing noise and failing to accurately reflect the degradation characteristics of real LDCT images. Secondly, we proposed a multi-level supervised U-net and designed frequency feature attention to enhance the model's learning of beneficial frequency information. Additionally, to address the issue of excessive smoothing in pixel-based loss functions and to strengthen frequency domain learning, we introduced frequency domain loss based on fast Fourier transform. Finally, through retraining and testing our proposed model and comparing it with baseline models, experiments demonstrated that our model achieved superior performance on our proposed dataset, and we achieve great improvement in both qualitative and quantitative experiments, exhibiting stronger noise suppression capability and clearer organizational edge representation. These achievements provide valuable references and insights for the development of LDCT image denoising.

References

1. Mathews, J.P., Campbell, Q.P., Xu, H., Halleck, P.: A review of the application of X-ray computed tomography to the study of coal. Fuel **209**, 10–24 (2017)
2. Seeram, E.: Computed Tomography: Physical Principles, Clinical Applications, and Quality Control. Elsevier (2015)
3. Brenner, D.J., Hall, E.J.: Computed tomography — an increasing source of radiation exposure. N. Engl. J. Med. **357**, 2277–2284 (2007). https://doi.org/10.1056/NEJMra072149
4. Xu, Q., Yu, H., Mou, X., Zhang, L., Hsieh, J., Wang, G.: Low-dose X-ray CT reconstruction via dictionary learning. IEEE Trans. Med. Imaging **31**, 1682–1697 (2012)
5. Wang, G., Ye, J.C., De Man, B.: Deep learning for tomographic image reconstruction. Nat. Mach. Intell. **2**, 737–748 (2020)
6. McCollough, C.H., et al.: Low-dose CT for the detection and classification of metastatic liver lesions: results of the 2016 low dose CT grand challenge. Med. Phys. **44**, e339–e352 (2017). https://doi.org/10.1002/mp.12345
7. Ding, Q., Long, Y., Zhang, X., Fessler, J.A.: Statistical image reconstruction using mixed Poisson-Gaussian Noise Model for X-Ray CT (2018). http://arxiv.org/abs/1801.09533
8. Du, W., Chen, H., Wu, Z., Sun, H., Liao, P., Zhang, Y.: Stacked competitive networks for noise reduction in low-dose CT. PLoS ONE **12**, e0190069 (2017)
9. Shiri Lord, I.: Ultra-low-dose chest CT imaging of COVID-19 patients using a deep residual neural network (2020)
10. Wu, D., Kim, K., Fakhri, G.E., Li, Q.: A cascaded convolutional neural network for X-ray low-dose CT image denoising (2017). http://arxiv.org/abs/1705.04267
11. Zhong, A., Li, B., Luo, N., Xu, Y., Zhou, L., Zhen, X.: Image restoration for low-dose CT via transfer learning and residual network. IEEE Access **8**, 112078–112091 (2020)
12. Kang, E., Chang, W., Yoo, J., Ye, J.C.: Deep convolutional framelet denosing for low-dose CT via wavelet residual network. IEEE Trans. Med. Imaging **37**, 1358–1369 (2018)
13. Ming, J., Yi, B., Zhang, Y., Li, H.: Low-dose CT image denoising using classification densely connected residual network. KSII Trans. Internet Inf. Syst. TIIS. **14**, 2480–2496 (2020)
14. Yang, L., Shangguan, H., Zhang, X., Wang, A., Han, Z.: High-frequency sensitive generative adversarial network for low-dose CT image denoising. IEEE Access. **8**, 930–943 (2019)

15. Arabi, H., Zaidi, H.: Improvement of image quality in PET using post-reconstruction hybrid spatial-frequency domain filtering. Phys. Med. Biol. **63**, 215010 (2018)
16. Lee, D.,Choi, S., Kim, H.: High quality imaging from sparsely sampled computed tomography data with deep learning and wavelet transform in various domains. Med. Phys. **46**, 104–115 (2019). https://doi.org/10.1002/mp.13258
17. Lal, A., et al.: A frequency domain SIM reconstruction algorithm using reduced number of images. IEEE Trans. Image Process. **27**, 4555–4570 (2018)
18. Uetani, H., et al.: A preliminary study of deep learning-based reconstruction specialized for denoising in high-frequency domain: use-fulness in high-resolution three-dimensional magnetic resonance cisternography of the cerebellopontine angle. Neuroradiology **63**, 63–71 (2021). https://doi.org/10.1007/s00234-020-02513-w
19. Park, N., Kim, S.: How do vision transformers work? (2022). http://arxiv.org/abs/2202.06709
20. Wang, H., Wu, X., Huang, Z., Xing, E.P.: High-frequency component helps explain the generalization of convolutional neural networks. In: Proceedings of the 2020 IEEE/CVF Conference on Computer Vision and Pattern Recognition (CVPR), pp. 8681–8691. IEEE, Seattle (2020). https://doi.org/10.1109/CVPR42600.2020.00871
21. Cui, Y., Knoll, A.: Exploring the potential of channel interactions for image restoration. Knowl.-Based Syst. **282**, 111156 (2023). https://doi.org/10.1016/j.knosys.2023.111156
22. Zhang, Z., Yu, L., Liang, X., Zhao, W., Xing, L.: TransCT: dual-path transformer for low dose computed tomography. In: De Bruijne, M., et al. (eds.) Medical Image Computing and Computer Assisted Intervention – MICCAI 2021, pp. 55–64. Springer International Publishing, Cham (2021)
23. Wang, D., Fan, F., Wu, Z., Liu, R., Wang, F., Yu, H.: CTformer: convolution-free Token2Token dilated vision transformer for low-dose CT denoising. Phys. Med. Biol. **68**, 065012 (2023). https://doi.org/10.1088/1361-6560/acc000
24. Liang, T., Jin, Y., Li, Y., Wang, T.: EDCNN: edge enhancement-based densely connected network with compound loss for low-dose CT denoising. In: Proceedings of the 2020 15th IEEE International Conference on Signal Processing (ICSP), pp. 193–198. IEEE, Beijing (2020)
25. Chen, H., et al.: Low-dose CT with a residual encoder-decoder convolutional neural network. IEEE Trans. Med. Imaging **36**, 2524–2535 (2017). https://doi.org/10.1109/TMI.2017.2715284

Research on Intelligent Recognition Algorithm of Container Numbers in Ports Based on Deep Learning

Zhehao Lin, Chen Dong(✉), and Yuxuan Wan

School of Computer Science and Engineering, Tianjin University of Technology, Tianjin 300380, China
dongc@tjut.edu.cn

Abstract. The identification of container number has important application value in the field of logistics and cargo transportation. A new container number recognition algorithm was proposed in this paper to solve the difficult problems such as different illumination conditions, blurred image, loud noise, damaged and polluted container number, zigzag deformation, etc. First, the low-light enhancement algorithm based on Retinex theory was used to process the container number image to deal with the problems of inconsistent port lighting conditions and background noise. The super-resolution reconstruction was used to deal with the problems of container surface contamination and container number damage. The backbone network was replaced by MobileNetv3 by improving the YOLOv5 algorithm. The ECA attention mechanism was added to achieve lightweight model and accurate location of box number area. STN is added before the convolutional layer of the CRNN to correct the image. Public images on Github and official images of Tianjin Port were used to generate samples through DCGAN network, and their data were enhanced. The obtained 6961 container number images were used as data sets to train the improved CRNN model. The mAP of the proposed method in container number location using the improved YOLOv5 reaches 93.7%, the accuracy rate reaches 94.5% in container number identification using the improved CRNN, and the average recognition speed reaches 29.1 frames/s. The method performs well in real-time performance and realizes the lightweight of the model. It can meet the requirements of port real-time and accurate identification of container number.

1 Introduction

With the continuous development of global trade and the rapid growth of logistics industry, container transport, as one of the main modes of cargo transport, has become an important part of the global trade and logistics field. However, in the process of container management and logistics tracking, the accurate location and identification of container number has always been a challenging problem. For different port lighting conditions, container number damage pollution, tortuous deformation, blurred images, loud noise, accurate real-time identification of the box number and other problems, the traditional container number identification method was often difficult to meet the actual needs.

With the development of artificial intelligence technology, algorithms based on deep learning are widely used in the field of object detection [1–4]. For example, Wang Zhenpeng et al. [5] improved Faster-RCNN and added the attention mechanism in the area generation network (RPN) to improve the detection speed of the case number while ensuring the accuracy. However, further improvement and verification were needed for complex environments such as the case number being seriously soiled and low light. Xu Zhengguang et al. [6] used YOLOv3 object detection algorithm and deeplabv3plus semantic segmentation algorithm to locate the character region of the display screen, which has good stability and real-time performance, but was limited to small samples. Zhang Ran et al. [7] adopted the average maximum suppression range (AMSR) algorithm to identify the boundary of the container code region, so as to reduce the interference of container images. This framework could meet the operating requirements in detection accuracy and processing speed, but it did not analyze the specific complex scene of the port.

In the field of character recognition, the application of deep learning has developed rapidly, and the use of neural networks for container number recognition [8–11] could solve some cases that could not be correctly recognized by humans. For example, Li Yanchao et al. [12] proposed an end-to-end box number recognition algorithm by locating regions and detecting characters and classifying them, which could cope with various factors such as uneven illumination, background changes and other image quality degradation factors, and the recognition accuracy has improved compared with other algorithms composed of character classifiers. However, there is no significant optimization for lightweight deployment and real-time recognition of the model. Chao Mi et al. [13] For problems such as container number inclination and deflection, the differential edge detection algorithm was used to binary segment the container number image, improved square method was used to locate the container number, BP neural network was used to identify the container number, and the comprehensive recognition rate was improved compared with traditional methods and yolov3. However, the defacement and character repair of the case number were not fully considered. Yang Dapeng et al. [14] used lightweight network as the trunk and added MRFPN feature extraction module to extract semantic information, which reduced the computational load and could meet the requirements of actual container number code recognition, but did not verify container numbers in various arrangements.

In this paper, a new container number identification method was proposed to address the requirements of accurate and real-time identification of container numbers due to different lighting conditions, blurred images, loud noise, damaged and polluted container numbers, zigzag deformation in ports: First, the low-light enhancement algorithm based on Retinex theory was used to reduce the impact of different port light on image quality, and super-resolution reconstruction was used to solve the problems of damaged, polluted, tortuous and deformed container number. MobileNetv3 was replaced by the backbone network of YOLOv5. In addition, ECA (Efficient Channel Attention) was added to Neck, and the improved YOLOv5 network was used to locate the container number area. DCGAN (Deep Convolutional Generative Adversarial Network) is used to generate the CRNN model after training the container number sample. Before CRNN, the Spatial Transformer Network (STN) was added to correct the container number in the image, and the container number was finally identified. This method achieves a good balance between detection speed and accuracy, and could be applied to real-time detection of container number on embedded devices.

2 Container Number Localization and Recognition Workflow

The workflow of container number location and identification in the complex scenario of the port is shown in Fig. 1. For the task of container number identification, the data collection and processing were carried out first. A rich and diverse training dataset was constructed by using the on-site shooting of the port and the data set provided by the Tianjin Port official, and the expanded sample of the container number generated by DCGAN to train the improved YOLOv5 model and the improved CRNN model. For the image with container number to be processed, the low-light enhancement algorithm based on Retinex theory was first used to enhance the image sharpness and contrast. Then, the improved YOLOv5 algorithm was used to locate the container number area and crop out the valid container number area in the image. Finally, the improved CRNN model was used for text correction and character recognition. After identifying the character information in the container number, the verification code was used to verify the correctness of the recognition. Finally, the accurate recognition result of the container number was obtained.

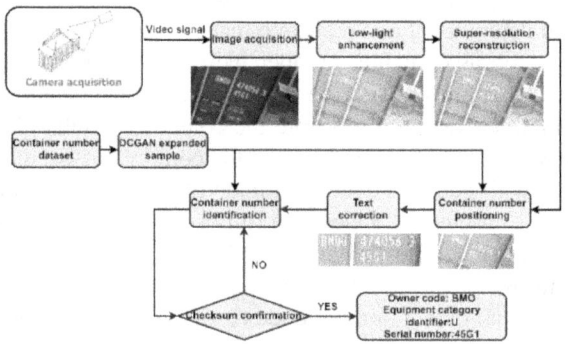

Fig. 1. Container number identification process in complex scenarios.

3 Low-Light Enhancement Method Based on Retinex Theory

In container number recognition, image quality directly affects the recognition accuracy. Under low light conditions, the image quality is poor, the noise is large, the color is distorted, and the recognition accuracy is affected. In this paper, low light enhancement algorithm based on Retinex theory is used to improve image quality. The specific process is shown in Fig. 2.

Initially, the original RGB image was converted into the HSV color space, and the luminance component V was processed using the Multi-Scale Retinex (MSR) algorithm,

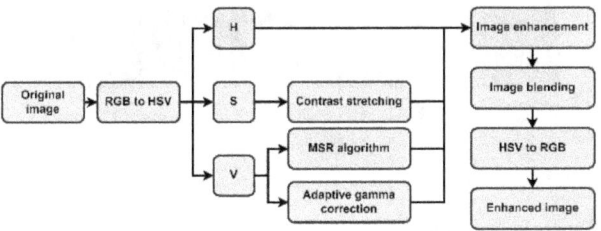

Fig. 2. Low-light enhancement process diagram Based on Retinex theory.

with the Retinex model described by Eqs. (1) and (2). Adaptive gamma correction was then applied to enhance the brightness and contrast of the image. This approach made the details in dark areas clearer, which aided in improving the recognizability of the container number image.

$$I(x, y) = R(x, y) \times L(x, y) \tag{1}$$

In the formula, $I(x,y)$ represents the original image, $R(x,y)$ denotes the object's reflection component, and $L(x,y)$ indicates the object's incident component.

$$V_{out} = GV_{in}^{\beta} \tag{2}$$

In the equation, V_{in} is the input luminance value, V_{out} is the output luminance value, and G is a parameter for Gamma correction.

Subsequently, after converting the saturation component S to the HSV color space, contrast stretching operations were conducted to enhance the vividness and visual impact of the image, with the specific stretching process described by Eq. (3). This aids in highlighting color features within the container number image, making it easier for recognition algorithms to capture key information.

$$S_{out} = (S_{in} - \min)\frac{N_{max} - N_{min}}{\max - \min} + N_{min} \tag{3}$$

In the equation, S_{in} represents the pixel value of the original image, *max* and *min* respectively denote the maximum and minimum pixel values of the original image, N_{max} and N_{min} respectively represent the maximum and minimum pixel values of the target image, and S_{out} is the pixel value of the image after contrast stretching treatment.

Finally, the processed HSV image components are fused and converted back to RGB to obtain the enhanced image. The brightness, contrast and clarity of the container number image after low-light enhancement are improved, effectively improving the accuracy of container number positioning and recognition, as shown in Fig. 3.

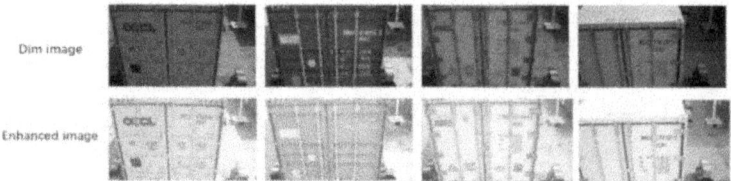

Fig. 3. Example of container images before and after low-light enhancement.

4 Character Super Resolution Reconstruction

In the identification of port container number, the problems such as ambiguity and distortion caused by damage and fouling affect the identification. The text super-resolution reconstruction technology can improve the clarity and readability of the carton number image, enhance the accuracy and stability of the recognition algorithm, effectively reduce the blur and noise interference, and help to accurately identify and extract the carton number information.

First, the high-resolution and corresponding low-resolution container number images in the dataset were used as training samples. Then, the image was preprocessed, including denoising and contrast enhancement. In the training stage, the SRCNN deep learning model was used. The specific network structure diagram of the model was shown in Fig. 4, where f_1 and f_3 respectively represent the convolution layer sizes corresponding to layers 1 and 3, n_1 and n_2 respectively represent the first and second nonlinear mapping layers.

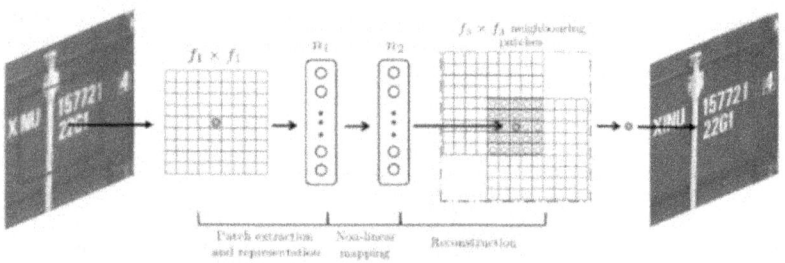

Fig. 4. Network structure of SRCNN

SRCNN model reconstructs high-resolution images by learning the mapping relationship between high-low resolution image pairs. By training and optimizing the model parameters, the model can accurately convert low-resolution images into high-resolution images. Figure 5 shows the comparison effect before and after reconstruction. This scheme significantly improves the clarity and identification accuracy of port container images, and thus improves the speed and accuracy of container number identification.

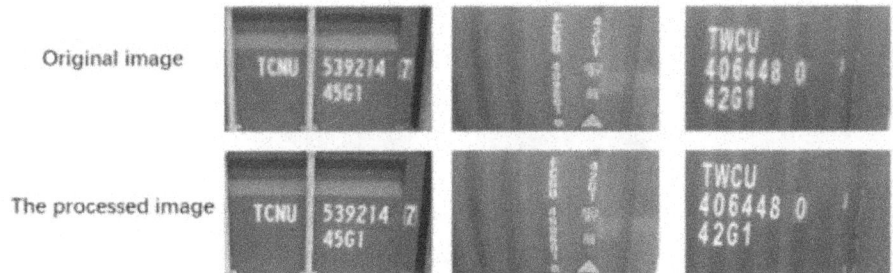

Fig. 5. Sample map of super resolution reconstruction.

5 Container Number Localization Method Based on YOLOv5

5.1 MobileNetv3 Module

MobileNetv3, a lightweight deep learning model, significantly improves its deployment efficiency in resource-constrained environments by adopting Bottleneck layer design (including linear bottleneck and depth-separable convolution) and adaptive activation functions. Its lightweight characteristics make it easier to deploy the model after replacing the YOLOv5 backbone network on mobile devices and embedded facilities in port terminals, meeting the real-time requirements of container number area detection while maintaining high detection accuracy. Global average pooling further reduces the number of parameters, improves model generalization ability, and ensures that both speed and accuracy requirements are met in container number positioning tasks.

5.2 ECA

The structure of the ECA attention mechanism was shown in Fig. 6. Initially, the feature map undergoes Global Average Pooling (GAP) to obtain aggregated features. The size of the one-dimensional convolution kernel was calculated based on the number of channels, followed by a one-dimensional convolution operation. Lastly, the Sigmoid activation function was used to learn the weight of each channel. ECA discarded the method of achieving channel communication through fully connected layers, focusing instead on each channel and its k adjacent channels to facilitate cross-channel information interaction, as shown in Eq. (4). By adding the ECA attention mechanism in the Neck, it is possible to effectively extract more information from the feature maps without significantly affecting the overall model parameters. This also avoided the impact of dimensionality reduction operations, thereby improving the accuracy of the model's detection.

$$K = \psi(C) = \left| \frac{\log_2(C)}{\gamma} + \frac{b}{\gamma} \right|_{odd} \quad (4)$$

In the equation, γ is set to 2, b is 1, K is the size of the convolutional kernel, C is the number of channels, and $|t|_{odd}$ represents the nearest odd number to t.

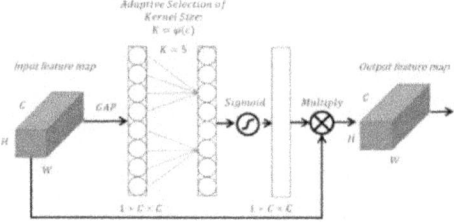

Fig. 6. ECA attention module.

5.3 Improvements to the YOLOv5 Model

YOLOv5 is composed of Backbone, Neck and Head, and is suitable for container number positioning. Backbone uses CSPDarknet53 to extract features, Neck fuses features of different levels through FPN, and Head predicts the position and category of the box number. Aiming at real-time, lightweight and small target detection requirements when deployed to embedded devices, this paper proposes an improved YOLOv5 algorithm, the specific structure of which is shown in Fig. 7.

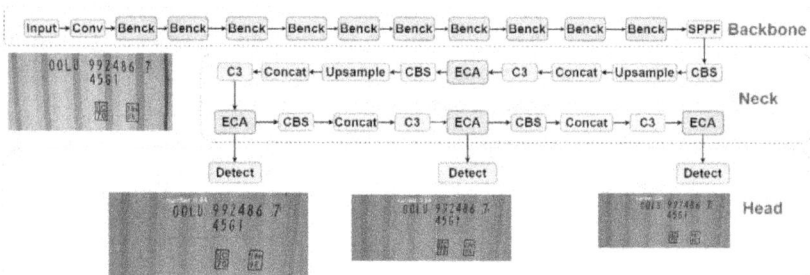

Fig. 7. Improved YOLOv5 network structure.

Firstly, the Backbone of YOLOv5 is replaced by Benck in MobileNetv3. MobileNetv3, as a lightweight network structure, has low parameter number and computational complexity, which was suitable for operation in resource-limited environments of embedded devices. At the same time, less computation was required, which could improve the reasoning speed. Secondly, adding ECA attention mechanism to Neck can effectively capture the dependencies between different channels in the feature map, and improve the model's ability to focus on the container number region and feature representation.

5.4 Generating Samples with DCGAN

DCGAN is an improvement of GAN, introducing convolutional neural network as the main architecture of generator and discriminator, which can capture spatial relationships and features of images and generate more realistic images. DCGAN eliminates the fully connected layer and uses convolution and deconvolution layers to reduce parameters and improve stability and generalization. It also introduces batch normalization and Leaky ReLU activation functions to speed up training, improve image quality, and avoid gradient disappearance. For container number generation, DCGAN can generate samples conforming to the characteristics of the real container number, expand the data set to improve the CRNN model, and improve the robustness and generalization ability of the model. Figure 8 shows a partial sample of the generated container numbers.

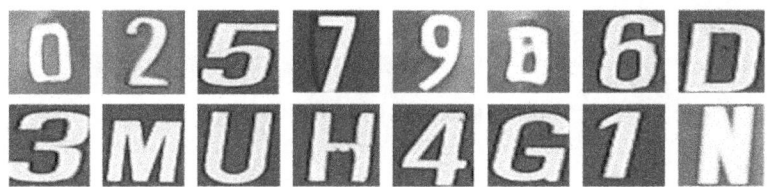

Fig. 8. Examples of sample images generated by DCGAN.

6 Improved CRNN for Container Number Identification

The task of port container number identification faces many challenges, such as fuzzy container number, soiling, surface deformation, etc. The traditional method is difficult to deal with effectively. In contrast, the CRNN model has significant advantages in this area. First, traditional methods require manual design of feature extractors or tedious pre-processing, while CRNN learns features directly from raw images through end-to-end learning, reducing the need for manual intervention. Secondly, CRNN combines the structure of convolutional layer and cyclic layer, which can make full use of spatial information of image and sequence information of text to understand and recognize the box number more comprehensively. In addition, by learning large amounts of data, CRNNs are better able to adapt to different forms and arrangements of box numbers without having to design specific rules or models for different situations. In order to improve the recognition accuracy of the CRNN model for the skewed container number image, this paper introduced the STN module, and the specific improved CRNN process was shown in Fig. 9.

In the CRNN model, feature extraction mainly relied on the convolutional layer, but the character recognition ability for distortion, tilt or Angle deviation was weak, which limited the robustness of the model. By learning the spatial transformation information of the image, STN module could make the model better adapt to the container number image of different scale, rotation and Angle of view. In the whole process, feature extraction and representation learning were firstly carried out through the localization network to capture the key feature points or feature regions in the image, which described the geometric structure and spatial transformation information of the image. Subsequently, the STN network predicted the parameters required to perform the spatial transformation, including rotation Angle, scaling ratio, and displacement, through the learned feature representation. These parameters were applied to the input image to implement geometric

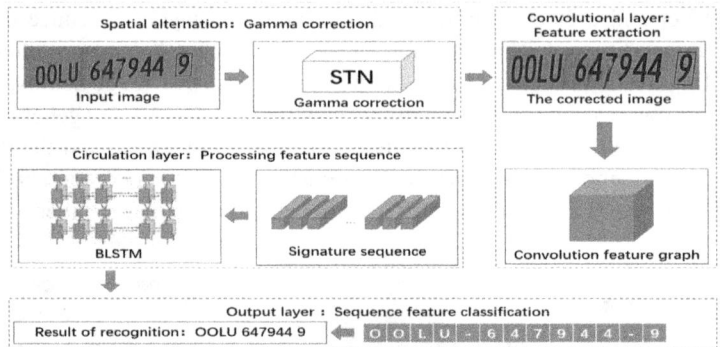

Fig. 9. Improved CRNN flowchart.

transformations of the image, such as rotation, scaling, and translation. Finally, the CRNN model recognizes characters on images transformed by STN space.

7 Experimental Results and Analysis

7.1 Dataset

By using a total of 2851 images with container number provided by Tianjin Port official and open data set on Github [15], data enhancement processing was carried out on them, including blurring, increasing brightness, reducing brightness, adding Gaussian noise, image offset and modifying size. A dataset containing 6961 images of damaged containers was constructed. The constructed dataset contained images of container numbers at multiple ports, under various extreme conditions, which correspond to the Obscure, Dim, Surface bending, Long-range shooting, High light, Dim, Foggy days, Contaminated or Angle skew images of container numbers in eight different environments and three different permutations of container numbers. The data set was divided into training set, verification set and test set according to the ratio of 8:1:1 to ensure that there is enough sample data in the training process, the verification process was effective, and the test evaluation was objective and accurate. The data enhancement legend was shown in Fig. 10.

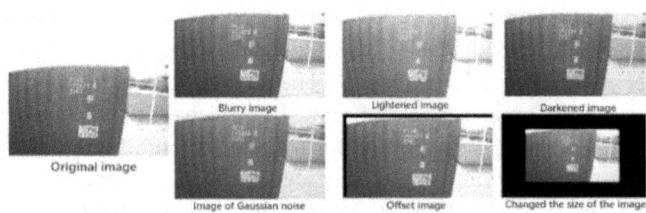

Fig. 10. Data enhanced image of container number.

7.2 The Improved YOLOv5 Was Used for Experimental Analysis of Container Number Region Positioning

In order to objectively evaluate the effectiveness of the improved YOLOv5 model, the model was evaluated in terms of Precision, Recall and mAP@0.5. After the common target detection algorithm Faster-RCNN YOLOv3, YOLOv4, YOLOv5 algorithm and the improved YOLOv5 model training, the training accuracy and recall rate, the mAP values for such as shown in Table 1.

Table 1. The results of container number location were compared by different target detection algorithm.

Algorithm	Precision	Recall	mAP@0.5
Faster-RCNN	78.9%	79.4%	76.1%
YOLOv3	70.2%	78.5%	72.5%
YOLOv4	83.7%	81.2%	82.1%
YOLOv5	85.2%	82.5%	88.4%
Improved YOLOv5	94.3%	86.2%	93.7%

By comparing the experimental data, it could be found that the detection accuracy of the improved YOLOv5 model is the highest, reaching 93.7%. In terms of detection speed, the original YOLOv5 model was the fastest, while the improved YOLOv5 model was the second fastest, but there was little difference, which met the standard of real-time port detection and met the real-time requirement.

Based on the analysis of three different arrangement of container number images and the detection of container number under eight extreme conditions, the optimized model could be used as a judgment standard for regional positioning of container number. The specific positioning and detection effects were shown in Fig. 11.

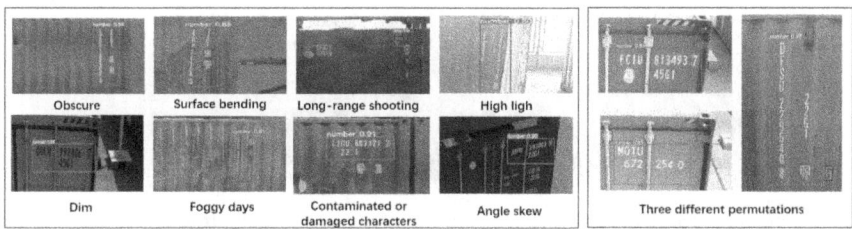

Fig. 11. Locating container numbers in various environments.

7.3 Analysis of the Improved CRNN for Container Number Recognition

In order to verify the effectiveness of lightweight and text recognition accuracy optimization of the proposed model, the proposed model was deployed on the embedded device

Jetson Nano to verify its performance. The deployment and recognition results are shown in Fig. 12. The traditional OCR model, YOLOv5 + CRNN model and the Improved YOLOv5 + Improved CRNN model were compared with the Improved YOLOV5 + Improved CRNN model, and the results were shown in Table 2.

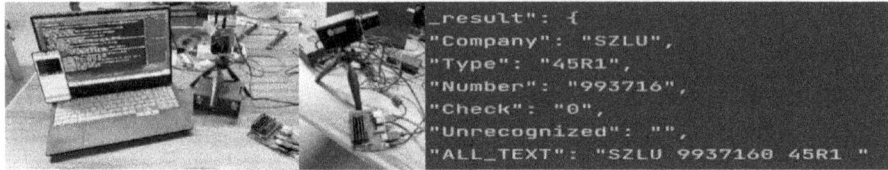

Fig. 12. Container number identification using Jetson Nano.

Table 2. Captions should be placed above the tables.

Algorithm	Model size	Recognition speed/(Frames/s)	mAP@0.5
Traditional OCR	14.5 MB	27.6	88.1%
YOLOv5 + CRNN	15.8 MB	30.4	91.9%
Improved YOLOv5 + Improved CRNN	14.2 MB	29.1	94.5%

By comparing the experimental data, it could be found that the accuracy rate of the improved CRNN model reaches 94.5%, and in terms of detection speed, the average recognition speed was 29.1 frames/s. Compared with the YOLOv5 + CRNN model, the speed of the improved model in this paper has decreased, but there was little difference. Moreover, the identification accuracy rate was improved to a greater extent, and the requirements of real-time container number identification in ports were better met. The specific identification effect deployed on embedded devices was shown in Fig. 13.

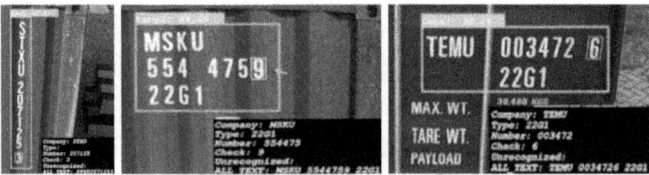

Fig. 13. Different arrangement of box number recognition effect.

8 Conclusion and Future Work

In view of the complex scenarios of container number recognition, such as different port lighting conditions, damaged and polluted container number, tortuous deformation, blurred image and loud noise, a new algorithm for container number recognition were proposed in this paper, and satisfactory results were obtained by using various technical means. First, the low light enhancement algorithm based on Retinex was used to process the image, which effectively solved the problems of insufficient light and background noise in the port, and the super-resolution reconstruction was used to deal with the situation of the container surface and the container number. Secondly, the improved YOLOv5 algorithm, by replacing the backbone network to MobileNetv3 and adding ECA attention mechanism to Neck, realized the model lightweight and accurate positioning of the box number region. Finally, the DCGAN network was used to generate samples, together with the public container number images of Github and the official container number images of Tianjin Port, to generate a dataset containing a total of 6961 container number images in three arrangements and eight extreme environments. Using this data set to train the improved CRNN model with STN network, the container number recognition was realized accurately, showing good real-time and recognition accuracy. Experimental verification showed that the improved algorithm could achieve 94.5% accuracy for container number recognition, and the average container number recognition speed is 29.1 frames/s, which was lower than the original YOLOv5 + CRNN model, but still met the real-time recognition requirements, which proved the effectiveness, robustness and generalization ability of the improved algorithm.

There are still some problems in this study. When the container number is damaged or dirty, the identification result is not accurate enough. In the future, the text recognition can be carried out after the text repair of the container number in the image. This is of great significance for the port to achieve automated container number identification and promote the rapid upgrade of port logistics. The current container number positioning model and container number recognition model adopt the strategy of separate training and optimization. In the future, we can consider integrating the two models to realize a new end-to-end method, so that the two can optimize each other during training.

References

1. Wang, A., Ren, C., Zhao, S., Mu, S.: Attention guided multi-level feature aggregation network for camouflaged object detection. Image Vis. Comput. **144**, 104953 (2024)
2. Zhang, J., Tian, M., Yang, Z., Li, J., Zhao, L.: An improved target detection method based on YOLOv5 in natural orchard environments. Comput. Electron. Agric. **219**, 108780 (2024)
3. Zhou, J., Yang, D., Song, T., Ye, Y., Zhang, X., Song, Y.: Improved YOLOv7 models based on modulated deformable convolution and swin transformer for object detection in fisheye images. Image Vis. Comput. **144**, 104966 (2024)
4. Zhu, P.F., Zhu, Q.L., Dong, X., Sun, M.C.: Flying target detection technology based on GNSS multipath signals. Sensors **24**(5), 1706 (2024). https://doi.org/10.3390/s24051706
5. Wang, Z., Wang, Y.: FRCA: High-Efficiency Container Number Detection and Recognition Algorithm with Enhanced Attention (2020)
6. Xu, Z.G., Wang, L., Niu, S., Kan, G.: A method of positioning and recognition of electronic scale characters based on deep learning. J. Phys. Conf. Ser. **1693**(1), 012122 (2020). https://doi.org/10.1088/1742-6596/1693/1/012122
7. Ran, Z., Zhila, B., Teng, W., Zheng, L.: An adaptive deep learning framework for shipping container code localization and recognition. IEEE Trans. Instrum. Meas. **70**, 1–13 (2021). https://doi.org/10.1109/TIM.2020.3016108

8. Capurro, C., Provatorova, V., Kanoulas, E.: Experimenting with training a neural network in transkribus to recognise text in a multilingual and multi-authored manuscript collection. Heritage **6**(12), 7482–7494 (2023)
9. Meng, F., Ghena, B.: Research on text recognition methods based on artificial intelligence and machine learning. Adv. Comput. Commun. **4**(5), 340–344 (2023). https://doi.org/10.26855/acc.2023.10.014
10. Shu, T., Zhu, K.-X., Qin, H.-B., Yang, C.: Dynamic receptive field adaptation for scene text recognition. Pattern Recognit. Lett. **178**, 55–61 (2024). https://doi.org/10.1016/j.patrec.2023.12.005
11. Yu, M.M., Zhang, H., Yin, F., Liu, C.L.: An approach for handwritten Chinese text recognition unifying character segmentation and recognition. Pattern Recognit. **151**, 110373 (2024)
12. Yanchao, L., Hao, L., Guangwei, G.: Towards end-to-end container code recognition. Multimedia Tools Appl. **81**(11), 15901–15918 (2022)
13. Mi, C., Cao, L., Zhang, Z., Feng, Y., Yao, L., Wu, Y.: A port container code recognition algorithm under natural conditions. J. Coastal Res. **103**(sp1), 822–829 (2020)
14. Yang, D., et al.: Lightweight container code recognition based on multi-reuse feature fusion and multi-branch structure merger. J. Real Time Image Process. **20**(6) (2023). https://doi.org/10.1007/s11554-023-01364-x
15. Bofan, L.: ContainerNumber-OCR. https://github.com/lbf4616/ContainerNumber-OCR?tab=readme-ov-file

Dr-SAM: U-Shape Structure Segment Anything Model for Generalizable Medical Image Segmentation

Xiangzuo Huo[1,2], Shengwei Tian[1(✉)], Bingming Zhou[3], Long Yu[1], and Aolun Li[1,2]

[1] School of Computer Science and Technology, Xinjiang University, Ürümqi, China
tianshengwei@163.com
[2] Xinjiang Key Laboratory of Signal Detection and Processing, Xinjiang University, Ürümqi, China
[3] School of Computer Science, Beijing University of Posts and Telecommunications, Beijing, China

Abstract. Medical image segmentation plays a pivotal role in computer-assisted medical diagnosis, contributing to precise diagnostics, treatment strategizing, and disease tracking. However, the availability of annotated data for medical image segmentation remains restricted, and conventional approaches predominantly rely on bespoke models with limited adaptability across diverse tasks. In this research, we introduce DrSAM, a foundation model for universal medical image segmentation. This model possesses two crucial attributes: (i) the retention and utilization of pre-trained SAM model weights, while introducing a minimal number of supplementary parameters and computations; (ii) the incorporation of a trainable U-shaped residual network and a Medical Output Token designed to capture the distinctive features at various levels within medical images and enhance mask granularity. DrSAM, a fine-tuned model with a subset of medical image datasets, surpasses existing state-of-the-art segmentation foundation models. DrSAM holds substantial potentials for automating medical image segmentation. Code is available at https://github.com/huoxiangzuo/Doctor-SAM.

Keywords: Medical Image Segmentation · Segment Anything Model · Fine Tuning · Feature Fusion

1 Introduction

In recent years, large-scale language models trained on massive corpora have demonstrated remarkable performance in both natural language understanding and generation tasks. Similarly, multimodal foundation models trained on vast amounts of text, images, videos, and other data have exhibited outstanding capabilities in visual content comprehension and generation. Leveraging their exceptional generalization capabilities and rich parameterized knowledge, these foundation models can swiftly adapt to new tasks through carefully designed instructions and fine-tuning techniques. Consequently, the utilization of these powerful, generalization-driven foundation models to address specialized problems across various domains has become a focal point of both research and application endeavors.

Medical image segmentation plays a critical role in modern medical diagnostics. By accurately delineating and identifying vital structures and pathologies within medical images, physicians can make more precise diagnoses, plan treatment strategies, and monitor disease progression [1, 2]. However, it is an expensive and time consuming task to obtain large-scale annotated medical image data in the medical domain, leading many existing methods to rely on custom models tailored for specific tasks, which lack generalizability across different tasks [3, 4, 14, 19].

Applying foundation model technology to specific vertical domains still faces challenges. The original foundation models trained on general domain corpora possess abundant common-sense knowledge but lack specialized knowledge in vertical domains. Conversely, vertical domain foundation models to some extent take on the role of domain experts. Exploring how to leverage existing domain knowledge representation methods such as knowledge graphs to enable vertical domain foundation models to learn, utilize, and integrate domain knowledge requires novel solutions. This endeavor aims to construct responsible, controllable, and interpretable domain expert foundation models.

The recent advancements in natural image segmentation have witnessed the emergence of segmentation foundation models [5, 6], showcasing remarkable versatility and performance across various segmentation tasks. However, their application in medical image segmentation has remained challenging due to substantial domain differences [7, 8]. SAM faces two key challenges: 1) coarse mask boundaries, often leading to the neglect of segmenting thin object structures. 2) Incorrect predictions, mask corruption, or significant errors in challenging cases (e.g., retinal vessels, sessile polyps). SAM and its fine-tuned models exhibit notably poorer performance in fully automatic mode for medical image segmentation. Further investigation reveals that the performance degradation is associated with the multiscale information fusion of adverse prompts and mask segmentation. In fully automatic mode, the inevitable presence of adverse prompts (such as points outside the mask or boxes significantly larger than the mask) may severely mislead the generation of masks.

Segment Anything Model (SAM), trained on over 1 billion masks, has demonstrated unprecedented generalization capabilities across various natural images. Some studies have shown promising results when applying SAM to segment certain medical images, indicating the promising utility of pre-trained SAM weights in the segmentation domain. There are two primary approaches to applying SAM to medical image segmentation: 1) Freezing SAM's image encoder and prompt encoder while only fine-tuning the mask decoder typically yields suboptimal results; 2) Utilizing adaptive [20, 21] or visual prompt [22] techniques to train the image encoder has improved the model's performance in specific domains. However, training such models incurs high GPU memory consumption due to the inability to pre-compute image embeddings. Additionally, these fine-tuning methods still require manually provided boxes or points, making fully automated medical image segmentation challenging to achieve.

To address the aforementioned challenges, we propose DrSAM (Doctor SAM) tailored for application in the medical segmentation domain. Specifically, two novel modules are designed and integrated into SAM: the first is the U-shaped fine-tuning fusion module, which establishes hierarchical skip connections between feature extraction and decoder layers in a U-shaped structure. Additionally, it leverages ViT pre-trained weights to retain domain knowledge feature fine-tuning learning under the basic structure of SAM. The second is the Med-Output Token, a learnable token incorporated alongside the Output Token and Prompt into the attention module. Within each attention layer, the Med-Output Token undergoes self-attention integration with other tokens (token to image) to enhance and refine SAM's performance on medical images. This study conducts segmentation and generalization experiments on publicly available datasets including Hyper Kvasir endoscopy dataset, Cell dataset, and Chase retinal vessel dataset. The results demonstrate that compared to the previously state-of-the-art domain generalization method MedSAM, DrSAM achieves a competitive level of performance. Moreover, DrSAM is trainable on personal devices with entry-level GPUs, thus facilitating the application of foundation models in primary healthcare settings.

Single-source domain generalization poses greater challenges considering training data from only one domain and extending it to an unknown domain, as the diversity of the training domain is limited. Hence, the mainstream solution to this problem involves utilizing data augmentation techniques to generate new domain data, thereby enhancing the diversity and information content of the training data. This approach has led to the design of various generation strategies for single-source domain generalization in computer vision tasks. Chen et al. [23] employed random bias fields to enhance data, which are common image artifacts in clinical MRI, or combined style information from randomly selected instances of different domains, along with additional noise and worst-case combinations to expand the domain space. Ouyang et al. [24] proposed a simple causality-inspired data augmentation method, significantly improving the cross-domain robustness of deep models. In contrast to previous methods, DrSAM enhances the generalization capability of deep models without requiring complex data augmentation, making it more competitive in practical applications.

Many studies have applied the SAM model to typical medical image segmentation tasks [27, 28] and other challenging scenarios [25, 26]. For instance, SAM's comprehensive evaluation across various medical images highlights its high-quality segmentation results for targets with diverse boundary features. However, SAM exhibits significant limitations when segmenting typical medical targets with weak boundaries or low contrast. Consistent with these observations, MedSAM [30], a direct fine-tuning of SAM as the foundation model, significantly enhances SAM's segmentation performance on medical images. MedSAM achieves this goal by fine-tuning SAM on a dataset comprising over one million pairs of medical image-mask pairs. The aforementioned work involves fine-tuning both the mask decoder and the image encoder [20, 29, 30]. Compared to these methods, the proposed DrSAM strikes a balance between performance and efficiency, yielding satisfactory results in fully automatic segmentation.

U-Net [9] holds an unassailable position as a classic medical image segmentation model, emphasizing the importance of extracting features at various levels of medical images by merely connecting encoder features with the decoder features through residuals. SAM [5] not only exhibits higher versatility in terms of model capacity but also may benefit from shared underlying architecture and training processes, yielding more consistent results across different tasks. Ma et al. proposed MedSAM [30], directly fine-tuning medical images on the SAM model, achieving favorable results. However, directly fine-tuning SAM's decoder or introducing numerous new decoder modules disrupts SAM's architecture, severely compromising foundation zero-shot segmentation performance [10]. Ke et al. designed the HQ-SAM architecture, featuring a learnable HQ-output token input alongside the original prompts and output tokens into SAM's mask decoder, training only the proposed modules. This transfer learning fine-tuning approach can generate higher-quality masks while preserving zero-shot capabilities.

Motivation. In this study, we were inspired by classic medical segmentation model U-net [9] and foundation model HQ-SAM [10] to propose a versatile foundation model for medical image segmentation, named DrSAM. DrSAM is capable of predicting highly accurate segmentation masks even in exceedingly challenging scenarios without the need for extensive data and computational resources, demonstrating robust zero-shot capabilities and flexible prompt handling. Specifically, we leverage and retain the pre-trained model weights of SAM while introducing minimal additional parameters and computations, thereby enhancing model efficiency. Furthermore, we devised a trainable U-shaped residual network coupled with a Medical Output Token, which effectively captures features at various levels within medical images, thereby further improving the precision of segmentation masks.

To validate the effectiveness of DrSAM, quantitative and qualitative experimental analyses were conducted. The experiments compared SAM, MedSAM, and the proposed DrSAM on three different segmentation datasets. Evaluation results demonstrate that, compared to other foundation models, DrSAM generates higher-quality masks while retaining zero-shot capability.

2 Method

2.1 DrSAM Architecture Design

In order to fully leverage the underlying architecture of the foundation model and its well-trained weights, we made no alterations to the SAM model's structure. And then, we designed the U-shaped structure on top of it to extract and fuse hierarchical encoder features, as depicted in Fig. 1. Shallow features with high frequency play a crucial role in medical image segmentation [15], and accurate segmentation results depend on both the global semantic context of the input image and local boundary details. Within the ViT encoder, we extract features from different stages of the encoder and fuse them into the corresponding scale of the decoder through residual connections, thereby obtaining advanced object semantics and low-level boundary information within the image. DrSAM comprises three main components: the SAM foundation model, the U-shaped fine-tuning fusion structure, and the Med-Output Token.

SAM Foundation Model. The encoder part of DrSAM still employs the pre-trained ViT-B model of SAM, with the image and prompt encoders frozen during training.

DrSAM does not make any adjustments to the image encoder, allowing image embeddings to be pre-computed before the training phase. Therefore, the training process of DrSAM does not require loading the image encoder. This ensures high GPU efficiency for the proposed method.

U-Structure Feature Extraction. Inspired by the U-Net architecture [9], we adopt the classic encoder-decoder structure. Multi-scale features are extracted from the global attention layer of the image encoder to obtain image embeddings. The early layers of the ViT encoder excel at capturing local features that are essential for capturing high-frequency details. Following the global attention block in the ViT encoder (i.e., with a window size of 0), we extract hierarchical features from various stages. Taking ViT-B as an example, we output features from the 2nd, 5th, 8th, and 12th blocks (in total, there are 12 blocks). The original features from these four stages have shapes of 64×64, and as we progress through the stages, they are upsampled successively to 512×512, 256×256, and 128×128. Through shortcut residual connections, these features are concatenated with the corresponding decoder features, and dimensionality reduction is performed using dual convolutions, akin to the upsampling operation in U-Net. It's noteworthy that in the concatenation of the decoder corresponding to stage 2, we include the transposed convolution upsampled features from SAM, aiming to maximize the retention of SAM's original zero-shot capabilities and prevent catastrophic forgetting.

As illustrated in the Fig. 1, the final hierarchical feature, having dimensions of 512×512, is dot product with the Med-Output Token processed through an MLP to obtain the mask results for DrSAM.

Med-Output Token. In SAM's original design, mask prediction is carried out using an output token, which is jointly inputted into the mask decoder along with the prompt, culminating in a dot product with the mask features. As depicted within the red box in the diagram, we introduce a new component called the Med-Output Token (size of 1×256) to enhance and refine SAM's performance on medical images.

The Med-Output Token, in conjunction with the output token and prompt, is fed into the attention module. In each attention layer, the Med-Output Token undergoes self-attention alongside other tokens (token-to-image), and this information is utilized for weight updates. Furthermore, before performing dot product with the U-shaped hierarchical features, we incorporate a new MLP structure to generate dynamic convolutional kernels from the Med-Output Token. This ensures that the model does not overfit to the new dataset, thereby preserving SAM's zero-shot segmentation capability.

2.2 Training of DrSAM

We exclusively train the proposed U-shaped structure, Med-Output Token, and its associated MLP. Unlike SAM, the prompt section employs a hybrid type of prompts. We keep the weights of the SAM section frozen during training. The initial learning rate is set to 0.001, and we utilize the AdamW optimizer [16] with a batch size of 6. The training is conducted for 20 epochs, and fine-tuning can be trained using a single NVIDIA RTX 3090 GPU.

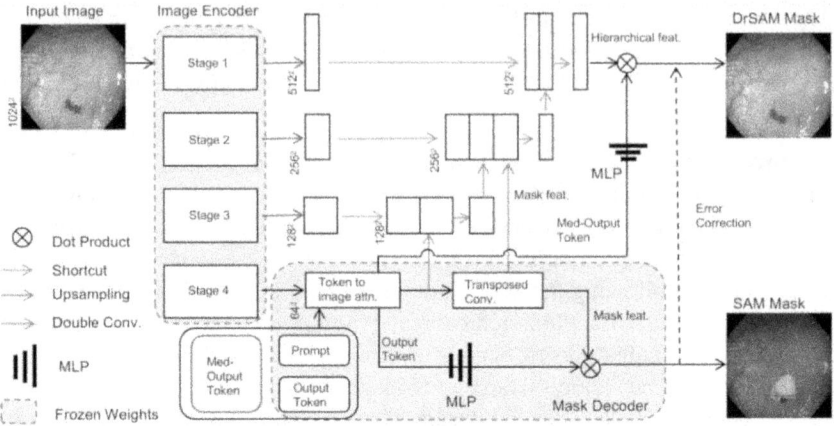

Fig. 1. DrSAM introduces U-structure and Med-Output Token into SAM to achieve high-quality mask prediction more suitable for medical images. In order to maintain the zero-sample capability of SAM, Med-Output Token reuses the mask decoder of SAM, passes through a new MLP layer, and performs dot product with the hierarchical features extracted by U-structure. When training, we fix the model parameters of the pretrained SAM.

For supervising DrSAM's mask predictions, we employ both BCELoss (Binary Cross-Entropy Loss) and Dice Loss, which are two commonly used loss functions in image segmentation tasks. They are typically used in combination to strike a balance between binary classification loss and segmentation accuracy. The formulas are as follows:

$$\text{BCELoss}(y, \hat{y}) = -\frac{1}{N} \sum_{i=1}^{N} [y_i \cdot \log(\hat{y}_i) + (1 - y_i) \cdot \log(1 - \hat{y}_i)] \quad (1)$$

The combined loss function is defined as:

$$\text{Dice Loss}(y, \hat{y}) = 1 - \frac{2 \cdot \sum_{i=1}^{N} y_i \cdot \hat{y}_i}{\sum_{i=1}^{N} y_i^2 + \sum_{i=1}^{N} \hat{y}_i^2} \quad (2)$$

$$\text{Loss}(y, \hat{y}) = \text{BCELoss}(y, \hat{y}) + \text{Dice Loss}(y, \hat{y}) \quad (3)$$

2.3 Inference of DrSAM

DrSAM follows the same inference process as SAM but incorporates mask predictions from the Med-Output Token for medical image mask prediction. During inference, the predicted masks generated by SAM are added to the mask predictions of DrSAM to perform mask correction at a spatial resolution of 512 × 512. Subsequently, the corrected masks are upsampled to the original resolution of 1024 × 1024 for output.

2.4 Advantages of DrSAM vs. SAM

The training and inference aspects of SAM and DrSAM are comprehensively compared in Table 1. DrSAM not only yields superior segmentation quality but also demonstrates remarkably fast and cost-effective training, requiring only a single consumer-grade GPU for fine-tuning. Moreover, DrSAM is lightweight and efficient, with negligible increases in model parameters, GPU memory usage, and inference time per image.

2.5 Advantages of DrSAM vs. MedSAM

In comparison to the MedSAM, our DrSAM still exhibits certain advantages in vertical domains. As shown in Table 1, while both MedSAM and DrSAM are compared in terms of training and inference, MedSAM requires substantial computational resources for fine-tuning through extensive medical image data, posing significant challenges for implementation in primary healthcare facilities and educational institutions. Conversely, DrSAM does not necessitate overall fine-tuning of the SAM foundation model; rather, it fine-tunes only the U-shaped multi-scale feature structure. Hence, it boasts lighter training speed and fewer learnable parameters, making it more suitable for deployment in scenarios with limited computational power and data capacity, such as primary healthcare facilities.

3 Experiments

3.1 Datasets

Medical images, as compared with natural images, possess distinct characteristics such as lower quantities and blurry boundaries. To efficiently adapt our model for medical image segmentation, we fine-tuned it on three typical endoscopy, pathology, and corneal vascular datasets: Cell, Chase, and Hyper Kvasir-Seg, which include fine-grained details such as blood vessels and inconspicuous sessile polyps. This significantly enhances the model's robustness in medical image segmentation. We merged the datasets and divided them into a 1/2 training and 1/2 testing split.

Cell Dataset [11]: This dataset originates from the 2018 Data Science Bowl Challenge and is designed for nucleus segmentation in different microscopic images. The challenge in this task lies in handling nucleus segmentation across various environments, including different cell types, magnification levels, and imaging modes. It comprises a total of 670 images. We combined single-cell labeled images to create complete labeled images.

Chase Dataset [12]: This dataset is dedicated to retinal vessel segmentation and includes 28 color retinal images, each of size 999×960 pixels, collected from the left and right eyes of 14 children. Every image is annotated by two independent human experts.

Hyper Kvasir-SEG [13]: This dataset consists of 1,000 images, providing both the original images and segmentation masks. In the masks, pixels representing polyp tissue (the region of interest) are indicated by foreground (white mask), while background (black) does not include polyp pixels.

3.2 Performance Comparisons

We compared the baseline foundation segmentation model SAM [5], the improved medical segmentation foundation model MedSAM [30], and our DrSAM. Except for SAM, all these models were trained using the same datasets and training strategies. We evaluated these models on the three datasets using metrics such as mIoU (mean Intersection over Union), mBIoU (mean Background Intersection over Union), and mDice.

As shown in the Table 2, these models, as foundation segmentation models, demonstrate excellent performance in segmenting medical images with clearly defined targets, even SAM without fine-tuning. DrSAM outperforms the other models on all three trained datasets, particularly excelling on the Chase dataset, indicating its superior segmentation capability for narrow objects.

Table 1. Segmentation qualitative performance comparison. *Indicates the performance of the model on the zero-shot dataset.

Method	Learnable Params (M)	GPU	Batch Size	FPS	Mem.
SAM	1191	128	128	5	7.6G
MedSAM	93.8	20	160	5	7.6G
DrSAM(Our)	33.1	1	6	4.3	8.2G

Table 2. Segmentation quantitative performance comparison.

Model	Cell			HyperKvasir-SEG			Chase		
	mIoU	mBIoU	mDice	mIoU	mBIoU	mDice	mIoU	mBIoU	mDice
SAM	0.7518	0.7127	0.8571	0.7677	0.5708	0.8686	0.1424	0.1271	0.2493
MedSAM	0.7677	0.7213	0.8686	0.8146	0.6148	0.8807	0.4272	0.421	0.5986
DrSAM	**0.7831**	**0.7709**	**0.8784**	**0.8573**	**0.7105**	**0.9231**	**0.7167**	**0.6911**	**0.7029**

In the qualitative experiments, we observe that while the SAM model is a foundation segmentation model for natural images and can provide good segmentation results for medical images with well-defined cell boundaries without specific training, reaffirming SAM's robust zero-shot capability. However, SAM struggles to accurately segment finer objects (e.g., blood vessels) and objects with blurry boundaries (e.g., sessile polyps) in medical images. After fine-tuning on medical datasets, MedSAM demonstrates improved segmentation performance for fine-grained objects. DrSAM performs well on all three datasets, providing more accurate segmentation for fine-grained objects and object boundaries.

In addition, we also conducted zero-shot experiments on the GlaS [17] and ISIC2018 [18] datasets. As shown in * in Fig. 2, DrSAM also has good zero-shot capabilities, which shows that DrSAM has the capabilities that a foundation model should have. The improvement of the U-shaped structure can enhance the ability to fine-tune the data set and has the potential to generalize to more medical image segmentation tasks.

3.3 Ablation Studies

As shown in the table, we conducted ablation experiments on the Hyper Kvasir-SEG dataset. By adding the trainable Med-Output Token and its corresponding MLP layer, fine-tuning training yields improved results, with mIoU and mDice reaching 0.8161 and 0.8956, respectively. However, it still struggles with the boundaries. The inclusion of the U-shaped structure design results in a relative improvement of 8.2% in mIoU and 3.7% in mDice compared to the baseline. When both components are incorporated, DrSAM achieves the best results (Table 3).

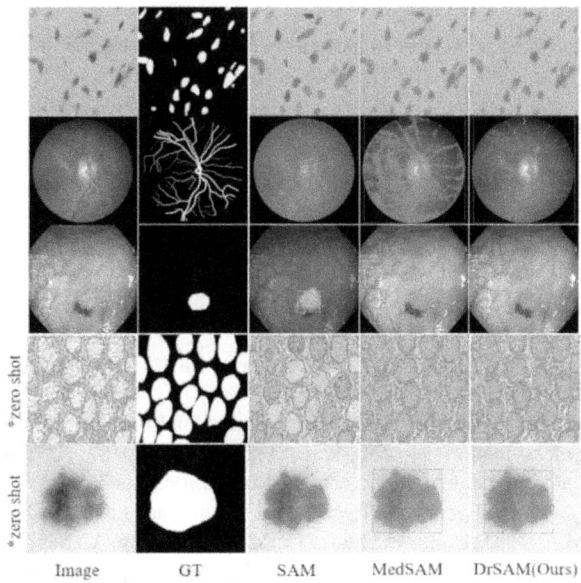

Fig. 2. Segmentation qualitative performance comparison. *Indicates the performance of the model on the zero-shot dataset.

Table 3. DrSAM ablation experiment results on HyperKvasir-SEG dataset.

Component	mIoU	mBIoU	mDice
SAM(baseline)	0.7677	0.5708	0.8686
Add Med-Output Token	0.8161	0.5156	0.8956
Add U-structure	0.8309	0.6158	0.9007
DrSAM(ours)	**0.8573**	**0.7105**	**0.9231**

4 Conclusion

In this paper, we introduce a foundation model, DrSAM, for medical image segmentation that necessitates minimal fine-tuning with only a small amount of data. Our purpose-built U-shaped structure effectively extracts and integrates features across different levels within medical images, while the trainable Med-Output Token refines the mask results. Building upon the foundation of the SAM universal foundation model, we retain its zero-shot capability and foundation segmentation performance. Experimental results demonstrate DrSAM's outstanding versatility in medical segmentation tasks, showcasing substantial potential in the realm of automated medical image segmentation.

Acknowledgements. This work was supported by the National Natural Science Foundation of China under Grant 62162058, and the Tianshan Talent Training Program 2023TSYCLJ0023.

References

1. De Fauw, J., et al.: Clinically applicable deep learning for diagnosis and referral in retinal disease. Nat. Med. **24**(9), 1342–1350 (2018)
2. Ouyang, D., et al.: Video-based AI for beat-to-beat assessment of cardiac function. Nature **580**(7802), 252–256 (2020)
3. Zhao, F., Xie, X.: An overview of interactive medical image segmentation. Ann. BMVA **2013**(7), 1–22 (2013)
4. Huo, X., Sun, G., Tian, S., et al.: HiFuse: hierarchical multi-scale feature fusion network for medical image classification. Biomed. Signal Process. Control **87**, 105534 (2024)
5. Kirillov, A., et al.: Segment Anything (2023). arXiv:2304.02643
6. Zou, X., et al.: Segment Everything Everywhere All at Once (2023). arXiv:2304.06718
7. Mazurowski, M., Dong, H., Gu, H., Yang, J., Konz, N., Zhang, Y.: Segment anything model for medical image analysis: an experimental study. Med. Image Anal. **89**, 102918 (2023)
8. Huang, Y., et al.: Segment Anything Model for Medical Images? (2023). arXiv:2304.14660
9. Ronneberger, O., Fischer, P., Brox, T.: U-net: convolutional networks for biomedical image segmentation. In: Medical Image Computing and Computer-Assisted Intervention – MICCAI 2015: 18th International Conference, Munich, Germany, October 5–9, Proceedings, Part III 18, pp. 234–241 (2015)
10. Ke, L., et al.: Segment Anything in High Quality (2023). arXiv:2306.01567
11. Caicedo, J., et al.: Nucleus segmentation across imaging experiments: the 2018 Data Science Bowl. Nat. Methods **16**(12), 1247–1253 (2019)
12. Fraz, M., et al.: An ensemble classification-based approach applied to retinal blood vessel segmentation. IEEE Trans. Biomed. Eng. **59**(9), 2538–2548 (2012)
13. Borgli, H., et al.: HyperKvasir, a comprehensive multi-class image and video dataset for gastrointestinal endoscopy. Sci. Data **7**(1), 283 (2020)
14. Zhang, C., et al.: A Comprehensive Survey on Segment Anything Model for Vision and Beyond (2023). arXiv:2305.08196
15. Liu, Y., Zhang, S., Chen, J., Yu, Z., Chen, K., Lin, D.: Improving Pixel-Based MIM by Reducing Wasted Modeling Capability (2023). arXiv:2308.00261
16. Loshchilov, I., Hutter, F.: Decoupled weight decay regularization (2017). arXiv:1711.05101
17. Sirinukunwattana, K., et al.: Gland segmentation in colon histology images: The GlaS challenge contest. Med. Image Anal. **35**, 489–502 (2017)

18. Codella, N., et al.: Skin Lesion Analysis Toward Melanoma Detection 2018: A Challenge Hosted by the International Skin Imaging Collaboration (ISIC) (2019). arXiv:1902.03368
19. Huo, X., Tian, S., Yang, Y., Yu, L., Zhang, W., Li, A.: SPA: Self-Peripheral-Attention for central–peripheral interactions in endoscopic image classification and segmentation. Expert Syst. Appl. **245**, 123053 (2024)
20. Wu, J., et al.: Medical SAM Adapter: Adapting Segment Anything Model for Medical Image Segmentation (2023). arXiv:2304.12620
21. Zhang, K., Liu, D.: Customized Segment Anything Model for Medical Image Segmentation (2023). arXiv:2304.13785
22. Chen, T., et al.: SAM fails to segment anything? SAM-Adapter: Adapting SAM in Underperformed Scenes: Camouflage, Shadow, and More (2023). arXiv:2304.09148
23. Chen, C., et al.: Realistic adversarial data augmentation for MR image segmentation. In: MICCAI 2020. LNCS, vol. 12261, pp. 667–677. Springer, Cham (2020). https://doi.org/10.1007/978-3-030-59710-8_65
24. Chen, C., Li, Z., Ouyang, C., Sinclair, M., Bai, W., Rueckert, D.: MaxStyle: adversarial style composition for robust medical image segmentation. In: Wang, L.W., Qi Dou, P., Fletcher, T., Speidel, S., Li, S. (eds.) Medical Image Computing and Computer Assisted Intervention – MICCAI 2022: 25th International Conference, Singapore, September 18–22, 2022, Proceedings, Part V, pp. 151–161. Springer Nature Switzerland, Cham (2022). https://doi.org/10.1007/978-3-031-16443-9_15
25. Chen, J., Bai, X.: Learning to "Segment Anything" in Thermal Infrared Images Through Knowledge Distillation With a Large Scale Dataset SATIR (2023). arXiv:2304.07969
26. Tang, L., Xiao, H., Li, B.: Can SAM Segment Anything? When SAM Meets Camouflaged Object Detection (2023). arXiv:2304.04709
27. Deng, R., et al.: Segment Anything Model (SAM) for Digital Pathology: Assess Zero-Shot Segmentation on Whole Slide Imaging (2023). arXiv:2304.04155
28. Hu, C., Li, X.: When SAM Meets Medical Images: An Investigation of Segment Anything Model (SAM) on Multi-Phase Liver Tumor Segmentation (2023). arXiv:2304.08506
29. Li, Y., Hu, M., Yang, X.: Polyp-SAM: transfer SAM for polyp segmentation. In: Medical Imaging 2024: Computer-Aided Diagnosis, pp. 759–765 (2024)
30. Ma, J., He, Y., Li, F., Han, L., You, C., Wang, B.: Segment anything in medical images. Nat. Commun. **15**(1), 654 (2024)

Aerial Multi-object Tracking via Information Weighting

Pengnian Wu[1], Bangkui Fan[2(✉)], Ruiyu Zhang[3], Yulong Xu[3], and Dong Xue[4(✉)]

[1] School of Software, Northwestern Polytechnical University, Shaanxi, China
[2] Chinese Academy of Engineering, Beijing, China
wpn.ttup@foxmail.com
[3] Intelligent Collaborative Perception and Analytical Cognition Laboratory, Beijing, China
[4] School of Aeronautics, Northwestern Polytechnical University, Shaanxi, China
xuedong@nwpu.edu.cn

Abstract. Multi-object tracking from an aerial perspective often faces typical challenges such as small objects, dual-source motion, and appearance similarity. This often results in low tracking accuracy. In this paper, we propose an Aerial multi-object Tracking method via Information Weighting (ATIW), which comprises four main components: adaptive weighting, distribution feature extraction, prediction box correction, and spatiotemporal feature enhancement. Adaptive weighting involves a dynamic fusion of distribution, motion, and appearance information, tailored to the object's scale and velocity. Distribution feature extraction utilizes the spatial distribution information of objects and their neighbors to facilitate identity association. The purpose of prediction box correction is to mitigate the negative impact of camera rotation on IoU matching. Spatiotemporal feature enhancement aims to fuse corresponding features based on the object's feature similarity in adjacent frames and the object's unique feature differences. The experimental results from the UAVDT dataset demonstrate that the proposed method can effectively improve the performance of aerial multi-object tracking. In particular, the IDF1 metric is improved by 0.5% without retraining the model.

Keywords: Multi-object tracking · Information weighting · Aerial perspective

1 Introduction

Recently, owing to the booming development of the unmanned aerial vehicle (UAV) industry, multi-object tracking technology from an aerial perspective has been gradually gaining widespread use [1]. Compared with the objects captured by common surveillance cameras, those viewed from an aerial perspective are generally small, low-resolution, and feature similar characteristics [2]. Moreover, the motion trajectory of an object in the video is influenced not only by the object itself but also by the motion of the UAV [3]. One of the most representative aerial multi-object tracking datasets is the UAVDT [3]. Existing multi-object tracking methods primarily utilize three types of information: spatial distribution [4], motion [5], and appearance features [6]. In terms of information extraction, ATIW enhances the method of extracting spatial distribution features as outlined in [4]. Additionally, ATIW refines the predicted object bounding box using Kalman filtering [7] and achieves feature enhancement through the method outlined in [8]. Although models based on single-dimensional information can effectively track objects in standard scenarios, their tracking capabilities significantly diminish in complex or dynamic environments. Tracking methods such as those in [5, 9] combine object appearance and motion information. The approach of combining object appearance with distribution information is utilized for tracking in [4, 10].

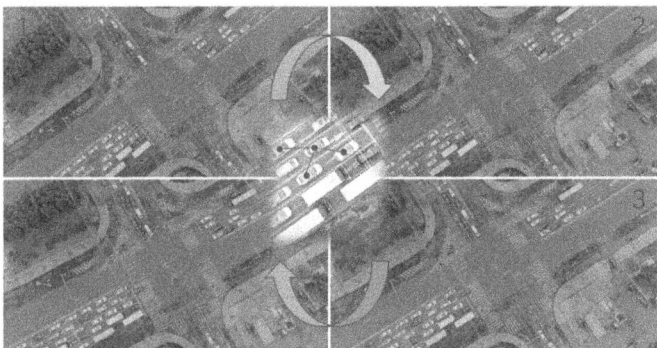

Fig. 1. Motivation Behind Our ATIW. Images numbered 1 to 4 were captured by a drone during its counterclockwise rotation. The magnified section in the center illustrates the overlapping regions among the four images. These images reveal that the target appears diminutive from the drone's perspective, offering very limited pixel information. Furthermore, while a significant number of targets exhibit similar appearances, their spatial distribution is relatively consistent in the short term. The non-linear nature of the target movement within the frame stems from the drone's own motion.

As shown in Fig. 1, the primary motivation of this research is to optimize the single-dimensional feature extraction method, focusing on the distribution, motion, and appearance characteristics of objects from an aerial perspective. Additionally, from the perspective of multi-level information fusion, this approach comprehensively utilizes the information of numerous objects through dynamic weighting to enhance the accuracy of object tracking. A series of experiments were conducted on the UAVDT dataset [3], demonstrating the efficacy of the proposed ATIW algorithm in enhancing aerial multi-object tracking. The main contributions of this paper are composed of the following four parts:

- Considering the scale and velocity characteristics of the object, we have designed an adaptive weighted fusion scheme that integrates distribution, motion, and appearance information to enhance the tracker.
- To address the challenge posed by small objects with limited information, we have incorporated the object's size and the number of neighbors into the existing distributed feature extraction method.

- To tackle the issue of object identity association failures due to UAV rotation, we propose an object prediction box correction method relying on an enhanced correlation coefficient.
- To address the challenge of similar appearance features, we have further improved the differentiation of appearance features between objects by utilizing the spatio-temporal context information of each object.

2 Introduction

The overall framework of the ATIW is depicted in Fig. 2. The main steps of the ATIW tracker are outlined in Algorithm 1. First, during the pre-processing stage (steps 2 to 8), parameters corresponding to the three types of object features are calculated. Subsequently, in the cost acquisition stage (steps 9 to 11), the identity matching cost for each of the three object feature types is calculated based on the previously determined parameters, culminating in the derivation of a comprehensive cost through adaptive weighting. Finally, during the identity matching stage (steps 12 to 14), the initial matching is conducted using the comprehensive cost, followed by a secondary matching based on the motion cost.

Algorithm 1: The Main Steps of ATIW Tracker

Input: An UAV video sequences $\{I_t\}_{t=1}^{T}$

Output: The tracked bounding box of objects B_t

1 while $t < T$ do
2   Input two adjacent images: I_t, I_{t+1}
3   Calculate the warp matrix according to (13)
4   Correct the prediction box obtained by Kalman filtering according to (14), (15)
5   Calculate the feature enhancement coefficient according to (24), (25)
6   Enhance the appearance feature according to (26)
7   Obtain the distribution feature matrix by R_t according to (8), (9)
8   Update the radius according to (10)
9   Obtain three types of cost matrices according to (19), (23), (27) and (12)
10   Obtain the velocity and size weight matrix according to (3), (6)
11   Adaptive weighting according to (7)
12   Synthesis matching: $matches_1 = Hungarian(C_{Total})$
13   Motion matching for the unmatched tracks and detections:
       $matches_2 = Hungarian(C_{IOU'})$
14   Obtain the tracked bounding box or initialize a new one
15 Return

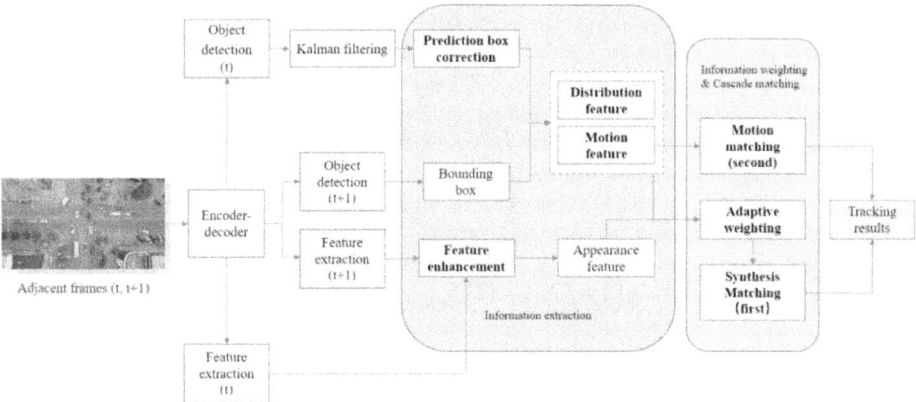

Fig. 2. The framework of our proposed ATIW tracker. The parts marked in bold are our key modules. The ATIW algorithm concentrates on post-processing for tracking by enhancing the model's ability to extract features of three types: distribution, motion, and appearance. It enhances the information fusion and cascade matching mechanism to comprehensively improve the tracking performance of small targets, particularly from the perspective of aerial imagery.

2.1 Adaptive Weighting

Existing methods, including [8, 11], combine object appearance and motion information for multi-object tracking but typically employ a fixed weighting approach. However, the size and velocity of objects vary across different scenes, times, and categories. As demonstrated in formulas (1)–(7), x_i and y_i denote the horizontal and vertical coordinates of the tracking box's center point, respectively. w_j and h_j represent the width and height of the new detection box, respectively. And the values of the parameters α, β, δ, μ are 2.118426, 1.1566297e−06, 0.22828, 0.089536, respectively. W and H denote the width and height of the image containing the newly detected object, respectively. When the object scale is small, resulting in sparse appearance features, the corresponding weight for these features should be reduced, while increasing the weights for the other two types of information. Conversely, when the object's velocity is low, resulting in consistent distribution information in adjacent frames, an increase in the corresponding weight for this information is warranted, while the weight for motion information should be correspondingly reduced.

$$v_i = \sqrt{(x_i - x_i')^2 + (y_i - y_i')^2} \tag{1}$$

$$\omega_{ij}^v = e^{-v_i} \tag{2}$$

$$\Omega^v = \begin{pmatrix} \omega_{11}^v & \cdots & \omega_{m1}^v \\ \vdots & \ddots & \vdots \\ \omega_{1n}^v & \cdots & \omega_{mn}^v \end{pmatrix} \tag{3}$$

$$s_j = \sqrt{\frac{w_j \cdot h_j}{W \cdot H}} \tag{4}$$

$$\omega_{ij}^s = \frac{\alpha}{1 + \left(\frac{s_j}{\beta}\right)^\delta} - \mu \tag{5}$$

$$\Omega^s = \begin{pmatrix} \omega_{11}^s & \cdots & \omega_{1n}^s \\ \vdots & \ddots & \vdots \\ \omega_{m1}^s & \cdots & \omega_{mn}^s \end{pmatrix} \tag{6}$$

$$C_{Total} = \frac{C_{Feature} + C_{GIOU'}}{2} g(1-\Omega^s) + C_{Distribution} g\Omega^s g\Omega^{v唯} + C_{GIOU'} g\Omega^s g(1-\Omega^v) \tag{7}$$

2.2 Distribution Feature Extraction

The method in [4] neglects the information of other neighbors around the object and the object's own scale information. Furthermore, when the farthest neighbor exceeds the detection range or the nearest neighbor is occluded, applying this method for object identity association may result in significant errors. Therefore, we introduce a method that calculates the distances between the object and its three nearest neighbors, as well as the minimum angle information using the object as a vertex. This method also incorporates the object's scale information and the count of remaining neighbors to construct a unique distribution information vector, thereby enhancing the accuracy of object identity association. Additionally, in identifying neighboring objects, the fixed radius is replaced with a dynamic radius that adjusts automatically based on the number of surrounding neighbors. However, it is crucial that this radius remains consistent when calculating the object's distribution information vector across adjacent frames. The methodology for constructing the object distribution feature vector and the dynamic radius update process are detailed in Formulas (8)–(11). Upon acquiring the object distribution feature vectors for both the previous and current frames, the cosine distance is calculated as per Formula (12) to derive the corresponding distribution cost matrix.

$$d_t' = \left(l_{\min}^t, l_{s\min}^t, l_{t\min}^t, \theta_1^t, \theta_2^t, \theta_3^t, s^t, q^t\right) \tag{8}$$

$$d_{t+1} = \left(l_{\min}^{t+1}, l_{s\min}^{t+1}, l_{t\min}^{t+1}, \theta_1^{t+1}, \theta_2^{t+1}, \theta_3^{t+1}, s^{t+1}, q^{t+1}\right) \tag{9}$$

$$R_{t+1} = \lambda R_t \tag{10}$$

$$\lambda = \begin{cases} \lambda_1 = 0.8, \hat{q}_t > 5 \\ \lambda_2 = 1.2, \hat{q}_t \leq 5 \end{cases} \tag{11}$$

$$C_{Distribution} = 1 - \cos\left(D_{track_t}', D_{\det_{t+1}}\right) \tag{12}$$

2.3 Prediction Box Correction

Traditional tracking methods based on the Kalman filter are ineffective in addressing the substantial deviation between the prediction box and the new detection box, a deviation caused by the sudden self-rotation of the UAV in aviation scenarios. Consequently, drawing inspiration from [12, 13], we propose utilizing the enhanced correlation coefficient [14] to adjust the prediction box, thereby minimizing its deviation from the new detection box. The detailed procedure for prediction box correction is delineated in Formulas (13)–(15). First, the coordinates of the other two vertices are calculated based on the top-left and bottom-right vertices of the prediction box. Subsequently, these coordinates, along with those of the initial vertices, are multiplied by the rotation parameters to derive the modified coordinates for all four vertices. Following this, the coordinates for the four vertices of the new prediction box are computed based on the adjusted vertex coordinates. The top-left and bottom-right coordinates of this new box are then determined, culminating in the completion of the prediction box correction. Subsequently, as delineated in Formulas (16)–(22), the GIOU and IOU costs between the corrected prediction box and the new detection box are calculated and then compared to their respective costs prior to correction. In $GIOU'$, post-correction information predominates, whereas in IOU', pre-correction information is more prominent. Ultimately, the motion cost matrix is derived based on Formulas (19) and (23).

$$M_{wrap} = ECC(I_t, I_{t+1}) \tag{13}$$

$$b_w = M_{wrap} \cdot b'_{track_t} \tag{14}$$

$$b''_{tract_t} = \left[\min_y(b_w), \min_x(b_w), \max_y(b_w), \max_x(b_w)\right] \tag{15}$$

$$GIOU_1 = GIOU\left(b'_{track_t}, b_{det_{t+1}}\right) \tag{16}$$

$$GIOU_2 = GIOU\left(b''_{tract_t}, b_{det_{t+1}}\right) \tag{17}$$

$$GIOU'\left(b'_{track_t}, b_{det_{t+1}}\right) = \max(GIOU_1, GIOU_2) \tag{18}$$

$$C_{GIOU'} = 1 - GIOU'\left(B'_{track_t}, B_{det_{t+1}}\right) \tag{19}$$

$$IOU_1 = IOU\left(b'_{track_t}, b_{det_{t+1}}\right) \tag{20}$$

$$IOU_2 = IOU\left(b''_{tract_t}, b_{det_{t+1}}\right) \tag{21}$$

$$IOU'\left(b'_{track_t}, b_{det_{t+1}}\right) = \min(IOU_1, IOU_2) \tag{22}$$

$$C_{IOU'} = 1 - IOU'\left(B'_{track_t}, B_{det_{t+1}}\right) \tag{23}$$

2.4 Spatial-Temporal Feature Enhancement

The image-based ReID method in [8] fails to fully exploit the spatio-temporal distribution characteristics of object appearance information for feature enhancement, thereby limiting improvements in feature similarity for identical objects. Given that prominent object features are crucial for differentiating between objects, we draw on the concept of utilizing spatio-temporal information for feature enhancement from [15]. Consequently, we propose spatio-temporal feature enhancement coefficients, which are derived from object feature similarity in adjacent frames and the object's intrinsic feature variance. Formula (24) illustrates the calculation method for the spatial feature enhancement coefficient, where f^a represents the a-dimensional feature of a specific object post-feature extraction. Formula (25) delineates the calculation method for the time series feature enhancement coefficient, with F_t denoting the feature vector of the specified object in frame t. Salient areas within the object's features are identified through computation, after which these features are amalgamated with their respective weights and superimposed onto the original features, thereby completing the enhancement process. Formula (26) depicts the process of executing feature fusion using the spatio-temporal feature enhancement coefficient, and the appearance cost matrix is finally constructed by Formula (27).

$$\Omega^{f_{spatial}} = \frac{\left(\sum_{a=1}^{A}(f^1 - f^a)^2 \ldots \sum_{a=1}^{A}(f^A - f^a)^2\right)}{\max\left(\left(\sum_{a=1}^{A}(f^1 - f^a)^2 \ldots \sum_{a=1}^{A}(f^A - f^a)^2\right)\right)} \quad (24)$$

$$\Omega^{f_{temporal}} = \frac{(F_{t+1} - F_t) \cdot (F_{t+1} - F_t)}{\max((F_{t+1} - F_t) \cdot (F_{t+1} - F_t))} \quad (25)$$

$$f'_{t+1} = \left(1 - \Omega^{f_{temporal}}\right) \cdot f'_t + \Omega^{f_{temporal}} \cdot \left(f_{t+1} \cdot \left(1 + \Omega^{f_{spatial}}\right)\right) \quad (26)$$

$$C_{Feature} = 1 - \cos\left(F'_{track_t}, F_{det_{t+1}}\right) \quad (27)$$

3 Experimental Setup and Results

The UAVDT dataset [3] was selected for model training and testing, with all objects being cars. Performance evaluation indicators were adopted from [17, 18]. The experimental framework is based on FairMOT [8], ensuring consistency in experimental details. The DLA34, pre-trained on the COCO dataset, was utilized as the backbone network, with the number of epochs set to 30. The training and testing platform was configured with a Gold 5218 CPU@2.10GHz × 80 and 2 × (RTX 3090 24G) GPUs.

Table 1 presents the comparison results. The AW module's comprehensive utilization of motion, appearance, and distribution information significantly improves tracking consistency and enhances the IDF1 indicator, as observed in the results. Further, the DFE module enhances the IDF1 metric using target distribution information, and the PBC module improves the model's overall tracking performance by correcting predicted boxes. Additionally, the STFE module, leveraging the capabilities of the preceding modules, employs strengthened features for target identity matching, thereby improving certain non-key tracking metrics. The DFE, PBC, and STFE modules each enhance the model's capacity to extract the three types of information, collectively optimizing tracking performance.

The essence of the proposed algorithm is to enhance target tracking consistency, evidenced by excellent performance in metrics like IDF1 and IDSW, while showing moderate results in the MOTA metric. Hence, Table 2 is dedicated to the comparative analysis of the IDF1 and IDSW metrics. While the new method does not achieve state-of-the-art results in FP and FN metrics, it exhibits improvements over baseline algorithms. In the area marked by a red arrow in Fig. 3, it is evident that in FairMOT's [8] tracking process, there are multiple identity switches in a short period, whereas ATIW maintains consistent object identity throughout. The analysis demonstrates that our proposed method effectively enhances multi-target tracking from an aerial perspective.

Table 1. Ablation study on UAVDT test dataset. Values in bold highlight the best results. The data in the table shows that with the stacking of various modules, the overall tracking performance of the model steadily improves.

Method	IDF1↑	MOTA↑	IDP↑	IDR↑	IDs↓	FP↓	FN↓	FM↓
Baseline	59.1	36.3	71.0	50.7	453	59543	157174	5128
+1	59.4	36.3	71.3	51.0	322	59660	157033	5113
+12	59.6	36.3	71.5	**51.1**	**316**	59689	**157014**	5130
+123	59.6	36.4	71.5	51.0	321	59487	157099	5103
+1234	**59.6**	**36.4**	**71.5**	51.0	323	**59477**	157107	**5100**

Table 2. Results of different trackers on UAVDT benchmarks. Values in bold highlight the best results. The information of the ignored region is not used. Our method performs well on multiple indicators that reflect tracking performance.

Method	IDF1↑	IDs↓	FP↓	FN↓	FM↓
[16]	23.7	9938	42245	163881	10463
[5]	43.7	2350	**33037**	172628	5787
[5]	58.2	2061	44868	**155290**	6432
[8]	59.1	453	59543	157174	5128
Ours	**59.6**	**323**	59477	157107	**5100**

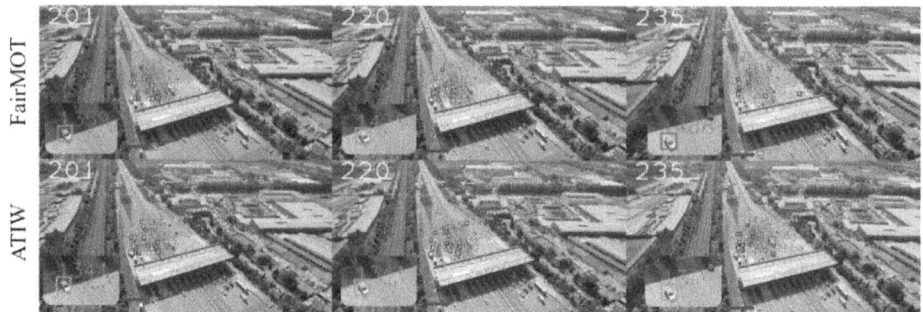

Fig. 3. The comparison of tracking performance between FairMOT and ATIW on the UAVDT test dataset. ATIW is still able to continuously track the target during the UAV maneuvering process without undergoing identity switching.

4 Conclusion

This study introduces a novel aerial multi-object tracking algorithm, ATIW, encompassing adaptive weighting, distribution feature extraction, prediction box correction, and spatio-temporal feature enhancement. Experimental results demonstrate that the ATIW algorithm fully leverages the distribution, motion, and appearance information of objects, thereby significantly enhancing aerial multi-object tracking performance. In particular, the IDF1 metric is improved by 0.5% without retraining the model. Future work will concentrate on consistently optimizing the fusion of object distribution, motion, and appearance information, aiming to substantially improve the operational efficiency and robustness of the algorithm on actual UAV platforms.

References

1. Xu, X., et al.: Stn-track: Multiobject tracking of unmanned aerial vehicles by swin transformer neck and new data association method. IEEE Journal of Selected Topics in Applied Earth Observations and Remote Sensing **15**, 8734–8743 (2022)
2. Zhu, P., et al.: Detection and tracking meet drones challenge. IEEE Trans. Pattern Anal. Mach. Intell. **44**(11), 7380–7399 (2021)
3. Du, D., Qi, Y., Yu, H., Yang, Y., Duan, K., Li, G., Zhang, W., Huang, Q., Tian, Q.: The unmanned aerial vehicle benchmark: Object detection and tracking. In: Proceedings of the European conference on computer vision (ECCV). pp. 370–386 (2018)
4. Liu, S., Li, X., Lu, H., He, Y.: Multi-object tracking meets moving uav. In: Proceedings of the IEEE/CVF Conference on Computer Vision and Pattern Recognition. pp. 8876–8885 (2022)
5. Wojke, N., Bewley, A., Paulus, D.: Simple online and realtime tracking with a deep association metric. In: 2017 IEEE international conference on image processing (ICIP). pp. 3645–3649. IEEE (2017)
6. Meinhardt, T., Kirillov, A., Leal-Taixe, L., Feichtenhofer, C.: Trackformer: Multi-object tracking with transformers. In: Proceedings of the IEEE/CVF conference on computer vision and pattern recognition. pp. 8844–8854 (2022)
7. Welch, G., Bishop, G., et al.: An introduction to the kalman filter (1995)
8. Zhang, Y., Wang, C., Wang, X., Zeng, W., Liu, W.: Fairmot: On the fairness of detection and re-identification in multiple object tracking. Int. J. Comput. Vision **129**, 3069–3087 (2021)

9. Yin, J., Wang, W., Meng, Q., Yang, R., Shen, J.: A unified object motion and affinity model for online multi-object tracking. In: Proceedings of the IEEE/CVF Conference on Computer Vision and Pattern Recognition. pp. 6768–6777 (2020)
10. Liang, T., Lan, L., Zhang, X., Peng, X., Luo, Z.: Enhancing the association in multi-object tracking via neighbor graph. Int. J. Intell. Syst. **36**(11), 6713–6730 (2021)
11. Zhang, Y., Sun, P., Jiang, Y., Yu, D., Weng, F., Yuan, Z., Luo, P., Liu, W., Wang, X.: Bytetrack: Multi-object tracking by associating every detection box. In: Computer Vision–ECCV 2022: 17th European Conference, Tel Aviv, Israel, October 23–27, 2022, Proceedings, Part XXII. pp. 1–21. Springer (2022)
12. Yu, H., Li, G., Su, L., Zhong, B., Yao, H., Huang, Q.: Conditional gan based individual and global motion fusion for multiple object tracking in uav videos. Pattern Recogn. Lett. **131**, 219–226 (2020)
13. Yang, J., Ge, H., Su, S., Liu, G.: Transformer-based two-source motion model for multi-object tracking. Applied Intelligence pp. 1–13 (2022)
14. Evangelidis, G.D., Psarakis, E.Z.: Parametric image alignment using enhanced correlation coefficient maximization. IEEE Trans. Pattern Anal. Mach. Intell. **30**(10), 1858–1865 (2008)
15. Fu, Y., Wang, X., Wei, Y., Huang, T.: Sta: Spatial-temporal attention for large scale video-based person re-identification. In: Proceedings of the AAAI conference on artificial intelligence. vol. 33, pp. 8287–8294 (2019)
16. Bochinski, E., Eiselein, V., Sikora, T.: High-speed tracking-by-detection without using image information. In: 2017 14th IEEE international conference on advanced video and signal based surveillance (AVSS). pp. 1–6. IEEE (2017)
17. Milan, A., Leal-Taixé, L., Reid, I., Roth, S., Schindler, K.: Mot16: A benchmark for multi-object tracking. arXiv preprint arXiv:1603.00831 (2016)
18. Ristani, E., Solera, F., Zou, R., Cucchiara, R., Tomasi, C.: Performance measures and a data set for multi-target, multi-camera tracking. In: Computer Vision–ECCV 2016 Workshops: Amsterdam, The Netherlands, October 8–10 and 15–16, 2016, Proceedings, Part II. pp. 17–35. Springer (2016)

Optimization Method for Fractal Image Compression Based on Self-similarity Evaluation and Gradient Bisection Algorithm

Caixu Xu[1], Di Xie[1], Hui Guo[1,2(✉)], Jie He[1,3], and Minglang Chen[1]

[1] Guangxi Key Laboratory of Machine Vision and Intelligent Control, Wuzhou University, Wuzhou 543000, Guangxi, China
3220002921@student.must.edu.mo
[2] Macao University of Science and Technology, Macao 999078, China
[3] College of Computer Science and Electronic Engineering, Hunan University, Changsha 410000, Hunan, China

Abstract. Fractal Image Compression (FIC) is a spatial domain compression technique with high compression ratio and good image quality. It is widely used in the fields of image restoration, denoising and watermarking. However, in terms of coding time, traditional fractal coding takes a certain amount of time for coding due to its need to find the best matching block traversal for sub-blocks. The long coding time is one of the main problems of fractal coding to be solved, which has a certain impact on the efficiency of fractal coding in practical applications. Meanwhile, since fractal coding itself is the application of self-similarity of images, the self-similarity of different categories of images also has a certain impact on the coding effect. To address the above problems, we first designed an algorithm based on SSIM to evaluate the overall self-similarity of images. Secondly, by analyzing the distribution of low-frequency coefficients of the image, we realize the dynamic classification of the sub-blocks to be coded based on the discrete cosine transform (DCT). And an adaptive threshold adjustment mechanism based on gradient bisection is proposed. Through comparative experiments, our optimization method significantly reduced encoding time (i.e., 96.12%) with only a 0.01 dB decrease in PSNR compared to the original FIC. The proposed scheme in this paper increases the usability of fractal coding, and provides a certain reference value for the subsequent fractal coding optimization research.

Keywords: FIC · Self-similarity evaluation · DCT · Dynamic codebook classification

1 Introduction

Fractal image compression method (FIC) [1] uses the self-similarity of the image to remove redundant information, and uses the iterative function system to reconstruct the image. It has the characteristics of high compression ratio, fast decoding speed, and decoding is independent of image resolution. It has been applied to media software such as Microsoft Encarta multimedia encyclopedia and Genuine Fractals plug-in of Photoshop. As a powerful spatial domain compression encoding method, the algorithm principles of FIC are also widely applied in image restoration, image denoising, digital watermarking, and face recognition fields [2–7]. The encoding process of FIC can be understood as a statistical process of similar regions in the image, thus, there is a drawback of long encoding time. Reducing the search range in the coding and matching process is an effective measure to shorten the coding time. Since the low-frequency coefficients after DCT transformation can effectively reflect the energy distribution characteristics of the image, many scholars classify the FIC codebooks based on this and have achieved good optimization results. However, such methods often rely on manually determined classification thresholds, which can impact both the coding efficiency and decoding quality, indicating that there is still room for improvement. Moreover, the effect of FIC essentially depends on the degree of self-similarity of the image, and images with poor structural similarity often exhibit block artifacts during decoding. Therefore, the evaluation of image self-similarity should be studied as a preliminary step in FIC research, enabling individuals to choose the application fields of FIC more accurately. To address these issues, we have refactored the application process of FIC. First, we calculate the self-similarity of the image and then use the calculation results to determine the FIC method to be used. By conducting experiments on two types of datasets, the average coding time of traditional fractal coding is greater than 96 s, while the average coding time of our proposed fractal coding optimization algorithm is only 48.34 s. Our main contributions include (Fig. 1).

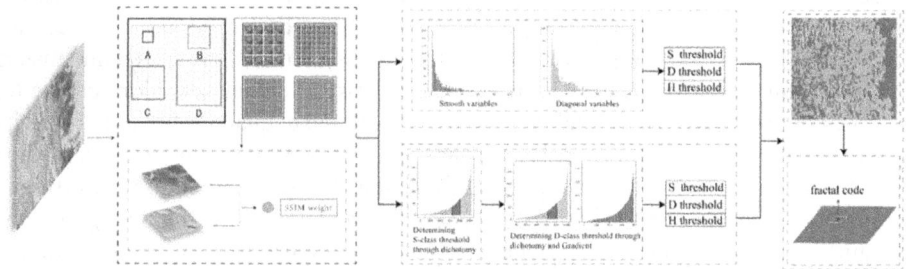

Fig. 1. Overview of the proposed FIC optimization method.

- Introducing the SSIM method to evaluate the self-similarity degree of a single image. We divide the image into various sub-blocks of different scales to cover a wide range of self-similar structures and use SSIM comparison to obtain the similarity relationship between sub-blocks. We also adjust the sub-blocks using downsampling to achieve cross-scale structural similarity comparison of sub-blocks with different sizes.
- Based on the distribution of low-frequency coefficients of multi-class images within the image, we have improved the codebook classification criteria based on DCT low-frequency coefficients to align the codebook clustering with the energy distribution of the image. Furthermore, we have proposed a new coefficient gradient method based on the bisection method on the sorting curve of the low-frequency coefficients. This

method enables the adaptive selection of the classification threshold, resulting in more accurate codebook clustering.
- We improved FIC using the above method and experimentally verified it on random regular images and various microscopic images. Theoretical proof was provided that microscopic images exhibit stronger self-similarity, aligning with human visual perception. Our method significantly enhances coding efficiency while maintaining decoding quality.

2 Related Work

2.1 Evaluation of Image Self-similarity

The degree of self-similarity in an image directly affects the effectiveness of fractal encoding, but there is currently no standard method for evaluating the self-similarity degree of an image. In fact, there have been some mature studies on assessing the similarity between images. Ref. [8] optimize the method for solving the image super-resolution problem using SSIM. The reference [9] optimized the PSNR evaluation method using weighted blur. The above methods are effective for measuring the similarity between images but are unable to directly assess the self-similarity within a single image. In recent years, scholars have quantified some structural properties within a single image using fractal dimension. In reference [10], the analysis of environmental detection images is conducted using fractal dimension. Literature [11] studies the application of fractal dimension in the initialization of recurrent neural networks. Fractal dimension is more suitable for measuring the complexity within an image, with limited effectiveness in expressing the self-similarity of the image. There is still some difference between the degree of self-similarity observed in the human visual system and the fractal dimension. To address this issue, Mu et al. [12] proposed a contrast sub-block selection scheme for the case where the self-similar region has its neighborhood to quantify the self-similarity property of the image. Yuan et al. [13] proposed a self-similarity quantization method for selecting sub-blocks with two-scale comparison. However, literature [12] did not consider the potential self-similarity structure at different scales in different regions, and literature [13] only divided the potential similarity structure into two scales, causing some degree of loss in capturing similarity structures across multiple scales. Therefore, we regard each fractal coding sub-block of a single image as an image, introduce and improve the similarity comparison method between images, and evaluate the self-similarity by combining the structure and brightness of the image in both multi-scale and global aspects.

2.2 DCT-Based Fractal Coding

The internal properties or laws of the image are particularly important for FIC coding rate and decoding quality. The method of neural networks has been widely used in video image compression optimization in recent years [14–16]. In recent years, some scholars have also applied neural network methods to improve fractal coding [17–19]. However, due to the dependence of fractal compression on the self-similarity characteristics of each image, the optimization effect of combining neural networks is relatively limited, and its versatility is poor. In the proposal of local feature-based shape models by [17], it is also mentioned that the annotation process remains a major challenge when neural networks are applied to fractal encoding. Due to the dependence of neural network on image annotation, and different images have different self-similar structures, it is difficult to have a unified and clear target annotation, which leads to its poor performance in fractal coding. DCT transform can better reflect the internal properties of the image, and many scholars have conducted extensive research on the fractal coding optimization scheme based on DCT transform. Among them, Duh et al. proposed a method of classifying the codebook by tripartition according to the low frequency coefficients of the image [20], which can effectively reduce the coding time. However, due to its equal division method for sub-blocks, it may lead to the loss of the optimal matching block in different images due to the different internal properties of the image, so there is still some room for optimization. Rawat et al. also proposed a method combining DCT with fractal encoding [21]. This method compresses color images using DCT to optimize the encoding quality issues caused by blocky artifacts. However, due to the fixed nature of its classification division, it may affect the optimal selection of similar sub-block regions for fractal encoding. Therefore, we choose to optimize the classification method and inter-class threshold dynamic selection based on the [20], aiming to strike a balance between time consumption and decoding quality.

3 Method

3.1 Self-similarity Evaluation Algorithm Based on SSIM

Most natural images exhibit a certain degree of self-similarity in their structure, implying that similar structures may exist at different or the same scales, in close proximity or at a distance. In microscopic images, this property is particularly obvious. As shown in Fig. 2, there may be a large number of cells and microorganisms with the same structure in the same biological microscopic image, which can be directly observed by the human eye.

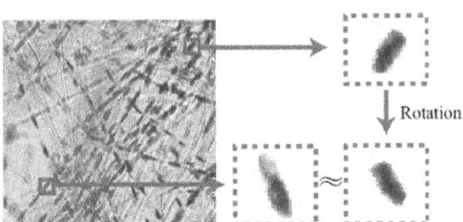

Fig. 2. The self similar structure appearing in bird feather tissue.

Calculating the self-similarity index of an image is the mainstream method for theoretically evaluating the degree of self-similarity. When the original image is segmented into several sub-blocks, each sub-block can be treated as a small-scale image. Therefore, we use SSIM for similarity calculation between sub-blocks, and standardize the scale of sub-blocks through downsampling during the comparison process to capture structural similarities at different scales across regions. Our method operates as shown in Fig. 3, where the image is first divided into a collection of sub-blocks of four different sizes. Define a minimum size block set and create a base block diagram set. Finally, take the coefficients of all the base blocks, and calculate the weighted average based on their global importance proportions to obtain the final self-similarity evaluation coefficient. The SSIM algorithm is as follows:

$$SSIM(x, y) = l(x, y)^\alpha * c(x, y)^\beta * s(x, y)^\gamma \quad (1)$$

where x and y are two image blocks of the same size. l, c, and s correspond to brightness comparison functions, contrast comparison functions, and structure comparison functions, where α, β, and γ are their weights respectively, all set to l by default in this paper. We calculate the weight of different base blocks by the variance of the gray values of the sub-blocks, and the weight represents the structural complexity ratio of the graph structure in the base block in all the base blocks. The calculation method is as follows:

$$W_n = \frac{V_n - V_{min}}{V_{max} - V_{min}}. \quad (2)$$

V_{max} is the maximum variance, V_{min} is the minimum variance, and V_n is the variance of the NTH basis block. After weighting the basis block in the weight of the image itself, the final self-similarity evaluation coefficient of the image is obtained by accumulating the coefficients of all basis blocks. We refer to this method as self-similarity evaluation based on Cross-scale SSIM (SECS) method, and the specific algorithm as Algorithm 1.

Algorithm 1 Image self-similarity evaluation coefficient algorithm.

Input: Image $= [[11, 12, \ldots, 1N], \ldots, [N1, N2, N3, \ldots, NN]]$, $B_1 =$ Subblock set 1, $B_2 =$ Subblock set 2, $B_3 =$ Subblock set 3, $B_4 =$ Subblock set 4.
Output: Self-similarity evaluation coefficient R.
1: **for** $b = B_{1,\ldots}, 2, 1$ **do**
2:      Perform SSIM calculations on b separately with B_1, B_2, B_3, and B_4.
3:      Calculate the weighting coefficients of each base block.
4:      Calculate the top 8 maximum coefficients in each set.
5:      $C_b =$ The product of the weighted coefficients of block b and the ssim coefficients.
6: **end for**
7: **for** $b = B_{1,\ldots}, 2, 1$ **do**
8:      $R = R + C_b$.
9:      **if** $b == 1$ **then**
10:          $R = mean(R)$.
11:          **return** Self-similarity evaluation coefficient R.
12:      **end if**
13: **end for**

3.2 Codebook Classification Based on Low-Frequency Coefficient Statistics

The energy of the image is mainly concentrated in the low-frequency region. By comparing the low-frequency coefficients of sub-blocks, it is possible to determine whether they

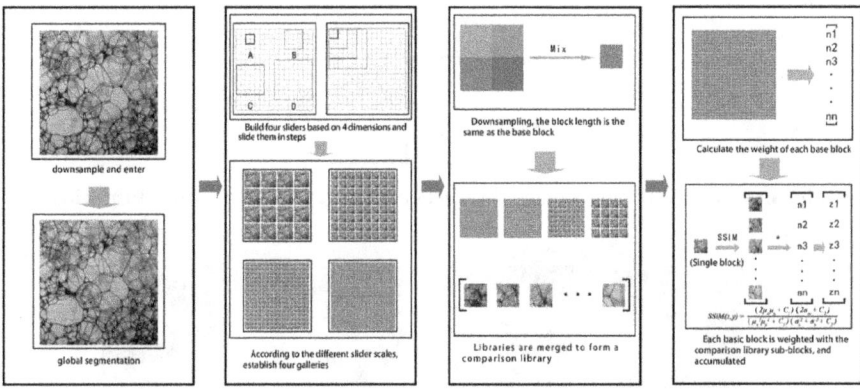

Fig. 3. Self-similarity Evaluation Method Process.

have similar texture distribution characteristics. The Discrete Cosine Transform (DCT) [22], with its excellent performance in aggregating frequency domain energy, has played a significant role in the field of digital image processing. After the image block undergoes DCT transformation, its low-frequency component mainly concentrates in the top-left coefficients of the transformed matrix, which can roughly reflect the energy distribution of the image block. Duh et al. [20] utilized this characteristic of DCT transformation to classify codebooks from the perspective of energy distribution, narrowing down the matching range between R blocks and D blocks. This not only shortens the encoding time but also ensures good decoding quality. Although this method has a clear classification strategy, it does not propose a calculation scheme for the classification threshold. Instead, it directly adopts a trisection method, which inevitably leads to inaccurate classification of some code blocks, affecting the quality of image reconstruction.

$$F(m, n) = \frac{2}{N} C_m C_n \sum_{i=0}^{N-1} \sum_{i=0}^{N-1} f(i, j) \cos\left(\frac{(2i+1)m\pi}{2N}\right) \times \cos\left(\frac{(2j+1)m\pi}{2N}\right). \quad (3)$$

In fact, since each image is different, inter-class thresholds should not be fixed and should be able to dynamically adapt to the texture distribution of each image. Therefore, based on the literature [20], we propose a statistical-based threshold dynamic adjustment method. Firstly, the image sub-block is transformed by DCT according to Eq. (3), and Fig. 4 is the low frequency coefficient matrix after transformation, where $F(0, 1)$ reflects the change of energy concentration in the vertical direction, and $F(1, 0)$ reflects the change of energy concentration in the horizontal direction. Therefore, according to $F(0, 1)$ and $F(1, 0)$ divides the image sub-blocks into three categories: smooth, diagonal/sub-diagonal, and horizontal/vertical.

Where N is the length of the image edge. $m, n = 0, 1, 2 \ldots, N - 1$, $C_k = \begin{cases} \frac{1}{\sqrt{2}}, & \text{if } k = 0 \\ 1, & \text{else} \end{cases}$.

When both $F(0, 1)$ and $F(1, 0)$ are smaller than the smooth threshold Ts, it indicates that the energy concentration changes in both the vertical and horizontal directions of

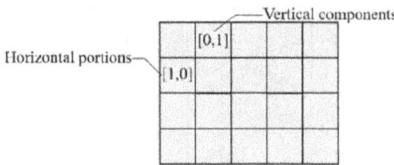

Fig. 4. Horizontal component and vertical component after DCT transformation.

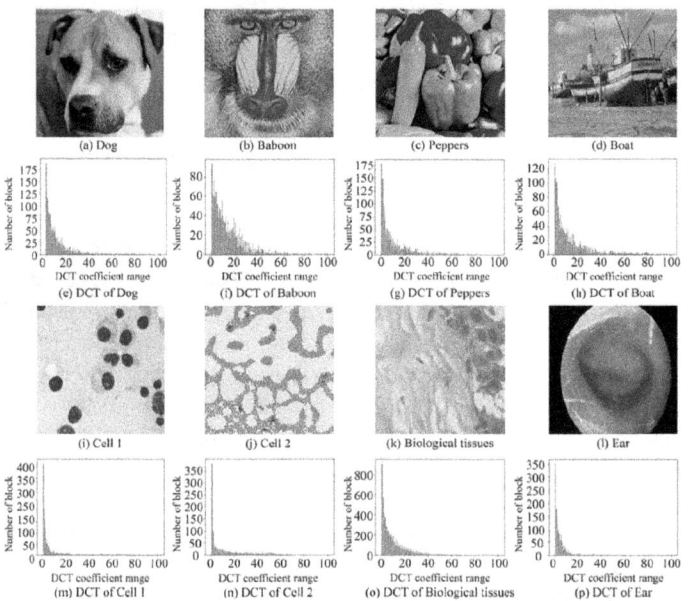

Fig. 5. Distribution of category parameters for images of different categories.

the block are relatively small. This suggests that the sub-block has uniform texture and is a smooth block, classified as the S category. When the absolute value of the difference between $F(0, 1)$ and $F(1, 0)$ is less than the diagonal threshold Td, it indicates that the difference between the vertical and horizontal energy changes and is small. At this time, the energy trend of the sub-block is diagonal or sub-diagonal distribution, and the sub-block belongs to the diagonal/sub-diagonal class, that is, the class D. The energy trend of the remaining domain blocks can be visualized as a horizontal or vertical distribution, belonging to Class H, namely the horizontal/vertical class. The thresholds Ts and Td are key to category classification. After dividing sub-blocks of different types of images, we calculate and sort their DCT horizontal coefficients, vertical coefficients, and their differences. As shown in Fig. 5, the majority of sub-blocks are concentrated in the range of smaller DCT coefficients.

We refer to this method as Fractal encoding based on Statistical histogram of low-frequency coefficients (FSHLC), the specific algorithm as Algorithm 2.

Algorithm 2 A fractal coding algorithm based on a statistical histogram of low-frequency coefficients.

Input: Image = [[11, 12,..., 1N], ..., [N1, N2, N3, ..., NN]], R_s, D_s.
Output: Fractal image encoding C.
1: D_{-list} = Generate Domain Atlas Based on D_s.
2: R_{-list} = Generate Range Atlas Based on R_s.
3: T_s, T_d = Calculate the target position after calculating the low-frequency distribution for the D_{-list}.
4: **for** $r - num = R_{-list}$ **do**
5:     Determine the category of R blocks based on T_s and T_d.
6:     **for** $d_{-num} = D_{-list-s} / D_{-list-d} / D_{-list-h}$ **do**
7:         C_{r-num} = Obtain the best matching block based on affine transformation.
8:     **end for**
9:     **if** $r - num = len(R_{-list})$ **then**
10:         return Fractal compression coding C.
11:     **end if**
12: **end for**

3.3 Adaptive Adjustment Methods for Inter-class Thresholds

For some cases where the image structure is not obvious, the threshold selection of the FSHLC method is completely based on statistical observation, which may still lead to the problem of inaccurate division, resulting in too many sub-blocks identified as smooth classes. Therefore, we further propose a dynamic adaptive classification algorithm combining the bisection method and the gradient difference method. For class S the threshold value is determined using the binary method. The DCT transformation is applied to each sub-block first, and $Max(F(0,1), F(1,0))$ is taken as the smoothness coefficient, F_S where F_{sn} for the nth D block is:

$$F_{sn} = \begin{cases} |F_n[1, 0]|, & if\,(|F_n[1, 0]| > |F_n[0, 1]|) \\ |F_n[0, 1]|, & else \end{cases}. \tag{4}$$

Then sort $F_{S0} - F_{S(m-1)}$ in ascending order, where m represents the total number of sub-blocks. The sorted sequence of F_S is denoted as F_{sl}. For the sorted sequence, calculate the median based on the maximum and minimum values of the smoothness coefficients, and the resulting median value at this point is the initial position, and its corresponding smoothing coefficient is the initial threshold value. Count the number of sub-blocks that are less than this median value and the number of sub-blocks that are greater than this median value, i.e., let $a = min(F_{sl})$, $b = max(F_{sl})$, $N_s(a, b)$ be the number of D blocks when F_s takes values in the range from a to b. Iterate the calculation of $S_n(a, b)$ to select the final binary interval, where:

$$S_n(a, b) = \begin{cases} b = \frac{a+b}{2}, & if\,N_s\left(a, \frac{a+b}{2}\right) > N_s\left(\frac{a+b}{2}, b\right) \\ a = \frac{a+b}{2}, & else \end{cases}. \tag{5}$$

When the difference between the two is less than 1/10 of the total number of sub-blocks, the median can be considered as the smoother position of the curve, which satisfies the convergence condition. At this point, a small number of extreme values are separated from a large number of small values. The smoothness coefficient at this median position is considered as the smooth class threshold T_S. Otherwise, an iterative operation is performed, i.e., the side with the smaller number of dichotomies is removed, and the judgment is continued by the method for the remaining portion until it stops when the difference between the two sides judgment condition is satisfied. When meet $\left| N_S\left(a, \frac{a+b}{2}\right) - N_S\left(\frac{a+b}{2}, b\right) \right| < \left(\frac{m}{10}\right)$ is met, take $F_{sl\left(\frac{a+b}{2}\right)}$ for S threshold T_s, less than D block as S class of T_s. Figure 6 shows the process of using binary partition method four times continuously on the codebook of dog.

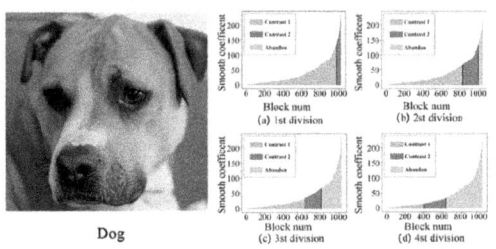

Fig. 6. The binary process of sub blocks.

For the remaining sub-blocks that have not been classified as S class, calculate their diagonal/secondary diagonal class coefficient as F_d, where the F_{dn} of the nth D block is:

$$F_{dn} = ||F_n[1, 0]| - |F_n[0, 1]||. \tag{6}$$

The same as T_s method, the dichotomy threshold T_{D1} of class D is determined by the dichotomy method. Since the sub-blocks corresponding to the coefficient interval of class S inevitably contain a part of the potential sub-blocks of class D, the parameter selection interval of the diagonal threshold will be narrowed and error will be caused. To address this issue, we construct a gradient map for each pair of adjacent coefficients after the binary process of the S class. Then, we select the position of the D class gradient threshold to minimize the error in the diagonal threshold caused by the missing D class sub-blocks. We set the gradient threshold as T_{D2}. When the number of S class blocks is s, we sort $F_{d(0)}$ to $F_{d(m-s-1)}$ in descending order and calculate the difference between each pair of adjacent coefficients, forming a gradient sequence F_{dl}. The gradient sequence has a total of m-s-1 elements, with the nth element denoted as $F_{dl(n)}$, where:

$$F_{dl(n)} = F_{d(n)} - F_{d(n+1)}. \tag{7}$$

Take the mean of the smallest 50% of elements to calculate the filtering value of the differences. Then, reassign each element in F_{dl} by subtracting the filtering value from the original value at that point in order to filter out a significant number of relatively low-gradient coefficients, where:

$$F_{dl(n)} = F_{d(n)} - F_{d(n+1)} - \frac{\sum_{v=\frac{m-s-1}{2}}^{m-s-1}\left(F_{d(v-1)} - F_{d(v)}\right)}{\frac{m-s-1}{2}}. \tag{8}$$

To reduce some noise, divide the sequence into intervals and reassign each element within each interval to the minimum value within that interval. When dividing into l interval every h elements, the elements within the l-th interval are assigned the value M_l. Among them, $lH = lh, lh+1, lh+2, \ldots, lh+9$.

$$M_l = min(F_{dl(lH)}), \tag{9}$$

Subsequently, iterate over F_{dl} from smallest to largest, select the corresponding F_d at the position of the first nonzero value as the gradient threshold T_{D2}. Take the average of the binary threshold T_{D1} and the gradient threshold T_{D2} as the final diagonal threshold T_D. Among them, $T_D = \frac{T_{D1}+T_{D2}}{2}$.

Then divide the sub-blocks with F_d less than T_D into class D, and define the remaining sub-blocks as class H. We refer to this method as the Fractal encoding based on Gradient dichotomy of low-frequency coefficients (FGDLC) method, the specific algorithm is as follows:

Algorithm 3 A fractal coding algorithm based on the gradient dichotomy of low-frequency coefficients.

Input: Image $= [[11, 12,\ldots, 1N], \ldots, [N1, N2, N3, \ldots, NN]]$, R_s, D_s.
Output: Fractal image encoding C.
1: $D_{-list} = $ Generate Domain Atlas Based on D_s.
2: $R_{-list} = $ Generate Range Atlas Based on R_s.
3: T_s, $T_d = $ Calculate the target position using gradient bisection method for the D_{-list}.
4: **for** $r-num = R_{-list}$ **do**
5:     Determine the category of R blocks based on T_s and T_d.
6:     **for** $d_{-num}=D_{-list-s}/\ D_{-list-d}/\ D_{-list-h}$ **do**
7:         $C_{r-num}=$ Obtain the best matching block based on affine transformation.
8:     **end for**
9:     **if** $r-num = len(R_{-list})$ **then**
10:         return Fractal compression coding C.
11:     **end if**
12: **end for**

Taking the codebook partition process of image with dog as an example, when the number of remaining D blocks is 100, the list of difference coefficients is built according to the difference between two adjacent coefficients. Then, the mean value of the first 50% difference is taken as the filter value, and the coefficient is subtracted from all the differences to eliminate the coefficient of the less volatile part. And take the minimum value from every h differences as their new value to eliminate individual spiky areas. Then, the position of the first non-zero value on the horizontal axis coordinates is used as the gradient threshold for the D class.

In Fig. 7(a), the horizontal axis represents the sequence number of D blocks after removing the S class, and the vertical axis represents the diagonal coefficient. In Fig. 7(b) and (c), the horizontal axis represents the difference index of sub-blocks, where n indicates comparing the nth sub-block with the (n+1)th sub-block. The vertical axis represents the difference between the two sub-blocks. The third image shows the difference coefficients after the above operation. A non-zero value appears close to 400. When

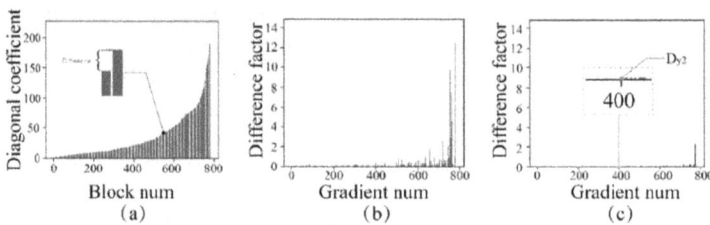

Fig. 7. Gradient selection process.

the non-zero value corresponds to a horizontal coordinate of m, the coefficient of the sub-block with a horizontal coordinate of m in the first image is taken as the gradient threshold. The final D class threshold is calculated as the average of the gradient threshold and the binary threshold. Sub-blocks in Fig. 7(a) with a vertical coordinate less than this threshold are defined as D class. The remaining D blocks are directly defined as H class. During the traversal process of R blocks, if a coefficient is greater than both the S class coefficient and the D class coefficient, it is searched in the H class.

4 Experiment

4.1 Data Sets and Evaluation Criteria

In order to verify whether our self-similarity evaluation method is consistent with human eye observations, and the effectiveness and generalizability of our proposed optimization method for codebook classification, two types of datasets are used in our experiments. The VOC dataset from PASCAL VOC Challenge, and the biomicroscopy dataset from Weakly Supervised Cell Segmentation in Multi-modality High-Resolution Microscopy Images, respectively. In the VOC dataset, different categories of images such as vehicles, portraits, landscapes, etc. are included. And in the biomicrography dataset, multiple categories of biomicrography images with different tissues, locations, and staining methods are included. Meanwhile, in order to avoid the influence of different image sizes or number of channels between different images on the experiments, this paper downsamples all the image sizes used in the experiments to 256 × 256 and converts them to grayscale images for the experiments.

In our proposed codebook classification optimization experiments for fractal coding, the above dataset is used to verify the effectiveness and universality of the coding scheme for different categories of images. In the self-similarity evaluation experiments, in order to verify the consistency of the self-similarity evaluation results proposed in this paper with the evaluation results derived from the human eye vision system, we similarly conduct comparison experiments by using the above VOC dataset, which contains images of a larger number of categories, with the biomicrographic dataset, which is self-similar to a larger number of images under the human eye vision system.

In the fractal coding experiments, we chose Peak Signal-to-Noise Ratio (PSNR) to verify the coding and decoding quality of different algorithms. PSNR is a common image quality evaluation method, which is often used to calculate the similarity of different images before and after coding, and the larger the PSNR is, the more similar the pictures are before and after decoding, and the better the quality of decoding is. The larger PSNR is, the more similar the images are before and after decoding, and the better the decoding quality is.

Where MAX^2 is the maximum pixel gray value and MSE is the mean square error. Generally, we think that the decoding quality is better when the PSNR is greater than or equal to 30 dB.

4.2 Results of Self-similarity Evaluation

Using SECS for calculation, the self similarity coefficient curves of 500 pieces each in these two types of datasets are shown in Fig. 8. Thereinto, the VOC dataset has the largest range of self-similarity evaluation coefficients, with a mean self-similarity of 0.1529. The dataset composed of biological microscopic images shows an overall improvement compared to regular images, with a higher self-similarity coefficient in a large number of images. The average self-similarity evaluation coefficient is 0.1867. As can be seen from Fig. 9, the biomicroscope image has more distribution in the region with larger coefficients than the ordinary image, indicating that the biomicroscope image has higher self-similarity. In addition, the overall span, extreme value and mean value of the self-similarity coefficient of the two types of data sets are shown in Table 1, and it can be found that the coefficient value of the biological microscopic image has smaller fluctuation and larger mean value. The above comparison results show that our method is consistent with the perception results of the human visual system, and can effectively verify the self-similarity of images.

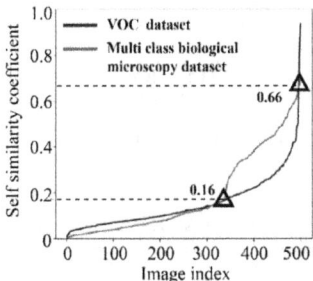

Fig. 8. Comparison of self similarity coefficients between multi class biological microscopy datasets and VOC datasets.

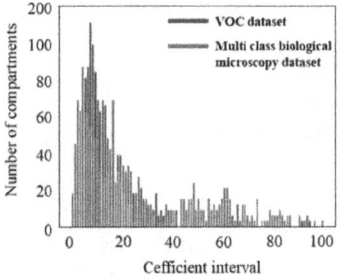

Fig. 9. Self-similarity coefficient distribution of three types of atlases.

4.3 Compression Performance Experiments

Figure 10 shows the visualization results of codebook classification using FSHLC and FGDLC methods. It can be observed that the FGDLC algorithm is more sensitive to the grayscale distribution of images and provides more accurate delineation of different categories.

Table 1. Extreme values, range, and mean of self-similarity evaluation for the three datasets after experimentation.

Correlation coefficient	Global maximum value	Global minimum value	Mean	Span
VOC	0.9325	0.0087	0.1529	0.9238
Microscopic images of multiple types of organisms	0.7140	0.0024	0.1867	0.7116

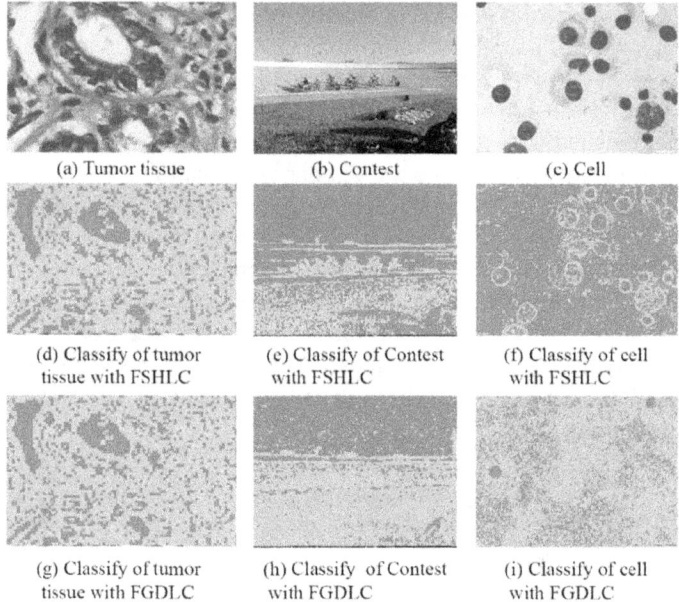

Fig. 10. Visualization of category division using FSHLC and FGDLC algorithms.

Figure 11 shows the overall encoding time curve for the VOC dataset under three algorithms. We used the original FIC as well as FGDLC and FSHLC to encode and decode two types of datasets. The average encoding time and average decoding quality obtained by different algorithms are shown in Table 2. From the table, it can be seen that compared to the original fractal coding, FGDLC optimizes the encoding time without a significant decrease in PSNR. The average encoding time for the VOC dataset decreased to 40.22 s, a speed improvement of 58.39%. For the multi-class biological microscopic dataset, the average encoding time decreased to 40.45 s, a speed improvement of 58.37%. We can also observe that although the FGDLC algorithm shows a minor improvement in decoding quality for the VOC dataset and the multi-class biological microscopic dataset, overall, it does not provide a significant optimization in terms of encoding time.

Therefore, we also conducted a statistical analysis of the minimum encoding time for each category, as shown in Table 3. Although the advantages of the FGDLC algorithm

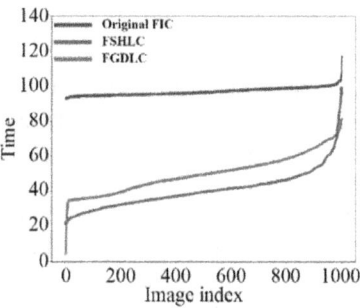

Fig. 11. The encoding time of the VOC dataset by the three types of algorithms.

Table 2. The average peak signal-to-noise ratio and average encoding time after fractal coding for three datasets.

Method	VOC		Microscopic images of multiple types of organisms	
	PSNR (dB)	Time (s)	PSNR (dB)	Time (s)
Original FIC	29.69	96.65	32.11	97.16
FSHLC	26.98(↓0.71)	40.22(↑58.39%)	31.32(↓0.79)	40.45(↑58.37%)
FGDLC	27.50(↓0.19)	49.60(↑48.68%)	31.83(↓0.28)	47.07(↑51.55%)

Table 3. Minimum time for three types of datasets after three types of fractal encoding, along with the corresponding peak signal-to-noise ratio (PSNR) for the image with the minimum time.

Method	VOC		Microscopic images of multiple types of organisms	
	PSNR (dB)	Minimal time (s)	PSNR (dB)	Minimal time (s)
Original FIC	20.41	92.75	33.00	93.66
FSHLC	24.88	20.95	27.75	17.42
FGDLC	37.93	3.88	43.19	6.51

are not significant in Table 2, it can be seen in Table 3, that the FGDLC algorithm only requires a minimum encoding time of 3.88 s for image encoding, while the same image requires 100.03 s for encoding using the original fractal encoding under the same hardware conditions. After decoding, the codebook encoded by the FGDLC algorithm achieves a PSNR of 37.93 dB, only 0.01 dB lower than FIC. This indicates that the FGDLC algorithm provides a very high acceleration ratio for certain images.

5 Conclusion

FIC is a compression method that can ignore the decoding image resolution, but fractal encoding inherently has issues with image adaptability, as well as time consumption problems due to the extensive traversal process during encoding. In our method, we first identify the self-similarity structure of different scales in the image, calculate the self-similarity coefficient of the image to analyze the degree of self-similarity in the image, in order to determine whether the image is suitable for fractal coding. Then, by observing the distribution pattern of low-frequency regions in the image, we improved the classification process of fractal codebooks based on DCT. Furthermore, we achieved dynamic adaptive sub-block classification through the binary gradient method, significantly enhancing the encoding speed. Additionally, by partitioning the codebook using dynamic thresholds, we also ensured a high decoding quality. We validated the effectiveness and universality of the above method on microscopic images and other datasets. We also consider introducing the idea of sparsity into the process of codebook classification to improved compression efficiency. Meanwhile, since our proposed algorithm is mainly based on the low-frequency distribution of the image itself, the algorithm will continue to be further attempted to be applied in some, e.g., video intra-frame data loss problems.

Acknowledgments. This work was supported by the National Natural Science Foundation of China under Grants (61961036), in part by the Natural Science Foundation of Guangxi, China under Grants (20GXNSFAA297259), the National Natural Science Foundation of China under Grants (62162054), in part by the Basic Ability Improvement Project for Young and Middle-aged Teachers in Guangxi, China (2024KY0694), and the Key Research Project of Wuzhou University (2023B001).

Disclosure of Interests. The authors have no competing interests to declare that are relevant to the content of this article.

References

1. Jacquin, A.E.: Image coding based on a fractal theory of iterated contractive image transformations. IEEE Trans. Image Process. **1**(1), 18–30 (1992)
2. Pi, M.H., Li, H.: Fractal indexing with the joint statistical properties and its application in texture image retrieval. IET Image Process. **2**, 218–230 (2008)
3. Zhuang, Z., Lei, N., Raj, A.N.J., Qiu, S.: Application of fractal theory and fuzzy enhancement in ultrasound image segmentation. Med. Biol. Eng. Comput. **57**(3), 623–632 (2019)
4. Cheul, Y.C., Shin, H.J.: A novel fast fractal super resolution technique. IEEE Trans. Consum. Electron. **56**(3), 1537–1541 (2010)
5. Ghazel, M., Freeman, G.H., Vrscay, E.R.: Fractal-wavelet image denoising revisited. IEEE Trans. Image Process. **15**(9), 2669–2675 (2006)
6. Pi, H., Li, H., Li, H.: A novel fractal image watermarking. IEEE Trans. Multimedia **8**(3), 488–499 (2006)
7. Tan, T., Yan, H.: The fractal neighbor distance measure. Pattern Recognit. **35**(6), 1371–1387 (2002)

8. Wang, C.Y., Li, J., Wu, J., Liu, J.: SSIM-based sparse image superresolution with rotation strategy and nonlocal regularization. In: 2022 China Automation Congress (CAC), pp. 2482–2486 (2022)
9. Jamali, M., Karimi, N., Samavi, S.: Weighted fuzzy-based PSNR for watermark visual quality evaluation. In: 2021 29th Iranian Conference on Electrical Engineering (ICEE), pp. 488–492 (2021)
10. Auccahuasi, W., Linares, O., Urbano, K., Sobrino-Mesias, J., Campos-Sobrino, M., Quispe-Peña, H.: Methodology for monitoring lagoon dimensions by means of fractal dimension analysis. In: 2024 2nd International Conference on Intelligent Data Communication Technologies and Internet of Things (IDCIoT), pp. 1722–1726 (2024)
11. Mayer, N.M., Obst, O.: Analyzing echo-state networks using fractal dimension. In: 2022 International Joint Conference on Neural Networks (IJCNN), pp. 1–8 (2022)
12. Mu, Z.C.W.X.M., Yang, Q.: Self-similarity studies of images. J. Zhengzhou Univ. Sci. Ed. **2**, 67–69 (2005)
13. Yuan, F.Z.: Research on image coding technology based on fractals (2009)
14. Lei, F., Ding, Y., Wang, Z.R., Tang, F.F.: Mixed distorted image restoration based on residual double deep Q network. In: 2023 42nd Chinese Control Conference (CCC), pp. 7918–7923 (2023)
15. Afro, P.-A., Strus, L., Bonnaud, L., Caplier, A., Robin, F.: Multi-QP rate distortion optimized quantization using deep learning. In: 2023 IEEE International Conference on Visual Communications and Image Processing (VCIP), pp. 1–5 (2023)
16. Usha Bhanu, N., Saravanakumar, C.: Investigations of machine learning algorithms for high efficiency video coding (HEVC). In: 2023 International Conference on Signal Processing, Computation, Electronics, Power and Telecommunication (IConSCEPT), pp. 1–5 (2023)
17. Xu, H.T., Yan, J.C., Persson, N., Lin, W.Y., Zha, H.Y.: Fractal dimension invariant filtering and its CNN-based implementation. In: 2017 IEEE Conference on Computer Vision and Pattern Recognition (CVPR), pp. 3825–3833 (2017)
18. Maha Lakshmi, G.V.: Implementation of image compression using fractal image compression and neural networks for MRI images. In: 2016 International Conference on Information Science (ICIS), pp. 60–64 (2016)
19. Guo, J.W., Sun, J.G.: An image compression method of fractal based on GSOFM network. In: 2008 Congress on Image and Signal Processing, vol. 1, pp. 421–425 (2008)
20. Duh, D.J., Jeng, J.H., Chen, S.Y.: DCT based simple classification scheme for fractal image compression. Image Vis. Comput. **23**(13), 1115–1121 (2005). https://doi.org/10.1016/j.imavis.2005.05.013
21. Wei Liu, et al.: SSD: single shot multibox detector. In: Computer Vision – ECCV 2016: 14th European Conference, Amsterdam, The Netherlands, October 11–14, 2016, Proceedings, Part I 14, pp. 21–37. Springer (2016)
22. Ahmed, N., Natarajan, T., Rao, K.R.: Discrete cosine transform. IEEE Trans. Comput. **C–23**(1), 90–93 (1974). https://doi.org/10.1109/T-C.1974.223784

DiffGIC: Diffusion Prior Based Null-Space Correction for High Resolution Grayscale Image Colorization

Yachao Li[1,2], Yutian Fu[3], Feng Dong[3], and Dong Liang[1,2(✉)]

[1] College of Computer Science and Technology, Nanjing University of Aeronautics and Astronautics, Nanjing, China
{liyachao,liangdong}@nuaa.edu.cn
[2] Shenzhen Research Institute, Nanjing University of Aeronautics and Astronautics, Nanjing, China
[3] Shanghai Institute of Technical Physics, Chinese Academy of Sciences, Beijing, China
{yutianfu,dongfeng}@mail.sitp.ac.cn

Abstract. Diffusion models have demonstrated exceptional abilities in colorizing grayscale images. To colorize high-resolution images, current methods use a strategy that combines super-resolution with hierarchical image processing (SR-HIPS). This approach involves shrinking the input images for the diffusion model to reduce computational resources. However, this can lead to the loss of detailed information in high-resolution grayscale images. To overcome this limitation, this paper introduces DiffGIC, a novel method leveraging color image decomposition via range-null space decomposition. DiffGIC takes color from low-resolution color images and details from high-resolution grayscale images. By adjusting the color using a pre-trained diffusion model and combining it with detailed grayscale information, our method produces high-quality, high-resolution colored images. Moreover, DiffGIC improves upon the SR-HIPS strategies by adding detailed grayscale details into the colorization process, marking a notable advancement over previous methods.

Keywords: Image Colorization · Diffusion Model · Super-Resolution

1 Introduction

Image colorization, transforming grayscale images into full color, is a thriving research topic within the field of low-level computer vision. Initially, this domain was dominated by studies that concentrated on employing specialized, small-scale datasets to train neural networks to achieve direct conversion from grayscale to color images [1]. However, these methods were constrained by the limited scale of the training datasets, which posed challenges in adapting these techniques to the diverse real-world scenarios. Recently, the focus has shifted towards leveraging the generative capabilities of pre-trained generators [2], known for their outstanding performance. Particularly, text-to-image generative models trained on large-scale datasets stand out for their extensive prior knowledge [3]. Leveraging this knowledge can markedly improve the accuracy and visual quality of image colorization.

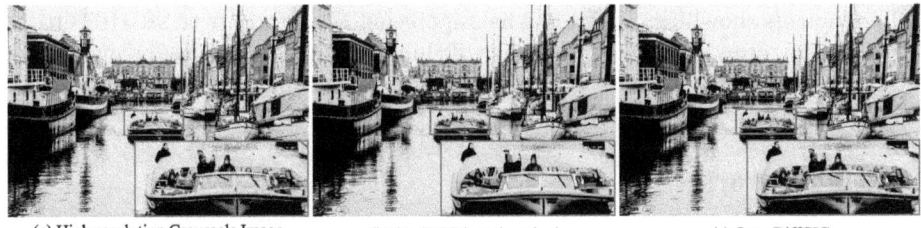

(a) High-resolution Grayscale Image   (b) SR-HIPS-based method   (c) Ours DiffGIC

Fig. 1. (a) The high-resolution (HR) grayscale image. (b) The HR color image generated by SR-HIPS-based method. (c) The HR color image generated by our DiffGIC.

Although diffusion models [4] offer considerable benefits for low-level tasks, the need for GPU memory grows with the size of the image. This poses a challenge when processing high-resolution images. Hierarchical image processing strategy (HIPS) [5], which utilizes super-resolution (SR) techniques, is widely used in practical situations to produce high-resolution color images on limited computational resources. It works by first reducing the resolution of images processed by diffusion models, producing low-resolution color images. These images are then upscaled to higher resolutions through super-resolution models powered by generative adversarial networks [6–9] or diffusion models [10, 11]. This approach often overlooks the finer details in high-resolution grayscale images. As a result, it may not accurately reproduce the nuances of the original high-resolution grayscale images.

In this paper, we introduce a novel diffusion-based method called DiffGIC, which leverages color image decomposition via range-null space decomposition [12] for HIPS-based image colorization. It extracts color from the low-resolution color images and details from the high-resolution grayscale images. Then, it adjusts the color using a pre-trained diffusion model and combines it with extracted details to produce high-resolution colored images. During the color adjustment, a patch-based noise prediction method is adopted to ensure small computational resources. Additionally, our method can be easily applied to SR-HIPS-based methods by adding detailed grayscale details into the colorization process. Experiments show that DiffGIC can produce high-quality, high-resolution color images using small computational resources. Figure 1 illustrates a comparison between DiffGIC and an SR-HIPS-based method. DiffGIC has significant advantages in retaining detailed information in high-resolution grayscale images.

The main contributions of this work are summarized as follows:

- We propose DiffGIC, a novel hierarchical diffusion-based high-resolution grayscale image colorization method that uses small computational resources to produce high-quality, high-resolution color images. Additionally, it can be easily applied to SR-HIPS-based methods to improve performance.
- We introduce a color image decomposition method based on range-null space decomposition. By extracting details from high-resolution grayscale images, we solve the problem of inconsistent details between high-resolution color results and grayscale images. In addition, we introduce a pre-trained diffusion model to adjust the color information in the low-resolution color results to resolve the difference from the expected color information.

- Experiments show that our method has significant advantages over SR-HIPS-based methods in terms of detail consistency with high-resolution grayscale images. At the same time, the proposed method can also be integrated with SR-HIPS-based methods to improve their upper performance bound.

2 Related Work

2.1 Grayscale Image Colorization

Grayscale image colorization aims to enhance grayscale images by adding vibrant colors, resulting in more visually appealing outputs. In recent years, deep learning-based image processing methods have proven very effective in many low-level color-related tasks [13]. Automatic colorization methods [14] focus on estimating the missing color channels in grayscale images to generate realistic color images without relying on text guidance. Although significant progress has been made in these works, automatic colorization still faces the challenge of uncertainty when dealing with real-world problems. Text-driven image colorization methods leverage the rich semantic information in text descriptions to drive colorization and reduce uncertainty. Recently, significant progress in text-to-image diffusion models [3] provides powerful tools for such methods. Some works, such as ControlNet [2], can produce colorization results that are highly consistent with text descriptions by fine-tuning these models.

2.2 Text-Driven Diffusion-Based Grayscale Image Colorization

Diffusion Models [4] learn the image generation process through iterative denoising steps initiated from an initial random noise. They have demonstrated superior performance in many low-level tasks, such as super-resolution [11], image despeckling [15], etc. For text-driven grayscale image coloring, ControlNet [2] colorizes images by introducing grayscale images as conditions to control the image generation process. DiffColor [16] inverses grayscale images into latent features for image generation and fine-tunes the diffusion model to align text descriptions and image colors.

Although these methods have superior performance, they require extensive computational resources, which limits their application in high-resolution grayscale image colorization. Hierarchical image processing strategy (HIPS) [5], which utilizes super-resolution (SR) techniques, is widely used in practical situations to produce high-resolution color images on limited computational resources.

2.3 Image Super-Resolution

Image super-resolution (SR) aims to recover high-resolution (HR) images from degraded low-resolution (LR) observations. ESRGAN [8] and SwinIR-GAN [9] assumed predefined degradation processes, such as bicubic downsampling and blurring using known parameters. BSRGAN [6] and Real-ESRGAN+ [7] propose using a combination of multiple degradation methods to synthesize LR-HR image pairs that mimic real-world data for the real-world blind SR task. Recent diffusion-based works, such as DiffBIR [10] and StableSR [11], have also shown competitive performance in real-world image

SR. However, the lack of utilization of the high-resolution grayscale images during the super-resolution process can result in inconsistencies between the details of color results and the high-resolution grayscale images.

In contrast to the high-resolution image hierarchical colorization based on SR, our approach focuses on leveraging the details in high-resolution grayscale images to address the issue of insufficient details in low-resolution color results. Additionally, it focuses on eliminating the differences between the color information in low-resolution color results and the color information in expected high-resolution color results.

3 DiffGIC

3.1 Preliminaries: Range-Null Space Decomposition

For image colorization and image super-resolution tasks, the degradation process is generally defined as:

$$y = \mathbf{A}x \tag{1}$$

where y denotes the degraded image and x represents the original image. $\mathbf{A}$ represents the degrade operator. To make it easy to understand, we use two operators, $\mathbf{A}_C$ and $\mathbf{A}_{SR}$, to denote the degrade operator for image colorization and image super-resolution. The operator $\mathbf{A}_C$ can be represented as a matrix $[\frac{1}{3}, \frac{1}{3}, \frac{1}{3}]$ that converts each RGB channel pixel $[r, g, b]^T$ to a grayscale value $[\frac{r}{3} + \frac{g}{3} + \frac{b}{3}]$. The operator $\mathbf{A}_{SR}$ can be designed as the average pooling downsampling. We can easily find their pseudo-inverse operators that $\mathbf{A}_C^\dagger$ is represented by the matrix $[1,1,1]$, while $\mathbf{A}_{SR}^\dagger$ is represented by the mean upsampling. Both degrade operators satisfy the equations $\mathbf{AA}^\dagger \mathbf{A}x \equiv \mathbf{A}x$ and $\mathbf{A}(\mathbf{I} - \mathbf{A}^\dagger\mathbf{A})x \equiv 0$.

According to $\mathbf{AA}^\dagger\mathbf{A}x \equiv \mathbf{A}x$, $\mathbf{A}^\dagger\mathbf{A}x$ can be seen as projecting x to the range-space of $\mathbf{A}$. In contrast, according to $\mathbf{A}(\mathbf{I} - \mathbf{A}^\dagger\mathbf{A})x \equiv 0$, $(\mathbf{I} - \mathbf{A}^\dagger\mathbf{A})x$ can be seen as projecting x to the null-space of $\mathbf{A}$. Any original image x can be decomposed into these two parts that satisfying:

$$x = \mathbf{A}^\dagger \mathbf{A} x + (\mathbf{I} - \mathbf{A}^\dagger\mathbf{A})x \tag{2}$$

Taking the image coloring task as an example, $\mathbf{A}_C^\dagger \mathbf{A}_C x$ can be regarded as the grayscale detailed information contained in x and $(\mathbf{I} - \mathbf{A}_C^\dagger\mathbf{A}_C)x$ can be seen as the color information contained in x.

3.2 Color Image Decomposition for Hierarchical Image Colorization

For high-resolution (HR) grayscale image colorization, current methods adopt the hierarchical image processing strategy (HIPS) to decrease the computational resource requirements. These HIPS-based methods first decrease the processed image size for text-to-image models and generate the low-resolution (LR) color image x_{lr}. Then, they utilize the super-resolution (SR) models to generate high-resolution image x based on $x_{lr} = \mathbf{A}_{SR}x$. The SR process neglects the detailed information in the HR grayscale image. Based on range-null space decomposition, we can solve this problem by converting the SR process to a new type of process. We generate the HR color image x by fusing the color information in x_{lr} and the detailed information in the HR grayscale image y. Specifically, according to Eq. 2, the color information, denoted as CI, can be extracted from x_{lr} as follows:

$$CI = \left(\mathbf{I} - \mathbf{A}_C^\dagger \mathbf{A}_C\right) x_{lr} \qquad (3)$$

According to Eq. 1 and Eq. 2, the detailed information, denoted as DI, can be extracted from y as follows:

$$DI = \mathbf{A}_C^\dagger \mathbf{A}_C x = \mathbf{A}_C^\dagger y \qquad (4)$$

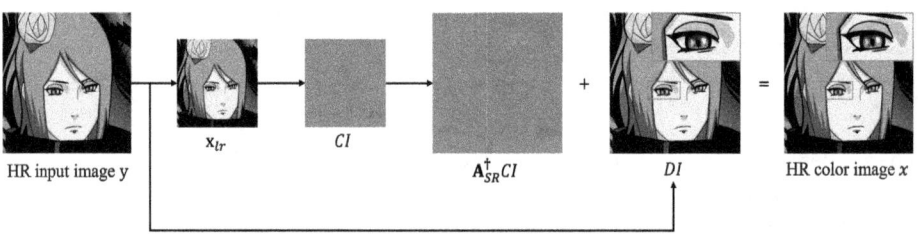

Fig. 2. Hierarchical grayscale image colorization based on range-null space decomposition. From the enlarged area, we can observe that the HR color image x retains the detailed information in HR input image y.

According to Eq. 2 and Eq. 3, we can find that CI is not the corresponding color information in x. So directly adding DI and CI can not generate the HR color image x. To obtain the corresponding color information in x, we first need to analyze the relationship between CI and x. According to $x_{lr} = \mathbf{A}_{SR} x$, we can deduce $CI = \left(\mathbf{I} - \mathbf{A}_C^\dagger \mathbf{A}_C\right) \mathbf{A}_{SR} x = \mathbf{A}_{SR} x - \mathbf{A}_C^\dagger \mathbf{A}_C \mathbf{A}_{SR} x$. According to the designs of $\mathbf{A}_C^\dagger$, $\mathbf{A}_C$ and $\mathbf{A}_{SR}$, we can deduce $\mathbf{A}_C^\dagger \mathbf{A}_C \mathbf{A}_{SR} x = \mathbf{A}_{SR} \mathbf{A}_C^\dagger \mathbf{A}_C x$, where $\mathbf{A}_C^\dagger \mathbf{A}_C x$ can be represented by DI. So the relationship between CI and x can be defined as follows:

$$CI = \mathbf{A}_{SR} x - \mathbf{A}_{SR} DI \qquad (5)$$

Now, let us assume that, which means that $\mathbf{A}_{SR}^\dagger \mathbf{A}_{SR} x = x$ does not lose any information during the downsampling and upsampling processes. The final HR color image can be obtained by:

$$x = DI + \mathbf{A}_{SR}^\dagger CI \qquad (6)$$

As shown in Fig. 2, the HR color image x generated by this new type of process maintains the color information in x_{lr} and the detailed information in the HR grayscale image y. However, since $\mathbf{A}_{SR}^\dagger \mathbf{A}_{SR} x = x$ does not hold in practice, there are some differences in details between the generated result and the original color HR image corresponding to y. According to Eq. 6, we can observe that these differences originate from

$\mathbf{A}_{SR}^{\dagger}CI \neq \left(\mathbf{I} - \mathbf{A}_{C}^{\dagger}\mathbf{A}_{C}\right)x$. As shown in Fig. 3, these differences appear as color distortion, which becomes increasingly obvious as the upsampling factor increases. Inspired by DDNM [17], we leverage the prior knowledge of a pre-trained diffusion model to eliminate these differences.

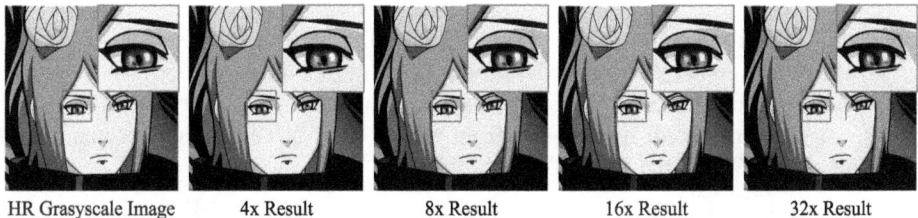

Fig. 3. Hierarchical grayscale image colorization based on range-null space decomposition with different upsampling factors.

3.3 Null-Space Diffusion Prior for Color Information Correction

Diffusion models generate images through T-step iteratively denoising. The generation starts by sampling a noise x_T from an i.i.d. Gaussian distribution and finishes by generating a clean image x_0. Prior knowledge of the diffusion model is included in every image generated during the denoising process. To use the prior knowledge for color correction, we adopt a pre-trained pixel-level diffusion model, allowing us to control the process explicitly. Specifically, we can get a predicted clean image $x_{0|t}$ from noisy image x_t at each timestep t. This operation can be simply represented as follows:

$$x_{0|t} = \frac{1}{\alpha_t}(x_t - \sigma_t \epsilon_\theta) \qquad (7)$$

where α_t and σ_t are predefined scale factors, $t \sim \{0, ..., T\}$. To ensure small computation resources, ϵ_θ is defined as the noise fused by weighting noises predicted by the diffusion model in a patch-based manner as described in Mixture of Diffusers [18].

To eliminate the differences originating from $\mathbf{A}_{SR}^{\dagger}CI \neq \left(\mathbf{I} - \mathbf{A}_{C}^{\dagger}\mathbf{A}_{C}\right)x$, we extract the color information in $x_{0|t}$ and use it to correct $\mathbf{A}_{SR}^{\dagger}CI$ through the null-space of $\mathbf{A}_{SR}$. Similar to Eq. 3, the color information in $x_{0|t}$ can be defined as $CI_{x|t} = \left(\mathbf{I} - \mathbf{A}_{C}^{\dagger}\mathbf{A}_{C}\right)x_{0|t}$. According to Eq. 2, the corrected color information $\widehat{CI}$ can be defined as follows:

$$\widehat{CI} = \mathbf{A}_{SR}^{\dagger}CI + \left(\mathbf{I} - \mathbf{A}_{SR}^{\dagger}\mathbf{A}_{SR}\right)CI_{x|t} \qquad (8)$$

Now, we can replace $\mathbf{A}_{SR}^{\dagger}CI$ in Eq. 6 with $\widehat{CI}$ to obtain the HR color image $\overline{x}_{0|t}$. This process can be defined as follows:

$$\overline{x}_{0|t} = DI + \widehat{CI} \qquad (9)$$

Then, we follow the denoising process of the diffusion model to add noise to $\bar{x}_{0|t}$. To boost the speed, we adopt the fast sampler DDIM [19] and define this process as follows:

$$x_{t-1} = \alpha_{t-1}\bar{x}_{0|t} + \sigma_{t-1}\left(\eta_t \epsilon + \sqrt{1-\eta_t^2}\epsilon_\theta\right), \epsilon \sim N(0, \mathbf{I}) \quad (10)$$

where η_t is a factor that controls the ratio of the newly introduced noise ϵ.

By iteratively controlling the generation process of the diffusion model in the above way, we can obtain the final HR color image x_0. Compared with the results obtained by Eq. 6, x_0 contains color information from x_{lr} and color information corrected by the diffusion model. We name this method as DiffGIC.

4 Experiments

4.1 Implementation Details

We adopted the pre-trained diffusion model provided by [20]. It is trained on the ImageNet [21] dataset with a size of 512 × 512. To reduce the computational resources, we used the patch-based noise prediction and fusion method proposed by Mixture of Diffusers [18] during the inference process. We chose 512 × 512 as the patch size and left the smallest possible overlapping area when dividing patches to reduce the number of patches and minimize the time cost caused by the patch-based noise prediction. During the inference process, we used DDIM as the accelerated sampling algorithm. We set $\eta_t = 1.0$ and adopted 4 DDIM denoising steps for testing.

4.2 Experiment Setup

Dataset. We evaluate our method on real-world datasets. For real-world datasets, we choose the DIV2K [22] validation set and the Real40 dataset we collected from the Internet. Real40 contains 40 images with a 2K resolution covering various real-world scenes, such as faces, streets, buildings, etc. During the evaluation phase, we downsample all images by 4x to simulate LR color results. For DiffGIC, we degrade all images into grayscale images and use them with LR color results as input for HR color image generation. For the SR-HIPS-based methods, we directly take the LR color results as input for 4x SR.

Compared Methods. To verify the effectiveness of our method, we compared our DiffGIC with SR-HIPS-based methods using several most commonly adopted SR methods, i.e., BSRGAN [6], ESRGAN [8], Real-ESRGAN+ [7], SwinIR-GAN [9], StableSR [11] and DiffBIR [10]. To ensure the fairness of the comparison, we also apply the introduced color image decomposition for these SR-HIPS-based methods by replacing the detailed information in the HR color results with the information in the HR grayscale image. For all methods, we use official code and models for testing. For both StableSR and DiffBIR, we adopt the same settings as DiffGIC to reduce their demand on computational resources and set 50 denoising steps for fair comparison.

4.3 Comparing with SR-HIPS-Based Methods

Quantitative Comparisons. We first show the quantitative comparison on the DIV2K [22] validation set and the Real40 dataset. As shown in Table 1 and Table 2, all SR-HIPS-based methods achieve significant improvements in all metrics by utilizing the introduced color image decomposition. Compared with these improved SR-HIPS-based methods, our method achieves the best results on all consistency metrics. Specifically, on the DIV2K validation set, compared with the results of the best improved SR-HIPS-based method, our DiffGIC outperforms 4.23 and 0.0122 on PSNR and SSIM metrics and exhibits a reduction of 0.0232 and 2.51 in LPIPS and FID metrics. On the Real40 dataset, compared with the results of the best improved SR-HIPS-based method, our DiffGIC outperforms 3.63 and 0.013 on PSNR and SSIM metrics and exhibits a reduction of 0.0222 and 1.94 in LPIPS and FID metrics. This demonstrates the superiority of DiffGIC in retaining detailed information of the HR grayscale image.

Qualitative Comparisons. To demonstrate the effectiveness of our method, we present visual results on the DIV2K [22] validation set and Real40 dataset in Fig. 4 and Fig. 5. We can observe that DiffGIC outperforms all SR-HIPS-based methods regarding colorization quality and detail consistency with the HR grayscale image. Specifically, DiffGIC can generate the HR color image with detailed information that is highly consistent with the HR grayscale image, as shown in Fig. 4. The results generated by the SR-HIPS-based methods are not only different from the LR image in terms of color information but also different from the HR grayscale image in terms of detailed information. Furthermore, as shown in Fig. 5, DiffGIC can maintain a high degree of consistency with the HR grayscale image on facial images, while SR-HIPS-based methods generate results that are inconsistent with the details in HR grayscale image.

Table 1. Quantitative comparison with the most commonly used SR-HIPS-based methods on DIV2K [45] validation set. bold and italic represent the best and second best performance, respectively. *: results of the HIPS-based methods improved by the introduced color image decomposition.

Method	PSNR↑	SSIM↑	LPIPS↓	FID↓
BSRGAN [6]	24.92	0.7027	0.3498	36.11
ESRGAN [8]	21.64	0.5728	0.3178	39.80
Real-ESRGAN+ [7]	24.47	0.7021	0.3324	35.36
SwinIR-GAN [9]	24.69	0.7165	0.3187	30.91
DiffBIR [10]	24.00	0.6351	0.3660	31.76
StableSR [11]	21.73	0.5482	0.4071	34.70
BSRGAN*	34.37	0.9648	0.0868	6.82
ESRGAN*	**36.15**	0.9586	**0.0479**	**3.67**
Real-ESRGAN+ *	35.53	**0.9706**	0.0774	5.62
SwinIR-GAN*	34.60	0.9668	0.0785	7.26
DiffBIR*	35.20	0.9616	0.0921	4.28
StableSR*	32.89	0.9407	0.1131	6.02
DiffGIC	*40.38*	*0.9828*	*0.0247*	*1.16*

Table 2. Quantitative comparison with the most used SR-HIPS-based methods on the Real40 dataset. bold and italic represent the best and second best performance, respectively. *: results of the HIPS-based methods improved by the introduced color image decomposition.

Method	PSNR↑	SSIM↑	LPIPS↓	FID↓
BSRGAN [6]	26.88	0.7738	0.3392	40.08
ESRGAN [8]	24.67	0.6866	0.2877	31.90
Real-ESRGAN+ [7]	26.17	0.7748	0.3188	37.36
SwinIR-GAN [9]	26.62	0.7905	0.3024	33.17
DiffBIR [10]	25.11	0.6648	0.4070	27.71
StableSR [11]	23.37	0.6067	0.4122	40.32
BSRGAN*	35.46	0.9651	0.0932	7.94
ESRGAN*	**38.15**	0.9674	**0.0478**	**2.75**
Real-ESRGAN+ *	36.34	**0.9704**	0.0844	5.17
SwinIR-GAN*	35.71	0.9676	0.0855	6.73
DiffBIR*	35.19	0.9473	0.1262	4.15
StableSR*	34.18	0.9376	0.1282	5.02
DiffGIC	*41.78*	*0.9834*	*0.0256*	*0.81*

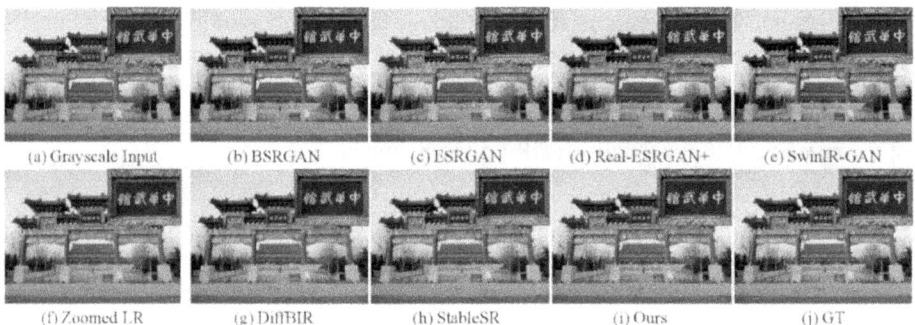

Fig. 4. Qualitative comparisons on the DIV2K [22] validation set. (Zoom in for details)

4.4 Comparison of Computational Resource Requirements

To evaluate the computational resource advantages of DiffGIC, we conducted a comparative analysis using ControlNet [2] based on Stable Diffusion 1.5 [23] as the baseline. Our measurements focused on the maximum GPU memory usage during the coloring process of 100 grayscale images, each sized 2048 × 2048 pixels. To begin, we downscaled all images to a resolution of 512 × 512 pixels and recorded the maximum GPU memory requirements using ControlNet. Subsequently, we measured the maximum GPU memory requirements of all HIPS-based methods for upscaling these low-resolution color results back to 2048 × 2048 pixels. Table 3 shows that using ControlNet to directly colorize grayscale images at high-resolution requires extensive computing resources. Adopting the HIPS-based methods reduces the required computing resources. Furthermore,

Table 3. Computational resource requirements comparison on 100 high-resolution grayscale images, each sized 2048 × 2048 pixels.

Method	Image Size	GPU Memory (GB)
ControlNet [2]	512 × 512	3.34
ControlNet [2]	2048 × 2048	15.5
ControlNet [2] + BSRGAN [6]	2048 × 2048	3.38
ControlNet [2] + ESRGAN [8]	2048 × 2048	3.38
ControlNet [2] + Real-ESRGAN + [7]	2048 × 2048	3.90
ControlNet [2] + SwinIR-GAN [9]	2048 × 2048	3.66
ControlNet [2] + DiffBIR [10]	2048 × 2048	11.76
ControlNet [2] + StableSR [11]	2048 × 2048	12.12
ControlNet [2] + DiffGIC	2048 × 2048	3.66

compared with the diffusion-based methods, our DiffGIC has significant advantages in reducing computing resources.

Table 4. Ablation studies of information sources on DIV2K [22] and Real40 dataset.

Datasets	Information Sources			PSNR↑	SSIM↑	LPIPS↓	FID↓
	LR Color Image x_{lr}	Grayscale Image y	Diffusion Prior				
DIV2K	✓	✓		26.48	0.7494	0.3843	28.08
	✓	✓	✓	38.94	0.9784	0.0296	1.59
	✓	✓	✓	40.38	0.9828	0.0247	1.16
Real40	✓	✓	✓	26.48	0.7494	0.3843	28.08
	✓	✓	✓	40.48	0.9791	0.0318	1.22
	✓			41.78	0.9834	0.0256	0.81

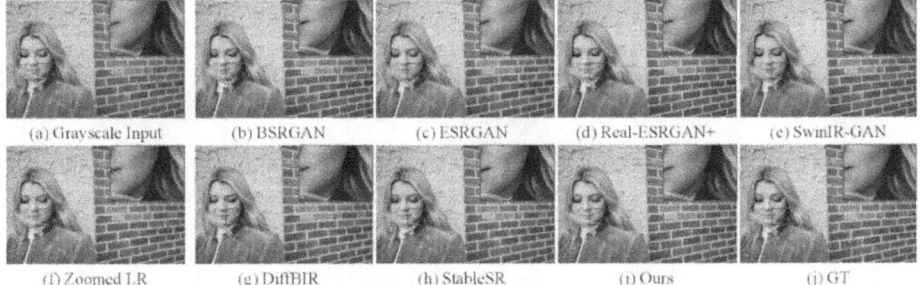

(a) Grayscale Input (b) BSRGAN (c) ESRGAN (d) Real-ESRGAN+ (e) SwinIR-GAN
(f) Zoomed LR (g) DiffBIR (h) StableSR (i) Ours (j) GT

Fig. 5. Qualitative comparisons on real-world images in the Real40 dataset. (Zoom in for details)

4.5 Ablation Study

Our DiffGIC utilizes three sources of information for hierarchical HR grayscale image colorization: the HR grayscale image y, the LR color image x_{lr}, and the diffusion prior of the pre-trained diffusion model. To verify the impact of different information sources on the results, we construct experiments on the DIV2K [22] validation set and Real40 dataset. For hierarchical image colorization, x_{lr} contains the necessary color information and is retained in all settings. As shown in Table 4, removing y results in significantly worse metrics. By introducing diffusion prior knowledge for color information correction, all metrics can be optimized. This demonstrates the importance of detailed information in HR grayscale images for hierarchical image colorization and the effectiveness of using diffusion prior for color information correction.

5 Conclusions

Motivated by the development of text-to-image models and their widespread application in image colorization tasks, this work discusses a common but underexplored problem, namely, how to use the information in HR grayscale images for HIPS-based image colorization. In this paper, we introduce the color image decomposition method based on range-null space decomposition and propose a diffusion-based color information correction method called DiffGIC. Compared with SR-HIPS-based methods, DiffGIC can generate HR color images that are highly consistent in details with the HR grayscale images at a low computational cost. Additionally, the introduced color image decomposition method can be easily applied to SR-HIPS-based methods, improving the consistency between the results and the HR grayscale images.

Acknowledgments. This work is supported in part by the National Natural Science Foundation of China under grant 62272229, the Natural Science Foundation of Jiangsu Province under grant BK20222012, and Shenzhen Science and Technology Program JCYJ20230807142001004.

References

1. Lee, J., Kim, E., Lee, Y., Kim, D., Chang, J., Choo, J.: Reference-based sketch image colorization using augmented-self reference and dense semantic correspondence. In: Proceedings of the IEEE/CVF Conference on Computer Vision and Pattern Recognition, pp. 5801–5810 (2020)
2. Zhang, L., Rao, A., Agrawala, M.: Adding conditional control to text-to-image diffusion models. In: Proceedings of the IEEE/CVF International Conference on Computer Vision, pp. 3836–3847 (2023)
3. Rombach, R., Blattmann, A., Lorenz, D., Esser, P., Ommer, B.: High-resolution image synthesis with latent diffusion models. In: Proceedings of the IEEE/CVF Conference on Computer Vision and Pattern Recognition, pp. 10684–10695 (2022)
4. Song, Y., Sohl-Dickstein, J., Kingma, D.P., Kumar, A., Ermon, S., Poole, B.: Score-based generative modeling through stochastic differential equations. In: International Conference on Learning Representations (2021)

5. Ho, J., Saharia, C., Chan, W., Fleet, D.J., Norouzi, M., Salimans, T.: Cascaded diffusion models for high fidelity image generation. J. Mach. Learn. Res. **23**(47), 1–33 (2022)
6. Zhang, K., Liang, J., Van Gool, L., Timofte, R.: Designing a practical degradation model for deep blind image super-resolution. In: Proceedings of the IEEE/CVF International Conference on Computer Vision, pp. 4791–4800 (2021)
7. Wang, X., Xie, L., Dong, C., Shan, Y.: Real-Esrgan: training real-world blind super-resolution with pure synthetic data. In: Proceedings of the IEEE/CVF International Conference on Computer Vision, pp. 1905–1914 (2021)
8. Wang, X., et al.: ESRGAN: enhanced super-resolution generative adversarial networks. In: Proceedings of the European Conference on Computer Vision Workshops, p. 0 (2018)
9. Liang, J., Cao, J., Sun, G., Zhang, K., Van Gool, L., Timofte, R.: SwinIR: image restoration using Swin transformer. In: Proceedings of the IEEE/CVF International Conference on Computer Vision, pp. 1833–1844 (2021)
10. Lin, X., et al.: DiffBIR: towards blind image restoration with generative diffusion prior. arXiv preprint arXiv:2308.15070 (2023)
11. Wang, J., Yue, Z., Zhou, S., Chan, K.C., Loy, C.C.: Exploiting diffusion prior for real-world image super-resolution. arXiv preprint arXiv:2305.07015 (2023)
12. Wang, Y., Hu, Y., Yu, J., Zhang, J.: GAN prior based null-space learning for consistent super-resolution. In: Proceedings of the AAAI Conference on Artificial Intelligence, vol. 37, pp. 2724–2732 (2023)
13. Li, L., Liang, D., Gao, Y., Huang, S.J., Chen, S.: ALL-E: aesthetics-guided low-light image enhancement. arXiv preprint arXiv:2304.14610 (2023)
14. Wang, Yi., Menghan Xia, Lu., Qi, J.S., Qiao, Yu.: PalGAN: Image Colorization with Palette Generative Adversarial Networks. In: Avidan, S., Brostow, G., Cissé, M., Farinella, G.M., Hassner, T. (eds.) Computer Vision – ECCV 2022: 17th European Conference, Tel Aviv, Israel, October 23–27, 2022, Proceedings, Part XV, pp. 271–288. Springer Nature Switzerland, Cham (2022). https://doi.org/10.1007/978-3-031-19784-0_16
15. Li, S., Higashita, R., Fu, H., Li, H., Niu, J., Liu, J.: Content-preserving diffusion model for unsupervised AS-OCT image Despeckling. In: Greenspan, H., et al. International Conference on Medical Image Computing and Computer-Assisted Intervention, vol. 14226, pp. 660–670. Springer (2023). https://doi.org/10.1007/978-3-031-43990-2_62
16. Lin, J., Xiao, P., Wang, Y., Zhang, R., Zeng, X.: Diffcolor: toward high fidelity text-guided image colorization with diffusion models. arXiv preprint arXiv:2308.01655 (2023)
17. Wang, Y., Yu, J., Zhang, J.: Zero-shot image restoration using denoising diffusion null-space model. In: The Eleventh International Conference on Learning Representations (2023). https://openreview.net/forum?id=mRieQgMtNTQ
18. Jiménez, Á.B.: Mixture of diffusers for scene composition and high resolution image generation. arXiv preprint arXiv:2302.02412 (2023)
19. Song, J., Meng, C., Ermon, S.: Denoising diffusion implicit models. arXiv preprint arXiv:2010.02502 (2020)
20. Dhariwal, P., Nichol, A.: Diffusion models beat GANs on image synthesis. Adv. Neural. Inf. Process. Syst. **34**, 8780–8794 (2021)
21. Russakovsky, O., et al.: ImageNet large scale visual recognition challenge. Int. J. Comput. Vision **115**, 211–252 (2015)
22. Agustsson, E., Timofte, R.: Ntire 2017 challenge on single image super-resolution: dataset and study. In: Proceedings of the IEEE/CVF Conference on Computer Vision and Pattern Recognition workshops, pp. 126–135 (2017)
23. Ramesh, A., Dhariwal, P., Nichol, A., Chu, C., Chen, M.: Hierarchical text-conditional image generation with clip latents. arXiv preprint arXiv:2204.06125 (2022)

Chinese Character Image Inpainting with Skeleton Extraction and Adversarial Learning

Di Sun[1], Tingting Yang[1], Xiangyu Pan[2], Jiahao Wang[2], and Gang Pan[2](✉)

[1] College of Artificial Intelligence, Tianjin University of Science and Technology, Tianjin 300222, China
[2] College of Intelligence and Computing, Tianjin University, Tianjin 300350, China
pangang@tju.edu.cn

Abstract. Chinese character image inpainting aims to restore the missing textual regions with realistic contents. Existing algorithms for text image inpainting are primarily designed for English characters, however, their performance is suboptimal when applied to Chinese characters. The primary challenge in Chinese character image inpainting lies in the scarcity of open-source datasets for this task. Additionally, conventional image inpainting algorithms fail to account for the guiding significance of the stroke topology structure inherent in Chinese characters during the inpainting process. In this paper, we propose a skeleton extraction algorithm based on line thinning, and contribute a dataset of Chinese character images and their skeleton images accordingly. In particular, we propose a skeleton extraction guided generative framework skeletonGAN for Chinese character inpainting, where the skeleton of Chinese characters is used as prior knowledge to guide the inpainting process. The whole framework comprises two parts: an SE network for skeleton-based Chinese character skeleton extraction and inpainting, and an SR network dedicated to Chinese character image inpainting. Experimental results demonstrate that the proposed method successfully fills the missing character information and achieves significant image inpainting results.

Keywords: Adversarial learning · Chinese character image inpainting · skeleton extraction

1 Introduction

The task of natural image inpainting has been extensively studied, but there are still few researches on Chinese character image inpainting. As a kind of ideographic characters, Chinese characters have a huge number and styles compared with English letters, and each character has a different and complex structure, which makes the task of Chinese image inpainting more difficult.

Due to the unique topological structure of Chinese characters, some methods treat this task as a line extraction and restoration problem [1, 2]. These methods are effective when the stroke has a clear structure, but they cannot handle multiple intersections when dealing with complex structures. In order to generate more realistic results, some studies [3] utilize generative adversarial networks (GANs) to restore Chinese character images. While these methods can yield smoother strokes, the lack of morphological constraints limits their effectiveness in repairing larger defect areas. As the field of image style transfer continues to evolve, some alternative methods [4–6] are presented for Chinese character font generation based on pairwise datasets. However, the creation of paired training datasets often requires significant human resources. Because the Chinese character image dataset is scarce, how to create a Chinese character image dataset with sufficient data quantity and rich data content is a problem.

Inspired by the idea image inpainting technology based on prior knowledge and text style transfer technology based on skeleton extraction, this paper aims to propose a Chinese character image inpainting method based on text skeleton extraction, which better combines the structural features of the text itself to complete the task of Chinese character image inpainting.

One challenge is shared with all the supervised methods: the training process needs paired data as ground truth. But the Chinese character image dataset is scarce, collecting a large scale Chinese character image dataset needs a lot of efforts. In addition, it has two unique scientific challenges: (i) The data set needs to provide a text skeleton image corresponding to the Chinese character image, and (ii) How to better use the structural information provided by the text skeleton image to guide the inpainting process, to ensure that the repaired Chinese character image has a better consistency in strokes.

We address the above challenges by contributing a large scale dataset and developing a deep supervised approach for Chinese character image inpainting. For the dataset, we introduce line thinning to generate datasets of Chinese character images and their skeleton images. For the network, we propose a two-branch image inpainting network inspired by GANs, called skeletonGAN. SkeletonGAN divides the inpainting process of Chinese character images into two stages. The first stage, known as the Character Skeleton Extraction Network (SE), aims to extract the skeleton information from the input defective image of Chinese characters, ultimately obtaining a completed text skeleton. SE employs the concept of text image style transfer to extract structural information from the input defective image of Chinese characters, eliminating stroke style characteristics such as stroke thickness and writing strength, and repairing the extracted defective skeleton structure. The second stage is referred to as the Chinese Characters Image Inpainting Network Based on Text Skeleton (SR). The purpose is to use the complete text skeleton information obtained in the previous stage as a prior knowledge to guide the inpainting of Chinese character images. This process can also be regarded as assign the style of the input Chinese character image to the text skeleton style transfer task.

In summary, the main contributions of this paper are summarized as follows:

- We offer a new perspective into Chinese character inpainting. The combination of adversarial training with skeleton extraction strengthens the perception of structural areas, allowing the model to synthesize the accurate contents.
- We design a skeleton extraction algorithm model based on line thinning, and contribute a Chinese character image dataset with corresponding skeleton images.

- We propose a Chinese character image inpainting framework (skeletonGAN) based on skeleton extraction and adversarial learning, which consists of an adversarial learning-based text skeleton extraction and restoration network SE and a Chinese character image inpainting network SR based on the text skeleton image.

2 Related Work

2.1 Chinese Character Inpainting

Compared with general image inpainting, Chinese characters have complex structures and styles, which make the work of Chinese character image inpainting very attractive and challenging. Recent years, there have also been some works on Chinese character inpainting. For example, CGAN [7] has been used to remove grids from images to recover Chinese characters. Li et al. [8] propose an improved architecture of GoogLeNet, extracting directional Gabor features as prior knowledge and incorporating the obtained feature maps into both the input layer and the original image. Ge et al. [9] pose an occlusion offline handwritten Chinese character inpainting method using a self-attention mechanism. This mechanism effectively addresses this problem, which can use the information of the whole image by using clues from all feature locations. Wang et al. [10] introduce a framework for the generation of semantically enhanced Chinese character inpainting, incorporating a Global Semantic Supervision Module to regulate context semantics. Li et al. [11] propose a prototype-feature-based structure guided generation framework, which is not only capable of adapting to multiple font styles, but also can comprehensively recover the font structures and strokes without the need for masking information through inference on the representations of styles. Zhao et al. [12] dish a character autoencoder based on the branch convolutional channel attention module, which replaces the traditional down-sampling module with BCCAM, gives different weights to repair occluded and unoccluded areas. Zheng et al. [13] put forward the EA-GAN network, which can accurately restore text structure when the damage area is large by introducing the attention mechanism of example texts, for repairing damaged texts in ancient Chinese books. Li et al. [14] develop a diffusion model based method DiffACR to automate the inpainting of eroded ancient Chinese characters. The method simulates erosionfication as a form of cold diffusion and uses a prior mask extracted directly from the damaged image to guide the inpainting process.

2.2 Character Image Style Transfer

Text image style transfer task is a branch of image style transfer task research, which aims to change the stylistic attributes of text while preserving its text content. In recent years, there has been a gradual emergence of research specifically focusing on image style migration for Chinese characters. Tian et al. [15] utilize the pix2pix model [16] by the paired training data to address the issue of image style migration in Chinese character font generation. Chang et al. [17] innovatively adapt the CycleGAN model, to migrate the stylistic feature patterns of images to Chinese font generation using unpaired training data. However, this method may encounter the pattern collapse problem due to the

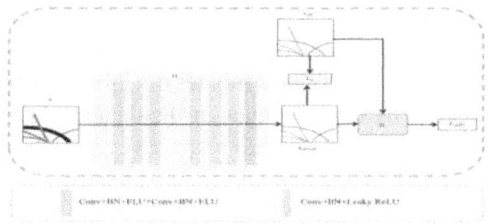

Fig. 1. The skeleton extraction architecture for dataset manufacture. It consists of a generator G and a discriminator D. The generator is based on constant size long convolution follows the ConvBatchNorm-ReLU architecture.

presence of Chinese characters with numerous highly similar strokes [18], which significantly reduces the diversity and quality of the generated results. Zeng et al. [19] pose the StrokeGAN model, which incorporates stroke coding to capture the pattern information of Chinese characters, thereby alleviating the pattern collapse problem of CycleGAN and enhancing the stylistic diversity of its generated characters. Subsequently, Gao et al. [20] present ChiroGAN, a multi-style Chinese character image style migration model based on skeleton transformation and stroke drawing. While these methodologies offer versatile approaches to the Chinese character inpainting task, they fail to yield the anticipated outcomes, indicating that significant challenges persist in our Chinese character inpainting endeavors.

3 Datasets

At present, there is no publicly available dataset specifically for Chinese character inpainting. To address this limitation, we design a skeleton extraction network to extract the skeleton structure from the input image and generate a dataset of Chinese character skeleton images.

Because the Chinese character image and the line image have a similar pair of line structure, inspired by the related research on line vectorization, we use randomly generated lines with different thicknesses and corresponding uniform line images as the training set, and train a line thinning network through adversarial training. Then the model after training is applied to the Chinese character image to generate the corresponding skeleton image, as shown in Fig. 1. The skeleton extraction architecture for dataset manufacture. It consists of a generator G and a discriminator D. The generator is based on constant size long convolution follows the ConvBatchNorm-ReLU architecture. We posit that the skeleton image corresponding to a Chinese character image can effectively remove calligraphic style attributes, such as aspect ratio, radical interval, and stroke density, while preserving skeletal structure elements like thickness, inclination, writing intensity, and the initial and final shape. These skeleton structures can offer prior knowledge during inpainting, thereby facilitating the generation of correctly structured Chinese character images.

We utilize this random masked image to process the Chinese character skeleton images used in the Chinese character image pairs, thereby providing data support for training. The dataset encompasses 3755 commonly used Chinese characters as per the first-level national standard of Chinese characters, and contains a variety of font styles including printed, handwritten, and stylised images of Chinese characters to adapt actual usage. Figure 3 shows some example images in the dataset. The first row depicts the images of Chinese characters paired with their respective text skeletons, while the second rows display the corresponding masked ones shows some images in our dataset.

4 Method

skeletonGAN has two subnetworks, Skeleton Extraction (SE) and Character Restoration (SR). The overview of the network is depicted in Fig. 2.

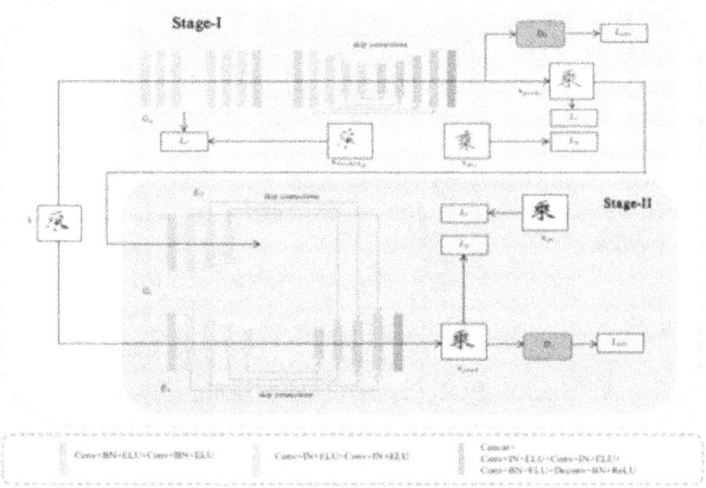

Fig. 2. The overview of skeletonGAN network, SE is used to extract the text skeleton image, in the second stage, SR uses the repaired text skeleton image as a prior knowledge to guide the inpainting process.

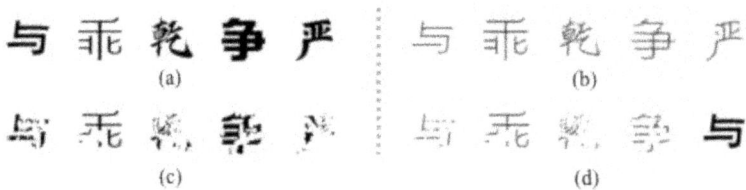

Fig. 3. Some example images in the dataset. The first row depicts the images of Chinese characters paired with their respective text skeletons, while the second rows display the corresponding masked ones.

4.1 Generator

The initial stage SE entails the extraction of incomplete features of Chinese character skeletons from defective images. Subsequently, the restored text skeleton images serve as prior knowledge to direct the restoration process in the next stage. The generator *Ge* extracts skeleton features and synthesizes incomplete Chinese character skeleton images, which are bifurcated into two distinct parts. This method improves the quality of the synthesis results, especially for the connection details of the Chinese character skeleton image. The first segment of *Ge* employs a long convolution structure, primarily refining the input image, eliminating stroke style information, and yielding an incomplete feature of the Chinese character skeleton image. Conversely, the second segment of *Gr* utilizes an encoder-decoder framework to synthesize a comprehensive skeleton image of Chinese characters. To preserve more intricate details, a skip connection structure is incorporated between the encoder and decoder. Instead of employing pooling operations, we adopt convolution with 3 × 3 pixel strides for downsampling, ensuring greater spatial support for masked region generation. The skeleton information can well retain the structure and arrangement information of the character strokes and at the same time eliminate all the stroke style information. We believe that the use of text skeleton images to guide the process of Chinese character images inpainting can be regarded as giving the calligraphy style to the character skeleton. So in the second stage SR, the generator *Gr* employs two encoders, E_1 and E_2, to extract features of incomplete Chinese character images and character skeleton images respectively. A decoder is then used to amalgamate and decode these two encoded features. The function of encoder E_1 is to extract features from input images as the primary encoder, while encoder E_2 extracts features from Chinese character skeleton images. The input image can provide calligraphy style features, and using Chinese character skeleton images as prior knowledge to guide the process of Chinese character image repair can be viewed as assigning the style of the input image to the Chinese character skeleton image.

4.2 Discriminator

To further promote the generation of more realistic results, we introduce a discriminator *D* as a binary classifier to distinguish real images from fake ones in both stages. The discriminator in the first stage functions to enhance the quality of the output Chinese skeleton image, ensuring that the stroke structure closely aligns with the actual Chinese image. The discriminator in the second stage is designed to encourage the generator to effectively integrate the structural information from the Chinese skeleton image, resulting in smoother and clearer outcomes.

4.3 Loss Function

The input masked Chinese character images of the network are represented as $\tilde{x}$ and the target output images of the network are represented as x_{gt}, the final output of the generator is expressed as x_{pred}. We first introduce a per-pixel reconstruction loss L_r to the generator, which is the L_2 between the generated Chinese character image and the ground truth image x_{gt}.

$$L_r = \|x_{gt} - \tilde{x}\|_2^2 \tag{1}$$

In order to make the generated image have a high structural similarity with x_{gt}, we then adopt a perceptual loss L_{p_e} to enhance the detailed features. L_{p_e} solves the problem of the influence of multiple fonts, which is the L_1 distance between the output image and the ground truth image, the formula for L_{p_e} can be expressed as:

$$L_{p_e} = \sum_{l=L-2}^{L-1} \beta_l \|\phi_l(x_{gt}) - \phi_l(x_{pred})\|_1 \tag{2}$$

when the mean square error loss function is used, the output image will be relatively smooth, the details are not real enough, and part of the high-frequency information is lost, the formula for L_{p_r} can be expressed as:

$$L_{p_r} = \sum_{l=L-2}^{L-1} \beta_l \|\phi_l(x_{gt}) - \phi_l(x_{pred})\|_2^2 \tag{3}$$

We further employ the adversarial loss. The adversarial loss judges the ability of discriminator to predict whether the character image is real or not. We use x_{pred} and x_{gt} as inputs, where the generator G is trained to minimize this objective against the adversarial D that tries to maximize it. The adversarial losses of SR and SE are expressed by the formulae respectively as

$$L_{adv_e}(G_e, D_e) = E_{(x_{gt})}\log(D_e(x_{gt})) + E_{(x_{pred})}\log(1 - D_e(x_{pred})) \tag{4}$$

$$L_{adv_r}(G_r, D_r) = E_{(x_{gt})}\log(D_r(x_{gt})) + E_{(\tilde{x})}\log(1 - D_r(x_{pred})) \tag{5}$$

The overall loss is defined as follow:

$$L_{skeletonGAN} = L_{SE} + L_{SR} \tag{6}$$

where the loss metric of LSE is denoted as:

$$L_{SE} = \lambda_r L_r + \lambda_{p_e} L_{p_e} + \lambda_{adv} L_{adv_e} \tag{7}$$

where the loss metric of LSR is denoted as:

$$L_{SR} = \lambda_r L_r + \lambda_{p_r} L_{p_r} + \lambda_{adv} L_{adv_r} \tag{8}$$

5 Experimental Results

SkeletonGAN is implemented based on python and pytorch. In training, we set the value of λ_r, λ_{p_e}, λ_{p_r} and λ_{adv} to 1.2, 0.5, 1 and 0.1. We also employ batch normalization in most convolutional blocks to encourage stability of the proposed model. In the experiment, our model perform a complete end-to-end training using the Adam optimizer. The batch size is set to 128. We train it on NVIDIA GeForce RTX 2080Ti GPU with 12GB GPU memory.

5.1 Quantitative Analysis

Figure 4 shows Chinese character inpainting results on the proposed dataset. It can be seen that the proposed algorithm yields satisfactory results, both at the level of text skeleton images and in the final restoration outcomes. Particularly when the style of Chinese character images is strong and the strokes are thicker, it can still generate relatively correct restoration results for Chinese character images. This is because at the first stage, the stroke style features in the input Chinese character images have been eliminated, which can simplify the restoration process of text skeleton images. This part can also be regarded as a restoration task similar to fine-line text images. The complete text skeleton image is used as a priori knowledge, combined with the tasks of image restoration and text style transfer, to ultimately obtain a complete Chinese character image. From the resultant image, it can be clearly seen that the direction of strokes and overall structure in the final restored Chinese character image are consistent with those in the text skeleton image. This also indirectly confirms the correctness of the skeletonGAN.

5.2 Qualitative Results

We compare the inpainting performance with the classic methods: the Examplar-Based Image Inpainting (EBII) [21], and HAN [3]. As illustrated in Fig. 5, the traditional method EBII synthesizes unrecognizable characters due to the large mask. HAN uses hierarchical discriminator to make the characters clear but it is easy to generate wrong characters. Our method can accurately capture visual information, the stroke lines are more smooth. Furthermore, a comparison of the inpainting results for the "Luo" character reveals that the proposed method is superior in preserving the stroke style of Chinese characters, with the stroke style being reapplied to the text skeleton image during the repair process.

5.3 Ablation Study

We show the influence of different factors of the proposed network by removing corresponding loss functions. The quantitative results are illustrated in Table 1. We find that these loss functions can all improve the effect of the model, but the action direction is slightly different. For example, L_{adv} is a crucial part by allowing the generator to avoid strange strokes and make the results semantically correct. Style consistency loss L_p reduces the artificial appearance, such as blurring, making the resulting image sharper overall.

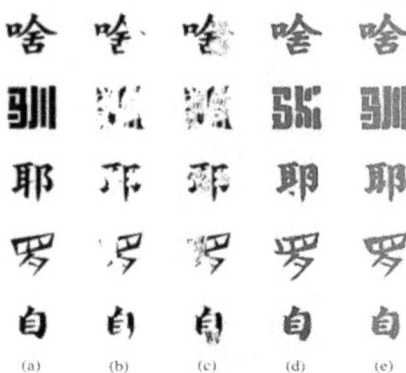

Fig. 4. Visual comparison with the classic methods: (a) ground truth images, (b) original input images, (c)–(e) are results from EBII, HAN, and our method, respectively.

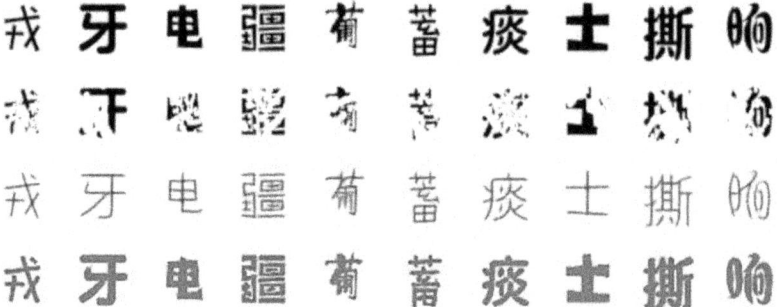

Fig. 5. Chinese character inpainting results on the proposed dataset. In each row from top to down: ground truth images, original input images, target skeleton images and our inpainting results.

Table 1. Inpainting results in terms of PSNR, SSIM, and OCR for ablation study. The values in bold means the best performances.

Methods	no-L_p	no-L_r	no-L_{adv}	skeletonGAN	Groundtruth
PSNR	24.803	23.5209	23.4820	**25.0472**	–
SSIM	0.7980	0.7148	0.7093	**0.8986**	–
OCR	0.7874	0.7642	0.6219	0.8384	**0.8510**

6 Conclusion

This paper demonstrates the effectiveness of introducing skeleton extraction into Chinese character image inpainting. Initially, we utilize paired line images to train a text skeleton extraction network based on line refinement. This effectively addresses the scarcity of skeleton image datasets for Chinese character images, leading to the creation of a new dataset comprising both image and skeleton images of Chinese characters, which are annotated with textual information. The dataset generation process is highly adaptable and can be modified and expanded according to specific requirements. Subsequently, we propose a skeleton extraction guided inpainting scheme that separates the structural characteristics of character images from stroke style attributes and employs the character skeleton as a foundational knowledge source to guide the inpainting process. The experimental results demonstrate that the proposed method outperformed compared models in subjective and objective comparisons.

Acknowledgments. This work was funded by the Natural Science Foundation of Tianjin (No. 21JCYBJC00640), 2023 CCF-Baidu Songguo Foundation (Research on Scene Text Recognition Based on PaddlePaddle).

References

1. Nazeri, K., Ng, E., Joseph, T., Qureshi, F.Z., Ebrahimi, M.: Edgeconnect: Generative image inpainting with adversarial edge learning (2019). arXiv:1901.00212
2. Sasaki, K., Iizuka, S., Simo-Serra, E., Ishikawa, H.: Joint gap detection and inpainting of line drawings. In: Proceedings of the IEEE Conference on Computer Vision and Pattern Recognition, pp. 5725–5733 (2017)
3. Chang, J., Gu, Y., Zhang, Y., Wang, Y.-F., Innovation, C.: Chinese handwriting imitation with hierarchical generative adversarial network. In: BMVC, p. 290 (2018)
4. Chang, J., Gu, Y.: Chinese typography transfer (2017). arXiv:1707.04904
5. Jiang, Y., Lian, Z., Tang, Y., Xiao, J.: DCFont: an end-to-end deep Chinese font generation system. In: SIGGRAPH Asia 2017 Technical Briefs, pp. 1–4 (2017)
6. Wu, S.-J., Yang, C.-Y., Hsu, J.Y.-J.: CalliGAN: style and structure-aware Chinese calligraphy character generator (2020). arXiv:2005.12500
7. Zhong, Z., Yin, F., Zhang, X.-Y., Liu, C.-L.: Handwritten Chinese character blind inpainting with conditional generative adversarial nets. In: 2017 4th IAPR Asian Conference on Pattern Recognition (ACPR), pp. 804–809 (2017). IEEE
8. Li, J., Song, G., Zhang, M.: Occluded offline handwritten Chinese character recognition using deep convolutional generative adversarial network and improved GoogleNet. Neural Comput. Appl. **32**, 4805–4819 (2020)
9. Song, G., Li, J., Wang, Z.: Occluded offline handwritten Chinese character inpainting via generative adversarial network and self-attention mechanism. Neurocomputing **415**, 146–156 (2020)
10. Wang, J., Pan, G., Sun, D., Zhang, J.: Chinese character inpainting with contextual semantic constraints. In: Proceedings of the 29th ACM International Conference on Multimedia, pp. 1829–1837 (2021)
11. Li, H., et al.: Generative character inpainting guided by structural information. Vis. Comput. **37**, 2895–2906 (2021)
12. Zhao, L., Yuan, Z., Lou, Y., Xu, Q., Qiao, X.: An auto-encoder of inscription character inpainting based on branch convolutional channel attention module (2023)
13. Wenjun, Z., Benpeng, S., Ruiqi, F., Xihua, P., Shanxiong, C.: EA-GAN: restoration of text in ancient Chinese books based on an example attention generative adversarial network. Herit. Sci. **11**(1), 42 (2023)

14. Li, H., Du, C., Jiang, Z., Zhang, Y., Ma, J., Ye, C.: Towards automated Chinese ancient character restoration: a diffusion-based method with a new dataset. In: Proceedings of the AAAI Conference on Artificial Intelligence, vol. 38, pp. 3073–3081 (2024)
15. Chen, J., Ji, Y., Chen, H., Xu, X.: Learning one-to-many stylised Chinese character transformation and generation by generative adversarial networks. IET Image Proc. **13**(14), 2680–2686 (2019)
16. Isola, P., Zhu, J.-Y., Zhou, T., Efros, A.A.: Image-to-image translation with conditional adversarial networks. In: Proceedings of the IEEE Conference on Computer Vision and Pattern Recognition, pp. 1125–1134 (2017)
17. Chang, B., Zhang, Q., Pan, S., Meng, L.: Generating handwritten Chinese characters using CycleGAN. In: 2018 IEEE Winter Conference on Applications of Computer Vision (WACV), pp. 199–207 (2018). IEEE
18. Goodfellow, I., et al.: Generative adversarial nets. Adv. Neural Inf. Process. Syst. **27** (2014)
19. Zeng, J., Chen, Q., Liu, Y., Wang, M., Yao, Y.: StrokeGAN: Reducing mode collapse in Chinese font generation via stroke encoding. In: Proceedings of the AAAI Conference on Artificial Intelligence, vol. 35, pp. 3270–3277 (2021)
20. Gao, Y., Wu, J.: GAN-based unpaired Chinese character image translation via skeleton transformation and stroke rendering. In: Proceedings of the AAAI Conference on Artificial Intelligence, vol. 34, pp. 646–653 (2020)
21. Criminisi, A., Perez, P., Toyama, K.: Region filling and object removal by exemplar-based image inpainting. IEEE Trans. Image Process. **13**(9), 1200–1212 (2004). https://doi.org/10.1109/TIP.2004.833105

The Weakly Supervised Network of Hierarchical Attention Mechanism for Fine-Grained Classification

Qian Long[1], Gaihua Wang[1,2(✉)], Hongwei Qu[3(✉)], Jingxuan Yao[1], and Bolun Zhu[1]

[1] College of Artificial Intelligence, Tianjin University of Science and Technology,
Tianjin 300457, China
{longqian,wanggh}@tust.edu.cn
[2] Hubei Key Laboratory of Optical Information and Pattern Recognition, Wuhan Institute of Technology, Wuhan 430205, China
[3] Wuhan Electronic Information Institute, Wuhan 430019, China
394139525@qq.com

Abstract. Fine-grained classification is challenging task to discriminate subtle and local differences from sub-categories. Many works improve the accuracy by relying heavily upon the use of the object or part annotations of images whose label are costly. In the paper, a weakly supervised network is proposed for fine-grained image classification without using expensive annotations. Firstly, it learns object detector by hierarchical attention mechanism automatically and localizes the objects or its parts to extract salient feature. Then, based on the theory of prototypical networks, it learns a metric loss function by computing distances to prototype representations of each class which is unsupervised clustering methods. Both are jointed to remove useless information or noise patches and retain discriminative features. Finally, we apply the proposed method to complete the classification of disaster-scene images. Compared with other methods, experimental results demonstrate our method is generalized and robust to different datasets.

Keywords: Fine-grained Classification · Hierarchical Attention Mechanism · Salient Feature · Metric Loss Function · Disaster-scene

1 Introduction

Fine-grained classification aims to recognize subordinate classes within basic-level categories, such as species of birds [1], flowers [2], animals [3], and models of cars [4]. Unlike general methods, the localization of objects and their parts is crucial for fine-grained image classification [5, 6]. It should be capable of localizing and representing the marginal differences within subordinate categories, which makes fine-grained recognition a challenging task.

Early works generally adopt a two-stage learning framework: firstly, they localize the discriminative regions of objects and extract discriminative features, then encode the discriminative features for training classifiers. These methods provide a way of encoding the salient features for distinguishing sub-categories. However, they also have some limitations: (1) the number of parts used is highly empirical, which limits flexibility and makes generalization to other datasets difficult. (2) They heavily rely on labor-consuming labeling, making them applicable only in domains where such annotations are difficult or expensive to obtain.

To address these problems, some researchers have begun to focus on recognizing sub-categories via weakly supervised part detection instead of using expensive annotations. Lin et al. [7] introduce bilinear pooling as the outer product of features, which can capture localized feature interactions from two CNNs. And it has been shown to achieve impressive performance on a wide range of visual tasks. However, bilinear features have high dimensionality, which makes them impractical for subsequent analysis. The compact bilinear representation [8] is derived through a novel kernelized analysis of bilinear pooling, providing insights into the discriminative power of bilinear pooling but with only a few dimensions. Dubey et al. [9] propose concepts from pairwise learning and label confusion, taking a step towards solving the problems of overfitting. Weakly Supervised Spatial Group Attention Network (WSSGA-Net) [10] highlights the correct semantic feature regions for more accurate classification by establishing a semantic enhancement mechanism. PHPQ [11] captures and retains fine-grained semantic information in multi-level features. GCA [12] uses clustering to divide the data into small clusters, and then aggregates them to get fine-grained information.

Object localization is very important for fine-grained image classification. To remove the influence of background noise and obtain meaningful global features, this paper proposes a hierarchical attention framework to localize subtle differences among different subcategories for fine-grained image classification.

2 The Proposed Method

The proposed method consists of four parts: plain CNN including Base conv-net and Conv Block, Attention Block including Attention Map and Max K Response Block, Interaction Model and total loss function. Figure 1 is the structure of network.

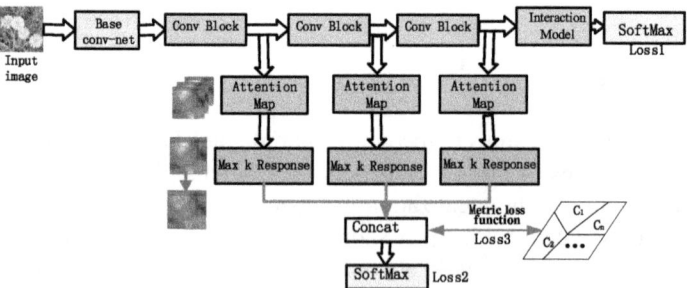

Fig. 1. The structure of network

2.1 Plain CNN

Given an image I, which is resized with $H \times W \times C$, H is the height of image, W is the width of image, C is the channel of image. Firstly, the input image I is passed by a plain CNN. CNN model is fine-tuned from the pre-trained CNN on ImageNet. In our experiments, our plain CNN models include VGG-16 and ResNet-18. Conv Blocks are composed of the conv3, conv4 and conv5 in VGG-16. For Resnet-18, Conv Blocks are con3_x, con4_x and con5_x. The original VGG-16 and Resnet-18 have 1000-class outputs. In this work, CNN model is fine-tuned on ImageNet. Then we get layers from conv1 to conv5 to train our datasets. The last fully-connected layer is reduced to related classes of datasets.

2.2 Attention Block

The whole framework generates a saliency map for input image from a hierarchical attention model. In hierarchical attention model, we extract attention features, which can filter out noisy patches and select the relevant objects. Given feature maps F from Conv Blocks. The outputs F of Conv Blocks are processed by attention mechanism $Mask_c(x, y)$. We define $f_c(x, y)$ at spatial location (x, y) of channel c. The saliency map of is expressed by

$$Mask_c(x, y) = sigmoid(f_c(x, y)) \qquad (1)$$

The output of Attention Map in each layer is computed by

$$M = F(1 + Mask_c) \qquad (2)$$

Multi-scale features are extracted by hierarchy layers. The output of saliency map can indicate the representative regions.

When get saliency feature from attention map, it is that some irrelevant region should be filter out and useful information should be retained. To complete the task, we add the Max K Response Block to find main objects or relevant region. The outputs of attention map are resized to column vector. Then we choose salient feature from the main objects. The max K saliency values are selected by Max K Response Block (Fig. 1). Given the output M of attention map. We select max k values from the M_i (i = 1,2,3). S is the concatenated vector from max k values. It can be expressed by

$$S = topk(M_1, M_2, M_3) \qquad (3)$$

2.3 The Total Loss Functions

Based on attention block, we get some salient features. In the training stage, each prototype C_k is the mean vector of the extracted salient features belonging to its class. N_k is the number of the kth class. Each epoch, When the input belongs to the kth class, we compute a distance between the output S of attention block and C_k. The distance is defined as the metric loss function. It is expressed by

$$Loss3 = MSELoss(S_k, C_k) \qquad (4)$$

After updating the gradient, we update the prototype C_k by

$$C_k = \frac{1}{N_k} \sum_k^S \qquad (5)$$

The total loss function has three parts. The first part is the loss of whole framework. It is loss1 in Fig. 1. The second part is the loss of the attention Block. It is the loss2 in Fig. 1. The third part is the metric loss function.

3 Experiments

All experiments are performed by PyTorch on NVIDIA GeForce RTX 2060 GPUs. The proposed approach is compared with different methods to verify its effectiveness. Accuracy is adopted as the evaluation metric to evaluate the classification performances. No extra annotation or object bounding box is used in the whole experiments.

3.1 Datasets and Baselines

Datasets. The CUB-200-2011 dataset comprises 11,788 images categorized into 200 subcategories, making it one of the most used datasets for fine-grained image classification. The Stanford Dogs dataset, constructed from images and annotations sourced from ImageNet, serves the purpose of fine-grained image classification tasks. It encompasses 20,580 images representing 120 breeds of dogs from diverse regions worldwide. The Oxford-Flower-17 dataset, on the other hand, contains 17 types of flowers, with each type consisting of 80 images.

Training deep neural networks directly on fine-grained datasets is often impractical, necessitating data preprocessing. In experiments, data augmentation techniques are commonly employed to augment the training image count, including random cropping, translation, and scaling. During training, images are typically randomly cropped to 224 × 224 patches to mitigate overfitting, with multiple patches extracted from the entire image for training purposes.

Baselines. We split state-of-the-art methods into two groups by the basic CNNs used in these methods: VGG-16 and ResNet-18, both of which achieved state-of-the-art performance on ImageNet. We initialize both network with the pre-trained network on the ImageNet and use a weight decay of 0.0001 with a momentum of 0.9 and set the initial learning rate to 0.1. The learning rate is divided by 10 every 20 iterations.

3.2 Comparison with All Kinds of Methods

We compare the proposed method with original BCNN, CBP and HBP. BCNN is a method which replaces the fully connected layers with bilinear pooling. CBP is a compact bilinear pooling method. In original paper of CBP, the features of CBP uses RM and TS projections. In our experiments, it uses TS projections. HBP is hierarchical bilinear pooling method which can integrate multiple cross-layer bilinear features to enhance their representation capability. We define the hierarchical attention model as HA model. We also test the performance of HA model. The model combining the hierarchical attention with prototypical networks is called as WSHA model.

The WSHA model is added on BCNN network, which is called as WSHA-BCNN. The WSHA model is added on CBP network, which is called as WSHA-CBP. The baseline is VGG-16 for BCNN and CBP. We add the proposed model on HBP network, which is called as WSHA-HBP. The baseline is ResNet-18 for WSHA -HBP.

Experiments on CUB-200-2011. Tables 1 and 2 show the comparison results on CUB-200-2011 dataset at the aspect of classification accuracy with 448 × 448 patches and 224 × 224 patches of images. CBP is a compact bilinear pooling method. We add the proposed method to CBP. WSHA-CBP offers the best accuracy that is 77.65%. We add the proposed HA model on HBP network which is called as HAHBP. The baseline is ResNet-18 for HAHBP. The accuracy is 74.82 higher than HBP network. We also test the accuracy of some recent methods, such as PHPQ [11], GCA [12]. PHPQ captures and retains fine-grained semantic information in multi-level features. GCA use cluster to divides the data into small clusters, and then aggregates them. In comparison, the WSHA-CBP achieves the highest classification accuracy among all methods without object and parts annotations.

We also resize original images. The training images are randomly cropped 224 × 224 patches. The test images are center cropped 224 × 224. The results are showed in Table 2. The accuracy also can be improved by using proposed model. If we use the VGG-16 to extract feature, the baseline method is higher than others baseline methods on CBP. Neither object nor parts annotations are used in these approaches, which leads fine-grained image classification to practical application. For different methods, it has an impressive boost when adding our attention model.

Table 1. Table shows the comparison results on CUB-200-2011 dataset with 448 × 448 patches.

Method	Base Model	Accuracy (%)
BCNN	VGG-16	70.34
PHPQ	Resnet-18	74.13
GCA	Vit-B/16	73.40
CBP	VGG-16	72.75
HACBP	VGG-16	73.50
WSHA-CBP	VGG-16	**77.65**
HBP	VGG-16	70.18
	Resnet-18	69.69
HAHBP	Resnet-18	74.82

Table 2. Table shows the comparison results on CUB-200-2011 dataset with 224 × 224 patches.

Method	Base Model	Accuracy (%)
BCNN	VGG-16	72.01
CBP	VGG-16	76.04
HACBP	VGG-16	**77.12**
HBP	VGG-16	72.71
	Resnet-18	72.95
The proposed model on HBP	Resnet-18	73.92

Experiments on Stanford Dogs. The classification accuracy on Stanford dogs is summarized in Table 3. The training images are randomly cropped 224 × 224 patches. The test images are center cropped 224 × 224. We can observe significant improvement for the proposed model compared with others methods. The proposed model on CBP has 80.03% accuracy. We add the HA model on HBP network. The accuracy of the proposed HA model is 78.26 higher than HBP network.

Table 3. Table shows the comparison results on Stanford dogs dataset.

Method	Base Model	Accuracy (%)
BCNN	VGG-16	60.29
PHPQ[19]	Resnet-18	79.83
CBP	VGG-16	78.71
HACBP	VGG-16	78.74
WSHA-CBP	VGG-16	**80.03**
HBP	VGG-16	74.65
	Resnet-18	77.55
HAHBP	Resnet-18	78.26

Experiments on Oxford-Flower-17. Table 4 shows the comparison results on Oxford-Flower-17 dataset. The training images are also randomly cropped 224 × 224 patches. The test images are center cropped 224 × 224. CBP has 89.12% accuracy. The performance of accuracy is 90.88% When adding the proposed model to CBP.

Table 4. Table shows the comparison results on Oxford-Flower-17 dataset.

Method	Base Model	Accuracy (%)
BCNN	VGG-16	84.71
CBP	VGG-16	89.12
HACBP	VGG-16	89.56
WSHA-CBP	VGG-16	**90.88**
HBP	VGG-16	87.52
	Resnet-18	88.09
HAHBP	Resnet-18	90.15

3.3 Applications

Disaster scenes include earthquakes, tsunamis and tornadoes are applied in ours experiments. The database contains approximately 1,757 color images, which have three different disaster types: 760 images are earthquake images; 556 images are tsunami images and the rest 441 images are tornado images. The earthquake data were from the Haitian earthquake in 2010 and the earthquake in Christchurch, New Zealand in 2011; the tsunami data came from the 2004 Tohoku tsunami in Japan and the 2004 Indonesian tsunami; and the tornado data was taken after the Moore tornado in Oklahoma, USA in 2013 [13]. We divide the dataset into different damage-level: DL1, DL2, DL3, which stands for no damage, mild damage, severe damage.

Sample images are cropped 224 × 224. When disaster-scenes are classified by three different disaster types. The experimental results are shown in Table 5. When the dataset is divided into different damage-level. There are three level of each disaster types. The results are shown in Table 6.

Table 5. The prediction of different disaster-scene

Method	Base Model	Type Accuracy (%)
CBP	VGG-16	86.58
HACBP	VGG-16	86.89
WSHA-CBP	VGG-16	**87.10**

In Table 5, we can see that HACBP is better than CBP. When combined HA model with metric loss function. The accuracy has a 1% boost. In Table 6, the first column is the prediction of Tornado level. The second column is the prediction of Earthquake level. The third column is the prediction of Tsunami level.

For Table 6, the prediction of Tornado level is best. The original CBP has 84.10% accuracy. The HACBP is 87.12%. WSHA-CBP has 88.23% accuracy. For the prediction of Earthquake and Tsunami, the accuracies are 61.58% and 59.12 respectively.

Table 6. The prediction of damage level in different disaster

Method	Level Accuracy (%) of Tornado	Level Accuracy (%) of Earthquake	Level Accuracy (%) of Tsunami
CBP	84.10	59.26	54.38
HACBP	87.12	60.52	57.66
WSHACBP	**88.23**	**61.58**	**59.12**

We also give some sample transformation with different stage in the Fig. 2. The first column is the original disaster-scene images. The second column is the images after data augmentation. The third column is the output of attention map. The fourth column is the region of selected features. From the Fig. 2, the salient features are extracted effectively and useless information are filtered out.

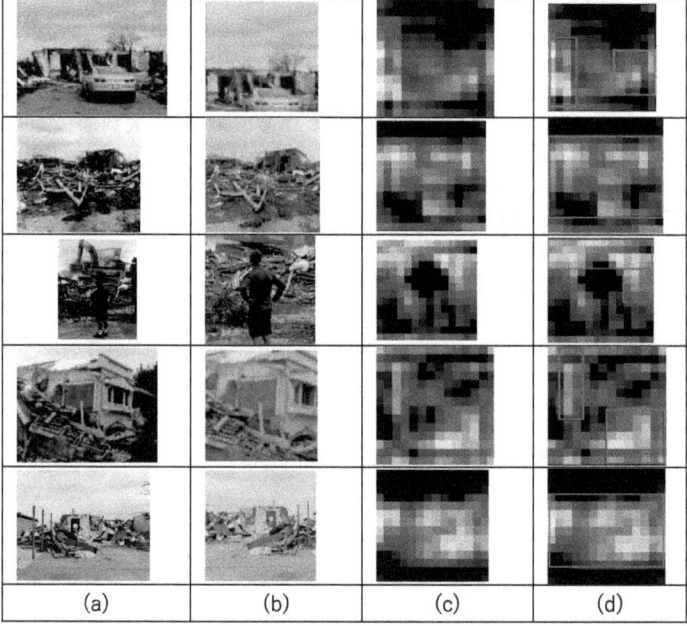

Fig. 2. Sample transformation with different stage: (a) Original images (b) images After the data augmentation (c) the output of attention map (d) The region of the selected feature

4 Conclusions

In this paper, the hierarchy attention model has been proposed for weakly supervised fine-grained image classification, which jointly integrates three level attention models. The hierarchy attentions jointly improve the multi-scale feature learning and have a progressive promotion. The metric loss function is based on clustering method which is unsupervised learning. The proposed approach is demonstrated to perform well on fine-grained image classification without requiring bounding box/part annotations. it should be beneficial to a wide variety of neural network models for applications.

Acknowledgments. This work is supported by the Open Foundation Project of Hubei Key Laboratory of Optical Information and Pattern Recognition, Wuhan Institute of Technology (Grant No. 202306).

References

1. Wah, C., et al.: The Caltech-UCSD Birds-200–2011 Dataset. Computation and Neural Systems Technical Report (2011)
2. OxFord Flowers 17. http://www.robots.ox.ac.uk/~vgg/data/bicos/
3. Khosla, A., et al.: Novel dataset for Fine-Grained Image Categorization. In: IEEE Conference on Computer Vision and Pattern Recognition (CVPR) (2011)
4. Krause, J., et al.: 3D object representations for fine-grained categorization. In: 4th IEEE Workshop on 3D Representation and Recognition, at ICCV 2013 (2013)
5. Wang, Y., Wang, Z.: A survey of recent work on fine-grained image classification techniques. J. Visual Commun. Image Represent. **59**, 210–214 (2019)
6. Cai, D., et al.: Convolutional low-resolution fine-grained classification. Pattern Recogn. Lett. **119**, 166–171 (2019)
7. Lin, T., Aruni, R., Maji, S.: Bilinear CNNs for Fine-Grained Visual Recognition (2017). arXiv:1504.07889v5
8. Gao, Y., et al.: Compact Bilinear Pooling (2016). arXiv:1511.06062v2
9. Dubey, A., et al.: Pairwise confusion for fine-grained visual classification. In: Computer Vision and Pattern Recognition (2018)
10. Xie, J.J., Zhong, Y.J., Zhang, J.G., et al.: A weakly supervised spatial group attention network for fine-grained visual recognition. Appl. Intell. **53**(20), 23301–23315 (2023). https://doi.org/10.1007/s10489-023-04627-z
11. Zeng, Z.Y., Wang, J.P., Chen, B., et al.: Pyramid hybrid pooling quantization for efficient fine-grained image retrieval. Pattern Recogn. Lett. **178**, 106–114 (2024). https://doi.org/10.1016/j.patrec.2023.12.022
12. Otholt, J., Meinel, C., Yang, H.J.: Guided cluster aggregation: a hierarchical approach to generalized category discovery. In: Proceedings of the IEEE/CVF Winter Conference on Applications of Computer Vision (WACV), pp. 2618–2627 (2024). https://openaccess.thecvf.com/content/WACV2024
13. Tang, S., Chen, Z.: Machine understanding of disaster-scene mechanics. IEEE J. Sel. Top. Appl. Earth Observ. Remote Sens. 21 (2019)

CS-KD: Confused Sample Knowledge Distillation for Semantic Segmentation of Aerial Imagery

Yue Sun[1,2], Lingfeng Huang[3], Qi Zhu[1,2], and Dong Liang[1,2(✉)]

[1] College of Computer Science and Technology, Nanjing University of Aeronautics and Astronautics, Nanjing, China
{sun.yue,zhuqi,liangdong}@nuaa.edu.cn
[2] Shenzhen Research Institute, Nanjing University of Aeronautics and Astronautics, Nanjing, China
[3] Shanghai Institute of Technical Physics, Chinese Academy of Sciences, Shanghai, China
huanglingfeng@mail.sitp.ac.cn

Abstract. Currently, semantic segmentation methods based on knowledge distillation (KD) mainly focus on transferring various structured knowledge to the student network and designing corresponding optimization goals to encourage the student network to imitate the output of the teacher network. However, these methods do not consider the impact of sample quality on model training. Especially for aerial images of complex scenes, problems such as object occlusion and boundary blur caused by factors such as illumination and imaging angle will introduce many confused samples. These confused samples can lead to labeling bias or incorrect predictions. Therefore, we propose a confused sample knowledge distillation method (CS-KD) and design an adaptive sample screening strategy. During the training process, CS-KD makes full use of the prediction capabilities of the teacher and student networks at all stages to screen confused samples pixel by pixel and adjust the importance of different training samples. Experiment results verify that, based on the Potsdam and Vaihingen benchmarks, CS-KD can achieve competitive performance compared with other state-of-the art KD methods. Additionally, our research showcases that CS-KD can integrate with existing KD methods to improve their upper performance bound.

Keywords: Semantic Segmentation · Knowledge Distillation · Sample Weighting · Confused Samples

1 Introduction

Semantic segmentation is one of the basic tasks of aerial remote sensing images, and its purpose is to classify each pixel in aerial images. It solves various practical problems through deep neural networks and is widely used in hazard assessment [1], urban planning [2], farmland detection [3], natural disaster detection [4] and other fields. It has important practical significance and application value.

The current deep neural networks, e.g., DeepLab [5, 6], PSPNet [7], HRNet [8], have achieved remarkable success and are widely used in semantic segmentation. However, these methods usually require a large number of pixel-level annotations to achieve good generalization performance, which incurs high storage and training costs. For devices with limited resources, there are significant challenges in deploying these models with high computational complexity and many model parameters. Therefore, model compression has become an important research topic. Model quantization [9] and pruning [10] help reduce inference costs. In contrast, knowledge distillation (KD) [11, 12] transplants the segmentation performance of cumbersome networks into lightweight networks, which is a simple but effective technique.

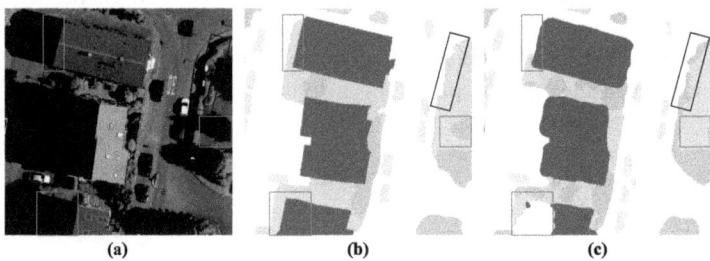

Fig. 1. The confused examples of problems existing from the Vaihingen datasets: (a) Image, (b) Ground Truth (GT), (c) Prediction.

Although semantic segmentation methods based on KD have been successful to a certain extent, there are still some limitations for large-scale aerial images of complex scenes. First, various interference factors may affect the aerial image, such as weather, occlusion, illumination and imaging angle changes. These factors may lead to reduced image quality and the appearance of many confused samples, thereby introducing labeling bias. The model's performance degrades due to learning this incorrect annotation information. As shown in Fig. 1, in the two red boxes on the left, the shadows of tall buildings (blue) block low vegetation (cyan). In the red box on the right, the shadows of tall trees (green) block low vegetation (cyan). This makes occluded vegetation invisible on aerial remote sensing images, causing labeling bias or model prediction errors. In addition, aerial remote sensing scenes have complex and special characteristics. Although there are differences between different types of objects, pixel features can easily be confused in complex backgrounds or situations where objects are intertwined. As shown in the black box in Fig. 1, the pixel features of trees (green) and low vegetation (cyan) are similar, so it is easy to confuse the pixel features, leading to incorrect category classification. These factors increase the challenge of semantic segmentation of aerial imagery.

To cope with the challenge of confused samples in complex aerial scenes and fully employ KD's advantages, we propose a new confused sample knowledge distillation (CS-KD) method. Specifically, in the CS-KD method, we design an adaptive sample screening strategy to measure the quality of samples through the weighting mechanism of teacher and student networks. This collaborative approach provides accurate sample quality assessment to identify confused samples. Then, CS-KD adopts the method of allocating low weights to alleviate the negative impact of confused samples on the student network, thereby improving its segmentation performance. In addition, as an independent KD training strategy, CS-KD can also be combined with existing KD methods to improve the model's upper performance bound.

The main contributions of this work can be summarized as follows:

- We propose a confused sample knowledge distillation (CS-KD) method. At the same time, the proposed CS-KD can also be integrated with existing KD methods to improve their upper performance bound.
- We propose an adaptive sample screening strategy to evaluate the samples' quality and allocate low weights to reduce the negative impact of confused samples on the student network, which is more conducive to stable training of the model in complex scenes.
- The proposed CS-KD can achieve effective segmentation performance in complex aerial remote sensing scenes, providing a reliable and efficient solution for aerial image segmentation tasks.

2 Related Work

2.1 Semantic Segmentation

Fully convolutional network (FCN) [13] was the cornerstone of deep learning technology applied to semantic segmentation problems. SegNet [14] utilized the Maxpooling indices to enhance location information and improve efficiency. PSPNet [7] employed the pyramid pooling module to integrate context and enhance the ability to obtain global information. DeepLabv3 [5] captured multi-scale context information using multiple parallel atrous rates of different proportions. Most efforts have focused on designing inexpensive, lightweight networks to solve this problem. Enet [15] utilized an asymmetric encoder-decoder structure to reduce parameters in a network. ICNet [16] utilized low-resolution semantic information and details of high-resolution images to recover and refine segmentation predictions with low computational cost progressively. BiSeNet [17] balanced speed and accuracy by designing spatial paths with small steps and a contextual path with fast downsampling.

2.2 Knowledge Distillation for Semantic Segmentation

Hinton et al. [18] first introduced the concept of knowledge distillation (KD). Most previous studies on KD, such as [19, 20], focused on image classification. However, image-level KD does not take the locally structured information for semantic segmentation into account, so it is with natural defects for pixel-level semantic segmentation. Most efforts have focused on defining the knowledge for the segmentation task to solve this problem. Liu et al. [12] extracted structured knowledge from teacher network to student network by using two structured distillation schemes. Wang et al. [21] put forward a new intra-class feature variation distillation (IFVD), which transformed the cumbersome teacher model into a compact student model. Shu et al. [22] introduced a new channel-wise KD method that minimized differences between teacher and student networks by utilizing asymmetric KL divergence. Feng et al. [23] improved the classification accuracy of existing compact networks by capturing similar knowledge in the pixel and category dimensions respectively. To solve the problem that the previous techniques ignore the global semantic relationship between pixels in different images, Yang et al. [11] attempted to model pixel–pixel and pixel–region comparison relationships in semantic segmentation tasks as knowledge and transfer global pixel correlation from teachers to students for semantic segmentation.

3 Proposed Method

3.1 Objective of Confused Sample Knowledge Distillation

Semantic segmentation is a dense pixel-level prediction task that assigns a specific class to each pixel in an image. Given an input image I with dimensions $W \times H \times 3$, the feature extractor of a segmenter first extracts a feature map F, where H and W represent the height and width of the input image and feature map, respectively. The categorical logit map Z is generated from feature map F by applying a classifier. Optimization is then performed using a cross-entropy loss:

$$L_{task} = \frac{1}{H \times W} \sum_{h=1}^{H} \sum_{w=1}^{W} CE\left(\sigma\left(Z_{h,w}\right), y_{h,w}\right) \tag{1}$$

where $y_{h,w}$ denotes the ground-truth label for the (h, w)-th pixel, and $Z_{h,w}$ denotes the output logits for the (h, w)-th pixel. The softmax function σ generates the category probability, and CE is the cross-entropy loss to measure the difference between the ground truth and category probability.

The existing KD methods usually use a pixel-wise alignment among class probabilities between a cumbersome teacher network t and a lightweight student network s to obtain a distillation loss, which can be formulated as

$$L_{kd} = \frac{1}{H \times W} \sum_{h=1}^{H} \sum_{w=1}^{W} KL\left[\sigma\left(\frac{Z_{h,w}^{s}}{T}\right) \| \sigma\left(\frac{Z_{h,w}^{t}}{T}\right)\right] \tag{2}$$

where $Z_{h,w}^{s}$ and $Z_{h,w}^{t}$ represent the output logits for the (h, w)-th pixel produced from the student and the teacher network, respectively. σ function calculates the category probability of the (h, w)-th pixel generated by the student and teacher networks, respectively. KL denotes the Kullback-Leibler divergence, which measures the difference between two probability distributions. The parameter T represents the temperature taken by distillation and reflects the label's softening degree. For a fair comparison with previous works [11, 12], we set $T = 1$ in our experiments.

To solve the problem of existing KD methods not considering sample quality in complex aerial remote sensing scenes, we propose an adaptive sample screening strategy based on sample quality assessment. This strategy is employed to generate quality scores for the samples. We utilize the quality score of each pixel as a weight to determine the contribution of each pixel. We use Eq. (3) to introduce the weight W_{cskd} into the loss function. The process of generating weight W_{cskd} will be described below.

$$L_{CSKD} = W_{cskd} \cdot L_{task} + L_{kd} \tag{3}$$

3.2 Confused Sample Knowledge Distillation (CS-KD)

In this section, we propose an adaptive sample screening strategy based on KD, and Fig. 2 shows the process of this strategy.

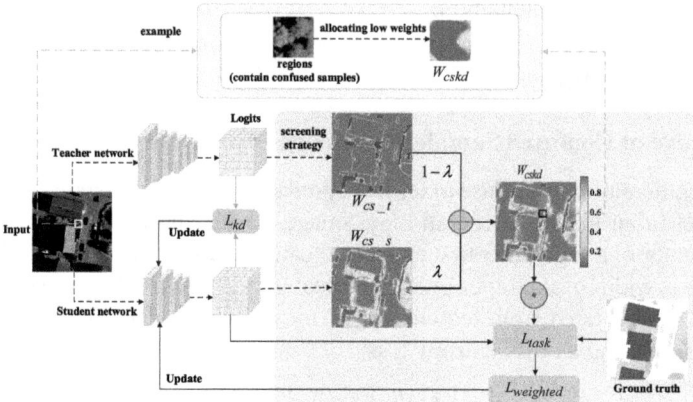

Fig. 2. The proposed distillation method. An illustrative example of allocating low weights to confused samples is provided above the method diagram.

Screening of confused samples requires measuring the sample quality score as a starting point. The original idea is to use the cross-entropy loss of the network as a criterion to evaluate the sample quality. After introducing KD, the most straightforward method is to use the cross-entropy loss of the teacher model as an evaluation criterion of sample quality. However, relying on the teacher to assess sample quality does not consider the student's needs and is inconsistent with the student's cognitive processes. Based on this motivation, we propose a teacher-student cooperation method to evaluate sample quality and dynamically adjust the collaboration weights between the teacher and student networks as the student network's cognitive levels increase. The sample quality score is calculated by a weighted combination of teacher and student networks. For each pixel in the image, first obtain the cross-entropy loss of the teacher and student networks respectively:

$$W_{cs\_s} = CE(\sigma(Z^s_{h,w}), y_{h,w}) \quad (4)$$

$$W_{cs\_t} = CE(\sigma(Z^t_{h,w}), y_{h,w}) \quad (5)$$

Then, utilize the CE loss weighting of the teacher and student networks to obtain the sample quality score of each pixel:

$$W_{cs} = \lambda \cdot W_{cs\_s} + (1 - \lambda) \cdot W_{cs\_t} \quad (6)$$

where λ is the parameter used to adjust the weight of the student and teacher networks. In the early stages of model training, relying on the student network to judge sample quality may transmit and amplify errors, posing challenges to correcting the student network. In contrast, the supervisory information provided by the teacher network is more accurate and reliable. Therefore, we introduce a warm-up strategy to ensure the stability and reliability of the weights. In practice, we set the initial value of λ to 0. After a warm-up period, the student network can generate more accurate pseudo-labels and calculate sample weights, and the value of λ gradually increases to 0.5. Then, after obtaining the W_{cs} of each pixel, normalize it within the [0, 1] range to obtain each pixel's relative weight W_{cskd}. The calculation formula is as follows:

$$W_{cskd} = \exp\{-W_{cs}\} \tag{7}$$

The value of W_{cskd} reflects the confusing degree of each pixel, with smaller values indicating that the pixel is more likely to be confused. These confused samples may cause the network to learn incorrect annotation information, thus affecting the network's performance. We allocate low weights to mitigate the negative impact of confused samples on the student network's performance, and apply the weight W_{cskd} to the loss function L_{task} of the semantic segmentation task:

$$L_{weighted} = W_{cskd} \cdot L_{task} \tag{8}$$

Finally, we use the CS-KD strategy to calculate the weighted segmentation loss $L_{weighted}$ for each pixel, and the student network updates the network's parameters by minimizing the L_{CSKD}:

$$L_{CSKD} = L_{weighted} + L_{kd} = W_{cskd} \cdot L_{task} + L_{kd} \tag{9}$$

3.3 Integrating with Other Approaches

Since CS-KD only affects L_{task} loss, it can be integrated with other KD methods without introducing additional optimization goals. In experiments, we integrate CS-KD with AT [19], CWD [22], DSD [23] and CIRKD [11] methods. Taking the CIRKD [11] methods as an example, we will demonstrate how to integrate CS-KD into CIRKD and derive the corresponding distillation loss formula.

The total loss defined by CIRKD [11]:

$$L_{CIRKD} = L_{task} + L_{kd} + \alpha L_{batch\_p2p} + \beta L_{memory\_p2p} + \gamma L_{memory\_p2r} \tag{10}$$

where L_{batch_p2p} represents distillation loss of mini-batch-based pixel-to-pixel, L_{memory_p2p} denotes distillation loss of memory-based pixel-to-pixel, L_{memory_p2r} denotes distillation loss of memory-based pixel-to-region. α, β and γ are the weight balance parameters. The further calculation details of L_{batch_p2p}, L_{memory_p2p} and L_{memory_p2r} are described in [11].

The distillation loss of CS-KD:

$$L_{CSKD} = W_{cskd} \cdot L_{task} + L_{kd} \tag{11}$$

After integrating CS-KD, the modified distillation loss of the CIRKD method is derived as follows:

$$L_{CIRKD\_CSKD} = W_{cskd} \cdot L_{task} + L_{kd} + \alpha L_{batch\_p2p} + \beta L_{memory\_p2p} + \gamma L_{memory\_p2r} \quad (12)$$

In this new loss term, we follow the default parameter settings in CIRKD [11], setting the weighting parameter α to 1, β to 0.1, and γ to 0.1. Moreover, CS-KD can seamlessly integrate with other semantic segmentation methods based on KD. This integration allows us to enhance the performance of the student network further from existing approaches.

4 Experiments and Results Analysis

4.1 Experimental Set

This paper carried out experiments on the two image sets of the ISPRS [26] 2D Semantic Labeling Challenge to validate the proposed method. We use DeepLabV3 [5] with ResNet-101 backbone [27] as the cumbersome teacher network for all experiments. For student networks, we use various segmentation architectures to verify the effectiveness of distillation methods. Specifically, DeepLabV3 and PSPNet [7] with different backbones of ResNet-18 and MobileNetV2 [28] are adopted. The networks are trained using mini-batch stochastic gradient descent (SGD) with a momentum of 0.9 and weight decay of 0.0005. We set the number of iterations to 40,000. The learning rate is initialized at 0.02 and is multiplied by $\left(1 - \frac{iter}{iter_{total}}\right)^{0.9}$ during training. In our experiments, we use a 512 × 512 patch size, which fits our memory budget. Normal data augmentation techniques such as random flipping and scaling in the [0.5, 2] range are applied during training. The temperature T is set to be 1. All experiments are conducted on two 3090 GPUs using mixed-precision training.

4.2 Comparing with Existing KD Methods

To verify the performance of CS-KD, we compare it with recent semantic segmentation methods based on KD, including AT [19], CWD [22], DSD [23] and CIRKD [11] on the above two representative datasets. The experimental results are shown in Tables 1 and 2. In experiments, we adopt DeepLabV3 with ResNet-101 backbone as the teacher network, denoted as "Teacher", and DeepLabV3 with ResNet-18 backbone as the student network, denoted as "Student".

The experimental results on the Potsdam dataset are shown in Table 1. All structured KD methods improve the segmentation performance of the student network compared to training without KD. Our CS-KD outperforms other KD methods regarding mIoU, mF_1, and OA, with significant advantages. The highest IoU were obtained by identifying four categories except Car. In addition, the qualitative results are shown in Fig. 3. The validity of our proposed approach is intuitively demonstrated, and the semantic labels produced by CS-KD are more consistent with the ground truth. In order to further verify the effectiveness of our network, we conducted experiments on the Vaihingen dataset, and the experimental results are shown in Table 2. The highest IoU were obtained in identifying the three categories of low vegetation, trees, and cars. The qualitative results are shown in Fig. 4.

Table 1. Experimental results on the Postdam dataset.

Method	IoU					mIoU (%)	mF_1 (%)	OA (%)
	Imp.Surf	Building	Low veg	Tree	Car			
Teacher	84.46	92.56	75.47	74.83	81.64	81.79	84.83	96.16
Student	81.16	89.97	72.69	73.25	76.12	78.62	81.95	95.53
+KD [18]	81.83	89.77	73.51	74.26	75.85	79.05	82.67	95.64
+AT [19]	82.73	90.69	74.20	74.40	78.01	80.01	83.40	95.85
+CWD [22]	83.55	91.06	73.79	72.85	78.71	79.99	83.84	95.81
+DSD [23]	83.44	91.13	73.59	73.42	**79.10**	80.14	83.65	95.82
+CIRKD [11]	83.40	91.48	74.22	74.20	78.74	80.41	83.91	95.91
+Ours	**83.97**	**91.55**	**75.14**	**74.76**	79.08	**80.90**	**84.14**	**96.02**

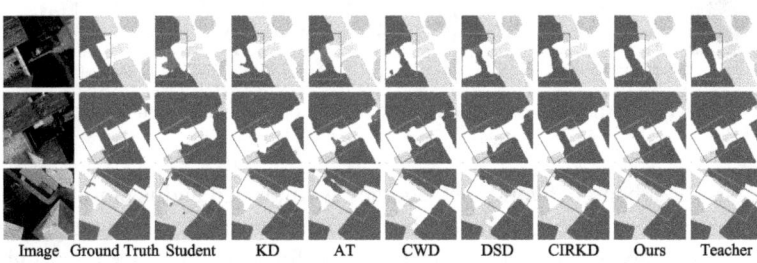

Fig. 3. Examples of segmentation results on the Potsdam dataset. Legend—white: impervious surfaces, blue: buildings, cyan: low vegetation, green: trees, yellow: cars, red: clutter/background (best viewed in color) (color figure online).

4.3 Ablation Study

Ablation Study About the Different Student Networks. To verify the effectiveness and robustness of our CS-KD, we evaluated different student networks on the Potsdam dataset. The experimental results are shown in Table 3. It can be observed from the experimental results that CS-KD achieved considerable results in all student networks, proving the robustness of CS-KD to changes in student network architecture. When using

Table 2. Experimental results on the Postdam dataset.

Method	IoU					mIoU (%)	mF_1 (%)	OA (%)
	Imp.Surf	Building	Low veg	Tree	Car			
Teacher	84.16	88.62	68.12	77.05	69.13	77.42	83.73	95.61
Student	82.58	85.82	64.91	76.04	63.95	74.66	81.56	95.10
+KD [18]	82.84	87.11	67.30	76.05	63.38	75.34	82.11	95.24
+AT [19]	82.80	**87.58**	66.47	75.99	64.64	75.50	82.14	95.27
+CWD [22]	82.81	86.48	66.62	75.70	64.81	75.28	82.04	95.20
+DSD [23]	82.79	86.79	66.28	76.30	65.04	75.44	82.08	95.21
+CIRKD [11]	**83.00**	86.70	66.72	76.07	65.24	75.55	82.34	95.26
+Ours	82.92	87.25	**67.70**	**76.35**	**66.22**	**76.09**	**82.95**	**95.36**

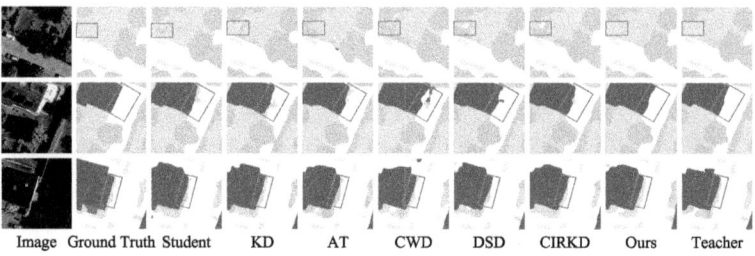

Image Ground Truth Student KD AT CWD DSD CIRKD Ours Teacher

Fig. 4. Examples of segmentation results on the Vaihingen dataset.

a more robust backbone network, the accuracy is improved and is closer to the performance of the teacher network. It should be noted that we use lightweight MobileNetV2 as the backbone network, aiming to verify the performance of CS-KD on lightweight networks to explore the possibility of deploying our method on mobile devices.

Ablation Study About the Effect of λ. We conducted ablation experiments on λ to explore its impact on CS-KD. λ is a parameter used to adjust the weight ratio of student and teacher networks. In Table 4, "[0,0]" means that the value of λ is 0, and only the weight of the teacher network participates in the calculation of loss; "[1,1]" means that only the weight of the student network participates in the loss calculation; "[0.5,0.5]" means that the value of λ is always 0.5, and the weights of the teacher and student networks participate in the calculation of loss in the same proportion; "[0,0.5]" means that the value of λ changes from 0 gradually rises to 0.5, and the weight of the student network gradually participates in the calculation; "[0,1]" means that the value of λ gradually increases from 0 to 1; "[0,0,0.5]" is the method used by CS-KD. A warm-up

Table 3. Ablation study about backbone. * denotes that we do not initialize the backbone with ImageNet [29] pre-trained weights.

Method	mIoU (%)	mF_1 (%)	OA (%)
T: DeepLabV3-Res101	81.79	84.83	96.16
S: DeepLabV3-Res18 +CS-KD	78.62 80.90	81.95 84.14	95.53 96.02
S: DeepLabV3-Res18* +CS-KD	76.76 77.65	80.95 81.79	95.18 95.36
S: DeepLabV3-MBV2 +CS-KD	78.68 79.73	82.83 83.35	95.59 95.84
S: PSPNet-Res18 +CS-KD	79.27 80.18	82.83 83.51	95.78 95.94

Table 4. Ablation study about the effect of λ in our CS-KD method.

λ	[0,0]	[1,1]	[0.5,0.5]	[0,0.5]	[0,1]	[0,0,0.5]
mIoU (%)	80.44	80.41	80.56	80.64	80.50	**80.90**

phase accounting for 10% of the total iterations is added. The experimental results are shown in Table 4. It can be observed that under the setting of "[0,0,0.5]", the mIoU of the network reaches the highest. The analysis shows that the sample weights provided entirely by the teacher network do not consider the needs of the student network, and the sample weights wholly provided by the immature student network easily transmit and amplify errors, which brings challenges to the correction of the student network. Therefore, the two methods' mIoU is the worst result among these sets of experiments. On the contrary, first giving the model a warm-up stage, the supervision information from the teacher network in the early stage of training is more conducive to the convergence of the student network. The student network acquires judgment ability as the training phase develops and gradually increases the proportion of sample weights provided by the student network to 0.5, reaching the highest mIoU.

4.4 Integrating with Existing KD Methods

We evaluate the performance impact of integrating CS-KD into existing KD methods on the Postdam dataset. We use DeepLabV3-Res18 as the student network and explore the effectiveness of CS-KD in the simplest integrated way under the experimental settings of the original method without changing any hyperparameters. The experimental results are shown in Table 5. Among the five baseline methods, CS-KD effectively improves the performance of all methods and further narrows the performance gap between the student and teacher networks.

Table 5. Integrating with existing KD methods.

Method	mIoU (%)	mF_1 (%)	OA (%)
T: DeepLabV3-Res101	81.79	84.83	96.16
S: DeepLabV3-Res18	78.62	81.95	95.53
+AT [19]	80.01	83.40	95.85
+AT [19]+CS-KD	80.34	83.69	95.87
+CWD [22]	79.99	83.84	95.81
+CWD [22]+CS-KD	80.40	83.88	95.91
+DSD [23]	80.12	83.65	95.82
+DSD [23]+CS-KD	80.36	83.81	95.89
+CIRKD [11]	80.41	83.91	95.91
+CIRKD [11]+CS-KD	80.86	84.21	96.01
+KD [18]	79.04	82.67	95.64
+KD [18]+CS-KD	80.90	84.14	96.02

5 Conclusions

We propose the CS-KD method for complex aerial image semantic segmentation tasks. Unlike previous feature-based and response-based distillation methods, we utilize weight scores that measure the degree of confusion of samples as knowledge to transfer from the teacher network to the student network and adjust the learning process accordingly, effectively improving the overall performance of the student network. CS-KD is easily integrated with existing distillation methods. Experimental results show that CS-KD outperforms existing KD methods. In future research, we will further explore the effectiveness of CS-KD in more complex scenes or other segmentation tasks.

Acknowledgments. This work is supported in part by the National Natural Science Foundation of China under grant 62272229, the Natural Science Foundation of Jiangsu Province under grant BK20222012, and Shenzhen Science and Technology Program JCYJ20230807142001004. The authors would like to thank all the anonymous reviewers for their constructive comments.

References

1. Pham, H.N., et al.: A new deep learning approach based on bilateral semantic segmentation models for sustainable estuarine wetland ecosystem management. Sci. Total Environ. **838**, 155826 (2022)
2. Trenčanová, B., Proença, V., Bernardino, A.: Development of semantic maps of vegetation cover from UAV images to support planning and management in finegrained fire-prone landscapes. Remote Sens. **14**(5), 1262 (2022)
3. Sheng, H., Chen, X., Su, J., Rajagopal, R., Ng, A.: Effective data fusion with generalized vegetation index: evidence from land cover segmentation in agriculture. In: Proceedings of the IEEE/CVF Conference on Computer Vision and Pattern Recognition Workshops, pp. 60–61 (2020)

4. Ji, C., Zhou, W., Lei, J., Ye, L.: Infrared and visible image fusion via multiscale receptive field amplification fusion network. IEEE Signal Process. Lett. (2023)
5. Chen, L.C., Papandreou, G., Schroff, F., Adam, H.: Rethinking atrous convolution for semantic image segmentation (2017). arXiv:1706.05587
6. Chen, L.C., Zhu, Y., Papandreou, G., Schroff, F., Adam, H.: Encoder-decoder with atrous separable convolution for semantic image segmentation. In: ECCV (2018)
7. Zhao, H., Shi, J., Qi, X., Wang, X., Jia, J.: Pyramid scene parsing network. In: Proceedings of the IEEE/CVF Conference on Computer Vision and Pattern Recognition (2017)
8. Wang, J., et al.: Deep high-resolution representation learning for visual recognition. TPAMI **43**(10), 3349–3364 (2020)
9. Wu, J., Leng, C., Wang, Y., Hu, Q., Cheng, J.: Quantized convolutional neural networks for mobile devices. In: Proceedings of the IEEE/CVF Conference on Computer Vision and Pattern Recognition, pp. 4820–4828 (2016)
10. He, W., Wu, M., Liang, M., Lam, S.K.: CAP: context-aware pruning for semantic segmentation. In: Proceedings of the IEEE/CVF Winter Conference on Applications of Computer Vision, pp. 960–969 (2021)
11. Yang, C., Zhou, H., An, Z., Jiang, X., Xu, Y., Zhang, Q.: Cross-image relational knowledge distillation for semantic segmentation. In: Proceedings of the IEEE/CVF Conference on Computer Vision and Pattern Recognition (2022)
12. Liu, Y., Chen, K., Liu, C., Qin, Z., Luo, Z., Wang, J.: Structured knowledge distillation for semantic segmentation. In: Proceedings of the IEEE/CVF Conference on Computer Vision and Pattern Recognition (2019)
13. Long, J., Shelhamer, E., Darrell, T.: Fully convolutional networks for semantic segmentation. In: Proceedings of the IEEE Conference on Computer Vision and Pattern Recognition, pp. 3431–3440 (2015)
14. Badrinarayanan, V., Kendall, A., Cipolla, R.: SegNet: a deep convolutional encoder-decoder architecture for image segmentation. IEEE Trans. Pattern Anal. Mach. Intell. **39**(12), 2481–2495 (2017)
15. Paszke, A., Chaurasia, A., Kim, S., Culurciello, E.: ENet: a deep neural network architecture for real-time semantic segmentation (2016). arXiv:1606.02147
16. Zhao, H., Qi, X., Shen, X., Shi, J., Jia, J.: ICNet for real-time semantic segmentation on high-resolution images. In: ECCV (2018)
17. Yu, C., Wang, J., Peng, C., Gao, C., Yu, G., Sang, N.: BiSeNet: Bilateral segmentation network for real-time semantic segmentation. In: ECCV (2018)
18. Hinton, G., Vinyals, O., Dean, J.: Distilling the knowledge in a neural network. In: NeurIPS (2015)
19. Zagoruyko, S., Komodakis, N.: Paying more attention to attention: improving the performance of convolutional neural networks via attention transfer. In: ICLR (2017)
20. Peng, B., et al.: Correlation congruence for knowledge distillation. In: ICCV (2019)
21. Wang, Y., Zhou, W., Jiang, T., Bai, X., Xu, Y.: Intra-class feature variation distillation for semantic segmentation. In: ECCV (2020)
22. Shu, C., Liu, Y., Gao, J., Yan, Z., Shen, C.: Channel-wise knowledge distillation for dense prediction. In: ICCV (2021)
23. Feng, Y., Sun, X., Diao, W., Li, J., Gao, X.: Double similarity distillation for semantic image segmentation. TIP **30**, 5363–5376 (2021)
24. Yu, T., Kumar, S., Gupta, A., Levine, S., Hausman, K., Finn, C.: Gradient surgery for multi-task learning. Adv. Neural. Inf. Process. Syst. **33**, 5824–5836 (2020)
25. Kendall, A., Gal, Y.: What uncertainties do we need in Bayesian deep learning for computer vision? NeurIPS **30** (2017)
26. Rottensteiner, F., Sohn, G., Gerke, M., Wegner, J.D.: ISPRS Semantic Labeling Contest. ISPRS, Leopoldshöhe, Germany **1**(4), 4 (2014)

27. He, K., Zhang, X., Ren, S., Sun, J.: Deep residual learning for image recognition. In: Proceedings of the IEEE/CVF Conference on Computer Vision and Pattern Recognition (2016)
28. Sandler, M., Howard, A., Zhu, M., Zhmoginov, A., Chen, L.C.: MobileNetV2: Inverted residuals and linear bottlenecks. In: Proceedings of the IEEE/CVF Conference on Computer Vision and Pattern Recognition, pp. 4510–4520 (2018)
29. Russakovsky, O., et al.: ImageNet large scale visual recognition challenge. Int. J. Comput. Vis. **115**, 211–252 (2015)

CD-Font: One-Shot Font Generation via Conditional Diffusion Model with Disentangled Guidance

Siyi Chen, Zhenhua Li[✉], and Dong Liang

School of Computer Science and Technology, MIIT Key Laboratory of Pattern Analysis and Machine Intelligence, Nanjing University of Aeronautics and Astronautics, Nanjing, China
{csy624,zhenhua.li,liangdong}@nuaa.edu.cn

Abstract. One-shot font generation aims to create a new font library by extracting style information from the reference font. Most existing font generation methods rely on GAN-based image-to-image translation frameworks, which still suffer from unstable training and imprecise character structure generation due to the nature of adversarial training. In this paper, we propose a one-shot font generation framework named CD-Font, based on a conditional diffusion model with style-content disentangled guidance. Unlike existing methods, we use two different encoders to separate the representations for styles and contents and fuse them as conditions of the diffusion model. Specifically, we concatenate the content image with the noisy image throughout all denoising steps to improve the integrity of character structures. During inference, we present a disentangled guidance sampling strategy to enable the generated font images to exhibit strong correlations with both the reference image and the target character. Extensive experiments and user studies demonstrate that our CD-Font outperforms current methods in one-shot font generation. Furthermore, we apply our method to cross-lingual font generation, showing its promising cross-lingual capability.

Keywords: Automatic Font Generation · Diffusion Model · One-Shot Image Generation

1 Introduction

Automatic font generation is a challenging task that has gained great attention recently [1–3]. Its objective is to generate stylized images of various characters based on the style of reference samples. This approach can significantly save time and effort for expert designers when creating new font libraries, as they only need to manually design a few reference images. This is particularly useful for languages with complex character sets, such as Chinese, Korean, and Japanese. Font generation has a wide range of applications in real world scenarios. It empowers designers, advertisers, and publishers to create unique and visually captivating fonts, enhancing brand identities, print materials, and digital media. Moreover, it aids in preserving and studying ancient writing systems, contributing to academic research and cultural preservation.

With the advancements in deep neural networks, the quality of generated images has been dramatically improved [2–4]. In the early days, most font generation methods were based on Generative Adversarial Networks (GANs) [5]. Zi2zi [6] is the first to employ GANs for Chinese font generation. However, it can only handle fonts that appear in the training set and requires a substantial amount of paired data for supervised training. Numerous few-shot font generation (FFG) methods have been proposed to address these limitations. FFG approaches require only a few (few-shot) or even a single (one-shot) style image as a reference to generate font images. Meanwhile, many GAN-based FFG works [7, 1, 2] have verified that style-content disentanglement can efficiently combine the style features extracted from the reference images with the content features of the content images to generate unseen contents of the target font. Although GAN-based font generation methods have achieved impressive visual quality, their adversarial training nature often results in unstable training and less diversity in generation. Recently, diffusion models have gained great popularity, and many works [8, 9] have witnessed its powerful generative ability. Diff-Font [10] first employs a diffusion model to generate fonts by using predefined tokens to represent the content and extracting the font style from a reference sample. It incorporates strokes as a finer-grained condition to improve the integrity of the generated characters. However, Diff-Font [10] has limitations in its ability to handle unseen characters during inference. To generate a complete font library, it requires incorporating all characters into the training set which significantly impairs the model's generalization ability.

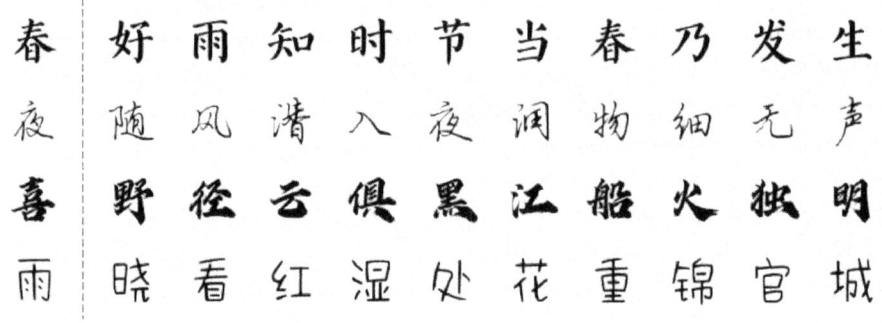

Reference　　　　　　　　　Imitation results generated by our method

Fig. 1. An ancient poem generated by our method, with each line representing a different font style. The font images in the first column serves as a reference for each style.

The limitations mentioned above highlight the need for further research and development in the field of font generation. Therefore, we propose a diffusion model-based framework for one-shot font generation. As shown in Fig. 1, our method can generate font images of the corresponding style only given one reference image. To achieve this, we use a pre-trained content encoder and a pre-trained style encoder to extract content features and style features, respectively. We also inject the content image into the denoising network to strengthen the control of the character structures. Once the model is trained, it can generate unseen styles with unseen contents, offering greater flexibility and efficiency in font generation task.

In summary, the main contributions of this paper are as follows:

- We propose a one-shot font generation framework based on the conditional diffusion model, which can preserve the structural integrity of the output images without using additional component data.
- During the sampling procedure, we introduce disentangled classifier-free guidance to effectively align the style and character of the generated image with the reference image and target content. It ensures a strong correlation between the input conditions and the output font images.
- Extensive experiments demonstrate competitive performance of our method compared to existing methods, further validating the efficacy of the proposed framework. Moreover, we apply our model to cross-lingual font generation, showing its generalization ability.

2 Related Work

2.1 Few-Shot Font Generation

Few-shot font generation aims to generate a new font library with only a few reference images. Most existing methods in this field adopt the style-content disentanglement paradigm to generate images with various style-content combinations. Based on the representation of style features, existing methods can be broadly categorized into two groups: global style representations and component-based feature representations. Methods using global representations [11, 12] typically model font styles as global statistic features extracted from reference images. On the other hand, component-based font generation approaches [13, 14] usually decompose the whole image into multiple parts or components to extract style information from local regions.

To reduce the dependency on components, MX-Font [7] uses multi-head encoders to implicitly extract different local concepts in a weakly-supervised manner. CG-GAN [15] employs a component-level discriminator to provide fine-grained supervision to the generator. However, these two methods still require component-level labels. FS-Font [16] learns the spatial correspondence between the content and reference glyphs and extracts fine-grained local styles from the references. However, the approach requires carefully selecting reference sets to cover as many specific components as possible. DG-Font [1] uses deformable convolutional networks (DCN) [17] instead of conventional convolutional networks to learn the spatial transformations from the source font to the target font, but suffer from artifacts and incomplete style transfer. CF-Font [2] introduces a content fusion module that uses fused content features to reduce the gap between the source and target domains.

Most of the mentioned methods are based on GANs, which can suffer from training instability issues. To further improve the quality of image generation, Diff-Font [10] introduces diffusion models to one-shot font generation. It treats different characters as different tokens, limiting its ability to generate unseen characters. In addition, Diff-Font uses a stroke dataset that costs human resources to label. These are extremely inconvenient in the few-shot font generation task.

3 Proposed Approach

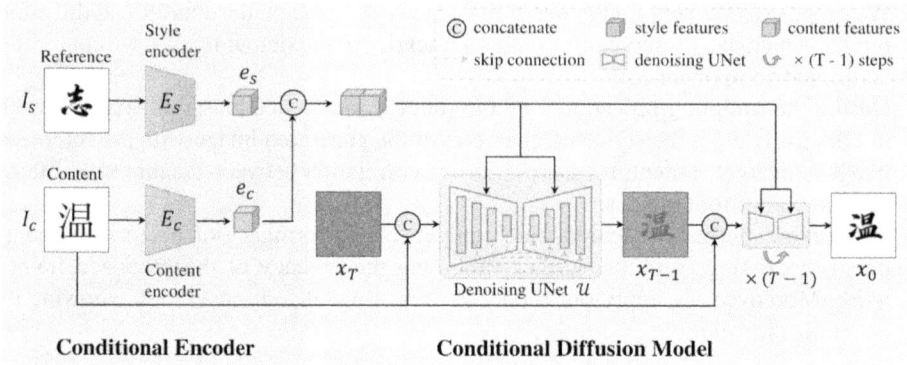

Fig. 2. Framework of our proposed method.

Overall Framework. Figure 2 presents an overview of the proposed approach, which consists of a conditional encoder module and a conditional diffusion module. The goal of our method is to train a conditional diffusion model $p_\theta(x|I_s, I_c)$ given a reference image I_s and a content image I_c. The trained diffusion model can generate a final result x that not only meets the character content matching requirement but also preserves the distinctive style of the reference image.

The denoising network $\mathcal{U}$ in our method adopts the architecture of UNet [18], comprising an encoder and a decoder. The style encoder E_s captures the style patterns of the reference image I_s, while the content encoder E_c extracts the content features from the content image I_c. By incorporating the concatenated features, the denoising network $\mathcal{U}$ effectively preserves crucial style information and structural details throughout the image generation process. To ensure precise control over unseen contents, we further concatenate the content image and the noisy image at each denoising step. This enables us to maintain the desired structure of the character and enhance the generation quality of font images.

3.1 Conditional Encoder

As shown in Fig. 2, the conditional encoder module consists of a style encoder E_s and a content encoder E_c. Both of the encoders are pre-trained and frozen during the training process of the conditional diffusion model. The pre-trained style encoder E_s and content encoder E_c are responsible for encoding the reference image I_s to style condition e_s and the content image I_c to content condition e_c, respectively. Specifically, e_s represents the unique style pattern of the reference image. e_c indicates the character structure of the input content image.

Style Condition. We use a pre-trained style encoder to extract style features. The style encoder is trained following DG-Font [1], which adopts the convolutional neural network architecture of VGG. The output of the convolutional layer is then flattened into a vector using the flatten operation. Subsequently, the flattened vector is passed through a linear layer, which produces the style features e_s. The extraction process can be summarized by the equation:

$$e_s = Proj(flatten(E_s(I_s))) \tag{1}$$

where E_s is the pre-trained style extractor, *flatten* represents unwrapping the multi-dimensional input data into a one-dimensional vector. A linear projection layer *Proj* is applied to unify the dimensionality with other conditions.

Content Condition. In contrast to Diff-Font [10], which uses predefined tokens to represent different characters and cannot handle font generation for unseen contents, we pre-train a content encoder with contrastive learning to encode content condition. Specifically, we feed an image as an anchor and select images with the same content but different styles as positive samples, while choosing images with different contents but same style as negative samples. This approach encourages the encoder to focus more on the content of the image and disregard the variations in font styles. As a result, the extracted features can better represent the structural information of characters. The training of the content encoder is guided by a Triplet Margin Loss, defined as follows:

$$L_{triplet} = max(d(a, p) - d(a, n) + margin, 0) \tag{2}$$

Here, a represents the latent features of the anchor, p represents the latent features of the positive sample, and n represents the latent features of the negative sample. The term $d(a, p)$ represents the distance between the anchor and the positive sample, and $d(a, n)$ represents the distance between the anchor and the negative sample. *margin* is a predefined value that controls the margin between positive and negative samples.

Similarly, we use the trained content encoder to extract features as the extraction process of style condition described above, which is formulated as:

$$e_c = Proj(flatten(E_c(I_c))) \tag{3}$$

where E_c is the trained content encoder, *flatten* represents the flatten operation, and *Proj* is a linear projection layer.

We concatenate the style condition and content condition at the channel level, and then add it with the time embedding of diffusion model to guide the generation process.

3.2 Conditional Diffusion Model

In conditional diffusion models, the forward process remains the same as that of the unconditional model. We adopt the diffusion model proposed in DDPM [19], which defines a Markov chain of diffusion steps to add gradually random noise to the data and then learn to reverse the diffusion process to construct desired data samples. The forward process is a Markovian process with the following conditional distribution:

$$q(x_t|x_{t-1}) = \mathcal{N}(x_t; \sqrt{1 - \beta_t}x_{t-1}, \beta_t \mathbf{I}) \tag{4}$$

where $t \sim [1, T]$ represents the time step, and $\beta_t \in (0, 1)\}_{t=1}^{T}$ is a fixed variance schedule. When $T \to \infty$, x_T becomes equivalent to an isotropic Gaussian distribution. Let $\alpha_t = 1 - \beta_t$ and $\overline{\alpha}_t = \prod_{i=1}^{t} \alpha_i$. We can sample x_t at any arbitrary time step t in a closed form:

$$x_t = \sqrt{\overline{\alpha}_t} x_0 + \sqrt{1 - \overline{\alpha}_t} \epsilon, \epsilon \sim \mathcal{N}(0, \mathbf{I}) \tag{5}$$

During the reverse process, we use a deep neural network p_θ to approximate the true posterior distribution $q(x_{t-1}|x_t)$. In our conditional diffusion model, we take the encoded style features e_s and content features e_c as conditions and input them into the diffusion model to guide the generation of target font images. To enhance control over the character structure in the generation process, we concatenate the noisy image x_t with the content image I_c in the channel-wise dimension. The concatenated image $x'_t = concat(x_t, I_c)$ is then passed through the denoising network $\mathcal{U}$, as illustrated in Fig. 2. The content image I_c will guide the denoising process and ensure that both the intermediate noise representations and the final image align with the given character. Hence, the denoising model is denoted as $p_\theta(x_t, t, e_s, e_c, I_c)$, and the reverse process can be formulated as:

$$\begin{aligned} p_\theta(x_{t-1}|x_t, e_s, e_c, I_c) &= \mathcal{N}(x_{t-1}; \mu_\theta(x_t, t, e_s, e_c, I_c), \beta_t \mathbf{I}) \\ &= \mathcal{N}(x_{t-1}; \mu_\theta(x'_t, t, e_s, e_c), \beta_t \mathbf{I}) \end{aligned} \tag{6}$$

For optimizing the parameters of the network θ, we use the simplified training objective of DDPM [20]. Specifically, we produce a noisy sample x_t corresponding to a time step t by adding Gaussian noise ϵ to x_0 and then predict the added noise according to the style features e_s and the content features e_c. We update the model parameters with a mean square error (MSE) loss, and our training objective can be defined as:

$$L_{mse} = \mathbb{E}_{t \sim [1,T], \epsilon \sim \mathcal{N}(0,I)} \left[\left\| \epsilon - \epsilon_\theta(x'_t, t, e_s, e_c) \right\|^2 \right] \tag{7}$$

3.3 Disentangled Guidance Sampling Strategy

After the diffusion model learns the conditional distribution, the inference process involves producing a random Gaussian noise $x_T \sim \mathcal{N}(0, I)$ and then sampling from $p_\theta(x_{t-1}|x'_t, e_s, e_c)$ iteratively from $t = T$ to $t = 1$. Although the generated images using the vanilla sampling technique appear acceptable, they often lack strong correlation with the conditional reference image I_s and content image I_c.

To enhance the influence of the conditioning signal e_s and e_c in the sampled images, we adapt the classifier-free guidance technique [9] into our disentangled guidance sampling procedure. We find that to sample images that not only meet the style requirement but also align perfectly with the target character requires disentangled guidance for both style and content. To perform this disentangled guidance, we employ the following equation:

$$\epsilon_{dis} = \epsilon_{uncond} + w_s \epsilon_{style} + w_c \epsilon_{content} \tag{8}$$

where $\epsilon_{uncond} = \epsilon_\theta(x'_t, t, \emptyset, \emptyset)$ is the unconditional prediction of the model. Here, $x'_t = concat(x_t, I_c)$ as mentioned in Sect. 3.2, and $\emptyset$ represents all-zeros tensor. The style-guided prediction and the content-guided prediction are represented by $\epsilon_{style} = \epsilon_\theta(x'_t, t, e_s, \emptyset) - \epsilon_{uncond}$ and $\epsilon_{content} = \epsilon_\theta(x'_t, t, \emptyset, e_c) - \epsilon_{uncond}$, respectively. w_s and w_c are guidance scales corresponding to style and content. In practice, we set the conditions e_s and e_c to $\emptyset$ with a probability of $\eta\%$ independently to get conditional and unconditional models during training.

By leveraging disentangled guidance, we can independently control and emphasize the effect of style and content during sampling. This approach enables us to generate images that not only exhibit the desired style but also maintain precise alignment with the target character, resulting in more faithful outputs.

4 Experiment

4.1 Experimental Setup

Datasets. To verify our one-shot font generation method, we collected a dataset consisting of 280 Chinese fonts. Each font in the dataset contains 1600 commonly used Chinese characters, and all images are resized to 80 × 80 pixels. In the training set, we randomly select 240 fonts, with each font containing 800 characters. The test set contains the remaining 40 unseen fonts with 800 unseen characters. We refer to this test set as the UFUC (Unseen Fonts Unseen Contents) dataset. We choose the *Song* font as our source font to generate content images.

Evaluation Metrics. To quantitatively compare the performance of different methods, we employ five commonly used evaluation metrics in font generation. These metrics can be categorized into pixel-wise metrics and perceptual metrics. Pixel-wise metrics include L1 distance, root mean square error (RMSE), and structural similarity index measure (SSIM). These metrics focus on calculating the pixel-level differences between the generated images and the ground truth. For the Perceptual metrics, we use FID [20] and LPIPS [21] which measure the similarity of features and align more closely with human vision.

Implementation Details. Our model has been trained with $T = 1000$ noising steps and a linear noise schedule. We use the AdamW optimizer with $\beta_1 = 0.9$, $\beta_2 = 0.999$, and a learning rate of $1e-4$. We train our model with 300,000 iterations, a batch size of 24, and a dropout rate of 0.1. To stabilize the model during training, we employ an exponential moving average rate of 0.9999. During inference, we adopt the DDIM [22] sampling strategy with only 15 steps to speed up sampling.

4.2 Experimental Results

Comparison Methods. We compare CD-Font with five state-of-the-art methods: FUNIT [23], MX-Font [7], DG-Font [1], CF-Font [2] and NTF-Loc [3]. For a fair comparison, we retrain all methods with our dataset based on their official codes. During inference, the same reference image of each font is employed for the one-shot setting.

Table 1. Quantitative comparison results on the UFUC dataset. The bold and underlined numbers denote the best and the second best, respectively.

Methods	Unseen Fonts Unseen Contents					User%
	L1 ↓	RMSE ↓	SSIM ↑	LPIPS ↓	FID ↓	
FUNIT [23]	0.0853	0.2408	0.6625	0.1911	48.7913	2.3
MX-Font [7]	0.0793	**0.2262**	0.6896	0.1632	51.1419	5.1
DG-Font [1]	0.0766	0.2425	0.6805	0.1281	42.3230	7.9
CF-Font [2]	0.0761	0.2406	0.6873	0.1277	42.8433	10.5
NTF-Loc [3]	0.0785	0.2332	0.6880	0.1389	40.3823	11.8
Ours	**0.0751**	0.2353	**0.6951**	**0.1266**	**31.0962**	**62.4**

Table 2. Quantitative comparison results on the UFSC dataset. The bold and underlined numbers denote the best and the second best, respectively.

Methods	Unseen Fonts Seen Contents				
	L1 ↓	RMSE ↓	SSIM ↑	LPIPS ↓	FID ↓
FUNIT [23]	0.0835	0.2380	0.6681	0.1877	49.5963
MX-Font [7]	0.0762	**0.2230**	0.6956	0.1605	51.6885
DG-Font [1]	0.0744	0.2388	0.6871	0.1263	44.3547
CF-Font [2]	0.0745	0.2381	0.6916	0.1265	43.7647
NTF-Loc [3]	0.0759	0.2286	0.6960	0.1357	41.3937
Diff-Font [10]	0.0768	0.2375	0.6910	0.1269	37.2524
Ours	**0.0722**	0.2298	**0.7044**	**0.1250**	**31.6030**

Quantitative Comparison. As shown in Table 1, our method outperforms the other compared methods. Although MX-Font [7] achieves the best RMSE on unseen fonts, it suffers a performance drop at the perceptual level. It is noted that RMSE focuses on pixel-wise differences between the generated image and the ground truth while ignores the feature similarity which is more closely related to human perception. We can observe that our method achieves state-of-the-art performance in perceptual-level metrics, i.e., FID [20] and LPIPS [21]. Since Diff-Font [10] cannot handle unseen contents, we also conduct comparative experiments on the testing fonts with seen contents. We refer to unseen fonts with seen contents as UFSC. The quantitative results are presented in Table 2, and our method also outperforms Diff-Font [10] by a margin.

Qualitative Comparison. Figure 3 provides a qualitative comparison of the results. We evaluate the generalization capability of all competitors by selecting five different fonts, including handwriting fonts, artistic fonts, and typewriter fonts. Our method generates characters with high quality in terms of style consistency and structural correctness.

However, FUNIT [23], MX-Font [7], and NTF-Loc [3] often produce results with structural errors, such as missing strokes and incomplete characters. FUNIT is originally an image-to-image translation framework for natural images, it may not perform well with font images. DG-Font [1] and CF-Font [2] tend to lose local details, especially when faced with large style differences between the source and the target fonts.

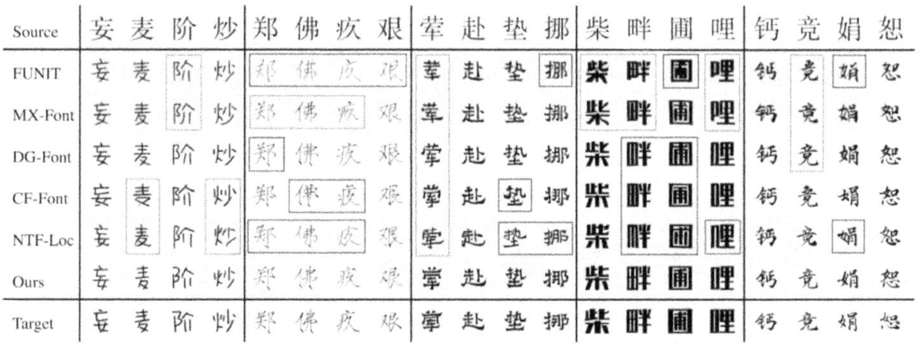

Fig. 3. Comparisons with the state-of-the-art methods for font generation on the UFUC dataset. We mark structural errors with red boxes, and mismatch styles with blue boxes (color figure online).

4.3 Ablation Study

Effectiveness of Each Module. Table 3 illustrates the effectiveness of different modules. The baseline uses a content encoder and a style encoder to extract content features and style features, respectively. These features are then concatenated and used as conditions for the diffusion model. This configuration is labeled as 'exp1' in Table 3. Then, we concatenate the content image with the noisy image as input to the diffusion model. This is denoted as 'exp2'. As shown in Fig. 4, 'exp2' is capable of generating characters with complete structures compared to 'exp1'. While the images generated using the vanilla sampling technique appear not bad, they often lack a strong correlation with the given content image and target style. To enhance this correlation, we introduce disentangled guidance sampling. As observed in Fig. 4, our model can generate images that preserve more local details of the target font.

Effectiveness of Guidance Scales. We further discuss the influence of the guidance scales w_s and w_c during inference. We gradually change w_s and w_c from 1 to 3 to perform ablation experiments on the UFUC dataset. As shown in Table 4, the setting $w_s = 3$, $w_c = 3$ achieves the best performance in our disentangled guidance sampling strategy. Therefore, we set the guidance scales w_s and w_c to 3 by default for other experiments of our method.

Table 3. Ablation study of different modules on the UFUC dataset. C and D represent concatenate operation and disentangled guidance in our proposed model. The bold and underlined numbers denote the best and the second best, respectively.

Methods	Settings		Unseen Fonts Unseen Contents				
	C	D	L1 ↓	RMSE ↓	SSIM ↑	LPIPS ↓	FID ↓
exp1	✗	✗	0.0770	0.2385	0.6913	0.1303	36.7729
exp2	✓	✗	<u>0.0763</u>	<u>0.2367</u>	<u>0.6932</u>	**0.1263**	<u>32.2503</u>
Ours	✓	✓	**0.0751**	**0.2353**	**0.6951**	<u>0.1266</u>	**31.0962**

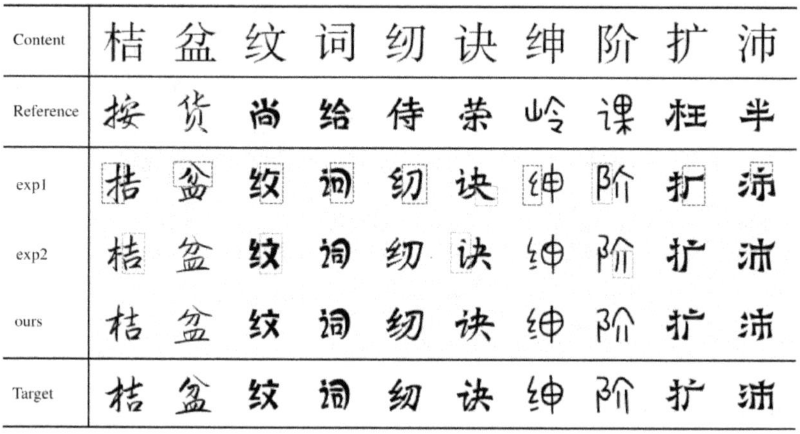

Fig. 4. Qualitative ablation results on the UFUC dataset. We mark structural errors with red boxes and mismatched styles with blue boxes (color figure online).

Table 4. Ablation study on the guidance scales.

Guidance Scales	Unseen Fonts Unseen Contents				
	L1 ↓	RMSE ↓	SSIM ↑	LPIPS ↓	FID ↓
$w_s = 1, w_c = 1$	0.0769	0.2387	0.6902	0.1311	<u>29.1867</u>
$w_s = 1, w_c = 3$	<u>0.0752</u>	**0.2353**	<u>0.6950</u>	<u>0.1267</u>	31.0977
$w_s = 3, w_c = 1$	0.0769	0.2386	0.6902	0.1312	**29.0889**
$w_s = 3, w_c = 3$	**0.0751**	0.2353	**0.6951**	**0.1266**	31.0962

4.4 Cross-Lingual Font Generation

CD-Font demonstrates the capability to decouple style and content and is able to effectively transfer styles to unknown content. To further validate the generalization of our model, we apply it to cross-lingual font generation. As depicted in Fig. 5, our model successfully generates Korean and Japanese characters without additional training, highlighting its impressive potential in the field of cross-lingual font generation.

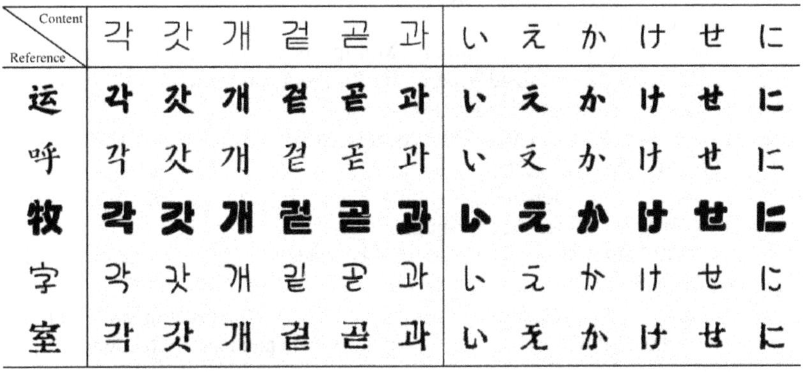

Fig. 5. Cross-lingual font generation (Chinese to Korean and Japanese).

5 Conclusion

In this paper, we propose a one-shot font generation framework based on the conditional diffusion model. We follow the style-content disentanglement paradigm, using two different encoders to extract style and content features for generating arbitrary combinations of style and content. To ensure precise control over the characters, we concatenate the content image with the noisy image as input to the model in each denoising step. During inference, we propose disentangled guidance sampling to enable the font images that exhibit strong correlations with both the reference image and the target character. Extensive experiments show the effectiveness of our approach.

Acknowledgments. This work was supported by the National Natural Science Foundation of China (NSFC) under Grants 62102178.

References

1. Xie, Y., Chen, X., Sun, L., Lu, Y.: DG-Font: deformable generative networks for unsupervised font generation. In: Proceedings of the IEEE/CVF Conference on Computer Vision and Pattern Recognition, pp. 5130–5140 (2021)
2. Wang, C., Zhou, M., Ge, T., Jiang, Y., Bao, H., Xu, W.: CF-Font: content fusion for few-shot font generation. In: Proceedings of the IEEE/CVF Conference on Computer Vision and Pattern Recognition, pp. 1858–1867 (2023)
3. Fu, B., He, J., Wang, J., Qiao, Y.: Neural transformation fields for arbitrary-styled font generation. In: Proceedings of the IEEE/CVF Conference on Computer Vision and Pattern Recognition, pp. 22438–22447 (2023)

4. Liang, D., et al.: Semantically contrastive learning for low-light image enhancement. Proc. AAAI Conf. Artif. Intell. **36**(2), 1555–1563 (2022)
5. Goodfellow, I., et al.: Generative adversarial nets. Adv. Neural Inf. Process. Syst. **27** (2014)
6. Tian, Y.: zi2zi: Master Chinese calligraphy with conditional adversarial networks (2017). https://github.com/kaonashi-tyc/zi2zi
7. Park, S., Chun, S., Cha, J., Lee, B., Shim, H.: Multiple heads are better than one: few-shot font generation with multiple localized experts. In: Proceedings of the IEEE/CVF International Conference on Computer Vision, pp. 13900–13909 (2021)
8. Dhariwal, P., Nichol, A.: Diffusion models beat GANs on image synthesis. Adv. Neural. Inf. Process. Syst. **34**, 8780–8794 (2021)
9. Ho, J., Salimans, T.: Classifier-free diffusion guidance. In: NeurIPS 2021 Workshop on Deep Generative Models and Downstream Applications (2021)
10. He, H., et al.: Diff-Font: diffusion model for robust one-shot font generation (2022). arXiv: 2212.05895
11. Zhang, Y., Zhang, Y., Cai, W.: Separating style and content for generalized style transfer. In: Proceedings of the IEEE Conference on Computer Vision and Pattern Recognition, pp. 8447–8455 (2018)
12. Gao, Y., Guo, Y., Lian, Z., Tang, Y., Xiao, J.: Artistic glyph image synthesis via one-stage few-shot learning. ACM Trans. Graph. **38**(6), 1–12 (2019)
13. Wu, S.J., Yang, C.Y., Hsu, J.Y.J.: CalliGAN: style and structure-aware Chinese calligraphy character generator (2020). arXiv:2005.12500
14. Cha, J., Chun, S., Lee, G., Lee, B., Kim, S., Lee, H.: Few-shot compositional font generation with dual memory. In: Vedaldi, A., Bischof, H., Brox, T., Frahm, J.-M. (eds.) ECCV 2020. LNCS, vol. 12364, pp. 735–751. Springer, Cham (2020). https://doi.org/10.1007/978-3-030-58529-7_43
15. Kong, Y., et al.: Look closer to supervise better: one-shot font generation via component-based discriminator. In: Proceedings of the IEEE/CVF Conference on Computer Vision and Pattern Recognition, pp. 13482–13491 (2022)
16. Tang, L., et al.: Few-shot font generation by learning fine-grained local styles. In: Proceedings of the IEEE/CVF Conference on Computer Vision and Pattern Recognition, pp. 7895–7904 (2022)
17. Dai, J., et al.: Deformable convolutional networks. In: Proceedings of the IEEE International Conference on Computer Vision (2017)
18. Ronneberger, O., Fischer, P., Brox, T.: U-Net: Convolutional networks for biomedical image segmentation. In: Medical Image Computing and Computer-Assisted Intervention, pp. 234–241 (2015)
19. Ho, J., Jain, A., Abbeel, P.: Denoising diffusion probabilistic models. Adv. Neural. Inf. Process. Syst. **33**, 6840–6851 (2020)
20. Heusel, M., Ramsauer, H., Unterthiner, T., Nessler, B., Hochreiter, S.: GANs trained by a two time-scale update rule converge to a local Nash equilibrium. Adv. Neural Inf. Process. Syst. **30** (2017)
21. Zhang, R., Isola, P., Efros, A.A., Shechtman, E., Wang, O.: The unreasonable effectiveness of deep features as a perceptual metric. In: Proceedings of the IEEE Conference on Computer Vision and Pattern Recognition, pp. 586–595 (2018)
22. Song, J., Meng, C., Ermon, S.: Denoising diffusion implicit models. In: International Conference on Learning Representations (2020)
23. Liu, M.Y., et al.: Few-shot unsupervised image-to-image translation. In: Proceedings of the IEEE/CVF International Conference on Computer Vision, pp. 10551–10560 (2019)

Image Super-Resolution Reconstruction Based on Dual-Branch Channel Attention

Jinyu Shi[✉], Zhanjun Si, Yingxue Zhang[✉], and Xinbin Yang

Tianjin University of Science and Technology, Tianjin 300457, China
{szj,yxzhang}@tust.edu.cn

Abstract. Image super-resolution reconstruction is an important technique for converting low resolution images into high-resolution images. High resolution images can provide more information and are crucial for advanced visual tasks. However, traditional methods cannot restore image details, resulting in blurring and not meeting practical requirements. In response to this, this paper proposes a dual-branch channel attention residual network (DCARN) for image super-resolution reconstruction, which focuses on the problem of multi-frequency information fusion. The proposed method first improve multi-spectral channel attention by adopting group convolution and discrete cosine transform to adapt to images of different sizes. In order to fully utilize channel and multi-spectral channel attention, a dual-branch channel attention residual block (DCARB) is further designed. Experiments on multiple public datasets show that the proposed method achieves improved performance and performs well on image reconstruction in terms of both subjective and objective quality, with richer stripe texture details.

Keyword: Image super-resolution · multi-spectral channel attention · Discrete cosine transform · Group convolution

1 Introduction

The rich emotional content and fine detail information conveyed by images make communication more vivid. However, images are subject to various influences during their passage, such as equipment limitations and processing methods, which can result in issues such as blurriness, color distortion, and low resolution. In recent years, the internet has been inundated with a profusion of low-resolution images that pose great challenges in terms of efficient utilization, especially in domains like medical imaging, satellite imaging, facial recognition, and surveillance. Therefore, there exists an acute demand for a rapid and effective means to enhance the resolution of such imagery. It is against this backdrop that the technology of image super-resolution reconstruction has emerged. Image super-resolution reconstruction is characterized as the employment of methodologies from disciplines such as signal processing and image processing, aimed at transforming low-resolution images into their high-resolution analogues. This approach serves to fulfill the objective of significantly improving the visual quality of these images.

Image super-resolution technology has undergone multiple stages of development. Early research predominantly relied on interpolation and filtering techniques, which, despite making some strides, often led to blurred and distorted images unsuitable for practical applications. The advent of machine learning and deep learning ushered ISR technology into a new era, with researchers beginning to explore the use of deep neural networks (DNNs) for image up-sampling. Dong et al. [1] marked a groundbreaking milestone by introducing the first convolutional neural network (CNN)-based ISR approach. Their SRCNN model employed a deep CNN to directly generate high-resolution images, pioneering the application of CNNs in ISR tasks. Shi et al. [2] proposed the end-to-end ESPCNN method, which introduced sub-pixel convolutions. This novel technique confined computational operations to the low-resolution domain throughout the network, only utilizing sub-pixel convolutions at the final stage to upscale feature maps into high-resolution images. Subsequently, researchers started incorporating attention mechanisms into visual problems to enhance existing ISR methods. In 2018, Jie et al. [3] introduced the SENet, a network featuring a two-stage mechanism to bolster the performance of crucial channels. Today, DNN-based super-resolution reconstruction has become the prevailing approach, unlocking immense potential in areas such as medical image processing, video surveillance, and smartphone photography.

Although image super-resolution method based on deep learning has been widely used in many fields, it still faces many challenges, such as computational complexity and image distortion. Therefore, it is of great significance to constantly explore new algorithms and improve the efficiency and reconstruction quality of image super-resolution methods. Therefore, this paper proposes an improved image super-resolution method based on improved multi-spectral channel attention mechanism and dual-branch design. The main contributions include:

1) To better incorporate multi-frequency domain information, we propose an improved Multi-Spectral Channel Attention (MSCA) mechanism.
2) To fully harness the advantages of both channel attention and multi-spectral channel attention in enhancing the quality of the high-resolution images, we propose a novel Dual-Branch Channel Attention Residual Block (DCARB).

2 Proposed Method

2.1 Overall Network Structure

In this paper, a dual-branch channel attention residual network (DCARN) is proposed for image super-resolution reconstruction by combining the dual-branch structure and improved multi-spectral channel attention mechanism. The overall structure is shown in Fig. 1.

The FEP is used to initially extract feature maps, which can provide support for the subsequent extraction of deep features. This part includes a convolutional layer and a ReLU activation layer, with a convolutional kernel size of 3×3, kernel number of C, a stride of 1, and padding of 1. The purpose of doing this is to ensure consistency in the size of the input and output. The process of preliminary feature extraction can be represented by the following formula:

$$F_{SF} = ReLU(Conv(L_{LR})) \qquad (1)$$

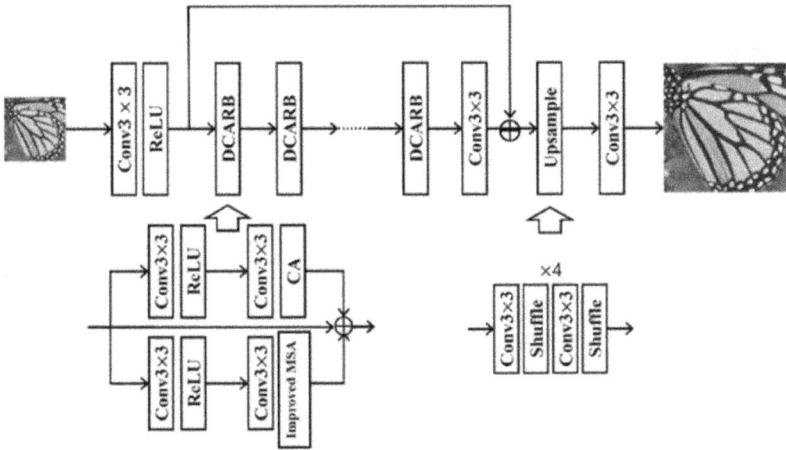

Fig. 1. Dual-branch Channel Attention Residual Network

The NFMP part is used to extract deep features. With the output of the FEP part as the input, more deep and abstract features are extracted for image reconstruction. This part is composed of N Dual-branch Channel Attention Residual Block (DCARB) modules and a convolution layer. The feature extraction process can be expressed by the following formula:

$$F_i = H_i(F_{i-1}) \tag{2}$$

$$F_{NF} = Conv(F_N) + F_{SF} \tag{3}$$

The RP part of this method uses sub-pixel layer for up-sampling, and then reduces the channel dimension to three channels through a convolution layer to obtain the reconstructed super-resolution image. The number of sub-pixel layers will be different when different scales of magnification are used. As mentioned earlier, using the sub-pixel layer can make the whole feature extraction and nonlinear feature extraction part be carried out in the low-resolution space, and at the same time, smaller convolution kernel size is used, which greatly reduces the computational complexity.

2.2 Improved Design of Multi-spectral Channel Attention

Previous implementations of the multi-spectral channel attention mechanism typically employed the Discrete Cosine Transform (DCT) [4] to compress channel information. A set of fixed-width and -height convolutions are constructed while using DCT for channel compression, leading to the limitation that this mechanism is effective in extracting rich information from channels only when the input size is known beforehand. However, the input sizes in image super-resolution reconstruction tasks are inherently variable, making the direct application of multi-spectral channel attention in such scenarios less applicable. This paper, therefore, sets out to improve the multi-spectral channel attention mechanism, adapting it for use in image super-resolution tasks where input dimensions are subject to variation.

This paper associates the principle of group convolution. Its advantage is that it does not need to know the size of the input data, it can more flexibly adapt to tasks with variable input size. For the task of image super-resolution reconstruction, the method of group convolution can make full use of the attention mechanism of multi spectral channels to incorporate more frequency domain information without worrying about the problem of input size. In addition, the use of group convolution also further accelerates the computation. Figure 2 demonstrates the improved multi-spectral channel attention mechanism in this paper.

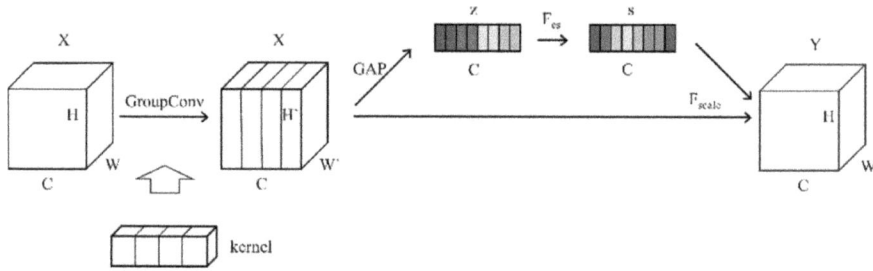

Fig. 2. Improved multi-spectral channel attention

2.3 Dual-Branch Channel Attention Mechanism

Branch structure is a very useful technique when designing deep learning networks. The classical deep learning networks ResNeXt [5], RepVGG [6] all use branch structure to improve the network performance, which enhances the representation ability of the model.

In this regard, this paper adopts the dual-branch structure to integrate the channel attention with the improved multi-spectral channel attention, and innovatively proposes the Dual-branch Channel Attention Residual Block (DCARB), whose structure is shown in Fig. 3. Specifically, considering the advantages of the idea of dual-branch attention in ResNeXt network, this paper also tries to design two branches in this module, each of which has a similar structure. The channel attention branch is responsible for compressing the low-frequency information in the channel to provide the global information of the feature map and generate the low-frequency attention feature map. The multi-spectral channel attention branch utilizes the proposed improved multi-spectral channel attention module, which is responsible for integrating information in other frequency domains into the channel compression process to provide details and edge information in the feature map and generate high-frequency attention feature map.

2.4 Loss Function

In image super-resolution reconstruction, the commonly used loss functions are l_1 and l_2 loss functions. l_1 loss function has better convergence performance, as shown in Fig. 4.

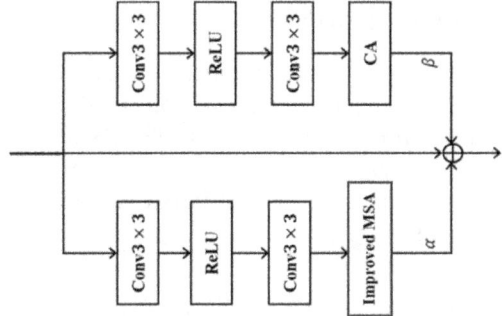

Fig. 3. Dual-branch Channel Attention Residual Block

Through comparison, it can be seen from the figure that in the initial and later stages of training, the loss value of training with l_1 loss function decreases faster and has better convergence performance. Therefore, this paper uses l_1 as the loss function.

The l_1 loss function can be expressed by the following formula:

$$L(\theta) = \frac{1}{N} \sum_{i=1}^{N} |y_i - \hat{y}_i| \tag{4}$$

Among them, θ represents the parameters in the network. The goal of training the network is to adjust the network parameters θ to make the loss value as small as possible. $\hat{y}_l$ represents the number of images in each batch of training samples. Represent high-resolution image; y_i represents the reconstructed image.

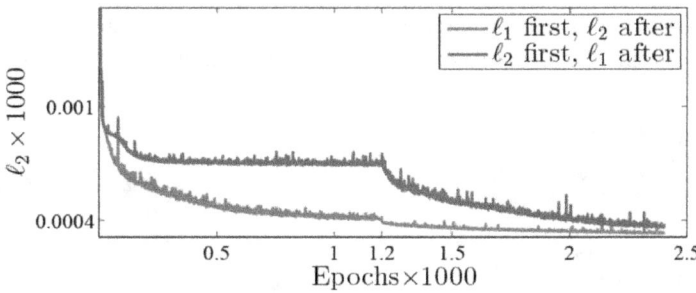

Fig. 4. Comparison of l_1 and l_2 loss function

3 Experiments

3.1 Experimental Setup

In order to fully verify the performance and generalization ability of the algorithm, DIV2K dataset [7], Set5 [8], Set14 [9], Urban100 [10] and Manga109 [11] are used for validation, where the training subset of DIV2K dataset is used as the training set of the network, and the others are used for testing.

3.2 Comparison with Existing Methods

The experiment in this section evaluates the performance from both subjective and objective aspects. Traditional super-resolution reconstruction algorithm Bicubic and four mainstream super-resolution networks SRCNN [12], SRResNet [13], DMCN [14], EDSR [15] are compared. A scaling factor of 4 is selected for validation.

Table 1 shows the performance in terms of PSNR and SSIM indicators of the five methods on four test datasets.

Table 1. Objective comparison with existing methods

Models	Set5 PSNR/SSIM	Set14 PSNR/SSIM	Urban100 PSNR/SSIM	Manga109 PSNR/SSIM
Bicubic	28.42/0.8104	26.00/0.7027	23.14/0.6577	24.89/0.7866
SRCNN	29.97/0.8556	27.20/0.7454	24.11/0.7091	26.63/0.8365
SRResNet	32.09/0.8973	28.55/0.7812	25.99/0.7829	30.31/0.9070
DMCN	32.33/0.8950	28.70/0.7845	26.31/0.7938	/
EDSR	32.46/0.8968	**28.80/0.7876**	**26.64/0.8033**	31.02/0.9148
Ours	**32.51/0.8993**	28.79/0.7870	26.61/0.8014	**31.06/0.9157**

3.3 Visualization of Reconstructed Images

This paper also compares the subjective quality of the reconstructed images. The following four representative images are presented to demonstrate the visual quality.

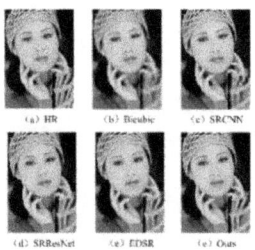

Fig. 5. Comparison of "woman" in Set5 dataset at 4 × SR

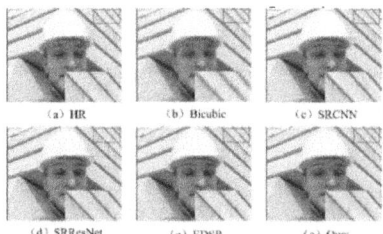

Fig. 6. Comparison of "foreman" in Set14 dataset at 4 × SR

3.4 Ablation Study

In order to verify the effectiveness of the proposed module, this paper compared and analyzed the effectiveness of the dual branch channel attention module. The experimental results are shown in Table 2.

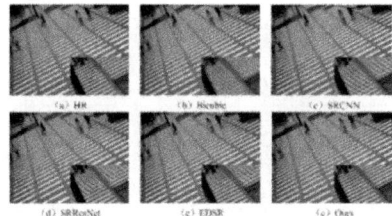

Fig. 7. Comparison of "img_093" in Urban100 dataset at 4 × SR

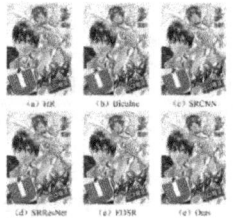

Fig. 8. Comparison of "DollGun" in Manga109 dataset at 4 × SR

Table 2. Objective evaluation index comparison

Dataset	Metric	Baseline	Baseline + CA	Baseline + MSA	Baseline + DCA
Set5	PSNR/dB	32.02	32.07	32.07	32.20
	SSIM	0.8936	0.8937	0.8941	0.8956
Set14	PSNR/dB	28.47	28.51	28.49	28.56
	SSIM	0.78	0.7804	0.7806	0.7818
Urban100	PSNR/dB	25.88	25.93	25.92	26.08
	SSIM	0.7796	0.7805	0.7807	0.7862
Manga109	PSNR/dB	30.22	30.25	30.27	30.46
	SSIM	0.9046	0.9051	0.9051	0.9081

From the experimental results, it can be seen that the addition of DCA can make the super division network obtain better reconstruction quality, and CA and MSA can also improve the reconstruction effect to varying degrees. From the characteristics of datasets, it can be found that Set14 and Urban100 data sets have more urban buildings and natural scenes than Set5 and Manga109 data sets, which indicates that CA and MSA will focus on different scenes, which on the other hand confirms that the proposed integration of CA and MSA can bring better generalization to the model to improve the network performance.

This paper designed a set of experiments to compare the effects of different attention levels on reconstruction performance. The experimental results are shown in Table 3, and it can be seen that different attention ratios do indeed affect the reconstruction effect, with C5M5 achieving a more balanced effect.

Table 3. Comparison of different combination strategies of the two channel attention

Dataset	Metric	C8M2	C5M5	C2M8
Set5	PSNR/dB	30.3727	**30.4045**	30.3816
	SSIM	0.8612	**0.8615**	0.8612
Set14	PSNR/dB	27.4364	**27.4473**	27.4379
	SSIM	0.7527	**0.7528**	0.7525
Urban100	PSNR/dB	24.3363	**24.3442**	24.3394
	SSIM	0.7175	**0.7177**	0.7174
Manga109	PSNR/dB	27.1716	27.1856	**27.1868**
	SSIM	0.8465	0.8463	**0.8466**

4 Conclusions

This paper proposes a dual-branch channel attention residual network (DCARN) for image super-resolution reconstruction task. By analyzing the characteristics of discrete cosine transform and group convolution, an improved multi-spectral channel attention is designed, solving the limitation of fixed image size. Based on the improvement of multi-spectral channel attention, a dual-branch structure is further proposed to fully integrating the advantages of multi-spectral channel attention and the traditional channel attention. The proposed method is able to take into account the various frequency domain features, helping the network build more rich details in the process of image reconstruction. Thorough experiments are designed to verify the effectiveness of the proposed method from both subjective and objective aspects. Considering the limitations, the downsampling method for low resolution images uses a simple bicubic interpolation method. In practical life, the generation of low resolution images is more complex, and when faced with noise, compression artifacts, or other image degradation, this can lead to a decrease in the performance of the network model in dealing with complex scenes. In the future, we will consider further optimizing the network structure, and continue to improve the robustness and generalization application capability.

References

1. Dong, C., Loy, C. C., He, et al. (2014). Learning a deep convolutional network for image super-resolution. European Conference on Computer Vision
2. Shi, W., Caballero, J., Huszár, F., et al. (2016). Real-time single image and video super-resolution using an efficient sub-pixel convolutional neural network. IEEE Conference on Computer Vision and Pattern Recognition
3. Shocher, A., Cohen, N., & Irani, M. (2018). "zero-shot" super-resolution using deep internal learning. IEEE Conference on Computer Vision and Pattern Recognition
4. Ahmed, N., Natarajan, T., Rao, K.R.: Discrete cosine transform. IEEE Trans. Comput. **100**(1), 90–93 (1974)
5. Yang, C. Y., Ma, C., & Yang, M. H. (2014). Single-image super-resolution: A benchmark. European Conference on Computer Vision

6. Chen, W., Rao, K.R.: Handbook of DCT-Based Audio Coding: Algorithms and Applications. Springer, Cham (2019)
7. Agustsson, E, & Timofte, R. (2017). NTIRE 2017 Challenge on Single Image Super-Resolution: Dataset and Study. IEEE Conference on Computer Vision and Pattern Recognition Workshops
8. Bevilacqua, M., Roumy, A., Guillemot, C., et al. (2012). Low-complexity single-image super-resolution based on nonnegative neighbor embedding. British Machine Vision Conference
9. Yang, J., Wright, J., Huang, T.S., et al.: Image super-resolution via sparse representation. IEEE Trans. Image Process. **19**(11), 2861–2873 (2010)
10. Huang, J. B., Singh, A., & Ahuja, N. (2015). Single image super-resolution from transformed self-exemplars. IEEE Conference on Computer Vision and Pattern Recognition, 5197–5206
11. Matsui, Y., Ito, K., Aramaki, Y., et al.: Sketch-based manga retrieval using manga109 dataset. Multimedia tools and applications **76**, 21811–21838 (2017)
12. Dong, C., Loy, C.C., He, K., et al.: Image super-resolution using deep convolutional networks. IEEE Trans. Pattern Anal. Mach. Intell. **38**(2), 295–307 (2015)
13. Ledig, C, Theis, L, Huszar, F., et al. (2016). Photo-realistic single image super-resolution using a generative adversarial network. IEEE Conference on Computer Vision and Pattern Recognition
14. Wang, X, Wang, C, Wang, C, et al.(2020).Dual-channel Multi-perception Convolutional Network for Image Super-Resolution. Journal of Northeastern University, 41(11), 1564–1576
15. Lim, B, Son, S. Kim, H. et al. (2017). Enhanced deep residual networks for single image super-resolution. IEEE Conference on Computer Vision and Pattern Recognition Workshops

A Flipped Reversible Information Hiding Method Based on AMP

Yaowen Fu, Haoshan Shi, Tianyang Qi$^{(\boxtimes)}$, Xueyan Gao, and Yifei Zou

College of Cyberspace Security, University of International Relations, Beijing 100091, China
qitianyang@uir.edu.cn

Abstract. Adaptive MSB Prediction is an effective technique to achieve Reversible Data Hiding in Encrypted Images(RDHEI). Specifically, the image is divided into 2 × 2 pixels blocks and encrypted to preserve pixel correlation, the shared MSB of pix-els in the block is extracted, only one of the four identical MSBs is saved, and the positions of the three vacated MSBs are embedded with data. However, the pixel blocks with poor correlation cannot embed data, in addition, the scheme has some blocks with very close pixel values but cannot embed data, which limits the embedding capacity. A new MSB prediction-based RDHEI framework is proposed, supporting an adaptive strategy. Flipping strategy makes some unavailable blocks available, enhancing embedding capacity. Experimental results show improved prediction accuracy and embedding capacity while ensuring reversibility.

Keywords: Reversible Data Hiding · Image Encryption · Adaptive Most Significant Bit Prediction · Image Encryption · Multimedia Security

1 Introduction

Reversible Data Hiding in Encrypted Images (RDHEI) is an emerging technique to achieve data hiding into cover image while protecting confidentiality of the content from being leaked [1–10]. Because of reversibility, the original image is able to be fully recovered once the embedded data is extracted. However, the implementation of such a property usually comes at the cost of reducing effective embedding capacity. How to improve capacity in this scenario is becoming a big challenge, which is crucial to the development of this technique.

Most Significant Bit (MSB) prediction is one of the most effective means to achieve RDHEI [11–14]. Even though effective, the existing MSB prediction schemes suffer from the problem of data extraction error [12], the reason is that proposed prediction formula is inaccurate. To deal with this limitation, Wang et al. [14] proposed Adaptive MSB Prediction (AMP), in which a flag with three bits is utilized to record the longest length of common MSBs. As a result, the reversibility can be achieved regardless of the value of length. Obviously, such kind of MSB prediction based RDHEI relies on the consistency of pixels within a selected block, which means once the consistency is not strong enough, the embedding capacity is restrained as a result. In particular, once the associate value of the flag is 0 or 1, which means the longest length of common MSBs is only 0 or 1, the corresponding block is considered to be an unavailable one.

Therefore, in this paper we are going to tackle how to improve the effective embedding capacity of AMP based RDHEI by introducing a flipping strategy with reversibility guaranteed. To the best of our knowledge, our scheme is the first to well improve the capacity of MSB prediction based RDHEI. For unavailable blocks in AMP scheme, we introduce flipping strategy to make most of them available again. The main contributions of this paper are summarized as the following three aspects:

(1) We propose a MSB prediction based RDHEI framework, which supports the proposed adaptive strategy. Specially, available blocks with $md > 1$ are employed to embed data using AMP scheme, while unavailable blocks with $md < 2$ using the proposed FAMP scheme. Moreover, a new 2×2 pixels structure as well as new location maps are also supported as preparations to construct the proposed flipping strategy.
(2) A flipping strategy as well as the novel location maps are introduced to improve the existing MSB prediction based RDHEI. Specially, because of the flipping strategy utilized, some of the unavailable blocks are turned to be available ones through flipping some of the pixels inside. The positions of corresponding pixels are recorded in the newly constructed location maps.
(3) We take experiments to compare the performance of proposed scheme with other schemes. Experimental results show that the proposed scheme is able to achieve better prediction accuracy and greater embedding capacity with reversibility guaranteed.

2 Proposed Scheme

2.1 Framework

Figure 1 depicts the FAMP scheme framework comprising three main modules: image encryption module, secret data embedding module, extraction and recovery module. The image encryption module encrypts and scrambles the original image for confidentiality. Next, the secret data embedding module utilizes the AMP algorithm for initial block selection and rearrangement. Unavailable blocks, indicated by green texture, undergo a second round of selection and rearrangement. Eligible blocks are converted into available ones using the FAMP strategy, while those failing predetermined conditions are placed at the image's end in reverse order. This strategy typically results in the first blocks being embeddable, while the last ones remain unavailable. To maintain reversibility, compressed location maps are generated after each round of block selection, recording the availability of original and flipped blocks. Blocks embedded with the AMP scheme are marked in blue, while those using FAMP are marked in orange.

After secret data embedding, the embedded image is sent to the receiver in the extraction and recovery module. This process is divided into three cases based on the key distribution state, each detailed in Fig. 6.

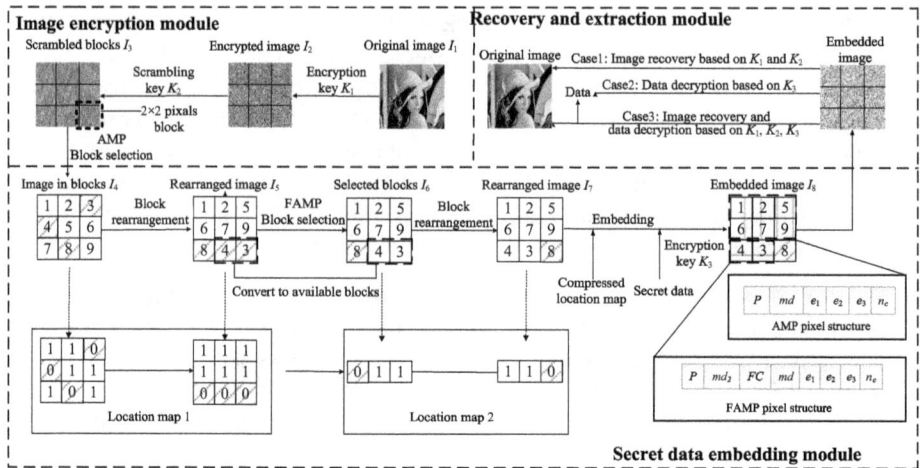

Fig. 1. Propose framework

2.2 Image Encryption

To ensure the security of image transmission, the original image I1 is protected before being transmitted by the image owner, using encryption key K1 and a scrambling key K2. Block-level encryption of the image after stream cipher encryption cannot resist complexity analysis. Attackers can perform complexity analysis on the image en-crypted with stream cipher to obtain partial original images. To enhance security, it is necessary to scramble the image after stream cipher encryption. The encryption method employed in this paper is the same as that described in References [14]. Block-level stream encryption: The process of block-level stream encryption is de-scribed as follows.

Fig. 2. The structure of 2×2 pixels block

Step 1: Image Segmentation. $M \times N$-sized original image is divided into pixel blocks of size 2×2. The number of pixel blocks is

$$n = \left\lfloor \frac{M}{2} \right\rfloor \times \left\lfloor \frac{N}{2} \right\rfloor \tag{1}$$

Step 2: Pixel decomposition. All pixels within each block are decomposed into 8 bits, denoted as

$$b_m^k(i,j) = \left\lfloor \frac{P_m(i,j)}{2^k} \right\rfloor \mod 2, k = 0, 1, 2, \cdots, 7. \tag{2}$$

where $P_m(i, j)$ represents the m-th pixel located in the i-th row and j-th column within the block, and $b_m^k(i, j)$ denotes the k-th bit of $P_m(i, j)$.

Step 3: Encrypting Block Pixels. Utilize an encryption key K_1 (e.g.RC4), along with the image I_1 to generate a pseudo-random matrix of size $\lfloor \frac{M}{2} \rfloor \times \lfloor \frac{N}{2} \rfloor$. Subsequently, decompose all values in the generated matrix into binary. Then, encrypt all original pixels in bit level using the formula (3)

$$e_m^k(i, j) = b_m^k(i, j) \oplus r^k(i, j), k = 0, 1, 2, \cdots, 7. \tag{3}$$

where $r^k(i, j)$ represents the k-th bit of the element located in the i-th row and j-th column of the pseudo-random matrix, and $e_m^k(i, j)$ represents the k-th bit of the m-th pixel within the block situated in the i-th row and j-th column. Finally, obtain the m-th encrypted pixel within the block located in the i-th row and j-th column as

$$E_m(i, j) = \sum_{k=0}^{7} 2^k \times e_m^k(i, j). \tag{4}$$

Step 4: Scramble Encryption. The encrypted images are once again divided into pixel blocks of size 2×2 by using the encryption key K_1. Subsequently, the scrambling key K_2 is employed to scramble the pixel blocks, altering the arrangement order and producing the final encrypted image. The purpose of scramble encryption is to prevent attackers from conducting complexity analysis to recover parts of the original image.

2.3 Generating Location Map Information

Figure 3 shows the process of location map generation. In scrambled image I_4, available and unavailable blocks are distinguished according to the value of *md*. Blank blocks with $md > 1$ are available and texture ones with $md < 2$ are unavailable. In block rearrangement, the third, fourth, and eighth blocks of image I_4 are arranged in reverse order to the end of the image I_5. The first location map is obtained from I_4 and I_5, in which available blocks are recorded as 0 and unavailable blocks as 1.

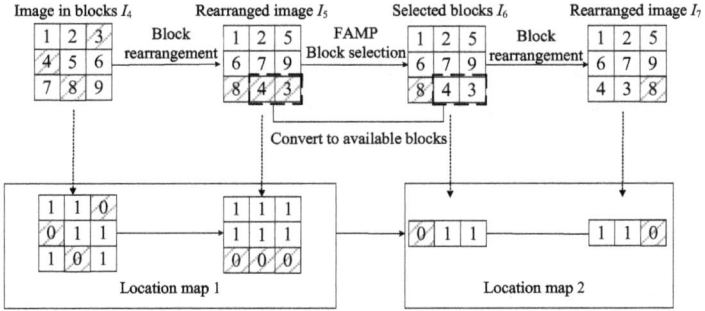

Fig. 3. The process of location map generation

Then, for I_5, FAMP block selection is performed to determine whether unavailable blocks could be turned to available ones according to whether md_2 is greater than 2. Specifically, the 3rd, 4th pixel blocks of I_5 are converted from unavailable blocks to available blocks in image I_6, the 8th pixel block is still an unavailable one. Then, blocks of I_6 are rearranged to generate I_7. In particular, the 8th pixel block of I_6 is arranged in reverse order to the end of I_7. The second location map is obtained from I_4 and I_5, in which available blocks are recorded as 0 and unavailable blocks as 1. The length of this location map just equals to the total number of pixel blocks with $md = 0$ and $md = 1$.

2.4 Flipping Based Adaptive MSB Prediction Scheme

In AMP scheme [14], pixel blocks with $md < 2$ cannot embed data, leading to the problem of low efficiency in pixels utilization. To solve this problem, we introduce FAMP scheme in this part. According to our design, for pixel blocks with $md > 1$, AMP scheme is utilized in data embedding. While for pixel blocks with $md < 2$, the FAMP is introduced to selected bits within corresponding pixel blocks. With the help of FAMP scheme, the number of common MSBs in most blocks is increased as a result, thus creating more space for data embedding. In this section, the detail of the proposed FAMP scheme is outlined.

As shown in Fig. 2, the encrypted image blocks are first divided into available blocks and unavailable blocks. Specifically, use formula (5) to calculate the longest different LSB bits for two pixels,

$$d_i = dif(P, C_i), i = 1, 2, 3. \tag{5}$$

and formula (6) to calculate the common MSB bits md for pixel blocks.

$$md = 8 - max(d_1, d_2, d_3) \tag{6}$$

Blocks with $md > 1$ are available blocks, otherwise they are unavailable blocks. For example, for pixels $P = 171$ and $C_1 = 180$, writing them in binary form yields $P = 171 = (10101011)_2$, $C_1 = 180 = (10110100)_2$. The 5th LSB of P and C_1 is different, indicating that $d_1 = dif(171,180) = 5$, which means that the longest different LSB digit between 171 and 180 pixels is 5. Similarly, using P, C_2 and C_3, calculate d_2 and d_3. Then, calculate the common number of MSB bits md using formula (6).

In this paper, the formula (7) is used to flip pixels C_i with $md < 2$ to obtain a new pixel block, where the first pixel P remains unchanged and C_i is updated as

$$C_i = \begin{cases} F(C_i, max(d_i)), & if\ d_i = max(d_1, d_2, d_3) \\ C_i, & other \end{cases}. \quad i = 1, 2, 3. \tag{7}$$

$F(C_i, max(d_i))$ indicates that the pixel bits corresponding to the maximum of d_1, d_2 and d_3 are flipped. Specifically, the 0 bit is flipped to 1 bit and the 1 bit is flipped to 0, leaving the unflipped pixel bits unchanged. For example, $F(191,7) = (1011\ 1111,7) = (1100\ 0000)$. In this case $d_1 = 7$ means that the 7th LSB to the 1st LSB of $191 = (1011\ 1111)$ is flipped, 0111111 is flipped to 1000000. After forming the new pixel block, formula (8) calculates the D_i between the first pixel P and the other three pixels(C_1, C_2, C_3).

$$D_i = \begin{cases} dif(P, C_i), & if\ d_i = max(d_1, d_2, d_3) \\ d_i, & other \end{cases} . \ i = 1, 2, 3. \qquad (8)$$

D_i represents the position of the first differing MSB between two pixels, where $D_i = dif(P, C_i)$ returns the maximum index of LSB that pixel P does not share with pixel C_i. For example, we have $dif(171, 180) = dif(10101011, 10110100) = 5$, the fifth LSB of 171 and 180 is different. At this time, a new 2 × 2 pixels block is formed after flipping, md_2 use formula (9) to calculate by using the D_i of the new pixel block.

$$md_2 = 8 - max(D_1, D_2, D_3). \qquad (9)$$

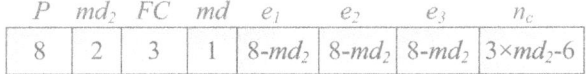

Fig. 4. The proposed 32 bits pixel

The proposed method flips the pixels, and the 32-bit structure of the pixel block is changed. The proposed 32-bit pixel structure is shown in Fig. 4, where pixel P length is 8 bits, the length of md_2 is 2 bits, the length of FC is 3 bits, and e_1, e_2 and e_3 are all (8-md_2) bits. Specifically, P is the first pixel of the original pixel blocks, the value range of md_2 calculate to range from 1 to 8, the available block range is from 3 to 8. After statistics, the number of pixel blocks is very small when $md_2 = 7$ and $md_2 = 8$. If length of md_2 use 3 bits to represent the 6 values of md_2, this will reduce the embedding capacity of the image. In order to improve the embedding capacity, $md_2 = 6$ is used to calculate the embedding capacity of pixel blocks with $md = 7$ and $md_2 = 8$ in this paper. The md_2 block has 4 values from 3 to 6, which are represented by only two bits in binary, effectively saving one bit per pixel block.

Table 1. Binary of md_2 value and embedding capacity

	md = 1	md = 2	md = 3	md = 4	md = 5	md = 6,7,8
md_2	-	-	00	01	10	11
n_c (bit)	-	-	3	6	9	12

Specifically, $md_2 = 3$ is represented by binary 00, $md_2 = 4$ is represented by binary 01, $md_2 = 5$ is represented by binary 10, and $md_2 = 6, 7$ and 8 is represented by binary 11. The length of FC is 3 bits, the 3-bit data from left to right indicates whether pixel C_1, C_2, and C_3 is flipped. If the pixel is flipped, the corresponding bit is denoted as 1, or it is denoted as 0. For example, $FC = 101$ represent that pixels C_1 and C_3 are flipped but pixel C_2 is not flipped. The length of *md* field is 1 bit which represents the *md* value of the original pixel block. If $md = 0$ before the original pixel block is flipped, it is recorded as 0 *md* field. If $md = 1$ before the original pixel block is flipped, it is recorded as 1 *md* field. This 1-bit data *md* is used when recovering the pixel block. e_1, e_2 and e_3 are the MSBs in the new pixel block that P does not share with C_1, C_2 and C_3. e_i has a length of ($8-md_2$) bits. The length of Nc is 32 bits minus the length of P, md_2, FC, md, e_1, e_2 and e_3:

$$n_c = 3 \times md_2 - 6 \qquad (10)$$

where n_c represents the embedding capacity of the flipped available pixel block and the Table 1 shows the binary representation of md_2 and its embedding capacity.

2.5 Data Embedding

For blocks with $md > 1$, we use AMP scheme to embed data. For blocks with $md < 2$, we utilize the FAMP scheme instead. The corresponding pseudocode is shown in Table 2.

Step 1: **Image encryption.** FAMP scheme adopts encryption key K_1 and scrambling key K_2 to achieve image encryption according to the process in Sect. 3.2.

Step 2: **Block selection using AMP.** Firstly, select pixel blocks with $md > 1$ as available ones to embed secret data. To ensure reversibility, generate a binary matrix of size $\lfloor \frac{M}{2} \rfloor \times \lfloor \frac{N}{2} \rfloor$ as Location Map 1. In particular, bit 1 in the map indicates an available block, and bit 0 an unavailable one.

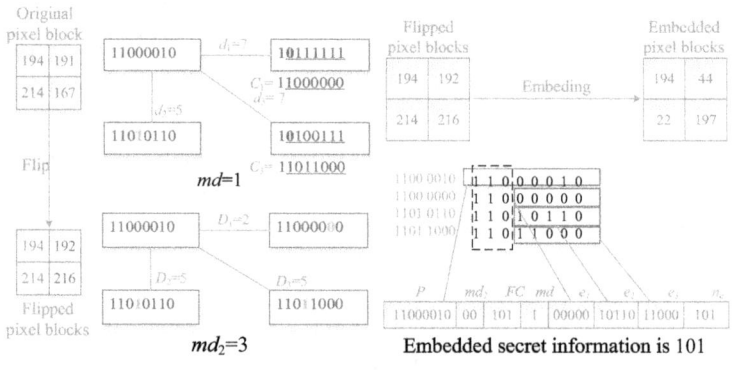

(a) Forming flipped pixel blocks (b) embedded data

Fig. 5. Four different flipped types of flips when $md = 1$

Step 3: **Rearranging blocks in AMP.** Arrange available blocks with $md > 1$ to first positions of the image, and unavailable ones to the end. Subsequently, compress Location Map 1 before embedding it into available blocks.

Step 4: **Block selection in FAMP.** Flipping the corresponding pixels in unavailable blocks to change their availability. Calculating the corresponding values of md_2, and blocks with $md_2 > 2$ are considered to be available blocks, while those with $md_2 < 3$

are unavailable ones. In Location Map 2, blocks with $md_2 < 3$ are recorded as 0, and blocks with $md_2 \geq 3$ are recorded as 1. The length of Location Map 2 just equals to the number chunks satisfies $md < 2$.

Step 5: **Rearranging blocks in FAMP.** Arrange blocks with $md_2 > 2$ for data embedding towards front position of the image, and reversing the order of the blocks with $md_2 < 3$ towards the back of the image.

Step 6: **Encryption of Embedded Information.** To prevent malicious access to the embedded confidential information, this paper employs classical symmetric encryption algorithms such as RC4 and AES. The embedded confidential information is encrypted using the data encryption key K_3.

Step 7: **Data Embedding.** To ensure reversibility, the lengths of Location Map 1 (lm_1), Location Map 1 (LM_1), the length of Location Map 2 (lm_2), and Location Map 2 (LM_2) are compressed and embedded into the available blocks towards the front of the image. Arithmetic coding is employed in this paper to compress the positional map information. Subsequently, the encrypted confidential data and the end marker are embedded into the remaining available blocks.

Figure 5 shows an example of using FAMP to embed data in a block with $md = 1$. As shown in the Fig. 5(a), this block is composed of pixels $P = 194 = (1100\ 0010)_2$, $C_1 = 191 = (1011\ 1111)_2$, $C_2 = 214 = (1101\ 0110)_2$, $C_3 = 167 = (1010\ 0111)_2$. This block is calculated to obtain $d_1 = 7, d_2 = 5, d_3 = 7$ and $md = 1$ and using the formula (5) and formula (6).

Figure 5(a) flip the pixel corresponding to the maximum value of d_i. In this case, $d_1 = 7, d_2 = 5, d_3 = 7$. Pixels C_1 and C_3 correspond to d_1 and d_3, because maximum value of d_i is 7. Therefore, flipping 7 bits LSB of pixels C_1 and C_3 by using the formula (7). The flipping rule is such that bit 1 is flipped to bit 0, and bit 0 is flipped to bit 1. The 7-bit LSB in pixel C_1 is the red part, 0111111 is flipped to 1000000, resulting in the pixel $C_1 = 192 = (1100\ 0000)_2$. Similarly, the 7-bit LSB in pixel C_3 is the red part, 0100100 is flipped to 1011000, resulting in the pixel $C_3 = 219 = (1101\ 1000)_2$. According to the formula (8), calculating $D_1 = 2$ for pixel C_1 and $D_3 = 5$ for pixel C_3. The new pixel block is composed of $P = 194$, $C_1 = 192$, $C_2 = 214$ and $C_3 = 219$.

Figure 5 (b) shows embedded data, C_1 and C_3 are flipped in Fig. 5 (a), so the FC field is 101. In this flipped pixel block, $md_2 = 3$ is an available block and record in binary as 00 in md_2 field, pixel block of $md_2 = 3$ shares 3 MSB with pixel P. e_1, e_2 and e_3 respectively record the MSBs not shared by C_1, C_2 and C_3 with P. e_1 represents the $(8-md_2)$ bits LSB of $C_1 = 192$, e_1 is 00000. e_2 represents the $(8-md_2)$ bits LSB of $C_2 = 214$, e_2 is 10110. e_3 represents the $(8-md_2)$ bits LSB of $C_3 = 219$, e_3 is 11011. The length of the embedded data n_c is $(3 \times md_2-6)$ bits. For the flipped block with $md_2 = 3$, the length of n_c is also 3 bits. In other words, 3 bits data can represent any binary number. In this example, $n_c = 101$. Combining P, md_2, FC, md, e_1, e_2, e_3 and n_c fields forms the pixel block after embedding the data is $P = 194 = (1100\ 0010)_2$, $C_1 = 44 = (0010\ 1100)_2$, $C_2 = 64 = (0101\ 0110)_2$, $C_3 = 167 = (1101\ 1101)_2$.

2.6 Data Extraction and Image Recovery

Depending on the availability of the image encryption key K_1, the scrambling key K_2, and the data encryption key K_3 held by the receiver, three types can be distin-guished:

Case1: For receivers with only keys K_1 and K_2, the original image and the secret information in encrypted form can be obtained.

Step1: Retrieve the position map and identify the embedding boundaries. Divide the embedded image into non-overlapping 2×2 pixels blocks, and extract lm_1, lm_2, LM_1, and LM_2 sequentially. The extracted LM_1 and LM_2 are decompressed to obtain the distribution of usable blocks for AMP and FAMP, along with the embedding boundaries.

Step2: For secret information extraction and pixel block restoration, the AMP-compressed blocks are first restored based on LM_1. The format of AMP blocks is shown in Fig. 2. Sequentially extract P and md, followed by e_1, e_2, and e_3, along with the secret information n_c, and restore the pixels according to the following formula (11).

$$C_i = Trunc(P, md) + e_i, i = 1, 2, 3. \tag{11}$$

Subsequently, restoring the FAMP-compressed pixel blocks based on LM_2. Sequentially extract P, md_2, FC, and md, then extract e_1, e_2, e_3, and the secret information n_c, and restoring the pixels according to the following formula (12).

$$C_i = \begin{cases} Trunc(P, md_2), & \text{if } C_i \text{ unchange} \\ C_i, & \text{if } C_i \text{ flip} \end{cases} . i = 1, 2, 3. \tag{12}$$

where $Trunc(P, md_2)$ represents the md_2 MSB of pixel P. "$+$" denotes the concatenation of the left and right operands, the $F(Trunc(P, md_2) + e_i, md)$ represents the (8-md) LSB of the reversal pixel $Trunc(P, md_2) + e_i$, with the remaining md MSB unchanged. Figure 8 shows an example of FAMP method for recovering pixels. It is known from the location map that this pixel block is embedded data using the FAMP method. Through the position map information, it is known that this pixel block is embedded data using the FAMP method, with pixels $P = 194$, $C_1 = 44$, $C_2 = 22$ and $C_3 = 197$. The four pixels are represented as a 32-bit pixel structure.

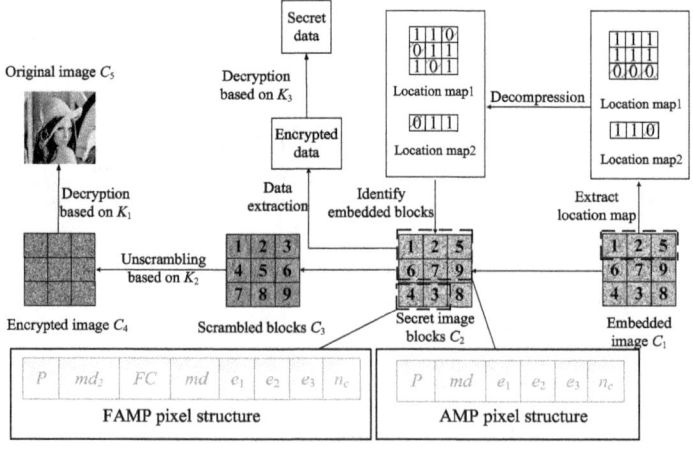

Fig. 6. Data extraction and image recovery

In Fig. 7, the receiver determines from $md_2 = 00 = 3$ that the first 3 bits of C_1, C_2, and C_3 match P, and identifies that e_1, e_2, and e_3 each occupy 5 bits. Thus, $C_1 = Trunc(P, md_2) + e_1 = 110 + 00000 = 11000000$, $C_2 = Trunc(P, md_2) + e_2 = 110 + 10110 = 11010110$, $C_3 = Trunc(P, md_2) + e_3 = 110 + 11000 = 11011000$. Subsequently, with $FC = 101$, it's noted that C_1 and C_3 were flipped while C_2 remained unchanged. Also, given $md = 1$, it is inferred that the 7 LSBs of C_1 and C_3 were flipped. Therefore, $C_1 = F(C_1, 1) = 10111111 = 191$, $C_2 = C_2 = 214$, and $C_3 = F(C_3, 1) = 10100111 = 167$.

Step3: To decrypt the recovered encrypted pixel blocks, decryption is performed sequentially using the scrambling key K_2 and the image encryption key K_1 to restore the original image.

Case2: For receivers with only the key K_3, they can only obtain the plaintext form of the secret information. Repeat Step 1 and Step 2 from Case 1, and decrypt the extracted secret information using the data encryption key K_3.

Case3: For recipients with keys K_1, K_2, and K_3, they can obtain the plaintext forms of both the original image and the secret information. Simply execute Case 1 and Case 2.

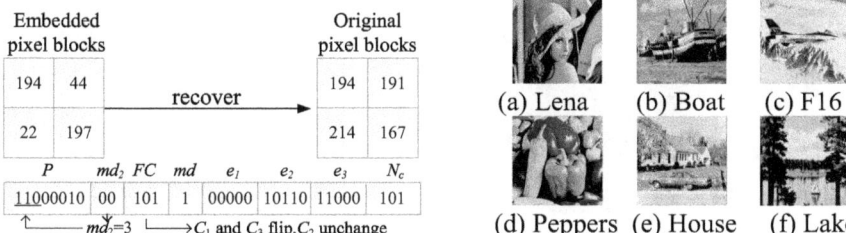

Fig. 7. Recovery of FAMP

Fig. 8. Test images

3 Experiment Result and Analysis

In this section, we compare the performance of the proposed FAMP scheme with AMP scheme [14] in terms of the number of available blocks and the overall embedding capacity. We perform experiments on six test images selected from the USC-SIPI image database [15], each of which is shown in Fig. 8 (a), (b), (c), (d), (e), and (f) respectively.

As is shown in Fig. 9, the number of available blocks obtained in our scheme is obviously more than that in AMP scheme, proportion of available blocks is 94.5%, 94.8%, 93.3%, 97%, 97.1% and 92.1% in six test images, each of which is greater than 81.8%, 80.6%, 82.3%, 83.8%, 76% and 72.4% in AMP scheme. This is because that once flipping strategy is introduced, the correlation of pixels within previously unavailable blocks turns to be stronger. Taking Lena for example, the proportion of available blocks is 94.5% in the proposed scheme, comparing with 81.8% in AMP scheme. The difference is even more obvious for textural images such as Lake and House, since textural images have more unavailable in AMP compared with smooth images.

We flip blocks of pixels with $md = 0$ and $md = 1$ so that the number of available blocs increases and the embedding capacity increases accordingly. The embedding capacity of a flipped block is related to the pixels within the block, and the embedding capacity usually depends on the smoothness of the image. The smoother the selected pixels are, the larger the embedding capacity is.

The overall embedding capacities are compared in Fig. 10. It is clear from the figure that the proposed scheme is better than its counterpart. In particular, the improvement in embedding capacity is 43,458, 27,252, 25,118, 34,884, 37,522 and 31,740 bits respectively, among which the average improvement value is 30,073 bits. We can find that in House and Lake the texture image, the embedding capacity increases significantly. Therefore, the proposed method is more effective for embedding capacity enhancement in texture images. But in Boat, F16 etc. the embedding capacity is also increased in smooth images. The reason is that smooth images have less overhead of location map information, so proposed scheme can improve embedding capacity for smooth images.

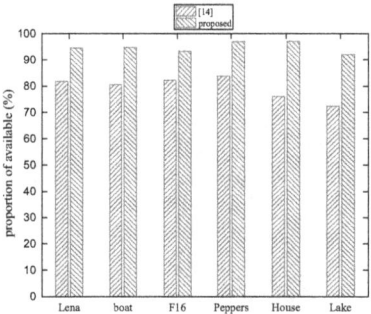

Fig. 9. Proportion of available blocks

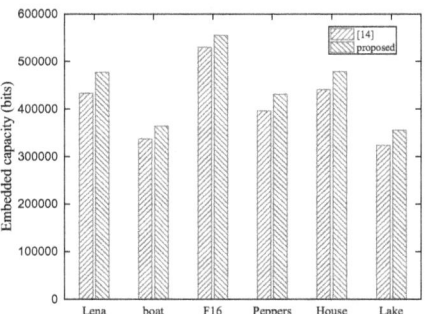

Fig. 10. Embedded capacity

4 Conclusion

This paper proposes a novel scheme base Adaptive MSB prediction in RDHEI. We improve embedding capacity while maintaining reversibility, which is crucial for the development of RDHEI techniques. we introduce FAMP scheme to make previously unavailable blocks available for data embedding. This is achieved by flipping pixels within the block, recording the positions of flipped pixels, and utilizing a new 2 × 2 pixels structure and novel location maps to support the proposed flipping strategy. Experimental results demonstrate the effectiveness of our proposed scheme compared to state-of-the-art techniques. The proposed approach achieves better prediction accuracy and greater embedding capacity while ensuring reversibility.

Acknowledgments. Supported by Student Academic Research Training Project of University of International Relations (No.3262024SWA01).

References

1. Tang, X., Zhou, L., Tang, G., et al.: Reversible data hiding based on improved block selection strategy and pixel value ordering. In: Proceedings of the 19th IEEE International Symposium on Dependable, pp. 619–627. Autonomic and Secure Computing, Canada (2021)
2. Tang, X., Zhou, Y., Cheng, Y., et al.: Weighted average-based complexity calculation in block selection oriented reversible data hiding. Secur. Commun. Netw., 1–15 (2022)
3. Tang, X., Zhou, L., Liu, D., et al.: Reversible data hiding based on improved rhombus predictor and prediction error expansion. In: Proceedings of IEEE 19th International Conference on Trust, pp. 13–21. Security and Privacy in Computing and Communications, China (2020)
4. Tang, X., Zhou, L., Tang, G., et al.: Improved fluctuation derived block selection strategy in pixel value ordering based reversible data hiding. In: Proceedings of the 20th International Workshop on Digital-forensics and Watermarking, pp. 163–177. China (2021)
5. Abdul Karim, M.S., Wong, K.: Universal data embedding in encrypted domain. Signal Process. **94**, 174–182 (2014)
6. Zhang, X.: Neversible data hiding in encrypted image. IEEE Signal Process. Lett. **18**(4), 255–258 (2011)
7. Hong, W., Chen, T.-S., Wu, H.-Y.: An improved reversible data hiding in encrypted images using side match. IEEE Signal Process. Lett. **19**(4), 199–202 (2012)
8. Liao, X., Shu, C.: Reversible data hiding in encrypted images based on absolute mean difference of multiple neighboring pixels. J. Vis. Commun. Image Represent. **28**, 21–27 (2015)
9. Khanam, F.-T.-Z., Song, K.-Y., Kim, S.: A modified reversible data hiding in encrypted image using enhanced measurement functions. In: 2016 Eighth International Conference on Ubiquitous & Future Networks, pp. 869–872 (2016)
10. Rupali, B., Aggarwal, A.: An improved block based joint reversible data hiding in encrypted images by symmetric cryptosystem. Pattern Recogn. Lett. **139**, 60–68 (2018)
11. Wu, X., Sun, W.: High-capacity reversible data hiding in encrypted images by prediction error. Signal Process. **104**, 387–400 (2014)
12. Puteaux, P., Puech, W.: An efficient MSB prediction-based method for high-capacity reversible data hiding in encrypted images. IEEE Trans. Inf. Forensics Secur. **13**(7), 1670–1681 (2018)
13. Wang, Y., Cai, Z., He, W.: High capacity reversible data hiding in encrypted image based on intra-block lossless compression. IEEE Trans. Multimedia **23**, 1466–1473 (2021)
14. Wang, Y., He, W.: High capacity reversible data hiding in encrypted image based on adaptive MSB prediction. IEEE Trans. Multimedia **24**, 1288–1298 (2022)
15. Image database of sipi. [EB/OL]. http://sipi.usc.edu/database/. Accessed Apr 2018

Decoupling Control in Text-to-Image Diffusion Models

Shitong Cao, Xuejie Zhang, Jin Wang, and Xiaobing Zhou(✉)

School of Information Science and Engineering,
Yunnan University, Kunming 650504, Yunnan, China
zhouxb@ynu.edu.cn

Abstract. Large text-to-image models allow for high-quality and diverse synthesis of images from a given text prompt. However, many scenarios require that the content creation be controllable. Recent methods add image-level controls, e.g., edge and depth maps, to manipulate the generation process together with text prompts to obtain desired images. In this work, we propose a decoupling control to disentangle one or multiple objects and individual objects' shapes and appearances in a given reference set while synthesizing novel renditions and rearranging them in different contexts. Given a set of images as input, we establish mapping relationships between the target's appearance and different "circles" through fine-tuning a pretrained text-to-image model. We achieve control over the local position of different "circles" by designing a novel local feature loss to decouple multi-targets. Extensive experiments demonstrate that our model can disentangle individual objects and allow for their translation within a scene, as well as arbitrary control over the combination of multiple targets while maintaining appearance consistency among the targets.

Keywords: Compositional and Consistent Generative · Disentangle Individual Objects · Local Feature Classification · Diversity Maintaining

1 Introduction

Have you ever imagined adding or removing elements in an image, wishing that only a specific object in the generated image could be moved a little to the left to meet the requirements better, or if it could be moved a bit to the right to be perfect? More complex scenarios, such as moving one object forward and another backward, without complex control conditions.

Recently developed large-scale text-to-image models have demonstrated unprecedented capabilities, enabling high-quality and diversified image synthesis through prompts written in natural language [1–3]. One of the main advantages of these models is the strong semantic priors learned from a large number of image-caption pairs. Though the ability of text-to-image synthesis models is becoming increasingly impressive, the quality of generated images is much worse when generating multiple objects. In text-to-image synthesis, there are some basic methods in text design [4, 5]. The text describes issues with the image generation pipeline, namely the lack of flexible user control to accurately guide generated images according to user ideas. To address this, descriptive information about objects in the images is needed. Some studies have attempted to use drawings, sketches, masks, or depth to control combined target creation, but these methods are mostly limited to single object scenarios and yield inconsistent results at higher resolutions and complexities. Currently, there are no methods that address the simultaneous generation and consistency of multiple targets. Thus, the paper proposes a decoupling control method based on categorizing targets, allowing independent control over different target categories. Additionally, control information is extracted from the text rather than being externally provided. The method aims to disentangle information between different targets [6, 7].

Our method can disentangle each target and the relationship between the targets and the background, allowing for independent control of each target. These attributes are crucial for various applications, such as film production, poster creation, dynamic generation of the target in videos, and the generation of complex object trajectories in a consistent manner. Therefore, our method has substantial practical value, enabling control over different targets while maintaining robust generation capabilities. It involves fine-tuning without the need for extensive computational resources or time.

2 Related Work

Conditional Image Synthesis: Generation based on diffusion models has achieved the best results [1-3]. Text-to-image synthesis has driven significant progress and has brought about tremendous changes. Text-to-image models, including Stable Diffusion (SD) [2], Dalle [3], and Imagen [8], have contributed largely to this advancement. There are also many methods emerging in the field of controllability research, using controls such as masks, human posture, depth maps, and sketches [9, 10]. These additional control conditions can be input into the model via a hypernetwork. The notion of hypernetworks originates from neural language processing methods [11, 12], where a smaller recursive neural network is trained to influence the weights of a larger neural network. By attaching a smaller neural network to a stable diffusion, the artistic style of its output image is altered [13-15].

In recent years, Transformer-based methods such as the GPT series [16, 17] and the BERT family [18, 19] have transformed the field of natural language processing. ChatGPT has excellent text parsing abilities, and Dalle3 has also been embedded within ChatGPT. Some methods use ChatGPT to generate intermediate control procedures to guide the generation process. Traditional studies on image layouts [20-22] tend to apply strategies like bounding boxes (bbox) or object categories for image synthesis. Neural network-based methods such as conditional GANs can generate controlled images with satisfactory results in specific scenes, but they lack generalizability and universality [23-25]. Some current research involves establishing a connection between specific targets and special characters, using the special character to express the specific target.

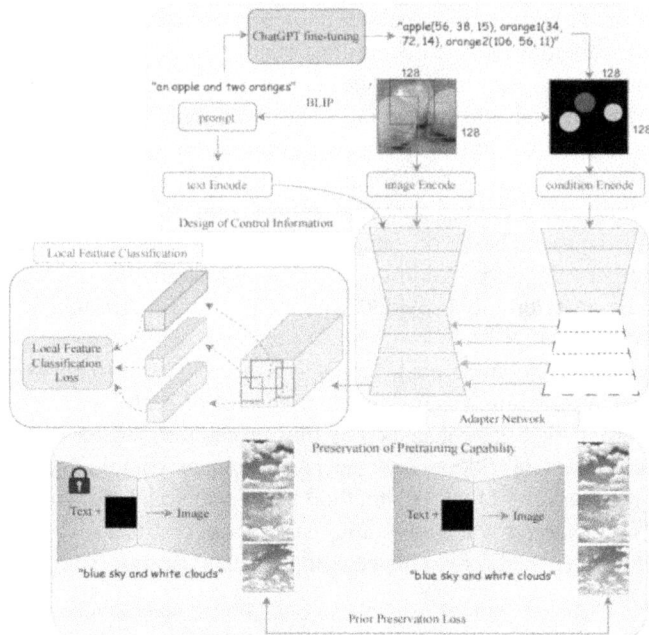

Fig. 1. Model architecture diagram, consisting of three components: the Control Condition Design Module, which automatically extracts control information from text and forms control conditions; the Adapter Network, which is a replicated version of the upper part of U-Net and is updated to be added to the corresponding lower part of U-Net; Local Feature Classification Network, which is used to supervise the position and category of the targets by classifying the features from U-Net locally.

3 Method

3.1 Adapter Network

Text-to-image models have achieved great success, allowing the generation of various images through text. We employ a small network to fine-tune the larger model, with a tiny adapter influencing the larger network. The adapter network allows for retaining the original pretrained model's knowledge, meaning one can capitalize on the extensive knowledge from training on large-scale datasets. This is particularly beneficial for scenarios with small datasets or a scarcity of data, allowing for the rapid fine-tuning of the model to suit new tasks or datasets.

The specific network model is depicted in Fig. 1. To incorporate the control module into Stable Diffusion, we transform the conditioned input image from an input size of 512×512 to a 64×64 feature space vector compatible with the size used by Stable Diffusion. Specifically, we use a tiny network $\varepsilon()$ consisting of four convolutional layers with 4×4 kernels and 2×2 strides. These layers are activated by ReLU and initialized with 16, 32, 64, and 128 channels, respectively. The network is initialized with Gaussian weights and trained jointly with the complete model. This is to encode the image space condition c_i into a feature space condition vector c_f. The formula is as follows.

$$c_f = \varepsilon(c_i) \tag{1}$$

The conditional vector c_f is passed to SD, forming the control.

Train the model by setting reconstruction loss between the denoised image and the real image. The reconstruction loss is for the entire image and is a global reconstruction loss. Given an initial noise map $\epsilon \sim \mathcal{N}(0, I)$, text prompts c_t, as well as a task-specific condition c_f, generates an image $X_{gen} = \widehat{X}_\theta(\epsilon, c_t, c_f)$.

They are trained using a squared error loss to denoise image or latent code $z_t := \alpha_t x + \sigma_t \epsilon$ as follows:

$$\mathcal{L}_{globe} = \mathbb{E}_{X,c_t,c_f,t,\epsilon}[W_t \|\widehat{X}_\theta(\alpha_t X + \sigma_t \epsilon, c_t, c_f) - X\|_2^2 \tag{2}$$

where X is the ground-truth image and α_t, σ_t, W_t are terms that control the noise schedule and sample quality, and are functions of the diffusion process time $t \sim \mu([0,1])$.

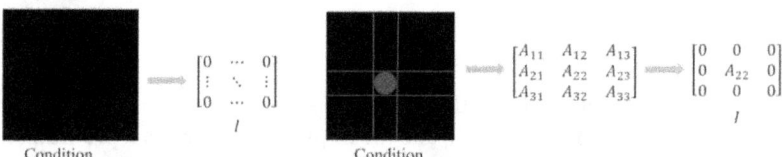

Fig. 2. Conversion of control conditions into a rectangular form.

3.2 Design of Control Information

In the previous section, the control conditions in the adapter network are generally edges, poses, depth, etc. However, it is not easy to obtain control conditions that meet user needs, and control conditions cannot be flexibly adjusted. Existing explicit control methods have resulted in models being biased towards visual control, significantly reducing their language control capabilities.

In this paper, we propose using different "circles" as conditions. The control conditions are simple and can be easily manipulated, allowing for a high degree of flexibility. By specifying the position and size of a circle, the corresponding image generation can be guided, ensuring that the generated results conform to specific layout or scene requirements. This decoupling allows individual control over each target, enabling composite and consistent generation.

As shown in Fig. 2, the control conditions are transformed into a matrix for analysis. The matrix, even after passing through the activation function, still contains a significant number of zeros. Therefore, its impact on the SD main network is minimal. When aiming to preserve the generation capabilities of the text-to-image model itself, where only text is used as input, the adapter network does not play a role. In this case, the adapter network receives a completely black image as input. The black image, where all the values in the matrix are set to 0, is passed as input to the pre-trained model without significantly affecting its pre-trained parameters, especially in a well-trained and robust model.

The information at the all-zero position does not add any additional information. When an all-black input is fed in, which means I is 0, $f(x) = I * W$ is approximately 0. Set I to 0, the gradient will also be 0, which means the parameters cannot be updated. Consequently, the standard deviation remains unchanged, effectively locking it. Once locked, it can generate the background as described by the text. The standard deviation combined with control represents the foreground, meaning that it generates this entity based on the foreground. We simply compute the gradients for the zero linear layer. Given an input map $I \in \mathbb{R}^{h \times w}$, the forward pass can be written as:

$$\mathcal{Z}(I; W, B) = B + I * W \tag{3}$$

When the matrix I is a zero matrix, the formula becomes as follows:

$$\mathcal{Z}(I; W, B) = B + 0 * W = B \tag{4}$$

When the matrix I is non-zero, the W matrix is also subjected to matrix partitioning, dividing W into nine corresponding smaller matrices. Thus, the formula becomes as follows:

$$\mathcal{Z}(I; W, B) = B + I * W = B + A_{22} * W_{22} \tag{5}$$

Using "circles" as control conditions, after passing through the adaptive network, the number of parameters is very small, and the impact on the original pre-trained model parameters is relatively small when sent to the stable diffusion. Still maintaining the prompt effect of the text, rather than relying solely on control conditions.

3.3 Local Feature Classification Loss

The global reconstruction loss minimizes the difference between the generated image and the input image, which leads to a lack of supervision and control over local information. Local classification loss can further improve the quality of generated samples. In the previous section, the control conditions are local, that is, the control condition circle, and the other black areas do not play a role. Enhance the control generation of local information based on local guidance.

In this paper, we propose the local feature classification loss, which addresses both the position and category loss. This approach stabilizes the generation of specific objects at fixed positions. Through experiments, we have observed that this local feature classification network does not create a jarring contrast between the target and the background. The local features are defined as w, and the category after passing through a linear function is denoted as $linear(W)$. The true category is defined as v, and the corresponding loss function is formulated as:

$$\mathcal{L}_{local} = MSE(v, linear(W)) \tag{6}$$

The U-Net part in the middle of the network is divided into an up-sampling layer, an intermediate layer, and a down-sampling layer, which are 64 * 64, 32 * 32, 16 * 16, and 8 * 8, respectively. We operate on the 16 * 16 features of the up-sampling layer, extract the corresponding local positions for classification calculation, and achieve supervision of local position targets.

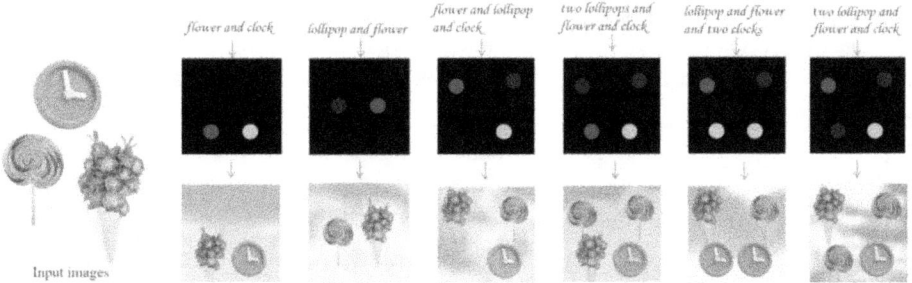

Fig. 3. Decontanglement control of multiple targets

3.4 Prior Preservation Loss

The loss of local feature classification is the control target, but to maintain the diversity of the background, we introduce the prior preservation loss in Dreambooth to maintain the strong generation ability of the large model. Specifically, we generate data $X_{pr} = \hat{X}(Z_{t_1}, C_{pr})$ by using the ancestral sampler on the frozen pre-trained diffusion model with random initial noise $Z_{t_1} \sim \mathcal{N}(0, I)$ and conditioning vector $c_{pr} := \gamma(f("abackgroundof"))$. The loss function is as follows.

$$\mathcal{L}_{pp} = \mathbb{E}_{X, c_t, c_f, t, \epsilon} \lambda W_{t'} \|X_\theta(\alpha_{t'} X_{pr} + \alpha_{t'} \hat{\epsilon}, c_{pr}, c_f) - X_{pr}\|_2^2 \qquad (7)$$

where X is the ground-truth image, $\epsilon \sim \mathcal{N}(0, I)$, c_t is a conditioning vector obtained from a text prompt, c_f is the information used for controlling the target, which is input to the model through an adapter network, and α_t, σ_t, W_t are terms that control the noise schedule and sample quality, and are functions of the diffusion process time $t \sim \mu([0,1])$. The second term is the prior-preservation term that supervises the model with its own generated images, and λ controls for the relative weight of this term.

$$\mathcal{L}_{total} = \mathcal{L}_{globe} + \mathcal{L}_{local} + \mathcal{L}_{pp} \qquad (8)$$

The three losses are combined as the overall loss function of the entire model. Guided by this loss function, the model can achieve control over the target positions while preserving the original generation capability of the pre-trained model.

4 Experiments

4.1 Experimental Design and Analysis

Stable Diffusion is an outstanding benchmark in text-to-image generation, providing a solid starting point for this research. We compute the similarity between the generated images and text using a pre-trained CLIP model to verify the alignment of the text with the generated images. The fidelity of the generated images is assessed by computing similarity with real images. To precisely evaluate the model's capability for target positioning control, we select texts from different categories containing positional relationship descriptions to generate images and calculate their similarity to the text. When target positional information is ambiguous, or the text does not specify target positioning, our model reverts to generative behavior on par with that of Stable Diffusion. This experiment was conducted on an NVIDIA 3090 GPU took approximately 5 h.

Table 1. Ablation studies on various components.

c_f	$\mathcal{L}_{globe}$	$\mathcal{L}_{local}$	$\mathcal{L}_{PP}$	Chat/Human operation	Clip-T C/H	Clip-I C/H
Stable Diffusion					0.3268	-
	√	√			0.2807	0.3314
	√		√		0.3269	0.3155
	√	√	√		0.3257	0.3281
√	√			√(C)/√(H)	0.3023/0.3022	0.3216/0.3204
√	√	√		√(C)/√(H)	0.2098/0.3011	0.3273/0.3273
√	√	√		√(C)/√(H)	0.3279/0.3292	0.3145/0.3164
√	√	√	√	√(C)/√(H)	0.3308/0.3312	0.3308/0.3312

4.2 Experimental Results

This study relies primarily on two evaluation metrics, namely Clip-T and Clip-I. Clip-T represents the similarity between generated images and text, while Clip-I measures the similarity between real images and generated images. The entire experiment is divided into two major blocks: one without control conditions and another with control conditions. The absence of control conditions is intended to assess whether the model retains its original ability to generate images from text. Through ablation studies (Table 1), we observed that our model still possesses the inherent image generation capability to produce diverse images. Moreover, our model can also perform controlled generation, which sets it apart from many explicitly controlled models. In explicit models, control conditions must be provided during the inference stage; otherwise, the model fails to generate normal images. Our model can switch between controlled and uncontrolled. When no control conditions are applied, the input for control conditions becomes entirely black, effectively removing any control, thus reverting the model to its initial state of text-to-image generation.

The ablation experiments also primarily discuss the impact of $\mathcal{L}_{loc}$ and $\mathcal{L}_{pp}$ on the model, both in uncontrolled and controlled scenarios. It can be observed that $\mathcal{L}_{loc}$ facilitates control over the target position, while $\mathcal{L}_{pp}$ promotes the generation of diverse images. This diversity manifests in the ability to alter the target's posture or the background of specific objects.

4.3 Visualization Results

Visualizing Circles as Control Conditions. As shown in Fig. 3, visualize circles as control conditions, with circles of different colors representing different targets. The

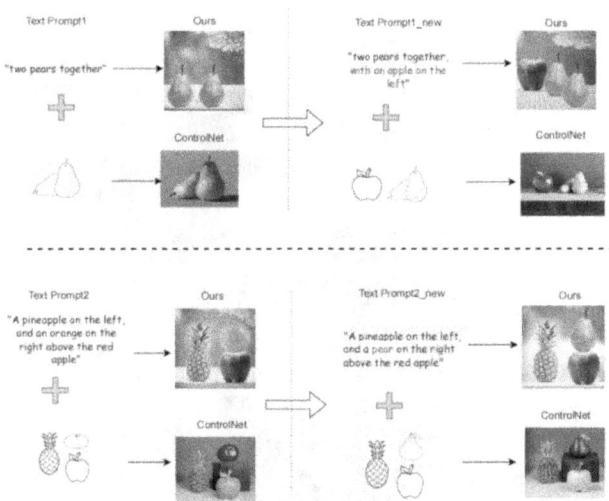

Fig. 4. Compare our method to the explicit information control model (ControlNet).

position of the circles can control the position of the targets generated. Through experiments, it can be seen that we can achieve any combination of these three goals, including understanding quantitative relationships. During the process of combining and generating images, it is possible to maintain consistency in the appearance of each target. In the subsequent visualization results, circles were not shown as implicit control conditions.

Comparison with Other Control Conditions. As shown in Fig. 4, preliminary experimental results indicate that our method outperforms the ControlNet network model in generating "complex" images with multiple object combinations. The advantage lies primarily in the simplicity and convenience of our approach to achieving controlled generation. Firstly, our method does not require additional control sketches. Instead, it extracts hidden information from textual cues to provide reasonable control over the spatial positions of individual objects. In contrast, ControlNet requires manual sketching, which significantly increases the complexity of user operations. Secondly, our project is also more straightforward in adjusting and modifying generated images. Modifying the text prompt can accomplish adjustments and modifications to the image. On the other hand, the ControlNet network model requires a new control sketch for such modifications.

Comparison with Existing Generative Models. The following compares this paper and wen xin yi ge, Stable Diffusion, Midjourney and DallE3 models regarding their generation performance. From the experimental results, it can be observed that these models achieve good results when generating images with relatively simple targets. However, when the generated scenes become "complex", the results generated by our model are more in line with the description in the text. As shown in Fig. 5, the description "Red cup, camera, desk lamp" denotes the need to generate multiple objects with a specific quantity relationship. "The camera is placed on the left side of the red cup" signifies the spatial relationship between different objects. "Desk lamp on the left, green bowl in the

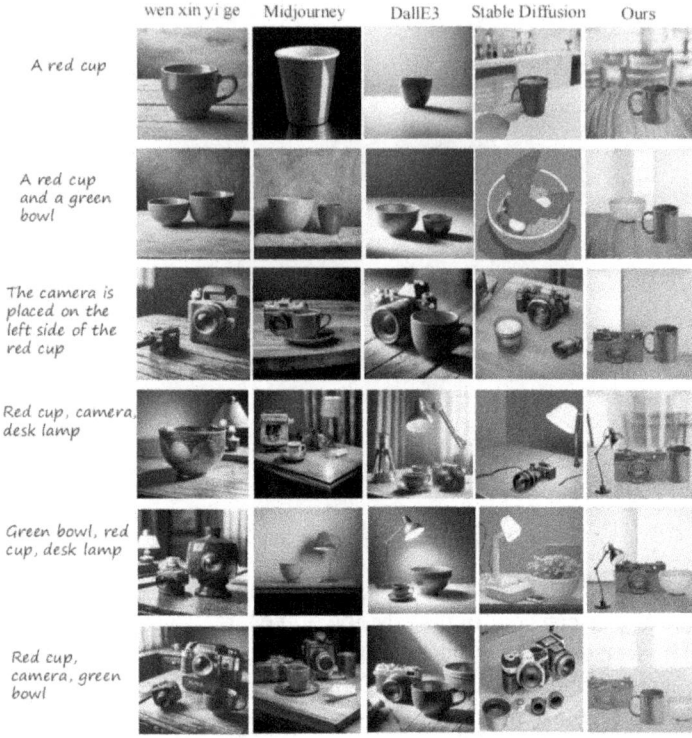

Fig. 5. The qualitative results of text-to-image generation from different models vary.

middle, and red cup on the right" represent combinations of multiple objects and their positional relationships with each other. Compared with the four models in this article, when faced with multiple target combinations, the generated results cannot match the text highly. The quantity relationships are not clearly expressed in the generated images, and the combinations of different objects are also inaccurately generated, with the absence of crucial objects. In contrast, our method achieves more accurate generation results by accurately expressing the information from the textual descriptions and providing reasonable spatial distribution.

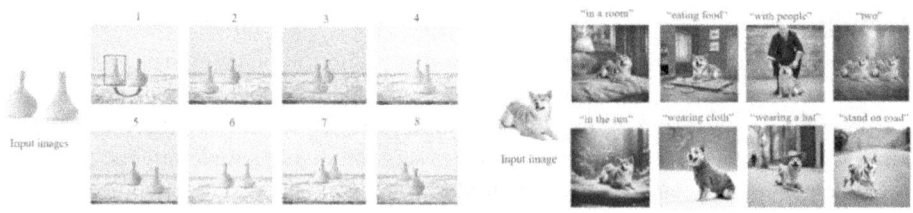

Fig. 6. Consistency generation of two objectives and one objective under different transformations.

Image Edit. As shown in Fig. 6, we complete consistency generation under different transformations for two targets and a single target. On the left side of the figure, we demonstrate controlled spawning of an object orbiting another object. In this process, you can maintain consistency in the appearance of two objects and understand that size and dimensions change as the distance between the objects changes. In the image on the right, when fed a specific image of a puppy, the model can generate consistent images of that specific puppy in different scenarios. The resulting image keeps the main subject as the input puppy, but the background, pose, number, and position change.

5 Conclusion

We propose a control method capable of orchestrating the arrangement and combination of multiple targets, whereby control over each target category is independent. This decoupling allows for the consistent generation of targets across various scenes. Additionally, our method facilitates seamless switching between controlled and uncontrolled scenarios. The cornerstone of our approach is the design of appropriate control conditions, which serve as a switch. Notably, this fine-tuning process requires only one image per category to generate high-quality pictures.

References

1. Shi, J., Wu, C., Liang, J., Liu, X., Duan, N.: DiVAE: photorealistic images synthesis with denoising diffusion decoder. arXiv preprint arXiv:2206.00386 (2022)
2. Rombach, R., Blattmann, A., Lorenz, D., Esser, P., Ommer, B.: High-resolution image synthesis with latent diffusion models. In: Proceedings of the IEEE/CVF Conference on Computer Vision and Pattern Recognition, pp. 10684–10695 (2022)
3. Ramesh, A., Dhariwal, P., Nichol, A., Chu, C., Chen, M.: Hierarchical text conditional image generation with clip latents. arXiv preprint arXiv:2204.06125 **1**(2), 3 (2022)
4. Liu, V., Chilton, L.B.: Design guidelines for prompt engineering text-to-image generative models. In: Proceedings of the 2022 CHI Conference on Human Factors in Computing Systems, pp. 1–23 (2022)
5. Pavlichenko, N., Ustalov, D.: Best prompts for text-to-image models and how to find them. In: Proceedings of the 46th International ACM SIGIR Conference on Research and Development in Information Retrieval, pp. 2067–2071 (2023)
6. Locatello, F., et al.: Challenging common assumptions in the unsupervised learning of disentangled representations. In: International Conference on Machine Learning, pp. 4114–4124. PMLR (2019)
7. Bengio, Y., Courville, A., Vincent, P.: Representation learning: a review and new perspectives. IEEE Trans. Pattern Anal. Mach. Intell. **35**(8), 1798–1828 (2013)
8. Saharia, C., et al.: Photorealistic text to image diffusion models with deep language understanding. Adv. Neural. Inf. Process. Syst. **35**, 36479–36494 (2022)
9. Zhang, L., Rao, A., Agrawala, M.: Adding conditional control to text-to-image diffusion models. In: Proceedings of the IEEE/CVF International Conference on Computer Vision, pp. 3836–3847 (2023)
10. Mou, C., et al.: T2I-Adapter: learning adapters to dig out more controllable ability for text-to-image diffusion models. arXiv preprint arXiv:2302.08453 (2023)

11. Alaluf, Y., Tov, O., Mokady, R., Gal, R., Bermano, A.: HyperStyle: StyleGAN inversion with hyper networks for real image editing. In: Proceedings of the IEEE/CVF conference on computer Vision and pattern recognition, pp. 18511–18521 (2022)
12. Dinh, T.M., Tran, A.T., Nguyen, R., Hua, B.S.: HyperInverter: improving StyleGAN inversion via hyper network. In: Proceedings of the IEEE/CVF Conference on Computer Vision and Pattern Recognition, pp. 11389–11398 (2022)
13. Chen, Z., et al.: Vision transformer adapter for dense predictions. arXiv preprint arXiv:2205.08534 (2022)
14. Stickland, A.C., Murray, I.: BERT and PALs: projected attention layers for efficient adaptation in multi-task learning. In: International Conference on Machine Learning, pp. 5986–5995. PMLR (2019)
15. Mallya, A., Davis, D., Lazebnik, S.: Piggyback: adapting a single network to multiple tasks by learning to mask weights. In: Proceedings of the European Conference on Computer Vision (ECCV), pp. 67–82 (2018)
16. Brown, T., et al.: Language models are few-shot learners. Adv. Neural. Inf. Process. Syst. **33**, 1877–1901 (2020)
17. Radford, A., Narasimhan, K., Salimans, T., Sutskever, I., et al.: Improving language understanding by generative pre-training (2018)
18. Devlin, J., Chang, M.W., Lee, K., Toutanova, K.: BERT: pre-training of deep bidirectional transformers for language understanding. arXiv preprint arXiv:1810.04805 (2018)
19. Liu, Y., et al.: ROBERTa: A robustly optimized BERT pretraining approach. arXiv preprint arXiv:1907.11692 (2019)
20. Li, Z., Wu, J., Koh, I., Tang, Y., Sun, L.: Image synthesis from layout with locality aware mask adaption. In: Proceedings of the IEEE/CVF International Conference on Computer Vision, pp. 13819–13828 (2021)
21. Zhao, B., Meng, L., Yin, W., Sigal, L.: Image generation from layout. In: Proceedings of the IEEE/CVF Conference on Computer Vision and Pattern Recognition, pp. 8584–8593 (2019)
22. Gafni, O., Polyak, A., Ashual, O., Sheynin, S., Parikh, D., Taigman, Y.: Make-A-Scene: scene-based text-to-image generation with human priors. In: European Conference on Computer Vision, pp. 89–106. Springer (2022). https://doi.org/10.1007/978-3-031-19784-0_6
23. Park, T., Liu, M.Y., Wang, T.C., Zhu, J.Y.: Semantic image synthesis with spatially-adaptive normalization. In: Proceedings of the IEEE/CVF Conference on Computer Vision and Pattern Recognition, pp. 2337–2346 (2019)
24. Chen, Q., Koltun, V.: Photographic image synthesis with cascaded refinement networks. In: Proceedings of the IEEE International Conference on Computer Vision, pp. 1511–1520 (2017)
25. Zhu, J.Y., Park, T., Isola, P., Efros, A.A.: Unpaired image-to-image translation using cycle-consistent adversarial networks. In: Proceedings of the IEEE International Conference on Computer Vision, pp. 2223–2232 (2017)

Arbitrary Scale Texture Synthesis with Feature Map Swapping

Di Sun[1], Yangde Lin[1], Sheng Shen[2], Zhiliang Zeng[2], Shizhao Zhang[2], and Qihang Wang[3](✉)

[1] College of Artificial Intelligence, Tianjin University of Science and Technology, Tianjin 300222, China
[2] Beijing Institute of Control and Electronic Technology, Beijing 100045, China
[3] College of Intelligence and Computing, Tianjin University, Tianjin 300350, China
164383983@qq.com

Abstract. Texture synthesis is a technique widely used in computer vision. Existing learning-based methods typically use fixed network structure, and they can only generate images that are the same size or integer multiples of the input sample. In this paper, we propose a swapping-aware texture synthesis method based on feature mapping using a deep generative model. To optimize the loss function, we conduct a dedicated exchange algorithm that operates directly in the feature map space. The texture matching is optimized by matching the feature map between the original image and the generated image. The model can generate texture images of any size based on input samples. The generated results can be extended from the inside of the image to the surrounding, resulting in an image larger than the original input size. The experimental results show that the proposed method effectively preserves more high-frequency details while maintaining the consistency of the generated content and texture, and obtains more realistic synthesized results.

Keywords: Textures synthesis · Arbitrary Size · GAN · Swap

1 Introduction

Texture synthesis (TS) is a process of taking a small texture and then make it larger in size, not by tiling, but by synthesizing it. Early example-based techniques [1–4] are widely used for creating perceptually similar, non-periodic textures from a single input. Due to the requirement of selecting samples for generating new textures, the selection of samples is a limitation. Furthermore, it is impossible to consider texture synthesis from the perspective of the global image, as it can only be synthesized from given samples. The recent research highlights the effectiveness of deep neural networks in image generation, with some using Convolutional Neural Networks (CNN) for texture synthesis [5–10]. These methods can roughly fall into single texture sample methods [5] and feed-forward network methods [7, 8].

More recently, Generative Adversarial Network (GAN)-based [9, 10] architectures gain significant traction in the realm of texture synthesis over recent years. This creates a competitive relationship between the two components, thereby enhancing the accuracy of the model's results. For instance, Zhou Yang et al. [9] use generative adversarial networks to synthesize textures. Given a texture sample, their model can generate integer multiples of the size of the input sample. These methods are suitable for images with small or large texture components. However, they typically have limitations in generating arbitrary size textures directly due to the fixed size input requirement, resulting in textures that match the input size or integer multiples of it.

The quality of image feature extraction has a significant impact on the performance of neural network models. The swapping is first proposed by Chen, T et al. [16]. They used it to accelerate the speed of Style Transfer to generate style images, but they only used the feature map of a certain layer of the CNN to swap. Inspired by them, we try to apply swapping to all layers of the loss network, and match and exchange the feature maps in the VGG-19 model of the loss network.

In this paper, we propose an algorithm capable of extrapolating to unknown areas with minimal neighboring information. Inspired by [12], we introduce an "arbitrary size generation texture network" based on the GAN architecture. Our model includes a generator for texture creation and a discriminator to compare the generator's output with the ground truth. During training, we use a patch-swap algorithm to optimize loss functions. The proposed approach can generate textures of any size, see Fig. 1. The swapping algorithm optimizes loss functions by calculating the similarity between feature maps and enhances texture synthesized results.

Our main contributions are: (1) We propose a GAN based texture synthesis framework. The combination of adversarial training with feature swapping allows the model to generate arbitrary textures directly from input images. (2) We design a patch-swap method to optimize loss functions and improve the synthesized contents.

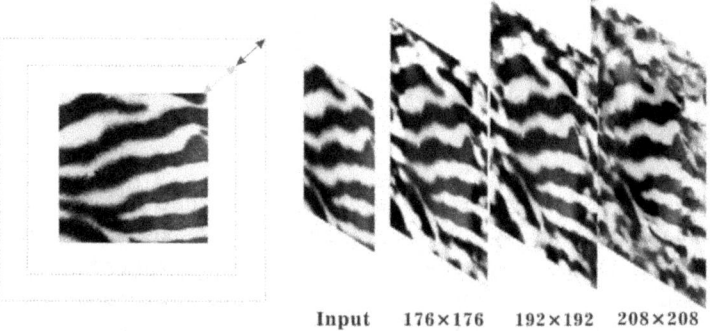

Fig. 1. Texture synthesis by the proposed method.

2 Related Work

In the early field of texture synthesis, sample-based methods are extensively used. Wei et al. [1] propose an effective example-based method to synthesize realistic textures quickly. Kwatra et al. [3] introduce an optimization-based method, while Darabui et al. [13] present the Image Melding method, which is based on patch-based optimization.

In recent years, there has been a growing focus on deep learning technologies [5, 8, 9, 14, 15]. Gatys et al. [5] demonstrate that CNN could generate textures from input samples by using feature maps to represent textures and calculating similarity between feature maps in different network layers. Their model introduces CNN as a new tool for texture synthesis. Li et al. [8] propose a texture synthesis method aimed at improving image quality, addressing issues such as generality, diversity, and suboptimality by designing a feed-forward network for synthesizing textures with meaningful interpolation. They improve the gram matrix loss by subtracting the feature mean. Ulyanov et al. [7] introduce texture networks based on the GAN model [11], capable of generating multiple samples from a single example of a texture and transferring artistic style from one image to another. Their model required training for a feed-forward Convolutional Network when given an input texture, with a loss function derived from [5]. Zhou et al. [9] use a GAN to synthesize textures, enabling their model to generate textures twice the size of the input sample, incorporating style loss and L1 loss into their GAN model.

Additionally, there are patch-based image synthesis methods. Chen et al. [16] achieve diverse style transfer, overcoming the limitations of existing methods. They use an inverse network to deterministically invert activation from stylized layers for stylized image generation and introduce a swap algorithm for style transfer. Li et al. [17] propose a Markov Random Field (MRF) loss function for optimizing image synthesis tasks applicable to style transfer and texture synthesis. Their MRF loss function calculates similarity from patches extracted from input samples. Song et al. [18] introduce a Convolutional Neural network-based image inpainting approach, enhancing results with a patch-swap algorithm that finds the closest-matching patch to fill missing information.

3 Method

Figure 2 shows the proposed framework that consists of a texture network and a loss network. For the texture network, the network structure is based on GANs network. The generator is used to extract visual features and synthesize the textural contents. The discriminator can improve the quality of synthesized results. For the loss network, the pre-trained VGG-19 serves as loss network. In addition, we design a swap module optimize the loss function.

3.1 Generator

The generator G follows the encoder-decoder fashion architecture. In contrast to [12, 21], we insert three residual blocks between them to increase network depth while preventing gradient disappearance, resulting in better generated images compared to models without these blocks. The generator comprises eight convolution layers and

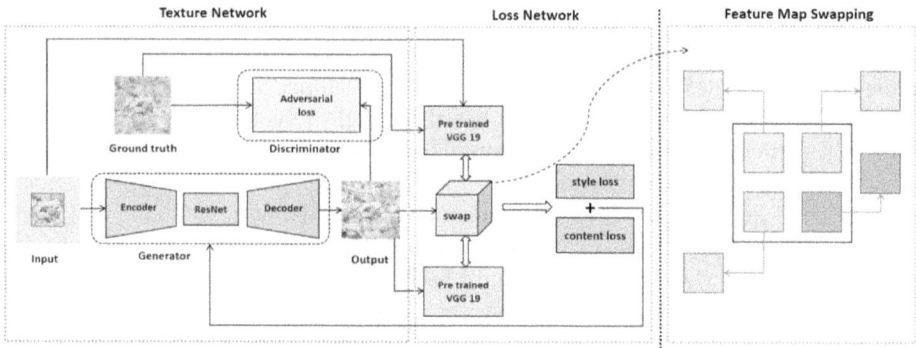

Fig. 2. Framework Overview. It includes a generator, a discriminator network, and a loss network. The generator's output serves as input for both the discriminator and the loss network, along with the texture samples. In the loss network, two input images traverse the network to calculate the style loss and content loss, with a swap operation matching the similarity of feature maps. In the Feature Map Swapping, squares represent the feature maps of different positions within the same layer of CNN, where different colors represent different feature maps at the same position. After calculation, the blue indicates that the feature map of this layer is most similar to the feature map of the input image, and then performs the exchange program, followed by further calculates style loss and content loss.

a deconvolution layer, with a 128 × 128 texture image as input. To enhance the quality of generated images, dilated convolution layers are added to increase the receptive field. Conv1 and decov7 layers employ 5 × 5 and 4 × 4 convolution kernels respectively, while the remaining convolution layers use 3 × 3 kernels. Conv2 and decov7 layers have a stride size of 2 × 2, whereas the rest have a stride size of 1 × 1. Except for conv9, which uses the Sigmoid activation function, ReLU activation function is applied in the other convolutional layers.

3.2 Discriminator

The discriminator is designed to use the output of itself and the generator to perform adversarial training to obtain the optimal results that the generator can obtain. To achieve this, we use the PatchGAN [20] network structure. In addition, Instance Norm and Max-pooling are utilized to enhance the stability of the training process.

3.3 Feature Map Matching Based on Swap

The swap algorithm is an operation on feature maps aimed at determining the similarity between input feature maps in the loss network. It's conceived as a specialized network layer for processing feature maps, comprising a convolutional layer and a deconvolutional layer. Unlike structures solely generating images within the original ones [16], our approach tackles image outpainting and applies the swap algorithm across all network layers.

The loss network could be divided into two models, $M_1(t_n)$ and $M_2(G)$. Model $M_2(G)$ extracts feature map patches of generated image, and model $M_2(G)$ extracts feature map patches of the ground truth I_{gt} which is similar as much as possible with those in generated images. The extract feature map patches should contain all channels. For feature map patches of generated image, the swap algorithm is defined by the following normalized cross-correlation measure, namely:

$$\alpha(G, t_n) := \underset{M_1(t_n)_i, i=1,2,\ldots,N}{\operatorname{argmax}} \frac{\langle M_2(G), M_1(t_n) \rangle}{\|M_2(G), M_1(t_n)\|} \quad (1)$$

3.4 Loss Function

In this section, we introduce three loss functions: style loss, content loss and GAN loss. **Style Loss and Content Loss.** Given a sample texture image I, the generator obtains the generated result I_0, then we feed I_0 into the loss network which is mentioned before to get the feature maps F_{I_0}. It is necessary to obtain the feature maps $F_{I_{gt}}$ of I_{gt} by using I_{gt} corresponding to I_0 as input for the loss network. Feature maps are extracted from $\{relu1\_2, relu2\_2, relu3\_3, relu4\_3, relu5\_4\}$ of loss network. We use both output of generator and ground truth as input for the loss network. The architecture of loss network is shown in Fig. 3.

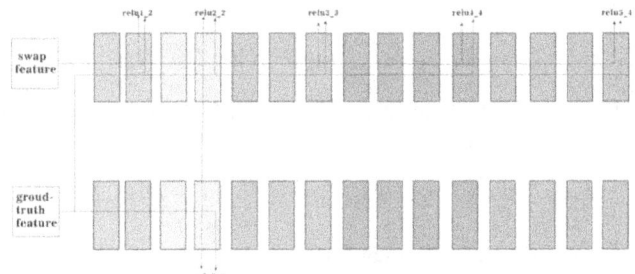

Fig. 3. Architecture of loss network. The loss network is based on VGG-19. The input of loss network is the swap feature and feature of ground truth. They go through the loss network and extract feature map from $\{relu1\_2, relu2\_2, relu3\_3, relu4\_3, relu5\_4\}$.

Assuming $F_{I_0} = \{F_{1_k}^l, F_{2_k}^l, \ldots, F_{n_k}^l\}$ represent the feature maps of I_0, $F_{I_{gt}}$ is extracted by I_0 from the loss network. $F_{I_{gt}} = \{F_{1_k}^l, F_{2_k}^l, \ldots, F_{n_k}^l\}$, where l and k represent the k_{th} feature map of the n_{th} position in the l layer. The feature maps of generated results I_0 and I_{gt} go through swapping to obtain a new feature map F_{swap}. $F_{swap} = \{F_{swap1_k}^l, F_{swap2_k}^l, F_{swap3_k}^l, \ldots, F_{swapj_k}^l\}$. Where l and k represent the k_{th} feature map of the j_{th} position in the l layer. Then G_{swap} and G_{gt} could be calculated as:

$$G_{\text{swap}} = \sum_k F_{\text{swap}\,i_k}^l F_{\text{swap}\,j_k}^l \quad (2)$$

$$G_{gt} = \sum k f_m^l f_n^l \quad (3)$$

By Eqs. (2) and (3), there is:

$$G_{\text{swap}} = G_{\text{swap}}^1, G_{\text{swap}}^2, \ldots, G_{\text{swap}}^L \qquad (4)$$

$$G_{gt} = G_{gt}^1, G_{gt}^2, G_{gt}^3, \ldots, G_{gt}^L \qquad (5)$$

where 1, 2, 3,..., L represents a layer in the loss network.

Then The style loss is calculated as the sum of the Euclidean distances between the gram matrix of the feature map after swapping and the ground truth's gram matrix.

$$L_{\text{style}} = \sum_{l=0}^{L} (G_{\text{swap}} - G_{gt})^2 \qquad (6)$$

The content loss is the Euclidean distances between feature maps at different positions in the same layer from the Convolutional Network. Here, the features of I_0 and $I_g t$ are extracted in *relu3_1* from the loss network. The function is as follows:

$$L_{\text{content}} = \sum_{i=0, l=0, j=0}^{i,j,l} (F_{I_0}(i,j,l) - F_{gt}(i,j,l))^2 \qquad (7)$$

In L_G, β is the tunable hyperparameter trading off the style loss and content loss with the standard generator GAN loss. The generator's loss function is defined as follows, where β is 4×10^{-4}:

$$L_G = L_{\text{style}} + L_{\text{content}} - \beta \log D(G(I_0)) \qquad (8)$$

Adversarial Loss. Adversarial loss is based on Generative Adversarial Networks (GANs) and is defined as follows:

$$L_D = \max_D E\big[\log(D(I_0, I_g t)) + \log(1 - D(I_0, I_1))\big] \qquad (9)$$

The input of discriminator are image pairs, the real image pair consisting of input image I_0 and ground truth I_{gt}, and the fake pair consisting of I_0 and image I_1 generated by generator, where γ is 1.0.

Therefore, the total loss function is defined as follows:

$$L_{\text{total}} = L_G + \gamma L_D \qquad (10)$$

4 Experiments

4.1 Implementation Details

The experiments are carried out on the TensorFlow framework. The generator is trained on 6500 images with 128 × 128 size. We conduct experiments on two datasets DTD (Describing Textures in the Wild) and Places365. During the training phase, we divide 6500 images into 6000 training datasets and 500 testing datasets. Our model is trained on NVIDIA Titan V GPU, and it took three days to train our network for iterating over 500,000. The optimizer we use is Adam. The learning rate is 10^{-6}.

4.2 Quantitative Evaluation

In the evaluation of synthesized results, the proposed method is compared with representative methods such as TSCNN [5], TSFFN [8] and NTS [9] for texture synthesis. These comparisons are conducted on testing datasets from DTD, and Places365. Consistent with standard practices in texture synthesis research, we employ Peak Signal to Noise Ratio (PSNR), Structural Similarity (SSIM) as quantitative metrics. As detailed in Table, comparative experiments show that the proposed method outperforms existing approaches on these metrics.

4.3 Qualitative Evaluations

To validate the synthesis performance, Fig. 4 present a comparative analysis of the predicted results from different methods. As illustrated in Fig. 4, the synthesized result from TSCNN seems to produce distorted structures, particularly noticeable edge regions. NTS tends to produce texture noise during the reconstruction of features. TSFNN is capable of recovering reasonable content but often ignores texture details. In contrast, our method enhances the perception of textural regions.

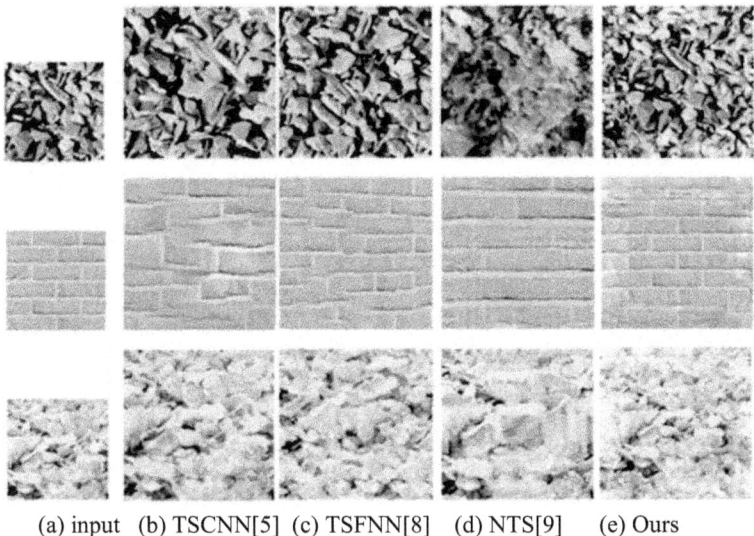

(a) input (b) TSCNN[5] (c) TSFNN[8] (d) NTS[9] (e) Ours

Fig. 4. Visual comparison of the proposed method with the others.

Figure 5 shows results for multi resolution images. The proposed method can generate different results from the original image. It can be seen that it is able to well preserve the important areas of input images and the overall structure over a large resolution span (176 × 176 to 208 × 208).

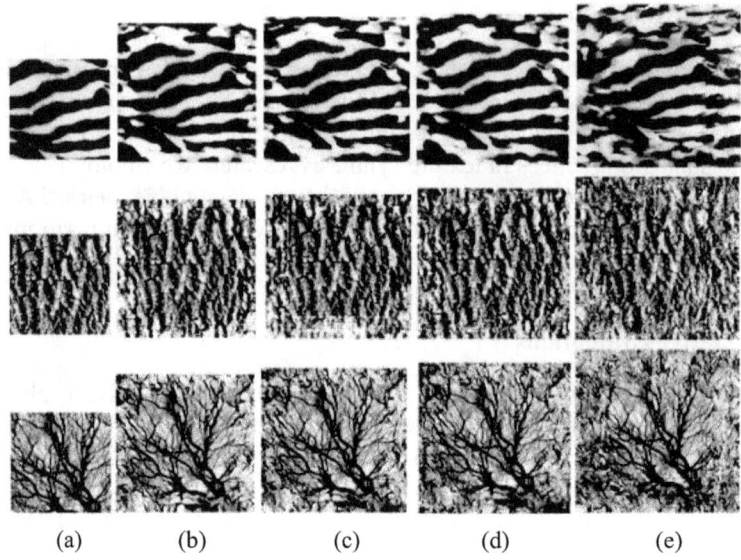

Fig. 5. Results for multi resolutions. (a) is the input with 128 × 128 size; (b) is the output with 176 × 176 size; (c) 184 × 184; (d) 192 × 192; (e) 208 × 208.

4.4 Ablation Study

In this subsection, we continue to analyze how the proposed modules contribute to the final performance of texture synthesis. Specifically, we verify the effectiveness of the backbone network by removing swap blocks. As can be seen from Fig. 6, the result with the swapping module is better than those without it. The reason is that after adding the swapping module, the generated feature map is compared with the reference image's feature map, and the optimal result is exchanged before calculating the loss function. This allows for the use of the optimal feature map to calculate the loss function, which is superior to directly using the extracted feature map for this purpose.In addition, PSNR, SSIM are all commonly used image evaluation. The larger their value, the better the image quality. It can be seen from Table 2 that when swap is added to the model, the evaluation result is the best (Table 1).

Table 1. Quantitative evaluations. ↑ means the higher the better.

Metric	TSCNN [5]	TSFNN [8]	NTS [9]	Ours
PSNR↑	17.39	17.75	18.62	**18.69**
SSIM↑	0.8988	0.9112	0.9010	**0.9187**

Table 2. Synthesized results in terms of PSNR, SSIM for ablation study.

Metric	w/o swapping	w swapping
PSNR↑	15.51	**16.65**
SSIM↑	0.39	**0.43**

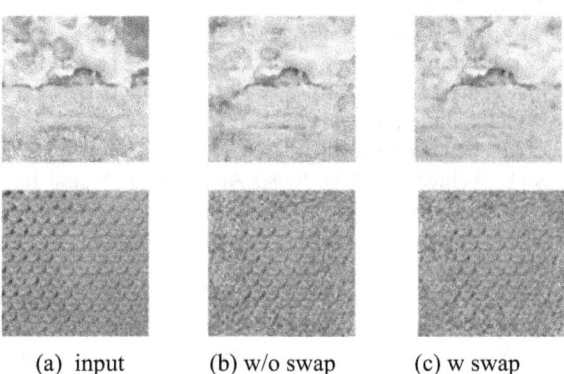

(a) input (b) w/o swap (c) w swap

Fig. 6. Ablation study.

5 Conclusion

In this paper, we have proposed a deep generative network for texture synthesis. The network is based on a GAN, with a feature mapping swapping strategy. Our method automatically synthesizes arbitrary texture images from input samples directly. We show that the feature swapping strategy significantly improves texture synthesized results. We provide in-depth comparisons with classic approaches and show visually plausible synthesized results.

References

1. Wei, L.-Y., Levoy, M.: Fast texture synthesis using tree-structured vector quantization. In: Proceedings of the 27th Annual Conference on Computer Graphics and Interactive Tecniques. SIGGRAPH '00, pp. 479–488. ACM Press/Addison Wesley Publishing Co., New York, NY, USA (2000)
2. Ashikhmin,M.: Synthesizing natural textures. In: Symposium on Interactive 3d Graphics (2001)
3. Kwatra, V., Essa, I., Bobick, A., Kwatra, N.: Texture optimization for example-based synthesis. ACM Trans. Graph. **24**(3), 795–802 (2005)
4. Efros, A.A., Freeman, W.T.: Image quilting for texture synthesis and transfer. In: Proceeings of the 28th Annual Conference on Computer Graphics and Interactive Techniques. SIGGRAPH '01, pp. 341–346. ACM, New York, NY, USA (2001)
5. Gatys, L., Ecker, A.S., Bethge, M.: Texture synthesis using convolutional neural networks. In: Cortes, C., Lawrence, N.D., Lee, D.D., Sugiyama, M., Garnett, R. (eds.) Advances in Neural Information Processing Systems 28, pp. 262–270. Springer, Heidelberg (2015)

6. Wilmot, P., Risser, E., Barnes, C.: Stable and controllable neural texture synthesis and style transfer using histogram losses. CoRR abs/1701.08893 (2017)
7. Ulyanov, D., Lebedev, V., Vedaldi, A., Lempitsky, V.: Texture Networks: feed-forward synthesis of textures and stylized images. arXiv e-prints (2016)
8. Li, Y., Fang, C., Yang, J., Wang, Z., Lu, X., Yang, M.-H.: Diversified texture synthesis with feed-forward networks. In: The IEEE Conference on Computer Vision and Pattern Recognition (CVPR) (2017)
9. Zhou, Y., Zhu, Z., Bai, X., Lischinski, D., Cohen-Or, D., Huang, H.: Nonstationary texture synthesis by adversarial expansion. CoRR abs/1805.04487 (2018)
10. Yu, N., Barnes, C., Shechtman, E., Amirghodsi, S., Lukac, M.: Texture mixer: A network for controllable synthesis and interpolation of texture. In: The IEEE Conference on Computer Vision and Pattern Recognition (CVPR) (2019)
11. Goodfellow, I., et al.: Generative adversarial nets. In: Ghahramani, Z., Welling, M., Cortes, C., Lawrence, N.D., Weinberger, K.Q. (eds.) Advances in Neural Information Processing Systems, vol. 27, pp. 2672–2680. Curran Associates, Inc., RedHook (2014)
12. Sabini, M., Rusak, G.: Painting outside the box: image outpainting with GANs. CoRR abs/1808.08483 (2018)
13. Darabi, S., Shechtman, E., Barnes, C., Dan, B.G., Sen, P.: Image melding: combining inconsistent images using patch-based synthesis. ACM Trans. Graph. **31**(4), 1–10 (2012)
14. Zhou, Y., Chen, K., Xiao, R., Huang, H.: Neural texture synthesis with guided correspondence. In: Conference on Computer Vision and Pattern Recognition (CVPR), pp. 18095–18104 (2023)
15. Ntavelis, E., Shahbazi, M., Kastanis, I., Timofte, R., Danelljan, M., Van Gool, L.: Arbitrary-scale image synthesis. In: Proceedings of the IEEE/CVF Conference on Computer Vision and Pattern Recognition, pp. 11533–11542 (2022)
16. Chen, T.Q., Schmidt, M.: Fast patch-based style transfer of arbitrary style. CoRR abs/1612.04337 (2016)
17. Li, C., Wand, M.: Combining markov random fields and convolutional neural networks for image synthesis. In: The IEEE Conference on Computer Vision and Pattern Recognition (CVPR) (2016)
18. Song, Y., et al.: Contextual-based image inpainting: infer, match, and translate. In: The European Conference on Computer Vision (ECCV) (2018)
19. He, K., Zhang, X., Ren, S., Sun, J.: Deep residual learning for image recognition. In: The IEEE Conference on Computer Vision and Pattern Recognition (CVPR) (2016)
20. Isola, P., Zhu, J.-Y., Zhou, T., Efros, A.A.: Image-to-image translation with conditional adversarial networks. In: The IEEE Conference on Computer Vision and Pattern Recognition (CVPR) (2017)
21. Iizuka, S., Simo-Serra, E., Ishikawa, H.: Globally and locally consistent image completion. ACM Trans. Graph. **36**(4), 107–110714 (2017)

A 3D-2D Hybrid Network with Regional Awareness and Global Fusion for Brain Tumor Segmentation

Wenxiu Zhao, Changlei Dongye(✉), and Yumei Wang

Shandong University of Science and Technology, Qingdao, China
dycl@sdust.edu.cn

Abstract. Accurate segmentation of brain tumors in MR images is crucial for their clinical diagnosis and treatment. Some existing methods do not adequately consider the relationship between tumor regions and the effect of fuzzy boundaries on segmentation. In this paper, we propose a 3D-2D Hybrid Network with Regional Awareness and Global Fusion for Brain Tumor Segmentation (HRGBTS). The model consists of three components: a hybrid encoder, a regional awareness module, and a feature fusion decoder. Specifically, the hybrid encoder uses 3D-2D hybrid convolutional blocks to extract multi-scale features from the brain tumor region. The regional awareness module (RAM) enhances the segmentation of tumor sub-regions by dynamically sensing the relationship between tumor cells and surrounding tissue cells through graph convolutional interactive inference. In the decoding stage, the feature fusion decoder, which consists of global fusion modules (GFMs) and cross-dimensional skip connections, is designed to improve boundary reconstruction. The GFM effectively fuses tumor information, enabling better tumor boundary reconstruction and addressing the challenge of boundary blurring. The cross-dimensional skip connections address the information mismatch problem caused by cross-dimensional changes. Extensive evaluations were made on three benchmark datasets, BraTS2018, BraTS2020, and BraTS2021, the Dice coefficients in the whole-tumor region (WT) were achieved to be 0.906, 0.917, and 0.903, respectively.

Keywords: Brain Tumor Segmentation · Global Fusion · Regional Awareness

1 Introduction

Brain tumors are the most prevalent and challenging primary tumors to treat, with varying degrees of invasiveness. Multimodal magnetic resonance imaging (MRI) technology [1] is widely used for diagnosing and surgically treating brain tumors. It plays a crucial role in monitoring, diagnosing, and predicting the prognosis of tumors. Therefore, accurate segmentation of gliomas from MRI images is a critical step in the diagnosis and treatment of this disease.

Automated MRI-based computerized segmentation not only means less time and cost, it also makes quantitative analysis more objective. In recent years, the widespread application of Convolutional Neural Networks (CNNs) in medical images has promoted the development of automatic segmentation of brain tumors [2, 3]. Fully Convolutional Neural Network (FCN) [4] achieves end-to-end semantic segmentation and shows a good performance in medical image segmentation. U-Net [5] has gained the most popularity for its ability to capture local characteristics in 2D or 3D space using its U-shaped structure. However, CNNs face challenges in effectively capturing global feature dependencies due to inherent limitations in the convolutional perceptual field. To address this limitation, researchers have proposed a two-stage approach that combines 3D and 2D networks to improve the extraction of single-layer contextual semantic information [6]. Specifically, this approach utilizes features learned by 2D convolutional neural networks (2D-CNNs) as input to the 3D-CNNs. This enables the acquisition of location information of the tumor from an even broader spatial environment. However, this method mainly focuses on the extraction and fusion of deep semantic features, without considering the relationship between different tumor regions and the importance of fuzzy boundaries for segmentation.

Xu et al. [7] proposed a multi-branch network that utilizes an attention mechanism to focus on each sub-region of the tumor so as to extract the tumor region. Wang et al. [8] incorporated a dynamic scale-aware context module that adapts contextual information dynamically. To deal with boundary-related information and effectively remove noise from MRI, they used an edge attention preserving (EAP) module. However, these efforts have ignored the critical role of global information in extracting tumor features.

In this paper, we present a new brain tumor segmentation model called HRGBTS, which consists of three components: a hybrid encoder, a region–aware module, and a feature fusion decoder. The hybrid encoder connects the 3DCNN and 2D MSCAN [9] in tandem, this combination effectively captures the spatial information of the tumor in 3D space. The regional awareness module is used to learn the texture and boundaries of tumor sub-regions by employing interactive graph inference. In the decoding process, we developed a feature fusion decoder that includes global fusion modules and cross-dimensional skip connections to reconstruct the tumor regions and address the boundary-blurring problem. To address the low percentage of tumor regions, we designed the Depth cropping algorithm and explored the impact of the normalization method in the cross-dimensional skip connections on the segmentation accuracy. Our research makes the following key contributions:

1. Hybrid encoder: This structure leverages multi-scale extraction of deep semantic features to effectively capture tumor shape and location information.
2. We designed a regional awareness module to extract texture features within the tumor to enable accurate segmentation of the sub-regions.
3. We introduce a feature fusion encoder during the decoding process. This encoder incorporates a global fusion module that effectively combines features from the tumor region, thereby reducing boundary ambiguity.
4. To mitigate the impact of low percentage of tumor regions on segmentation accuracy, we explored various data cropping methods aimed at balancing the dataset.

2 Method

2.1 Network Structure

The architecture of the 3D-2D Hybrid Network with Regional Awareness and Global.

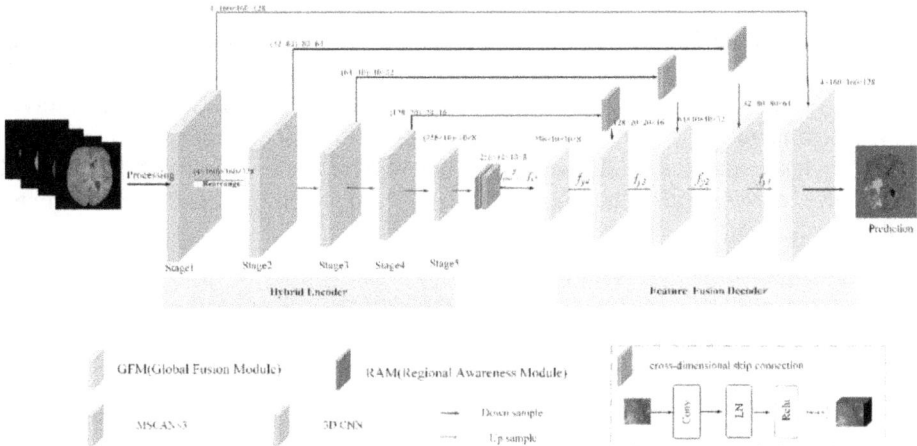

Fig. 1. Overview of the proposed network structure.

Fusion for Brain Tumor Segmentation(HRGBTS). This illustrated in Fig. 1. HRG-BTS comprises three key components: a hybrid encoder, a regional awareness module, and a feature fusion decoder. The hybrid encoder integrates both 2D and 3D convolutional blocks to extract deep semantic features from multimodal MRI scans. This hybrid design enables the network to capture comprehensive information from different dimensions of the input data. To address the challenge of distinguishing features from molecular regions, the regional aware-ness module (RAM) aggregates features from various regions. It employs inter-active graph inference to enhance the differentiation of molecular features, allowing for more precise segmentation. The feature fusion decoder consists of cross-dimensional skip connections and global fusion modules. The cross-dimensional skip connections act as a bridge between the hybrid encoder and the global fusion module, facilitating information interaction between the encoder and decoder. The global fusion module effectively fuses the semantic features of the different layers. This leads to better reconstruction of tumor boundaries, thus facilitating accurate and complete segmentation of brain tumors.

2.2 Hybrid Encoder

The hybrid encoder in our proposed model consists of a tandem structure that comprises a 3D convolutional blocks and a 2D Multi-Scale Convolutional Attention Network (MSCAN). This combination enables effective information capture in 3D space. To prevent overfitting, residual connectivity is integrated into the 3D convolutional block, as depicted in Fig. 2. We use rearranging to achieve dimensional transformation from 3D to 2D which solves the problem of dimensional mismatch. The encoder's four layers (stages 2–5) employ three Multi-Scale Convolutional Attention Network (MSCAN) structures to enhance feature extraction. The MSCAN structure uses a Multi-Scale Convolutional Attention (MSCA) module instead of multi-head attention for feature extraction (refer to Fig. 2 for the detailed structure). The MSCA module facilitates information exchange across multiple scales, thereby improving feature representation, particularly for capturing tumor location information. Furthermore, the MSCA module facilitates information sharing between different feature layers, enhancing the training efficiency of the model.

The hybrid encoder establishes a connection between 3D and 2D features and solves the problem of missing spatial information due to slice discontinuity, enabling information exchange and fusion. This approach can maximize the benefits of both 3D and 2D features, allowing for better capture of tumor shape and location information and facilitating accurate tumor segmentation.

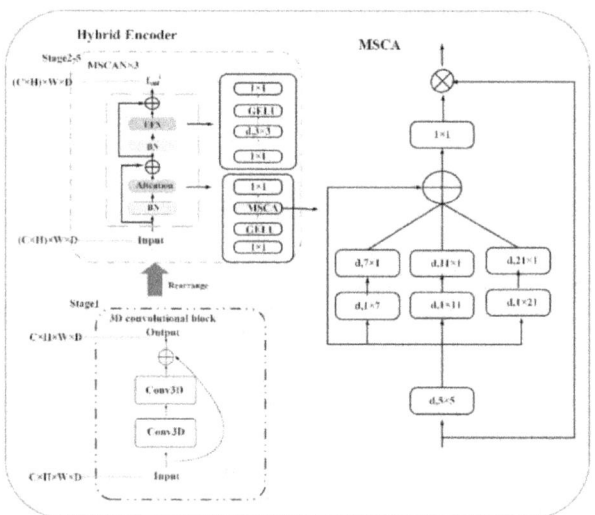

Fig. 2. Overview of the proposed network structure.

2.3 Regional Awareness Module

In order to be able to accurately segment the different subregions of a tumor (e.g. NCR/NET, ED and ET), we have designed a region awareness module. The mechanism of this module is shown in Fig. 2. The input features are given as $X \in R^{C \times H \times W}$, which $H \times W$ is the total number of features, and C denotes the feature dimension. The mapping of X is followed by contextual inference using the adjacency matrix A of the graph G (where the graph $G = (V, E, A)$ contains the set of nodes V, the edges E denotes the connection relationship between nodes and the adjacency matrix $A$is used to describe the degree of association between nodes.

Mapping method: The original feature $X \in R^{C \times H \times W}$ is mapped to the non-Euclidean interaction space to generate a mapping feature $G \in R^{C \times V}$. Then, pixels with similar features can be aggregated to a node, where the mapping feature vector X^{map} can be represented by a node in the interaction graph G as $v, v \in V$. Mathematically, this can be expressed as follows:

$$G = \mu_1(X) \times \mu_2(X) \tag{1}$$

where $\mu_1(X)$, $\mu_2(X)$ denote the convolution operation of the graph projection [10] and the feature dimensionality reduction convolution operation. Due to the fact that the shape, size and location of brain tumors in MRI images may vary significantly, we abandoned the traditional convolution approach and used a learnable (deformable convolution) method [11].

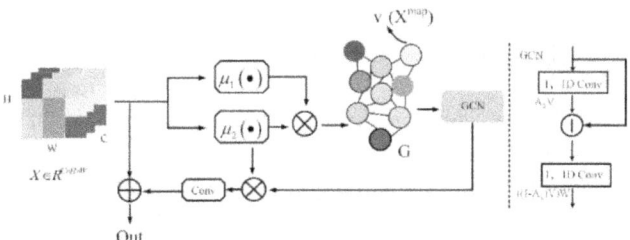

Fig. 3. Regional awareness module.

Graph convolutional region aware: After projecting The inference of the interaction graph is performed by learning the edge weights corresponding to the features of each node based on graph convolution [12]. The structure of the graph convolution is shown in Fig. 3, which performs a one-dimensional convolution operation in the channel and node directions. The graph convolution equation can be expressed as:

$$H = GCN(G) = \left((I - \hat{A}_g)V\right)W, \tag{2}$$

Back-projection: After the inference is complete, the non-Euclidean features are back-projected onto the original features using a linear interpolation algorithm. The final result is a set of $H \times W$ instances of *Out* features. Mathematically, this can be expressed as follows:

$$Out = X + Conv\left(\mu_2(X)^T \times H\right), \tag{3}$$

2.4 Feature Fusion Decoder

In this section, we design a feature fusion decoder aimed at reconstructing the tumor region and addressing the boundary blurring issue. The decoder consists of two parts: cross-dimensional skip connections and global fusion modules. Cross-dimensional skip connection(CSC) aims to bridge the semantic gap between the hybrid decoder and the global fusion modules by providing pixel-level features on features extracted from the hybrid decoder. The CSC can be mathematically represented as follows:

$$Y = Rearange(ReLU(LN(Conv(X)))), \tag{4}$$

where X represents the side output of the hybrid feature extraction network and Y represents the result of the transformation. $Conv$ represents a convolution with the 1×1 kernel, and $Rearange$ denotes the transformation function.

Global Fusion Module. The global fusion module involves multiple fusion operations, as depicted in Fig. 4. We define the feedforward features obtained from the aforementioned sampling and transformation connections as f_y and f_{out}^i, respectively, and the first fusion and convolution operations obtain the initial fusion features f_{fuse}. Then the process is represented by Eq. (6).

$$f_{fuse} = Conv_{3D}\left(Concat\left(f_y, f_{out}^i\right)\right) + f_y + f_{out}^i, \tag{5}$$

We employed a channel attention mechanism based on an attention vector $C_{weight} \in R^{C \times 1 \times 1 \times 1}$ learned from the initial fused features, The $C_{weight} \in R^{C \times 1 \times 1 \times 1}$ is learned through a sequence of operations, including global average pooling (GAP) and a fully connected layer (FC), with C denoting the number of channels. The output of the global fusion module, denoted as f_{out}, is obtained using the following equation:

$$C_{weight} = FC(GAP(f_{fuse})), f_{out} = (C_{weight} \times f_{fuse}) + f_y + f_{out}^i, \tag{6}$$

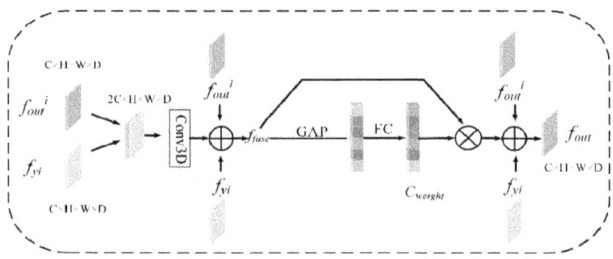

Fig. 4. Global fusion Module

2.5 Loss Function

We define the loss function L_{Seg} as a combination of a weighted binary cross-entropy loss L_{BCE}^w and a Dice coefficient loss L_{Dice}, with Laplace smoothing added to perform the task of segmenting brain tumors. The formula is as follows:

$$\begin{aligned} L_{Seg} &= L_{BCE}^w + L_{Dice}, \\ L_{BCE}^w &= w \times \left[-y\log(\hat{y}) + (1-y)\log(1-\hat{y}) \right], \\ L_{Dice} &= 1 - \frac{2|x \cap y| + 1e-5}{|x| + |y| + 1e-5} \end{aligned} \quad (7)$$

where $x, \hat{y}$ represents predicted output; y represents Ground truth. w is the weighting coefficient with a value of 2. L_{Seg} provides effective image-level and pixel-level supervision for precise segmentation, resulting in high-quality region segmentation.

3 Experiment

3.1 Experimental Details

Dataset. To evaluate the effectiveness of the HRGBTS network, we conducted experiments using three datasets obtained from BraTS (Brain Tumor Segmentation) challenges 2018, 2020, and 2021 [13]. The input data was cropped to a size of 160 × 160 × 128 along the D axis. We applied several data augmentation techniques during the training phase. These techniques included random scaling, random flipping in three directions, the addition of Gaussian noise, Gaussian blurring, and random contrast adjustments.

3.2 Ablation Experiments and Analysis

Table 1. Results of ablation experiments with different cutting methods. The best value for each metric is shown in bold.

Method	DICE		
	WT	ET	TC
Depth cropping	0.907	**0.765**	**0.830**
Center Cropping	0.904	0.762	0.814
Random cropping	**0.909**	0.750	0.799

First, we have analyzed the impact of different cropping methods on the segmentation results. We designed experiments and evaluated three methods: depth cropping, center cropping and random cropping. The results of our experiments, shown in Table 1, demonstrate the best overall performance of the model when Depth cropping is employed, suggesting that Depth cropping solves the problem of data imbalance to some extent. Therefore, we chose Depth cropping as the method to process the data in our experiments.

Secondly, we investigated the impact of three key components: the hybrid feature extraction encoder, the regional awareness module(RAM) and the feature fusion decoder. The experimental results for different models are shown in Table 2.

Table 2. Results of ablation experiments with different cutting methods. The best value for each metric is shown in bold.

Model	DICE		
	WT	ET	TC
(1) Baseline	0.907	0.765	0.830
(2) Baseline + Hybrid Encoder	0.916	0.777	0.840
(3) Baseline + RAM	0.915	0.771	0.838
(4) Baseline + Feature Fusion Decoder	0.917	0.773	0.841
(5) HRGBTS	**0.917**	**0.782**	**0.853**

Effectiveness of hybrid encoders. The effectiveness of the hybrid encoder is verified by comparing it with Baseline, called model (1).Model (2) employs a hybrid encoder and has a significantly higher Dice score compared to model (1). Our analysis of Fig. 5, Case 2 demonstrates that the hybrid encoder reduces erroneous segmentation, and these results show that the hybrid encoder is able to capture global information effectively.

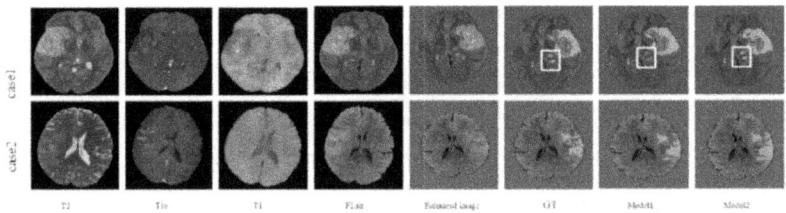

Fig. 5. Results of ablation experiment for model (2).

Effectiveness of the region awareness module. The results demonstrating the effectiveness of the region awareness module (model (3)) are given in Table 2. Compared to model (1), model (3) improves the Dice score by 0.6% for enhanced tumor segmentation and 0.8% for tumor core segmentation. This indicates that the use of the region awareness module can improve the performance of accurately segmenting tumor subregions Fig. 6 provides a visualisation of the segmentation results. In Case 1, it is clear that model (3) places more emphasis on the segmentation of sub-regions.

Effectiveness of feature fusion decoder. In this experiment, we replace the conventional CNN decoder with the global fusion module and utilized the cross-dimensional skip connection to connect it to the hybrid encoder. The inclusion of the feature fusion decoder in Model (4) further improved the segmentation results compared to Model(1). (Model (4): WT:0.917 ET:0.773 TC:0.841, Model (1) WT:0.907 ET:0.765 TC:0.830). As shown in Fig. 7, the segmentation results of Model (4), which benefits from the global fusion module, are more accurate. Conversely, Model (1) exhibited a tendency for over-segmentation (as indicated by the white box in Case 2. Consequently, the global fusion module facilitates the learning of tumor regions while suppressing redundant information.

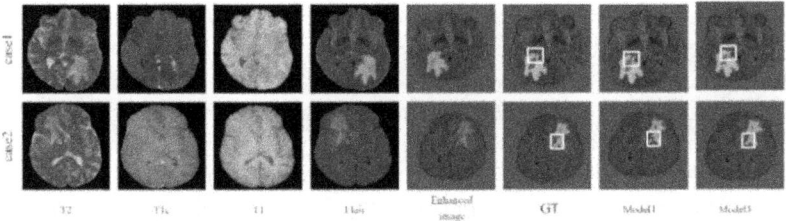

Fig. 6. Results of ablation experiment for model (3).

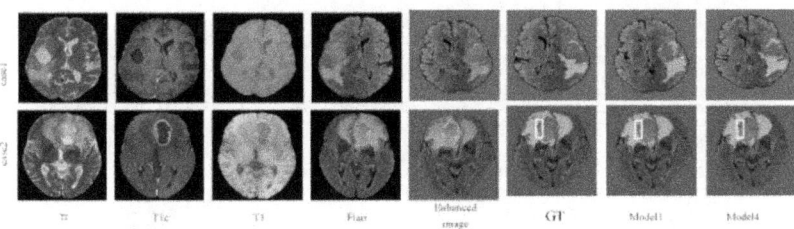

Fig. 7. Results of ablation experiment for model (4).

3.3 Comparison with State-of-the-Arts

To compare the performance of our model, we conducted a comprehensive analysis by comparing it with several classical brain tumor segmentation methods. HRGBTS is based on the architecture of 3DUNet, and our results demonstrate its superiority over 3DUNet in terms of average Dice scores for the three datasets and the three tumor regions.

Table 3. Comparison of this model with other SOTA models. (The best result for each metric is shown in bold.)

Method	BraTS2018				BraTS2020				BraTS2021			
	DICE				DICE				DICE			
	WT	ET	TC	Mean	WT	ET	TC	Mean	WT	ET	TC	Mean
3D-UNet	0.887	0.725	0.798	0.865	0.904	0.762	0.814	0.874	0.891	0.792	0.844	0.853
DMFNet	0.868	0.753	0.778	0.832	0.884	0.748	0.759	0.874	0.872	0.763	0.798	0.826
TransBTS	0.900	0.772	0.839	0.843	0.902	0.772	0.823	0.863	0.870	0.818	0.850	0.884
VNet	0.886	0.770	0.803	0.847	0.916	0.762	0.836	0.882	0.900	0.766	0.823	0.875
E1D3	0.892	0.742	0.832	0.825	0.902	0.781	**0.877**	0.891	0.894	0.816	**0.861**	0.891
AttU-Net	0.901	0.763	0.832	0.876	0.915	0.770	0.840	0.894	0.879	0.809	0.838	0.886
Kong et al	0.871	0.741	0.789	0.814	0.888	0.752	0.783	0.825	0.886	0.775	0.792	0.832
MISSFormer	0.893	0.744	0.820	0.868	0.906	0.775	0.792	0.872	**0.905**	0.802	0.836	0.874
Zhu et al	0.868	**0.773**	0.832	0.853	0.901	0.732	0.848	0.822	**0.905**	0.798	0.834	0.852
Ours	**0.906**	0.742	**0.858**	**0.891**	**0.917**	**0.782**	0.853	**0.899**	0.903	**0.821**	0.860	**0.893**

Specifically, HRGBTS achieved average improvements of 3.4%, 2.5%, and 4% across the three datasets, respectively. We also compared HRGBTS with VNet [14], which utilizes feature fusion from compressed and decompressed paths through stitching for medical image segmentation. As shown in Table 3, VNet obtained better results in segmenting the ET regions. Furthermore, we compared HRGBTS with AttU-Net [15], which incorporates a self-attention gating module to highlight features in local regions. HRG-BTS achieved a significant improvement of 1.5% in the mean Dice score for the BraTS2018 dataset when compared to AttU-Net.

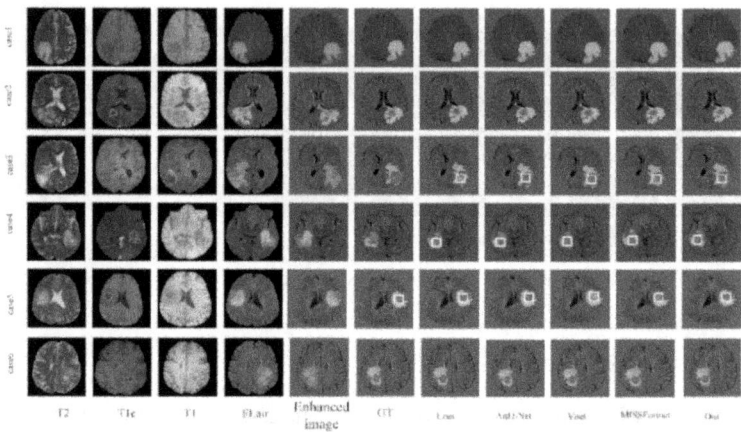

Fig. 8. Visualisation of segmentation results.

TransBTS [16] represents the first attempt to combine 3DCNN with Transformer for brain tumor segmentation. This method capitalizes on the spatial relationships of 3D images and leverages the features of the Transformer to predict both local and global brain tumor characteristics. As a result, TransBTS achieves the best Dice results in the ET region. E1D3 [17], consists of one encoder and three independent decoders, each specializing in a different tumor region. As demonstrated in Table 3, E1D3 achieves optimal performance in the core tumor region (TC). Kong et al. [18] introduce a dual attention mechanism, They assign weights to different sub-regions based this mechanism. Furthermore, MissFormer [19] introduces a novel hierarchical codec structure for medical image segmentation, incorporating both global dependency and local correlation. Notably, the average Dice improvement achieved by HRGBTS on the three datasets is 2.3%, 2.7%, and 1.9%, respectively. Zhu et al. [20] used Swin transformer as a feature extraction network and utilised graph convolution for feature inference. This combination effectively improves the segmentation accuracy, especially in the whole tumor region.

Figure 8 shows the qualitative results obtained by comparing our proposed model with several representative models. The regions in the white rectangles in all segmentation results indicate the dominance of HRGBTS. Notably, in Case 2 of Fig. 8, our model effectively avoids the false-positive results observed from other models (marked with white rectangles), and is much closer to the true labels in terms of the segmentation of peri-tumor oedema regions. In Cases 3 and 5, our model achieves more complete and precise boundaries, and even though MISSFormer applies the idea of global dependency, the segmentation results show that there is still mis-segmentation in the segmentation of necrotic regions.

4 Conclusion

In this paper, we propose a 3D-2D Hybrid Network with Regional Awareness and Global Fusion for Brain Tumor Segmentation (HRGBTS). HRGBTS consists of a hybrid encoder, a Regional awareness module, and a feature fusion decoder. The performance of HRGBTS has been extensively evaluated on the BraTS 2018, 2020, and 2021 datasets. The results unequivocally demonstrate the effectiveness of our approach in accurately segmenting tumor regions. In the future, we plan to investigate the impact of imaging modalities on tumor segmentation.

Acknowledgments. The authors did not receive support from any organization for the submitted work.

Disclosure of Interests. The authors declare that they have no known competing financial interests or personal relationships that could have appeared to influence the work reported in this paper.

References

1. Menze, B.H., et al.: The multimodal brain tumor image segmentation benchmark (brats). IEEE Trans. Med. Imaging **34**(10), 1993–2024 (2014)
2. Huo, Y., et al.: 3D whole brain segmentation using spatially localized atlas network tiles. NeuroImage **194**, 105–119 (2019)
3. Saouli, R., Akil, M., Kachouri, R., et al.: Fully automatic brain tumor segmentation using end-to-end incremental deep neural networks in MRI images. Comput. Methods Programs Biomed. **166**, 39–49 (2018)
4. Long, J., Shelhamer, E., Darrell, T.: Fully convolutional networks for semantic segmentation. In: Proceedings of the IEEE Conference on Computer Vision and Pattern Recognition, pp. 3431–3440 (2015)
5. Ronneberger, O., Fischer, P., Brox, T.: U-Net: convolutional networks for biomedical image segmentation. In: Medical Image Computing and Computer-Assisted Intervention–MICCAI 2015: 18th International Conference, Munich, Germany, October 5–9, 2015, Proceedings, Part III 18, pp. 234–241. Springer (2015). https://doi.org/10.1007/978-3-319-24574-4_28
6. Mlynarski, P., Delingette, H., Criminisi, A., Ayache, N.: 3D convolutional neural networks for tumor segmentation using long-range 2D context. Comput. Med. Imaging Graph. **73**, 60–72 (2019)
7. Xu, H., Xie, H., Liu, Y., Cheng, C., Niu, C., Zhang, Y.: Deep cascaded attention network for multi-task brain tumor segmentation. In: Medical Image Computing and Computer Assisted Intervention–MICCAI 2019: 22nd International Conference, Shenzhen, China, October 13–17, 2019, Proceedings, Part III 22, pp. 420–428. Springer (2019). https://doi.org/10.1007/978-3-030-32248-9_47

8. Wang, K., Zhang, X., Zhang, X., Yuting, L., Huang, S., Yang, D.: Eanet: Iterative edge attention network for medical image segmentation. Pattern Recogn. **127**, 108636 (2022)
9. Guo, M.-H., Lu, C.-Z., Hou, Q., Liu, Z., Cheng, M.-M., Hu, S.-M.: SegNext: rethinking convolutional attention design for semantic segmentation. arXiv preprint arXiv:2209.08575 (2022)
10. Chen, Y., Rohrbach, M., Yan, Z., Shuicheng, Y., Feng, J., Kalantidis, Y.: Graph-based global reasoning networks. In: Proceedings of the IEEE/CVF Conference on Computer Vision and Pattern Recognition, pp. 433–442 (2019)
11. Dai, J., et al.: Deformable convolutional networks. In: Proceedings of the IEEE International Conference on Computer Vision, pp. 764–773 (2017)
12. Li, Q., Han, Z., Wu, X.-M.: Deeper insights into graph convolutional networks for semi-supervised learning. In: Proceedings of the AAAI Conference on Artificial Intelligence, vol. 32 (2018)
13. Bakas, S., et al.: Identifying the best machine learning algorithms for brain tumor segmentation, progression assessment, and overall survival prediction in the brats challenge. arXiv preprint arXiv:1811.02629 (2018)
14. Milletari, F., Navab, N., Ahmadi, S.-A.: V-Net: fully convolutional neural networks for volumetric medical image segmentation. In: 2016 Fourth International Conference on 3D Vision (3DV), pp. 565–571. IEEE (2016)
15. Wang, S., Li, L., Zhuang, X.: AttU-NET: attention U-Net for brain tumor. In: Brainlesion: Glioma, Multiple Sclerosis, Stroke and Traumatic Brain Injuries: 7th International Workshop, BrainLes 2021, Held in Conjunction with MICCAI 2021, Virtual Event, September 27, 2021, Revised Selected Papers, Part II, pp. 302–311. Springer (2022). https://doi.org/10.1007/978-3-031-09002-8_27
16. Wang, W., Chen, C., Ding, M., Yu, H., Zha, S., Li, J.: TransBTS: multimodal brain tumor segmentation using transformer. In: Medical Image Computing and Computer Assisted Intervention–MICCAI 2021: 24th International Conference, Strasbourg, France, September 27–October 1, 2021, Proceedings, Part I 24, pp. 109–119. Springer (2021). https://doi.org/10.1007/978-3-030-87193-2_11
17. Bukhari, S.T., Mohy-ud Din, H.: E1D3 U-Net for brain tumor segmentation: submission to the RSNA-ASNR-MICCAI brats 2021 challenge. In: Brainlesion: Glioma, Multiple Sclerosis, Stroke and Traumatic Brain Injuries: 7th International Workshop, BrainLes 2021, Held in Conjunction with MICCAI 2021, Virtual Event, September 27, 2021, Revised Selected Papers, Part II, pp. 276–288. Springer (2022). https://doi.org/10.1007/978-3-031-09002-8_25
18. Kong, D., Liu, X., Wang, Y., Li, D., Xue, J.: 3D hierarchical dual attention fully convolutional networks with hybrid losses for diverse glioma segmentation. Knowl.-Based Syst. **237**, 107692 (2022)
19. Huang, X., Deng, Z., Li, D., Yuan, X., Fu, Y.: Missformer: An effective transformer for 2d medical image segmentation. IEEE Trans. Med. Imaging **42**, 1484–1494 (2022)
20. Zhu, Z., He, X., Qi, G., Li, Y., Cong, B., Liu, Y.: Brain tumor segmentation based on the fusion of deep semantics and edge information in multimodal MRI. Inf. Fus. **91**, 376–387 (2023)

GLAD: A Global-Attention-Based Diffusion Model for Infrared and Visible Image Fusion

Haozhe Guo[1], Mengjie Chen[1], Kaijiang Li[1], Hao Su[1(✉)], and Pei Lv[1,2,3]

[1] School of Computer and Artificial Intelligence, Zhengzhou University, Zhengzhou, China
ghzsqmr@stu.zzu.edu.cn, {chenmj,riversky}@gs.zzu.edu.cn,
{iesuhao,ielvpei}@zzu.edu.cn
[2] Engineering Research Center of Intelligent Swarm Systems, Ministry of Education, Zhengzhou, China
[3] National Supercomputing Center in Zhengzhou, Zhengzhou, China

Abstract. Infrared and visible image fusion (IVIF) is a widely used approach to enhance scenario understanding, which fuses the salience of infrared images and the texture details of visible images. Existing methods typically focus on extracting local feature maps between connected layers while ignoring the global features, which incurs the issue of fine-grained loss (e.g., texture and edge blurring) in the fused images. To address the issue, we propose *GLAD (GLobal-Attention-based Diffusion model)*, a novel IVIF approach to produce high-quality fused images with fine-grained. In GLAD, we first tailor a denoising network of the diffusion model to learn the joint distribution of multi-channel data. Next, we proposed a global attention fusion module to synthesize the global features extracted from the denoising network into a fine-grained fused image. Moreover, considering the influences of illumination factors, we design a fusion loss function to improve the denoising network for IVIF task. Qualitative and quantitative experiments demonstrate that our GLAD is 7.08% better than other state-of-the-art methods on the MSRS dataset.

Keywords: Image fusion · Diffusion process · Global attention

1 Introduction

Image fusion [1–5] is a longstanding task to integrate images from different sensors to enhance the scenario understanding. In the field of image fusion, infrared and visible image fusion (IVIF) is the most widely used method. Although infrared images can effectively capture objects and decrease the illumination influence, they focus on objects' heat salience and lack of texture details. In contrast, visible images contain rich texture and structural details but are sensitive to illumination influence. Therefore, their complementary nature allows IVIF to enhance the representations of object salience and texture details simultaneously.

Recently, IVIF techniques have been ubiquitously applied in fields of object detection [6], tracking [7], pedestrian re-identification [8], semantic segmentation [9], and so on.

Existing studies of IVIF have made remarkable achievements, which are mainly divided into traditional approaches and learning-based approaches [10]. Traditional approaches primarily consist of multi-scale transform-based approaches [11], sparse representation-based approaches [12], salience-based approaches [13], and hybrid approaches [14]. These approaches offer high interpretability but heavily rely on manual design. Specifically, these approaches lack versatility since they extract and fuse features by pre-defined algorithms that require manual adjustments for different fusion tasks [15]. Learning-based approaches can be further categorized into extraction-based approaches and generation-based approaches. Extraction-based approaches [17] extract features from source images using convolutional neural networks (CNN), and then fuse features from different source images using tailored rules. Next, the fused image is produced by combining the extracted features. Generation-based approaches are popular in computer vision, which aims to train a generative model (e.g., generative adversarial network (GAN) [18, 19], diffusion model [21, 22]) to generate fused images by simulating the sample distribution of the training dataset.

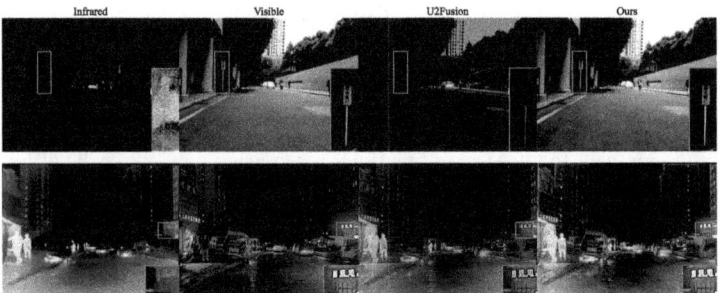

Fig. 1. Samples of IVIF results. Compared with related studies, our proposed GLAD generates better fine-grained fused images (red boxes). (Color figure online)

Although existing learning-based approaches have made considerable progress in IVIF, they focus on extracting local features without adequately considering global features. Specifically, these studies typically extract local feature maps between connected layers [21], which incurs the issues of fine-grained information loss (e.g., texture and edge blurring) in the fused images. For example, as shown in the red boxes of Fig. 1, U2Fusion [20] cannot produce a fine-grained fused image, and there are blurred edges and textures in signposts, and the text in the zoomed-in area.

To address the issues, we propose GLAD (GLobal-Attention-based Diffusion model), a novel IVIF approach that can produce high-quality fused images with fine-grained. In GLAD, we first tailor a denoising network of the diffusion model to learn the joint distribution of multi-channel information. Then, global features are extracted from the five steps of the denoising network, and we combine these global features into a fine-grained fused image by a proposed global attention fusion module (GAFM). Moreover, considering the influences of illumination environment factors, we design a fusion loss function to improve the diffusion model for the IVIF task. Qualitative and quantitative experiments demonstrate that our GLAD is 7.08% better than other related state-of-the-art methods on the MSRS dataset [17].

To summarize, our main contributions are three-fold:

- We propose a global-attention-based diffusion model, named GLAD, which is a novel IVIF approach that can produce high-quality fine-grained fused images.
- We propose a GAFM to effectively synthesize global features to fine-grained fused images, and design a novel fusion loss to improve the fusion performance by considering structure information and illumination factors.
- Extensive experiments demonstrate that GLAD can output impressive results and reach the state-of-the-art methods level.

2 Related Work

Below we summarize the representative studies most related to IVIF. In this field, researchers have made remarkable achievements, which are primarily categorized into the traditional methods [11–13] and the learning-based methods [10, 18, 19].

Traditional Method. The key of traditional methods lies in feature extraction and fusion, which can be roughly categorized into multi-scale transform-based approaches [11], sparse representation-based approaches [12], salience-based approaches [13], and hybrid approaches [14]. Although these approaches offer high interpretability, they heavily rely on manual design rule.

Learning-based Method. To solve the complexity problem of manually designing fusion rules in traditional methods, researchers introduce learning-based methods for the IVIF task. The representative learning-based methods can be further classified into extraction-based approaches and generation-based approaches.

Extraction-based approaches use CNN to extract features from source images and then fuse features with tailored rules. Next, the fused image is produced by combining the extracted features. Researchers modify the network architecture or combine multiple loss functions to improve the fusion performance of the network. Li et al. [16] propose DenseFuse, an IVIF approach based on CNN and dense connection. Tang et al. [17] consider the effect of the light factor and propose a light-aware CNN fusion approach called PIAFusion.

Generation-based approaches consider the image fusion task as a transformation from source images to target images. Ma et al. propose FusionGAN [18] to ingeniously frame the task as a competitive interplay between the generator and discriminator, treating it like a game. Then, Ma et al. [19] further used multi-classification GAN in GANMcC to estimate visible and infrared domain distributions simultaneously. However, GAN has the disadvantage of unstable training, and it is difficult to explain its internal mechanism. With the excellent performance of diffusion models [24] in visual tasks in recent years, some scholars have tried to apply diffusion models in this field. Yue et al. proposed [21] Dif-Fusion to produce fused images with high color fidelity, and DDFM [22] as a generalized image fusion model proposed by Zhao et al. achieved excellent performance.

In this paper, we propose a new IVIF approach, named GLAD, to produce high-quality fine-grained fused images. GLAD introduces a GAFM and fusion loss to the diffusion model [21], and reaches the state-of-the-art level.

3 Method

3.1 Overview

Given an infrared image I_{ir} and a visible image I_{vi}, our method GLAD is modeled as a function Ψ to generate a high-quality fine-grained fused image $I_{fu} = \Psi(I_{ir}, I_{vi})$, where $I_{ir} \in R^{H \times W \times 1}$, $I_{vi} \in R^{H \times W \times 3}$, and $I_{fu} \in R^{H \times W \times 3}$.

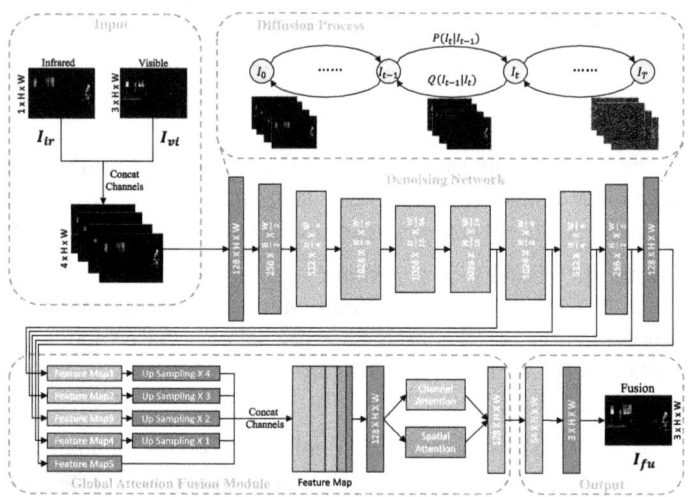

Fig. 2. System Pipeline. Given an infrared image I_{ir} and a visible image I_{vi}, our GLAD is modeled as a function Ψ to generate a high-quality fused image $I_{fu} = \Psi(I_{ir}, I_{vi})$.

Figure 2 shows the overall pipeline of GLAD. The proposed GLAD consists of two stages. In the first stage, we tailor a denoising network of diffusion model, and concatenate I_{ir} and I_{vi} along the channel dimensions and input them into the denoising network [21]. Through the diffusion process, we train the denoising network to learn the distribution of image data. In the second stage, we input the data into the trained denoising network, and utilize a designed fusion loss to train proposed GAFM. Finally, we extract global feature maps from five stages in the denoising network, and these global feature maps are constructed to a fine-grained fused image I_{fu}.

We will detail the diffusion model, the GAFM, and the fusion loss in Sect. 3.2, Sect. 3.3, and Sect. 3.4, respectively.

3.2 Diffusion Model

We tailor a diffusion model [21] to extract the image features more effectively. Specifically, we leverage the U-Net architecture in SR3 [23] as a denoising network to synthesize the distribution of infrared and visible image data through the diffusion process in the denoising diffusion probabilistic model [24].

Input. Unlike most fusion methods, aiming at learning the joint distribution and the underlying feature structures of infrared and visible image pairs, we concatenate a pair of aligned infrared image $I_{ir} \in R^{H \times W \times 1}$ and visible image $I_{vi} \in R^{H \times W \times 3}$ (H and W indicate the image height and width) in channel dimensions to form a four-channel input data fed into the denoising network and learn the data distribution [21].

Forward Diffusion Process. As shown in Fig. 2, we gradually add Gaussian noise to the input data during the forward diffusion process until the data approaches pure noise. From the DDPM [24], it is known that given the input data I_0, timestep t, variance schedule $\alpha_1, \ldots, \alpha_t$, and the sampled noise, the noise multi-channel distribution image I_t can be calculated by

$$P(I_t|I_0) = \mathcal{N}\left(I_t; \sqrt{\overline{\alpha_t}}I_0, (1-\overline{\alpha_t})Z\right) \qquad (1)$$

where Z represents the standard normal distribution, $\overline{\alpha_t} = \prod_{i=1}^{t} \alpha_i$.

Reverse Diffusion Process. In the reverse diffusion process, the denoising network performs a series of small denoising operations at each timestep to obtain the image of the previous timestep and obtains the original image by gradual denoising [25]. Similarly, given the noisy image I_t corresponding to timestep t, the probability distribution of It − 1 under the condition It can be calculated by

$$Q(I_{t-1}|I_t) = \mathcal{N}\left(I_{t-1}; \mu_\theta(I_t, t), \sigma_t^2 Z\right) \qquad (2)$$

where $\mu_\theta(I_t, t)$ is the mean value of $Q(I_{t-1}|I_t)$ and σ_t^2 is the variance, they also can be calculated.

3.3 Global Attention Fusion Module

After training the denoising network, to ensure that the model can focus on both global features and local details, we first utilize the trained denoising network to extract feature maps from each stage. Then, we design a GAFM to synthesize global feature maps to a fine-grained fused image.

As shown in the denoising network of Fig. 2, we use the backbone [21, 23] as our denoising network, there are five convolutional layers in the right part. We extract five stages of the feature maps and the size of five feature maps are $\frac{H}{16} \times \frac{W}{16}$, $\frac{H}{8} \times \frac{W}{8}$, $\frac{H}{4} \times \frac{W}{4}$, $\frac{H}{2} \times \frac{W}{2}$ and $H \times W$, each of which extracts features generated by the trained denoising network at three timesteps (i.e., 5, 50, 100). As shown in the GAFM in Fig. 2, for the model to pay attention to both global features and local details, after obtaining the diffusion feature maps, the feature maps of the five stages are enlarged into $H \times W$ dimensions by the corresponding upsampling operations. Then, the feature maps are concatenated in the channel dimension to obtain the global feature map, and the same channel attention mechanism and spatial attention mechanism as in scSE [26] are used for the global feature map to obtain the new feature map. Finally, the feature map is transformed into 128 channels by a fully connected layer, and the final 3-channel output fusion image is obtained through the 3 × 3 convolution layer.

3.4 Fusion Loss

To better focus on infrared images' salience and visible images' texture details while adapting to the influence of environmental illumination, we train our GAFM by a designed fusion loss $\mathcal{L}_{fus}$ that consists of illumination loss $\mathcal{L}_{ill}$, intensity loss $\mathcal{L}_{int}$, and gradient loss $\mathcal{L}_{gra}$.

Illumination Loss. Aiming to better adapt to the illumination conditions and preserve semantic information from the source image, we introduce an illumination loss [17]. Specifically, by using the light binary classification network to output the light probability P of the image, and then assigning the light weights $W_{ir} = P$ and $W_{vi} = 1 - P$. The illumination loss $\mathcal{L}_{ill}$ is finally defined as

$$\mathcal{L}_{ill} = W_{ir} \cdot \frac{1}{HW} ||I_{fu} - I_{ir}||_1 + W_{vi} \cdot \frac{1}{HW} ||I_{fu} - I_{vi}||_1 \tag{3}$$

where I_{fu}, I_{ir} and I_{vi} represent fused image, infrared image, and visible image respectively, and $||\cdot||_1$ represents $L1$ loss.

Intensity Loss. In order to maintain the best intensity distribution for the fused image obtained by GLAD, we employ an auxiliary intensity loss [21], defined as

$$\mathcal{L}_{int} = \frac{1}{HW} ||I_{fu} - max(I_{ir}, I_{vi})||_1 \tag{4}$$

Gradient Loss. Aiming to retain sufficient texture information in the final fused image while maintaining intensity distribution, we use a gradient loss [21], defined as

$$\mathcal{L}_{gra} = \frac{1}{HW} ||\nabla I_{fu} - max(\nabla |I_{ir}|, \nabla |I_{vi}|)||_1 \tag{5}$$

where ∇ indicates the gradient operator.

Finally, the total fusion loss $\mathcal{L}_{fus}$ utilized to train our model is defined as

$$\mathcal{L}_{fus} = \mathcal{L}_{ill} + \mathcal{L}_{int} + \mathcal{L}_{gra} \tag{6}$$

4 Experiments

In this section, we first present our experiment implementation, including datasets, metrics, and implementation details. Next, we perform some comparison and generalization experiments to show the superiority of GLAD. Finally, we reveal the effectiveness of using the global attention fusion module based on the ablation study.

4.1 Implementation

Datasets. To evaluate the performance of our framework, we conduct extensive experiments on three public datasets, i.e., **MSRS** [17], **KAIST** [27], and **M3FD** [6]. **MSRS** dataset is an multispectral dataset based on the MFNet dataset, containing 1444 pairs of high-quality aligned infrared and visible images. **KAIST** dataset captures a variety of regular traffic scenes, including campuses, streets, and countryside, both day and night, respectively. The image size is 640 × 480. **M3FD** dataset includes scenes such as campuses, resorts, roads, etc., and most of the images are 1024 × 768 pixels.

Metrics. In our comparative experiments, we utilize six metrics to comprehensively evaluate the fused effect: entropy (**EN** [28]), standard deviation (**SD**), mutual information (**MI**), visual information fidelity (**VIF** [29]), quality assessment based on blur and noise factors (**Qabf** [30]), and structural similarity index measure (**SSIM**). **EN** measures the amount of information the fused image contains. **SD** reflects the extent to which the values of individual pixels in the image are deviated from the average value. **MI** primarily evaluates how well the fused image aggregates information from the original image pairs. **VIF** measures the information fidelity of the fused image. **Qabf** quantifies the edge information and granularity level in the fused image. **SSIM** measures the structural similarity between source images and fused images [10].

Implementation Details. Our proposed GLAD is trained on the MSRS dataset and we adopt the training settings in Dif-Fusion [21]. During training, we randomly select 160 × 160 patches from both visible and infrared images and extract diffusion features from these patches produced at three time steps (e.g., 5, 50, 100) to construct multi-channel features. For training the fusion module, we employ the Adam optimizer to minimize loss, with a fixed learning rate of 0.0001. The training process utilizes a batch size of 24, and we iterate through 300 epochs to train the model. All of the training process is performed on a server equipped with an NVIDIA RTX3090 GPU.

4.2 Comparison with State-of-the-Art Methods

Below we compare our model with five state-of-the-art methods, FusionGAN [18], GANMcC [19], U2Fusion [20], TarDAL [6] and Dif-Fusion [21]. U2Fusion is based on CNN architectures, while FusionGAN, GANMcC, TarDAL, and Dif-Fusion are based on generative models and their variants.

Qualitative Comparison. The qualitative results of different fusion methods on the MSRS 00537D image are shown in Fig. 3. Overall, our method, TarDAL, and Dif-Fusion effectively preserve the texture details of the visible image while highlighting the salient targets of the infrared image. However, the fused image obtained by U2Fusion appears darker. In some details, as depicted in the zoomedin areas of the red and green boxes, the fusion results obtained by FusionGAN and GANMcC are slightly misaligned compared to the original image, with a significant loss of texture details in the zoomed-in areas. In contrast, our method preserves the texture details of the notice boards in the figure well, resulting in fine-grained fused images.

Quantitative Comparison. The quantitative results are shown in Fig. 4. Our method achieves superior performance across all six metrics. Particularly noteworthy is the significant improvement observed in four metrics (i.e., EN, SD, VIF, and Qabf). The highest SD and VIF values indicate that the fused images obtained by our method have high contrast and sizable visual effects. The highest MI and SSIM indicate that our method retains more structural information and features from the source images. Furthermore, thanks to our global attention fusion module, our method achieves the highest Qabf, indicating that our fusion results retain more edge information and achieve the finest level of granularity.

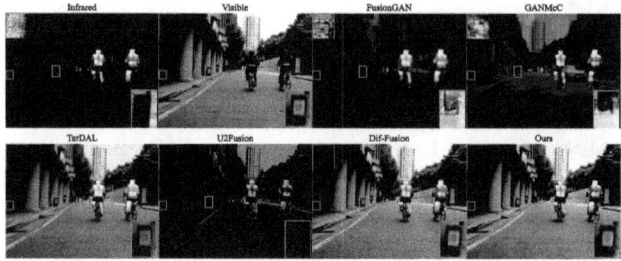

Fig. 3. Qualitative comparison on the 00537D image pair from the MSRS dataset.

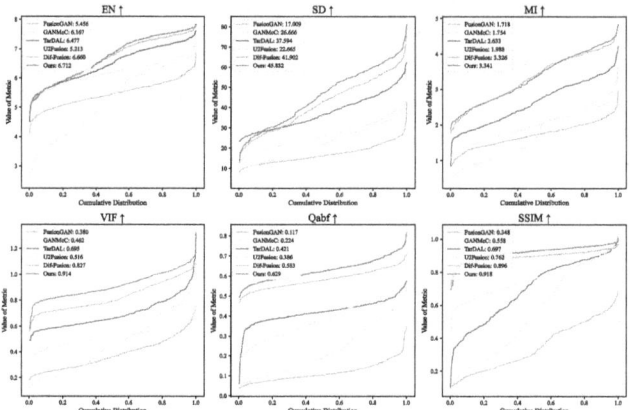

Fig. 4. Quantitative comparisons of the six metrics, i.e., EN, SD, MI, VIF Qabf and SSIM, on 361 image pairs from the MSRS dataset.

4.3 Generalization Experiment

Below we conduct experiments on the KAIST and M3FD datasets to assess GLAD's generalizability. Specifically, our fusion model was trained on the MSRS dataset and then directly evaluated on the KAIST and M3FD datasets.

Qualitative Comparison. The qualitative results of different fusion methods on the KAIST set09_V000_I02542 are shown in Fig. 5. From the red-boxed zoomed-in area in the figure, all six methods highlight the infrared pedestrian target, with FusionGAN having a more prominent target and U2Fusion having a darker target. However, from the zoomed-in area in the green box, FusionGAN and GANMcC lose the texture details of the visible image, such as the traffic sign. Figure 6 shows the fusion results of different fusion methods on M3FD00572. From the figure, all six methods can retain the infrared pedestrian targets well, but only our method and the Dif-Fusion method based on the diffusion model better retain the textual details in the zoomed-in area of the red box in the figure. Overall, benefiting from the learning of image features by the diffusion model and the application of the global attention fusion module, our method retains more feature details from the source images and gains finely-grained fused images.

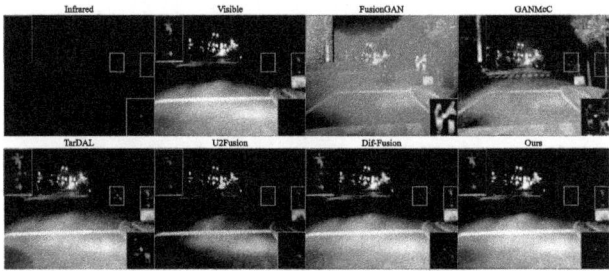

Fig. 5. Qualitative comparison on the set09_V000 _I02542 image pair from the KAIST dataset.

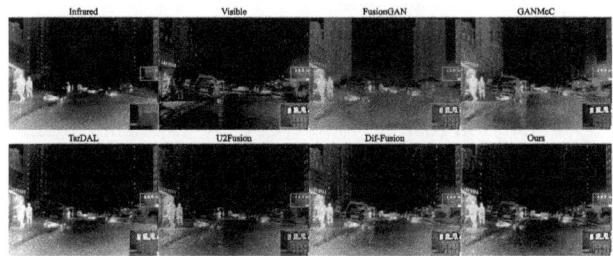

Fig. 6. Qualitative comparison on the 00572 image pair from the M3FD dataset.

Table 1. Fusion quality evaluation on 2257 aligned image pairs from the KAIST dataset. **Bold** represents the best results, and underlining represents the second-best results.

Methods	EN ↑	SD ↑	MI ↑	VIF ↑	Qabf ↑	SSIM ↑
FusionGAN	6.361	25.383	2.438	0.444	0.168	0.321
GANMcC	6.875	38.112	2.344	0.432	0.251	0.458
TarDAL	7.048	50.239	3.336	0.715	0.508	0.858
U2Fusion	6.559	32.623	2.537	0.689	0.521	**0.878**
Dif-Fusion	7.089	52.509	**3.916**	0.799	0.615	0.864
Ours	**7.109**	**57.921**	3.842	**0.832**	**0.638**	0.862

Quantitative Comparison. The fusion results on 2257 pairs of KAIST datasets are presented in Table 1. Compared with the other five methods, our approach achieves the highest EN, SD, VIF, and Qabf values, as well as the second-highest MI values. This indicates that the fusion results obtained by our method closely resemble the visual perception of the human eye and better retain both the local details and global information of the source images. Following the most work, we randomly select 25 pairs of M3FD datasets, and the test results of different fusion methods are shown in Table 2. Our method performs well across five metrics, namely EN, SD, MI, VIF, and Qabf, further validating the generalization ability of our proposed GLAD.

Table 2. Fusion quality evaluation on 25 image pairs from the M3FD dataset. **Bold** represents the best results, underlining represents the second best results.

Methods	EN ↑	SD ↑	MI ↑	VIF ↑	Qabf ↑	SSIM ↑
FusionGAN	6.907	32.707	2.102	0.256	0.158	0.482
GANMcC	6.997	35.838	1.735	0.332	0.168	0.595
TarDAL	7.493	47.750	2.471	0.447	0.407	0.871
U2Fusion	7.042	35.686	1.876	0.476	0.549	**0.973**
Dif-Fusion	7.390	43.829	2.820	0.498	0.570	0.869
Ours	**7.598**	**53.276**	**3.243**	**0.614**	**0.641**	0.856

4.4 Ablation Study

We propose a global attention fusion module(GAFM) to enable the model to focus on both local details and global features. We further conduct ablation experiments to confirm the effectiveness of the GAFM. Specifically, all other modules remain unchanged and are trained for 300 epochs under identical settings without the GAFM. The final results of the ablation experiments on the MSRS test set are presented in Table 3. 错误!未找到引用源。. It is evident that the removal of the global attention module results in a performance decrease in our method across five metrics (namely, EN, SD, VIF, Qabf, and SSIM). This further validates the capability of our proposed global attention module to effectively capture both the global and local information of the source image.

Table 3. The fusion performance with and without the GAFM on the MSRS dataset.

Methods	EN ↑	SD ↑	MI ↑	VIF ↑	Qabf ↑	SSIM ↑
w/o GAFM.	6.644	41.828	**3.344**	0.831	0.576	0.900
w GAFM.	**6.712**	**45.832**	3.341	**0.914**	**0.629**	**0.919**

5 Conclusion

In this paper, we propose GLAD, an IVIF method that can produce high-quality fused images with fine-grained. In GLAD, we tailor a denoising network of the diffusion model, propose a GAFM, and design a fusion loss function to improve our performance for the IVIF task. Through qualitative and quantitative experiments experiments conducted on multiple datasets, including MSRS, KAIST, and M3FD, we have demonstrated the superior performance of GLAD compared with other SOTA methods.

Acknowledgements. Thanks for the suggestion of reviewers. This work was supported in part by National Key R&D Program Project under Grant 2022YFC3803203, Joint Fund of the Ministry of Education for Equipment Pre Research with Grant 8091B032257, and National Natural Science Foundation of China under Grant 62372415.

References

1. Dogra, A., Goyal, B., Agrawal, S.: From multi-scale decomposition to non-multiscale decomposition methods: a comprehensive survey of image fusion techniques and its applications. IEEE Access **5**, 16040–16067 (2017)
2. Sun, C., Zhang, C., Xiong, N.: Infrared and visible image fusion techniques based on deep learning: a review. Electronics **9**(12), 2162 (2020)
3. Ma, W., et al.: Infrared and visible image fusion technology and application: a review. Sensors **23**(2), 599 (2023)
4. Tang, L., Zhang, H., Xu, H., Ma, J.: Rethinking the necessity of image fusion in high-level vision tasks: a practical infrared and visible image fusion network based on progressive semantic injection and scene fidelity. Inf. Fus. **99**, 101870 (2023)
5. Zhang, X., Demiris, Y.: Visible and infrared image fusion using deep learning. IEEE Trans. Pattern Anal. Mach. Intell. (2023)
6. Liu, J., et al.: Target-aware dual adversarial learning and a multi-scenario multi-modality benchmark to fuse infrared and visible for object detection. In: Proceedings of the IEEE/CVF Conference on Ccomputer Vision and Pattern Recognition, pp. 5802–5811 (2022)
7. Li, C., Zhu, C., Huang, Y., Tang, J., Wang, L.: Cross-modal ranking with soft consistency and noisy labels for robust RGB-T tracking. In: Proceedings of the European Conference on Computer Vision (ECCV), pp. 808–823 (2018)
8. Lu, Y., et al.: Cross-modality person re-identification with shared-specific feature transfer. In: Proceedings of the IEEE/CVF Conference on Computer Vision and Pattern Recognition, pp. 13379–13389 (2020)
9. Zhou, W., Liu, J., Lei, J., Yu, L., Hwang, J.N.: GMNet: Graded-feature multilabel-learning network for rgb-thermal urban scene semantic segmentation. IEEE Trans. Image Process. **30**, 7790–7802 (2021)
10. Ma, J., Ma, Y., Li, C.: Infrared and visible image fusion methods and applications: a survey. Inf. Fus. **45**, 153–178 (2019)
11. Liu, Y., Liu, S., Wang, Z.: A general framework for image fusion based on multiscale transform and sparse representation. Inf. Fus. **24**, 147–164 (2015)
12. Liu, Y., Chen, X., Ward, R.K., Wang, Z.J.: Image fusion with convolutional sparse representation. IEEE Signal Process. Lett. **23**(12), 1882–1886 (2016)
13. Bavirisetti, D.P., Dhuli, R.: Two-scale image fusion of visible and infrared images using saliency detection. Infrared Phys. Technol. **76**, 52–64 (2016)
14. Ma, J., Zhou, Z., Wang, B., Zong, H.: Infrared and visible image fusion based on visual saliency map and weighted least square optimization. Infrared Phys. Technol. **82**, 8–17 (2017)
15. Li, S., Kang, X., Fang, L., Hu, J., Yin, H.: Pixel-level image fusion: A survey of the state of the art. information Fusion **33**, 100–112 (2017)
16. Li, H., Wu, X.J.: DenseFuse: a fusion approach to infrared and visible images. IEEE Trans. Image Process. **28**(5), 2614–2623 (2018)
17. Tang, L., Yuan, J., Zhang, H., Jiang, X., Ma, J.: PIAFusion: a progressive infrared and visible image fusion network based on illumination aware. Inf. Fus. **83**, 79–92 (2022)
18. Ma, J., Yu, W., Liang, P., Li, C., Jiang, J.: FusionGAN: a generative adversarial network for infrared and visible image fusion. Inf. Fus. **48**, 11–26 (2019)
19. Ma, J., Zhang, H., Shao, Z., Liang, P., Xu, H.: GANMcC: a generative adversarial network with multiclassification constraints for infrared and visible image fusion. IEEE Trans. Instrum. Meas. **70**, 1–14 (2020)
20. Xu, H., Ma, J., Jiang, J., Guo, X., Ling, H.: U2Fusion: a unified unsupervised image fusion network. IEEE Trans. Pattern Anal. Mach. Intell. **44**(1), 502–518 (2020)

21. Yue, J., Fang, L., Xia, S., Deng, Y., Ma, J.: Dif-Fusion: towards high color fidelity in infrared and visible image fusion with diffusion models. IEEE Trans. Image Process. (2023)
22. Zhao, Z., et al.: DDFM: denoising diffusion model for multi-modality image fusion. In: Proceedings of the IEEE/CVF International Conference on Computer Vision, pp. 8082–8093 (2023)
23. Saharia, C., Ho, J., Chan, W., Salimans, T., Fleet, D.J., Norouzi, M.: Image superresolution via iterative refinement. IEEE Trans. Pattern Anal. Mach. Intell. **45**(4), 4713–4726 (2022)
24. Ho, J., Jain, A., Abbeel, P.: Denoising diffusion probabilistic models. Adv. Neural. Inf. Process. Syst. **33**, 6840–6851 (2020)
25. Baranchuk, D., Rubachev, I., Voynov, A., Khrulkov, V., Babenko, A.: Label-efficient semantic segmentation with diffusion models. arXiv preprint arXiv:2112.03126 (2021)
26. Roy, A.G., Navab, N., Wachinger, C.: Concurrent Spatial and Channel 'Squeeze & Excitation' in Fully Convolutional Networks. In: Frangi, A.F., Schnabel, J.A., Davatzikos, C., Alberola-López, C., Fichtinger, G. (eds.) MICCAI 2018. LNCS, vol. 11070, pp. 421–429. Springer, Cham (2018). https://doi.org/10.1007/978-3-030-00928-1_48
27. Choi, Y., et al.: Kaist multi-spectral day/night data set for autonomous and assisted driving. IEEE Trans. Intell. Transp. Syst. **19**(3), 934–948 (2018)
28. Qu, G., Zhang, D., Yan, P.: Information measure for performance of image fusion. Electron. Lett. **38**(7), 1 (2002)
29. Han, Y., Cai, Y., Cao, Y., Xu, X.: A new image fusion performance metric based on visual information fidelity. Inf. Fus. **14**(2), 127–135 (2013)
30. Xydeas, C.S., Petrovic, V., et al.: Objective image fusion performance measure. Electron. Lett. **36**(4), 308–309 (2000)

An Approach for Extracting Road Network from Remote Sensing Images

Zhihui Wang[1,2(✉)], Yu Wang[1,2], and Yuliang Ni[1,2]

[1] School of Computer Science, Fudan University, Shanghai, China
zhhwang@fudan.edu.cn
[2] Shanghai Key Laboratory of Data Science, Shanghai, China

Abstract. In recent years, the neural network architecture has developed rapidly and has been widely used in the semantic segmentation of remote sensing images. In this paper, we apply the neural network to the road network extraction of high-resolution remote sensing images. Subsequently, a series of single-pixel coordinate points are obtained by using the refinement method. Given the different lengths of road sections, our algorithm uses a double-loop mechanism to perform multi-scale fitting of them, which improves the rough results of the neural network and enhances the accuracy of road network extraction. For multiple line segments that may be on the same road, we also propose appropriate rules to classify and merge them. Our experimental results show that compared with other methods of road network extraction, our approach can obtain better results.

Keywords: Road Network · Deep Learning · Image Recognition

1 Introduction

Research related to high-resolution remote sensing images has developed into many fields, such as image classification, parcel segmentation, and semantic segmentation. Geographic information extracted by remote sensing images can be well applied in the valuable directions of life such as rail transit, meteorology, and agriculture. Therefore, road network extraction in remote sensing images is still an important direction [9]. Recently, China's urbanization process has got faster and faster. Road network construction and spatial layout development in first-tier cities are particularly important. In the big cities, the irregular shapes of the street blocks, the shadings of tall buildings and green plants, and other factors lead to a low contrast between road network features and non-road network features, which poses a great challenge to the road network extraction task.

In this paper, we use the convolutional neural network model to extracting road network from remote sensing images, and then perform further post-processing on the rough road network extracted by the model, including road network skeleton extraction, and the improved RANSAC [2, 6] algorithm for the vectorization of road network. Finally, the Ramer-Douglas-Peucker (RDP) [1, 7] algorithm is used for vector path compression.

Our contributions in this paper are mainly as follows: Firstly, through neural network training and parameter adjustment, our approach can handle the considerable large scale of remote sensing images and optimized them through model fusion. Secondly, based on the results of the neural network, our approach can further carry out a series of post-processing, especially for the improvement of the road fitting algorithm, so that our road network extraction approach can obtain a higher precision. Thirdly, compared with other methods of extracting the road network, we have proposed a set of practical methodology. Our approach can process the input of images and output the vectorized road network for further processing.

2 Our Approach

The structure of our neural network model is based on U-Net [8]. In order to obtain better result, we have fine-tuned the network structure, such as the use of the pre-training model, the alignment of the size of the up-sampled feature map, the fusion of multiple model results, etc. At the beginning of the road network post-processing, we introduced some morphological knowledge; in the task of road vector fitting, the improved RANSAC algorithm allows our experiments to proceed smoothly; for the road after fitting, classification reconstruction and vector compression are carried out, we combined some mathematical knowledge to make our method more convincing.

2.1 Model Structure and Model Fusion

U-Net is an improved version of fully convolutional network (FCN) [5]. We furtherly improve the idea of the U-Net structure and replace the down-sampling part with the pre-trained ResNet [3] structure in PyTorch. In addition, we use different variants of ResNet (ResNet50 / ResNet101 / ResNet152) as the up-sampling part for training different models, and select the models for each variant for prediction, then finally voted on the prediction of a single-pixel to achieve model fusion. For convenience, we call the model U-Net*.

2.2 Road Refinement

The choice of the refinement algorithm is determined according to the actual situation. Since the refinement algorithm has discontinuous results for skeleton extraction in the practical applications, we do not focus on the integrity and connectivity of the skeleton. Instead, we only need to obtain the discrete pixel feature map with the road network structure. We compared the effects of Hilditch's algorithm [4] and Zhang's algorithm [10] on road network skeleton extraction, and the results of these two algorithms are different. In our experiments, the Zhang's algorithm can get more suitable results, and the skeleton produced by Hilditch's algorithm is ambiguous.

2.3 DL-RANSAC Algorithm

By drawing the lessons from the idea of cyclically using RANSAC [2, 6], we made the improvement and presented the approach of Double Loop RANSAC (DL-RANSAC). This method can perform more robust multi-scale fitting and improve the road network coverage.

In RANSAC, the result returned by the fitting contains three parts: the coordinate point set, the slope k of the fitted line, and the offset b. To facilitate the representation and storage of line segments, we only retain the coordinates of the two endpoints of the straight line, so the data structure of the line segment is $line = [point_{left}, point_{right}]$.

A single loop RANSAC can fit multiple line segments in a binary image. However, the position of pixels is expressed based on the Cartesian coordinate system, the least-squares fit in RANSAC cannot fit the straight line that perpendicular to the x-axis, we fixed this problem in the algorithm. In addition, there is a fixed parameter N in RANSAC, which is the number of minimum pixels that meet the straight-line fit. If this parameter is too large, the shorter line segment will not fit. On the contrary, it is easy to fit the wrong line segment. So we improved the algorithm to achieve dynamic multi-scale fitting and called it double loop RANSAC(DL-RANSAC): nesting an outer loop and setting the dynamic parameter N (specifically, the outer loop gradually decreases, but will not fall below the minimum threshold). In this case, the longer line segment will be fitted first, and then the shorter line segment will be fitted. The specific algorithm is shown by Algorithm 1.

2.4 Segment Classification

In the process of circular line fitting using discrete pixels with a road network architecture, multiple similar lines will be fitted on the same road segment, so we set certain clustering rules to cluster the same line segment.

We consider using the angle of the straight lines as one of the similarity measures to cluster different straight lines. In the following, we will define the rule for the intersection of straight lines from the parallel and intersection of line segments.

Algorithm 1 Double Loop RANSAC Algorithm

Input:
    Binary image with road skeleton: $Image_{data}$
    The minimum number of pixels needed to fit a straight line: n
    Inner loop RANSAC iterations: k
    Error threshold of fitted model and external points: t
        The number of minimum demand points that meet the qualified straight line and the minimum threshold of the outer circle: $N_{miniFit}$, $N_{miniGap}$

Output:
    Set of line segments that are not perpendicular to the x axis $Lines_{Novx}$
    Set of line segments that are perpendicular to the x axis $Lines_{Vx}$

1: Initialize $Image_{data}$ and return the pixel coordinate set P_{XYs} of road features, and declare that a $P_{original}$ is equal to P_{XYs}
2: Initialization result coordinate point set $Lines_{Novx}$ and $Lines_{Vx}$ are empty
3: Initialize the outer loop number batch to 1
4: **while** $P_{XYs}/P_{original} \geq 0.1$ && $N_{miniFit}/batch \geq N_{miniGap}$ **do**
5:     $N_{miniFit}/ = batch$
6:     **while** $line_{Novx}$ is exist **do**
7:         Get $RANSAC_{fitmodel}$ and $RANSAC_{fitdata}$ from RANSAC($n, k, t, N_{miniFit}$)
8:         Obtain line segment endpoints from the fitted model and data to form a line segment representation $line_{Novx}$
9:         $P_{XYs} = P_{XYs} - RANSAC_{fitdata}$
10:         $Lines_{Novx}$.append($line_{Novx}$)
11:     **end while**
12:     **while** $line_{Vx}$ is exist **do**
13:         Get $line_{Vx}$
14:         $P_{XYs} = P_{XYs} -$ data in $line_{Vx}$
15:         $Lines_{Vx}$.append($line_{Vx}$)
16:     **end while**
17:     $batch += 1$
18: **end while**
19: **return** $Lines_{Novx}$ and $Lines_{Vx}$

Parallel Line Segments. If the slope k of the two straight lines is equal, but the offset b is inconsistent (shown in Fig. 1(a)), we set the threshold th_1 to determine the relationship between the distance D_1 of the two straight lines and the threshold. D_1 can be calculated by $D_1 = \frac{|b_1 - b_2|}{\sqrt{k^2+1}}$.

If the slope k and the offset b of the two straight lines are equal (shown in Fig. 1(b)), two cases are considered: (1) If two lines intersect directly, they are classified into the same category; (2) If the lines are parallel, we determine the relationship by comparing the distance D_2 with a predefined threshold th_2, where D_2 is calculated as $D_2 = min(distance(B_1, A_2), distance(A_1, B_2))$.

Intersecting Line Segments. If the angle θ between two straight lines is greater than the predefined threshold th_θ, they must not be of the same type. The angle θ can be

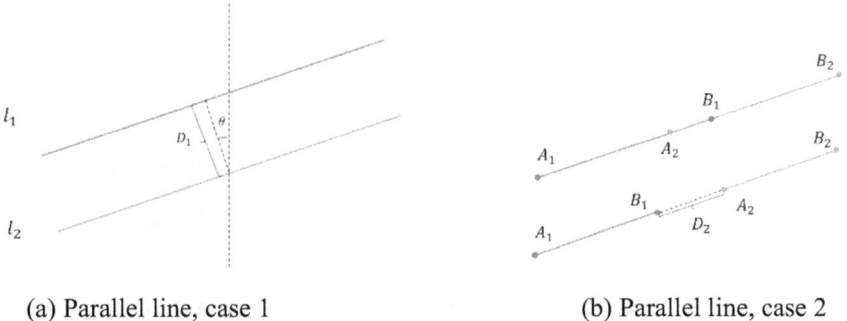

(a) Parallel line, case 1 (b) Parallel line, case 2

Fig. 1. Examples of parallel line segments.

obtained by $\theta = abs(arctan(\frac{k_1-k_2}{1+k_1*k_2}))$, where k_1 and k_2 are the slopes of the two lines, respectively.

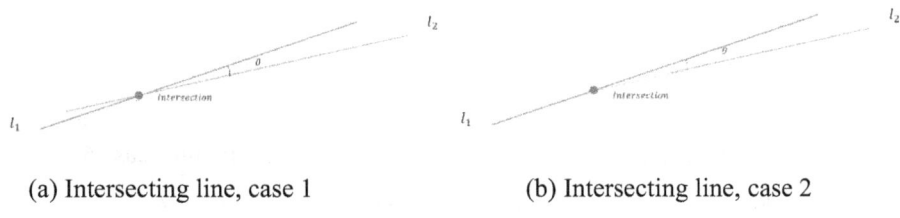

(a) Intersecting line, case 1 (b) Intersecting line, case 2

Fig. 2. Examples of intersecting line segments (case 1 & case 2).

If the angle between two straight lines is less than the threshold th_θ, consider the following situations:

1. If the intersection falls on two straight lines at the same time (shown in Fig. 2(a)), the lines are directly classified into the same category, and the coordinates of the intersection point are retained. The x and y of the intersection coordinate can be obtained by the following formula:

$$x = \frac{b_2 - b_1}{k_1 - k_2}, y = \frac{b_2 * k_1 - b_1 * k_2}{k_1 - k_2} \tag{1}$$

2. If the intersection point is located only on one of the straight lines, but the two straight lines intersect in the value range of x (shown in Fig. 2(b)), the lines are classified into the same category, but the coordinates of the intersection point are not retained.

3. If the intersection point is located only on one of the straight lines, and the two straight lines do not intersect in the value range of x (shown in Fig. 3(a)), we need another predefined distance threshold th_3. If the distance D_3 between the endpoints of the two straight lines is less than the threshold th_3, the lines are of the same type.

4. If the intersection point is not on any straight line, but is located in the middle of the two lines (shown in Fig. 3(b)), the threshold th_3 and the distance D_3 are also used to

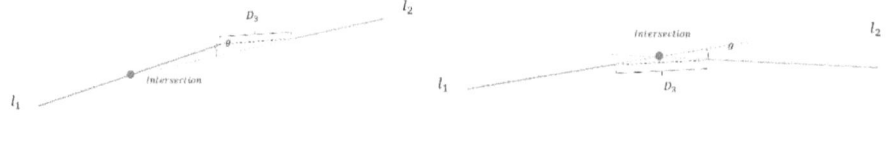

(a) Intersecting line, case 3   (b) Intersecting line, case 4

Fig. 3. Examples of intersecting line segments (case 3 & case 4).

determine whether the two lines are of the same type. However, the position of the intersection point needs to be further judged here. If the intersection point is within the range of the current image, the coordinates of the intersection point are retained. Otherwise, they are not retained.

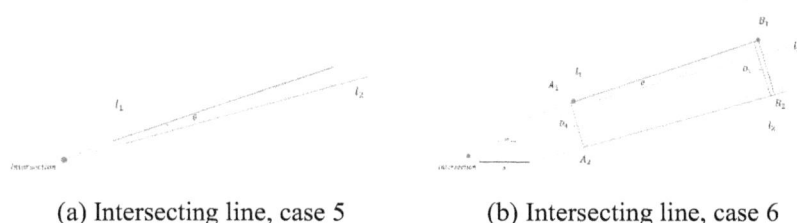

(a) Intersecting line, case 5   (b) Intersecting line, case 6

Fig. 4. Examples of intersecting line segments (case 5 & case 6).

5. Consider the last case, where the intersection point is not on any straight line. Ideally, the situation that satisfies the same category is shown in Fig. 4(a). However, it may be as shown in Fig. 4(b). That is, the intersection point of the two-line segments is far outside the picture range. At this case, we need a pre-define distance threshold th_4, and calculate the vertical distances D_4 and D_5 from A_1 and B_1 to another line. If both D_4 and D_5 are smaller than the threshold th_4, the lines are classified into the same category. Here D_4 (or D_5) can be obtained by the following formula:

$$D_4(\text{dis from } A_1 \text{ to } l_2) = \left| \overrightarrow{A_1A_2} - \frac{\overrightarrow{A_1A_2}\overrightarrow{A_2B_2}}{|A_2B_2|^2}\overrightarrow{A_2B_2} \right| \qquad (2)$$

2.5 Vector Path Compression

After we classify the line segments by the above line segment rules, the set of line segments of each category is $L = l_1, l_2, \ldots, l_n$, where l_i has two endpoints. We convert the line segment set into a point set and sort all the endpoints according to the coordinate size, then use the Ramer-Douglas-Peucker (RDP) [1, 7] algorithm to perform vector path compression on the ordered coordinate points. After that, we can delete unnecessary endpoints, and connect the retained points to obtain the final vectorization result of road network.

3 Experimental Results

3.1 Data Description

The road network source data we obtained is vector data stored in the format of GeoJSON. Each node of the road label is represented by the latitude and longitude coordinates based on the Mercator coordinate system. We use relevant toolkits in Python to convert these nodes into tiles annotate and download the corresponding tilemap on Google Maps. The downloaded annotations and data are as shown in Fig. 5, and the size is 256 * 256. Because the downloaded tile labels are single-pixel binary images, we performed morphological dilation preprocessing to better match the width of the roads in the map data. Similarly, before the neural network training, we conducted artificial screening and elimination of dirty data.

3.2 Model Training and Prediction

Through the experiment and parameter adjustment process, we found that adding loss weights has a critical effect on the experimental results. We regard the road network extraction task as a semantic binary classification task, using *CrossEntropyLoss* in PyTorch as a loss function, and the specific calculation method of the function is as the following formula.

$$\text{loss}(x, \text{class}) = -\log(\frac{\exp(x[class])}{\Sigma_j \exp(x[j])}) = -x[class] + \log(\sum_j \exp(x[j])) \quad (3)$$

When using *CrossEntropyLoss* without adding any parameters for model training, our binary prediction results account for almost 0% of the road network. Through analysis and thinking, we found that the ratio of the road network to the non-road network in the data has a large skew. In the case where the non-road network accounts for a large amount, the network tends to determine the pixels as non-road networks during the gradient descent optimization process. Because in this case, even if all road networks are predicted to be non-road networks, the accuracy of classification prediction will also be considerable.

Notice that in *CrossEntropyLoss*, the calculation formula with weight is (*default weight = None*): *loss(x, class) = weight[class](−x[class] + ($\sum_j exp(x[j])$))*. We use the following calculation method for the weight of determining the two-class (i.e., road and non-road), $weight = \frac{1}{log(w_b+P)}$, where *P* represents the ratio of the sum of road pixels (or the sum of non-road pixels) to the total number of pixels in the data, w_b represents a pre-defined bias parameter.

With the help of the weight, our approach can obtain quite impressive results especially for the experiments on the skew data of the test set. Several representative results are shown in Fig. 5. Each subgraph contains the original image of the test picture, the single-pixel annotated image, the experimental annotated image, and the predicted image (because we predict and return a probability of (0–1) for each pixel value *p*, so the value of a single-pixel in the prediction map comes from *p* * 255, not only 0 and 255).

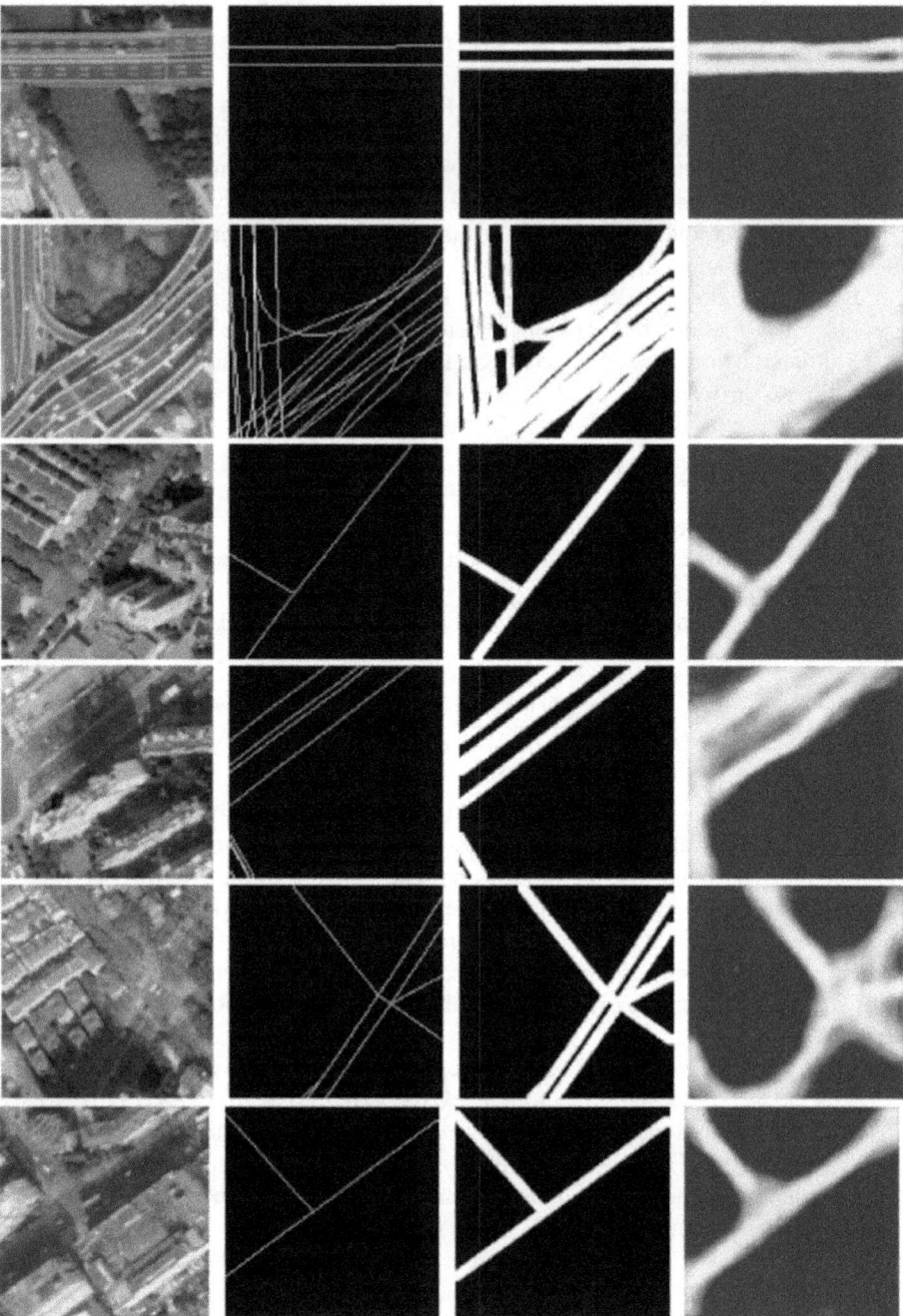

Fig. 5. Datasets and test predictions. There are six groups of sample pictures. From left to right, in each group are the original satellite image, the vector single-line road network label, the road network label after morphological expansion, and the U-Net* prediction result.

3.3 Road Refinement and DL-RANSAC

In our experiments, we set the number of pixels of randomly generated lines as 2. In addition, we set the random number k to 500, the distance threshold between the non-fitting point and the fitted line is set to 100, and the minimum number of pixels required to meet the required straight line is dynamically decreased from 125 in the outer loop of Algorithm 1 until it is less than the minimum threshold of 50.

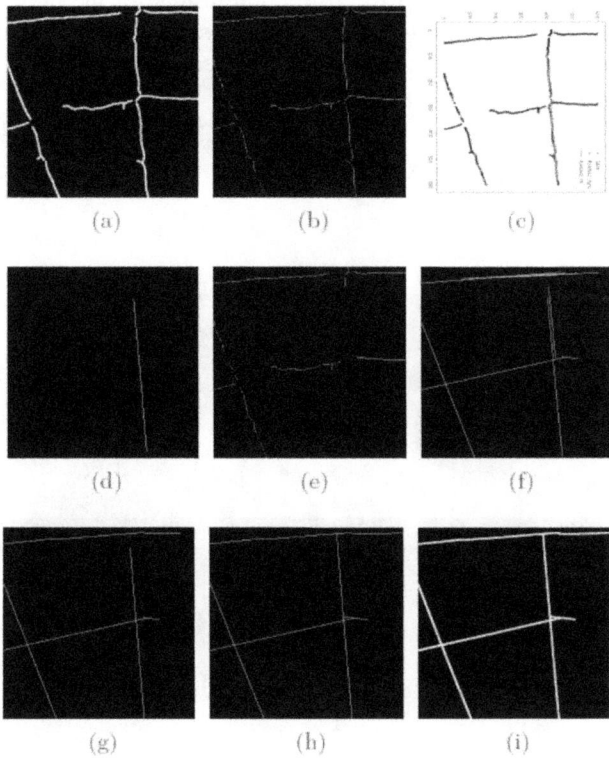

Fig. 6. The results of our DL-RANSAC: a) Filter results of U-Net*. b) Skeleton extraction results. c) RANSAC fitting. d) Fitted line. e) Skeleton after removing fitting results. f) After DL-RANSAC iterative fitting. g) Reconstruction result. h) The result after repairing. i) Final result.

Our fitting results on the sample data are shown in Fig. 6. It can be seen that we perform a route fitting on a binary image with a road skeleton, and the pixels of the fitting will be deleted before the next round of fitting until the final fitting is completed. Compared with the original results, the fitted straight line removed burrs and repaired the disconnection of the intersection to some extent.

3.4 Classification and Reconstruction

It can be seen that in the results of DL-RANSAC, we have multiple straight line fittings on the same road segment at the same time. Therefore, based on the line segment classification rules introduced in the previous section, we further reconstruct the fitting results of DL-RANSAC. It is worth mentioning that, with the help of vector path compression based on Ramer-Douglas-Peucker (RDP) algorithm, we can also repair some small line segments which are disconnected incorrectly.

The segment classification and reconstruction results for the previous picture are shown in Fig. 6. After the classification and reconstruction, the redundant lines of the same road segment disappeared, and the reconstructed road segments also retained the characteristics of the original set of road segments.

3.5 Experiments on the Road Network

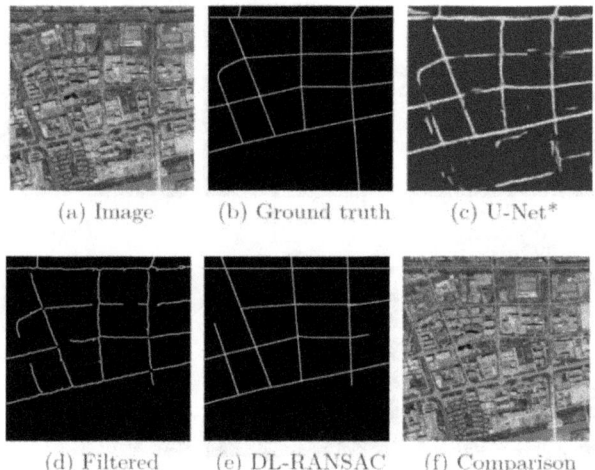

(a) Image (b) Ground truth (c) U-Net*

(d) Filtered (e) DL-RANSAC (f) Comparison

Fig. 7. The results of our approach.

In this set of experiments, we have conducted road network prediction experiments on the large size of maps that we grabbed. Some of the results are shown in Fig. 7. It can be seen that compared to the rough results of the neural network, the vector results fitted by DL-RANSAC look more comfortable, they do not have too much burr effect, and achieve connections for some broken intersections. However, the disadvantage is that due to the uncertainty defect of the RANSAC algorithm itself, a small part of the road network will be lost and the fitting errors will occur. A final road network coverage result is shown in Fig. 8.

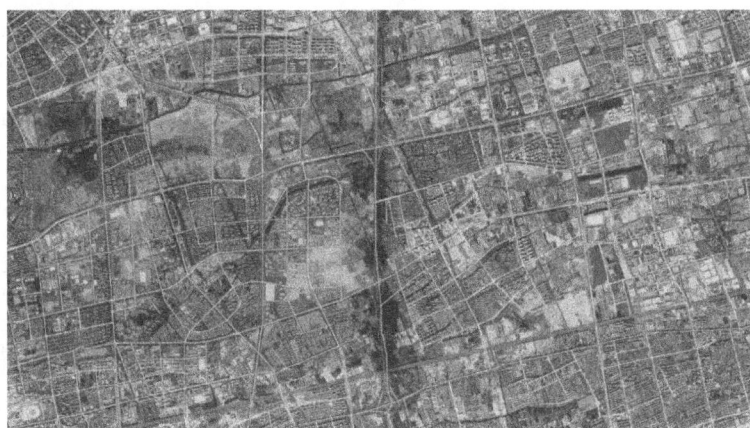

Fig. 8. The result of a road network.

4 Conclusion

In the road network extraction task, the data requirements using traditional mathematical methods are relatively more stringent, and the boundary conditions that need to be considered in a certain scene are also more detailed. For the road network extraction task for urbans, such as Shanghai, the traditional method is difficult.

In this paper, we present an approach for extracting road network from remote sensing images, and also provide the approach for processing the results of image recognition to improve the quality of extracted road network. The experimental results show that our approach can get better results, especially in the settings of an urban.

Acknowledgments. This work was supported in part by the Scientific & Technological Innovation 2030 - "New Generation AI" Key Project (No. 2021ZD0114001; No. 2021ZD0114000), and the Science and Technology Commission of Shanghai Municipality (No. 21511102200). Zhihui Wang is the corresponding author of this work.

References

1. Douglas, D.H., Peucker, T.K.: Algorithms for the reduction of the number of points required to represent a digitized line or its caricature. Cartographica Int. J. Geogr. Inf. Geovisualization **10**(2), 112–122
2. Fischler, M.A., Bolles, R.C.: Random sample consensus: a paradigm for model fitting with applications to image analysis and automated cartography. Commun. ACM **24**(6), 381–395 (1981)
3. He, K., Zhang, X., Ren, S., Sun, J.: Deep residual learning for image recognition. In: Proceedings of the IEEE Conference on Computer Vision and Pattern Recognition, pp. 770–778 (2016)
4. Hilditch, C.J.: Linear skeleton from square cupboards. Mach. Intell. **6**, 403–420 (1969)

5. Long, J., Shelhamer, E., Darrell, T.: Fully convolutional networks for semantic segmentation. In: Proceedings of the IEEE Conference on Computer Vision and Pattern Recognition, pp. 3431–3440 (2015)
6. Miao, Z., Shi, W., Samat, A., Lisini, G., Gamba, P.: Information fusion for urban road extraction from VHR optical satellite images. IEEE J. Sel. Top. Appl. Earth Observations Remote Sens. **9**(5), 1817–1829 (2016)
7. Ramer, U.: An iterative procedure for the polygonal approximation of plane curves. Comput. Graph. Image Process. **1**(3), 244–256 (1972)
8. Ronneberger, O., Fischer, P., Brox, T.: U-Net: convolutional networks for biomedical image segmentation. In: Proceedings of the 18th International Conference on Medical Image Computing and Computer-Assisted Intervention - MICCAI, Part III. Lecture Notes in Computer Science, vol. 9351, pp. 234–241. Springer (2015). https://doi.org/10.1007/978-3-319-24574-4_28
9. Soni, P.K., Rajpal, N., Mehta, R.: A comparison of road network extraction from high resolution images. In: Proceedings of the First International Conference on Secure Cyber Computing and Communication (ICSCCC), pp. 525–531. IEEE (2018)
10. Zhang, T., Suen, C.Y.: A fast parallel algorithm for thinning digital patterns. Commun. ACM **27**(3), 236–239 (1984)

Sparse Point Cloud Upsampling Based on Neural Implicit Functions

Wenjun Wang[1,2], Xiangyu Kong[2], Daole Wang[1,2], and Xiuyang Zhao[2(✉)]

[1] Shandong Provincial Key Laboratory of Network Based Intelligent Computing, University of Jinan, Jinan, China
[2] School of Information Science and Engineering, University of Jinan, Jinan, China
zhaoxy@ujn.edu.cn

Abstract. In this paper, we propose a novel point cloud representation method based on neural implicit functions - spatial fields. This method utilizes neural implicit functions to transform three-dimensional coordinate points into local spatial fields, converting the original "discrete-discrete" point cloud representation into a "discrete-continuous" geometric representation, thereby to obtain continuous point cloud representations and richer geometric detail expression. In this method, each three-dimensional coordinate point in the original sparse point set is transformed into a local spatial field embedding multi-layer neighborhood information by means of implicit functions. Eventually, multiple such local spatial fields are aggregated into a continuous high-resolution spatial field to approximate the object surface as closely as possible. At last, arbitrary-scale sampling can be conducted in the high-resolution spatial field for point cloud densification needs at arbitrary resolutions in downstream applications such as 3D medical image reconstruction and autonomous driving. This paper provides an example to illustrate how to utilize the results of the proposed solution for 3D model reconstruction.

Keywords: Sparse point cloud · neural implicit functions · upsampling · Three-dimensional reconstruction

1 Introduction

As one of the most commonly used 3D data formats, point clouds have extensive applications in various fields such as geometric analysis and autonomous driving. Point clouds can exist with extremely low or high densities and can provide both global shape and refined geometric information of objects. Common 3D scanning devices include LiDAR sensors, depth cameras, and specialized cameras. However, this method is susceptible to the influence of equipment and environment, resulting in sparse, noisy, and unevenly distributed points. The sparsity and non-uniformity of the clouds can adversely affect the performance of downstream tasks, including semantic classification [1], rendering [2], 3D reconstruction [3−5], virtual/augmented reality [6] [7], and autonomous driving [8] [9]. Additionally, point clouds can also be applied in traditional automotive industries, mechanical, or architectural designs. Therefore, converting point clouds into dense, uniform, and clean representations is crucial. The process is known as point cloud upsampling.

The purpose of point cloud upsampling is to increase the density of point cloud data while ensuring that the quality of the object's global shape and geometric details remains intact, thus obtaining a high-resolution regular point cloud. However, increasing the density of points implies adding interpolated information, which can make local edge details handing extremely challenging.

Existing point cloud upsampling methods [10−17] can broadly be divided into two types: optimization-based methods and deep learning-based methods. Optimization-based methods heavily rely on prior knowledge, such as fitting local geometric information. Though the optimization-based methods are demonstrated to have some effectiveness in upsampling smooth surfaces, they often encounter difficulties when dealing with complex corners and edge regions. Learning-based methods break though this limitation by using various networks [18−22] (such as convolutional neural networks and multi-layer perceptrons) to learn multi-scale and multi-feature structures [10−24], thereby significantly improving traditional optimization-based methods. However, the existing methods still face some challenges, such as unevenly distributed dense points generating or certain local edge features neglect, which will leading to a significant decrease in the quality of reconstructed point clouds. Furthermore, the existing methods mostly consider fixed-factor upsampling, such as 4x or 8x. When practical applications require point cloud densification at multiple different scales, training multiple models separately for different scales will results in inefficiency and resource wastage.

NePs [25] introduced a new point cloud representation method to address the upsampling issue with fixed factors, but simply combining the upsampled blocks into a complete point cloud as the prediction result ignores the inconsistency between local patches [27]: Firstly, without global shape information, it is difficult to determine the geometric shape of block boundaries, leading to outliers on dense point clouds. Secondly, combining inconsistent blocks can result in holes or uneven points in the predicted point cloud. This paper extracts multi-dimensional features from a given uneven sparse point set and embeds multi-scale features from the graph structure formed by neighborhood information and the neighborhood information of the neighborhood information, as a supplement to global shape information, to eliminate the problem of outliers in dense point clouds.

Addressing the aforementioned challenges, this paper introduces a novel and powerful point cloud upsampling method. By designing a simple and efficient multi-scale sampling model based on neural implicit functions, it generates accurate and uniformly dense point sets. This model converts sparse point clouds into high-quality dense point sets and can be applied to various downstream tasks such as point cloud object classification and segmentation. Traditional point cloud upsampling methods typically follow three steps: (1) feature extraction, (2) feature expansion, and (3) coordinate reconstruction. The limitation of this approach lies in the fact that, during feature extraction, only the central point and local features are usually considered, neglecting features from local neighborhoods and their adjacent points. Furthermore, during feature expansion, only simple operations like replication and convolution pooling are applied, resulting in unevenly distributed dense point sets often clustering together, making complete coverage of the object surface challenging.

This paper abandons the traditional three-step approach and proposes a point cloud upsampling method based on implicit functions. Specifically, this paper introduces the concept of spatial fields and designs a bidirectional neural implicit function, which achieves a dual mapping between the feature space of sparse point sets and the implicit spatial field, obtaining continuous spatial fields as information about the object surface. To ensure that the spatial fields approximate the object surface, this paper emphasizes the importance of features extracted from sparse point sets. Advanced semantic features and low-dimensional geometric features are extracted from the central points of sparse point sets, embedding local neighborhood features, while ensuring the final features are rich and expressive through the connection of local neighborhood information with different weights. Finally, this paper maps the features obtained from the central points of continuous spatial fields back to sparse point sets, generating dense and uniformly distributed target point sets. By using a comprehensive loss function, this paper ensures that the generated point sets approximate the original point cloud and are evenly distributed on the shape surface.

The contributions of this work can be described as follows:

- This paper introduces a novel point cloud representation method based on neural implicit functions called Spatial Fields. By utilizing neural implicit functions to transform three-dimensional coordinate points into local spatial fields, this method achieves continuous point cloud representation and richer geometric detail expression.
- This paper designs a point cloud upsampling network based on neural implicit functions to apply the proposed point cloud representation method to point cloud densification tasks. It achieves high-precision upsampling at arbitrary scaling factors.
- The method proposed in this paper achieves competitive upsampling results on public datasets, demonstrating its effectiveness in point cloud upsampling tasks.

2 Method

Assuming a sparse and unevenly distributed three-dimensional point cloud X, where N represents the number of points, and each point is associated with three-dimensional coordinates, the network model in this paper undergoes a series of processes to transform it into a dense and uniformly distributed point cloud Y. Additionally, it is expected that this dense point cloud can closely approximate the surface of the three-dimensional object as closely as possible while minimizing noise or outliers. Previous works often directly established a mapping between sparse point clouds and dense point clouds, leading to information overload and reduced accuracy. This paper utilizes a neural implicit function to learn a continuous mapping as shown in Eq. (1), transforming discrete point cloud information into a continuous geometric representation, enhancing the expressive power of the point set while reducing resource wastage caused by excessive storage costs.

$$\mathbf{P} = \{(p_i \in R^6)\}_{i=1}^n \xrightarrow{NIFs} \{p_i^r \in s_i\}_{i,r=1}^{n,R}, \tag{1}$$

where pi represents each point in the point cloud, including the three-dimensional coordinate information of the points.

The point cloud representation method based on neural implicit functions proposed in this paper can transform discrete pi into a continuous spatial field si. Si contains the multi-scale neighborhood information and global shape of pi, representing a continuous geometric surface. By transforming each point in the point set into a spatial field and aggregating them together, a continuous smooth high-resolution spatial field is eventually formed to approximate the object surface as closely as possible, as shown in Eq. (2).

$$S = \bigcup_{i=1}^{n} s_i \xrightarrow{\text{resample}} S' \in S \qquad (2)$$

Subsequently, upsampling at arbitrary resolution factors is performed on the high-resolution spatial field to achieve multi-scale point cloud densification.

Specifically, to generate a more accurate and uniformly dense point set, this paper extracts multi-dimensional features from the given unevenly sparse point set and embeds multi-scale features from neighborhood information and graph structures formed by the neighborhood information of the neighborhood information. Subsequently, a bidirectional mapping from sparse point sets to local spatial fields is established. By learning the final features obtained from the unevenly sparse point set, this paper generates a continuous spatial field in three-dimensional space, aiming to simulate the object's surface as closely as possible. The inverse mapping here maps the spatial field features meeting specific conditions back to the unevenly sparse point set to generate a dense and uniformly distributed point set.

Local Spatial Field: This paper proposes a point set representation based on neural implicit functions. It first assumes that each center point in 3D space can be linearly expressed through its neighboring points. Then, it transforms the three-dimensional coordinate point features in the point set into a latent implicit representation of embedded multi-scale neighborhood features with the three-dimensional coordinate point as the starting point. These latent implicit representations are defined as local spatial fields, as shown in Eq. (3).

$$\mathbf{s} = f_\theta(p_i, c_i, q) \qquad (3)$$

where pi represents any three-dimensional coordinate point in the point set, ci represents the k local neighborhood features of pi, and q is the input sparse point cloud set.

Meanwhile, to improve the accuracy of the spatial field, this paper sets distance constraints to select points with stronger semantic features, as shown in Eq. (4).

$$\mathbf{Dist}(\mathbf{c}_{(x,y,z)}, \mathcal{S}) \in [\mathbf{D}_l, \mathbf{D}_u] \qquad (4)$$

where c represents a point containing three-dimensional coordinate information (x, y, z), s represents the local spatial field centered at c, Dl and Du represent the lower and upper distance limits set in this paper, respectively.

Since it is not possible to calculate the distance from a three-dimensional coordinate point to an unknown local spatial field, this paper divides the input sparse point cloud into multiple overlapping patches centered at three-dimensional coordinate points. Three points are randomly selected within each patch to form a three-dimensional local surface, and the distance from the center point to the three-dimensional local surface is defined as the distance from the three-dimensional coordinate point to the unknown local spatial field.

The points that meet the distance constraints are selected and transformed into local spatial fields, as illustrated in Fig. 1.

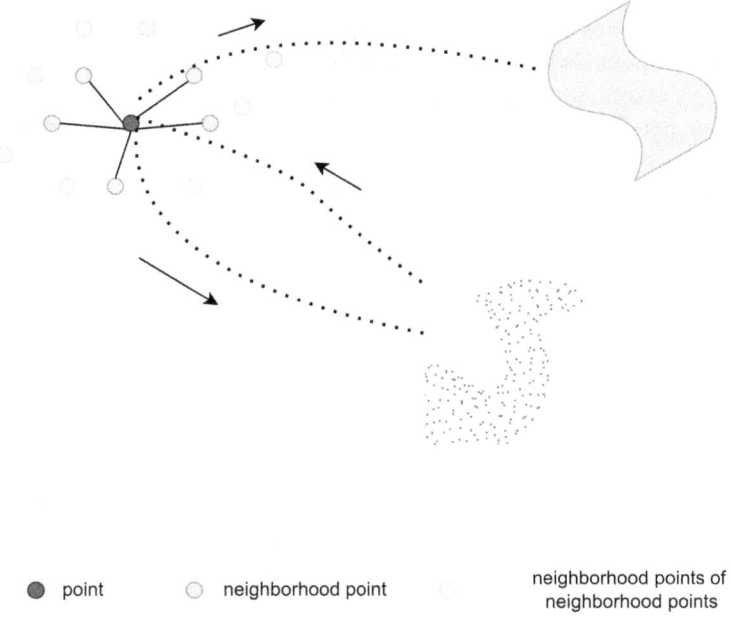

● point   ○ neighborhood point   neighborhood points of neighborhood points

Fig. 1. Local spatial field structure diagram.

The ultimate goal of point cloud upsampling is to obtain a densely distributed point set that uniformly covers the surface of an object. However, directly solving for the surface is a challenging task. Local spatial fields extend the representation range of point sets, enhance semantic features, and represent part of the object surface information composed of new points that do not exist in the sparse point set. When aggregated together, sufficiently large local spatial fields can be regarded as the object surface.

Surface Reconstruction: The method proposed in this paper based on neural implicit functions transforms each three-dimensional coordinate point in the sparse point cloud into a continuous local spatial field. By aggregating all local spatial fields, a sufficiently large continuous high-resolution spatial field is generated to simulate the object surface, thus achieving point cloud densification at arbitrary sampling factors. However, since different local spatial fields are based on different coordinate systems, this paper calculates a weight based on the features of the three-dimensional coordinate point and its neighborhood points. Continuous high-resolution spatial field generation is achieved through weighted aggregation of multiple local spatial fields, as shown in Eqs. (5) and (6).

$$w_k = e^{-\alpha_1 |x-x_k|_2^2}, \forall k \in N(x) \tag{5}$$

$$S = \left(\sum w_j \cdot s_j\right) / \left(\sum w_j\right) \tag{6}$$

The next step is the design of the network architecture.

Network Architecture Design: In the feature extraction stage, given the input sparse point cloud, this paper designs feature extraction modules at different levels. Lower-level network modules extract local features of points, while higher-level network modules capture global features of points. Finally, these features are aggregated to form multi-level features of points with stronger expressiveness. Specifically, for each point in the sparse point cloud, this paper utilizes the state-of-the-art method DGCNN to extract K multi-scale neighborhood features of the three-dimensional coordinate point. Subsequently, after passing through a max-pooling layer, the final features used for embedding in the dual mapping layer are obtained, as shown in Fig. 2.

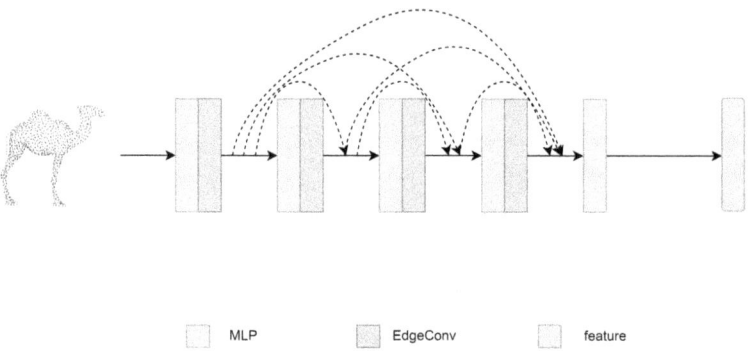

Fig. 2. Feature extraction architecture.

The generation of local spatial fields relies on the design of the bidirectional implicit functions. Here, this paper adopts an encoder-decoder approach. Points in the sparse point cloud act as center points, while random points in the spatial field are selected as query points. Local features, center points, and query points are concatenated as inputs to the implicit function. Through multiple blocks consisting of MLP layers, normalization layers, and ReLU activation layers, the final output forms the continuous high-resolution spatial field. Points features obtained through arbitrary sampling in the continuous high-resolution spatial field are mapped back to three-dimensional coordinate space to generate a densified point set with the desired sampling factor. The overall architecture is shown in Fig. 3.

Loss Function: To ensure that the generated dense point set is more evenly distributed on the object surface, this paper utilizes Chamfer Distance (CD) as shown in Eq. (7).

$$d_{\text{CD}}(S_1, S_2) = \frac{1}{S_1} \sum_{x \in S_1} \min_{y \in S_2} |x - y|_2^2 + \frac{1}{S_2} \sum_{x \in S_2} \min_{y \in S_1} |y - x|_2^2 \tag{7}$$

Hausdorff Distance (HD) as shown in Eq. (8).

$$d_{HD}(S_1, S_2) = max(h(S_1, S_2), h(S_2, S_1)) \tag{8}$$

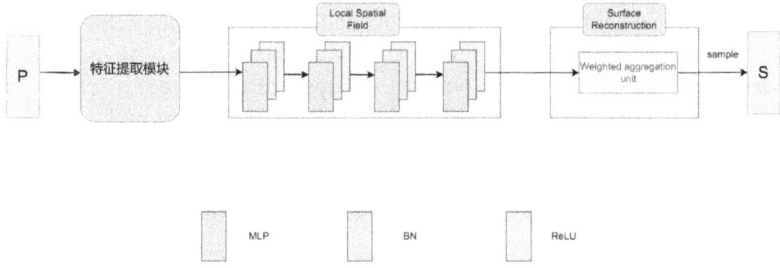

Fig. 3. Overall architecture.

and Point-to-Plane Distance (P2F) as shown in Eq. (9) to evaluate the reconstruction error between the generated point set S1 and the ground truth point set S2.

$$d_{P2F}(S_1, \beta) = \frac{1}{|S_1|} \sum_{x \in S_1} d(x, \beta) \tag{9}$$

3 Experiments

Dataset: This paper utilizes the PU-GAN dataset, which consists of 147 3D models of various shapes collected from the PU-Net, MPU dataset, and Visionair library. The dataset includes a diverse range of representative 3D models, such as smooth models like polyhedrons and models with complex and intricate details like sculptures. This enhances the robustness of the experiments conducted in this paper. 120 point cloud models were randomly selected for training, while the remaining were used for testing. From each training point cloud, 200 patches were randomly cropped, resulting in 24,000 patches used for training.

Training Details: To enhance the robustness of the network, this paper applies rotation, scaling, and Gaussian noise perturbation to the input point sets. In all experiments conducted on the PyTorch platform, the training duration was set to 200 epochs, the batch size was 64, the initial learning rate of the Adam optimizer was 0.0001, with a decay rate of 0.9.

Evaluation Metrics: This paper adopts Chamfer Distance (CD), Hausdorff Distance (HD), and Point-to-Plane Distance (P2F) as evaluation metrics. For all metrics, smaller values indicate better result quality.

Results and Comparison: We conducted comparisons of our proposed method with PU-Net, MPU, PU-GAN, PU-GCN, PU-EVA, and APU. Training was carried out separately at 4x and 16x to ensure fairness, maintaining identical batch sizes, iteration counts, and learning rates. The comparative results are as follows:

(1) Upsampling evaluation metrics on the PU-GAN dataset are presented in Table 1.
(2) Specific metric changes in terms of CD and HD are illustrated in Fig. 4.
(3) Visualization of large-scale sampling factors is shown in Fig. 5.
(4) Visual comparisons with baseline experiments on the PU-GAN dataset are depicted in Fig. 6.

Our method consistently demonstrates outstanding performance across all scenarios. Additionally, Fig. 7 showcases a reconstruction example designed by us, including the input sparse point cloud, the dense point cloud upsampled using our method, and the three-dimensional model reconstructed using Poisson reconstruction.

Ablation Study: We conducted ablation experiments by removing the CD loss, removing the HD loss, and replacing the final features extracted from local spatial fields with features extracted by PointNet to verify the effectiveness of the method. Specific results are shown in Table 2.

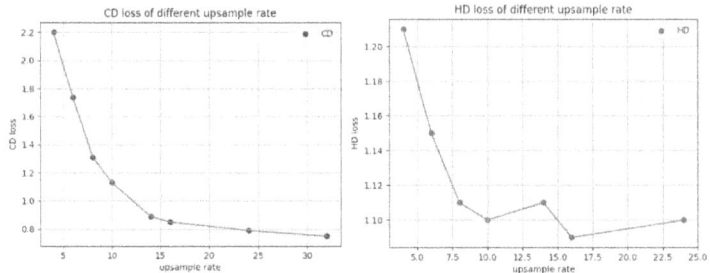

Fig. 4. CD and HD of differents upsample rate.

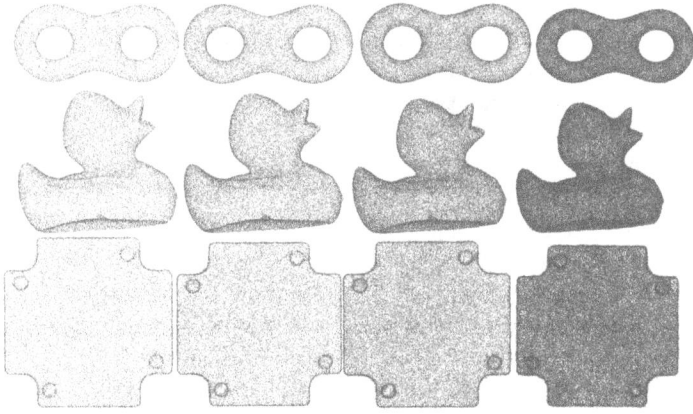

Fig. 5. Results of upsampling with a large scaling factor. From left to right, they are 8x upsampling, 16x upsampling, 32x upsampling, and 256x upsampling.

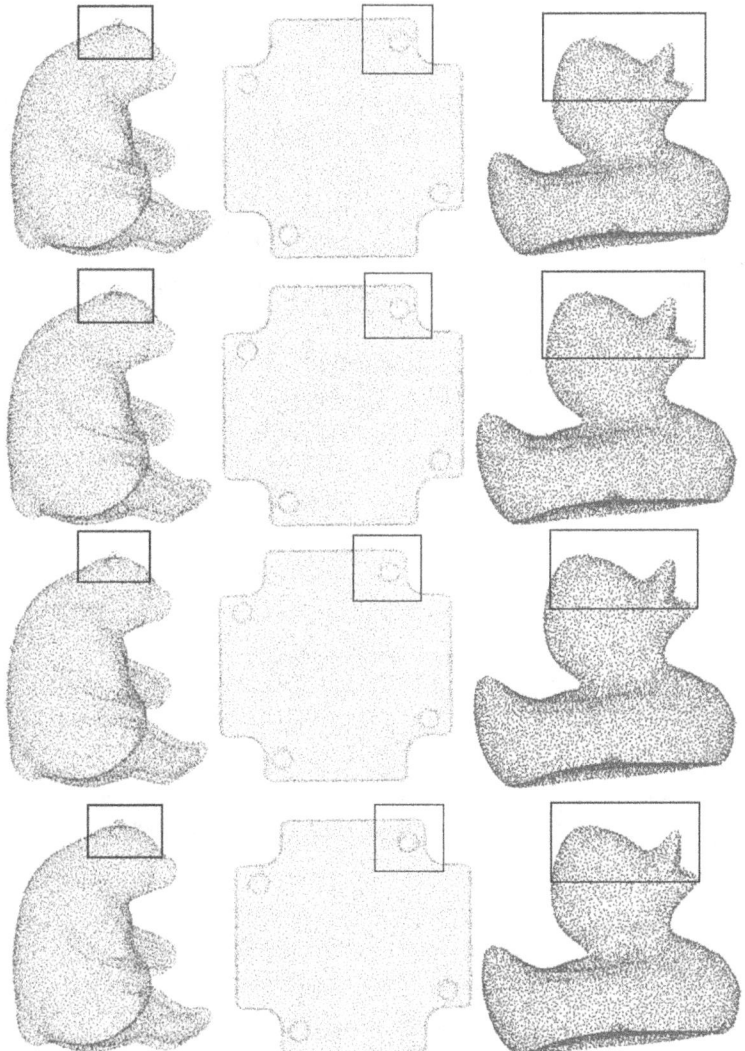

Fig. 6. Visualizing Experimental Results Comparison,The images from top to bottom are: PU-GCN, PU-EVA, APU and ours.

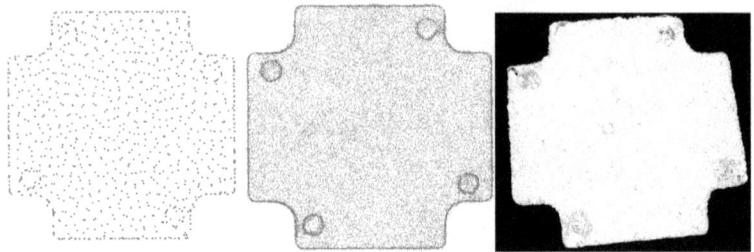

Fig. 7. One downstream application - Example of three-dimensional econstruction.

Table 1. Results and comparisons for 4 ×, 8 ×, and 16 × upsampling on PU-GAN dataset with supervised training.

Method	CD(r = 4) ↓	HD(r = 4)↓	P2F(r = 4) ↓	CD(r = 8) ↓	HD(r = 8)↓	P2F(r = 8) ↓	CD(r = 16) ↓	HD(r = 16)↓	P2F(r = 16) ↓
PU-Net[16]	4.04	3.53	12.74	3.97	3.26	9.92	3.98	3.03	8.92
MPU[14]	2.26	1.9	8.02	1.42	2.45	8.04	0.95	2.41	7.26
PU-GAN[10]	2.25	2.08	7.87	1.35	1.62	7.4	0.88	1.58	6.65
PU-GCN[24]	2.22	1.28	7.64	1.34	**1.11**	7.25	0.87	1.12	6.50
PU-EVA[12]	2.27	2.93	7.78	1.36	3.09	6.53	0.93	3.50	6.39
APU[26]	2.36	2.17	9.03	1.39	1.61	7.27	0.89	2.07	6.47
NePs[25]	2.49	2.39	**7.32**	1.52	2.31	7.14	0.94	2.43	6.52
Ours	**2.2**	**1.21**	**7.32**	**1.31**	**1.11**	**6.29**	**0.85**	**1.09**	**6.37**

Table 2. Results of the ablation study on PU-GAN dataset.

	CD↓	HD↓	P2F↓
w/o Lcd	2.37	1.42	8.68
w/o Lhd	2.25	1.81	7.94
w/o Fields	2.39	2.01	7.71
ours	**2.20**	**1.21**	**7.32**

4 Conclusion

This paper presents an innovative strategy for point cloud upsampling leveraging neural implicit functions, which possess the flexibility to handle arbitrary scaling factors. The methodology involves establishing bidirectional implicit functions that establish connections between the feature space and the implicit surface. This allows for the extraction of both high-level semantic features and low-dimensional geometric features from central points. Moreover, the process entails aggregating local spatial fields generated by each three-dimensional coordinate point, resulting in the derivation of a continuous and highly precise implicit spatial field of latent features.

Through random sampling within this spatial field, the method achieves point cloud densification across a spectrum of scaling factors. Experimental results provide compelling evidence of the robustness and generalization capabilities of our proposed approach. Consequently, our method emerges as a competitive alternative to existing state-of-the-art upsampling techniques.

References

1. Xiang, T., et al.: Walk in the cloud: Learning curves for point clouds shape analysis. In: Proceedings of the IEEE/CVF International Conference on Computer Vision, pp. 915–924 (2021)
2. Dai, P., et al.: Neural point cloud rendering via multi-plane projection. In: Proceedings of the IEEE/CVF Conference on Computer Vision and Pattern Recognition, pp. 7830–7839 (2020)
3. Hoppe, H., et al.: Surface reconstruction from unorganized points. Proceedings of the 19th Annual Conference on Computer Graphics and Interactive Techniques, pp. 71–78 (1992)
4. Kazhdan, M., Hoppe, H.: Screened poisson surface reconstruction[J]. ACM Trans. Graph. (ToG) **32**(3), 1–13 (2013)
5. Newcombe, R.A., et al.: Kinectfusion: real-time dense surface mapping and tracking. In: 2011 10th IEEE International Symposium on Mixed and Augmented Reality, pp. 127–136. IEEE (2011)
6. Held, R., et al.: 3D puppetry: a kinect-based interface for 3D animation. UIST. **12**, 423–434 (2012)
7. Santana, J.M., Wendel, J., Trujillo, A., et al.: Multimodal location based services—semantic 3D city data as virtual and augmented reality[C]//Progress in location-based services. Springer International Publishing **2017**, 329–353 (2016)
8. Lang, A.H., et al.: Pointpillars: fast encoders for object detection from point clouds. In: Proceedings of the IEEE/CVF Conference on Computer Vision and Pattern Recognition, pp. 12697–12705 (2019)
9. Wang, Y., et al.: Pseudo-lidar from visual depth estimation: Bridging the gap in 3D object detection for autonomous driving. In: Proceedings of the IEEE/CVF Conference on Computer Vision and Pattern Recognition, pp. 8445–8453 (2019)
10. Li, R., et al.: Pu-gan: a point cloud upsampling adversarial network. In: Proceedings of the IEEE/CVF International Conference on Computer Vision, pp. 7203–7212 (2019)
11. Li, R., et al.: Point cloud upsampling via disentangled refinement. In: Proceedings of the IEEE/CVF Conference on Computer Vision and Pattern Recognition, pp. 344–353 (2021)
12. Luo, L., et al.: Pu-eva: an edge-vector based approximation solution for flexible-scale point cloud upsampling. In: Proceedings of the IEEE/CVF International Conference on Computer Vision, pp. 16208–16217 (2021)
13. Qian, Y., Hou, J., Kwong, S., et al.: Deep magnification-flexible upsampling over 3d point clouds [J]. IEEE Trans. Image Process. **30**, 8354–8367 (2021)
14. Yifan, W., et al.: Patch-based progressive 3D point set upsampling. In: Proceedings of the IEEE/CVF Conference on Computer Vision and Pattern Recognition, pp. 5958–5967 (2019)
15. Ye, S., Chen, D., Han, S., et al.: Meta-PU: An arbitrary-scale upsampling network for point cloud [J]. IEEE Trans. Visual Comput. Graphics **28**(9), 3206–3218 (2021)

16. Yu, L., et al.: Pu-net: Point cloud upsampling network. In: Proceedings of the IEEE Conference on Computer Vision and Pattern Recognition, pp. 2790–2799 (2018)
17. Zhao, Y., Hui, L., Xie, J.: Sspu-net: Self-supervised point cloud upsampling via differentiable rendering. In: Proceedings of the 29th ACM International Conference on Multimedia, pp. 2214–2223 (2021)
18. Li, Y., et al.: Pointcnn: convolution on x-transformed points [J]. Adv. Neural Inf. Process. Syst. **31** (2018)
19. Wu, W., Qi, Z., Fuxin, L.: Pointconv: deep convolutional networks on 3D point clouds.In: Proceedings of the IEEE/CVF Conference on computer vision and pattern recognition, pp. 9621–9630 (2019)
20. Liu, Y., et al.: Relation-shape convolutional neural network for point cloud analysis. Proceedings of the IEEE/CVF Conference on Computer Vision and Pattern Recognition, pp. 8895–8904 (2019)
21. Maturana, D., Scherer, S.: Voxnet: a 3D convolutional neural network for real-time object recognition. In: 2015 IEEE/RSJ International Conference on Intelligent Robots and Systems (IROS), pp. 922–928. IEEE (2015)
22. Riegler, G., Osman Ulusoy, A., Geiger, A.: Octnet: learning deep 3D representations at high resolutions. In: Proceedings of the IEEE Conference on Computer Vision and Pattern Recognition, pp. 3577–3586 (2017)
23. Long, C., et al.: Pc2-pu: patch correlation and point correlation for effective point cloud upsampling. In: Proceedings of the 30th ACM International Conference on Multimedia, pp. 2191–2201 (2022)
24. Qian, G., et al.: Pu-gcn: point cloud upsampling using graph convolutional networks. In: Proceedings of the IEEE/CVF Conference on Computer Vision and Pattern Recognition, pp. 11683–11692 (2021)
25. Feng, W., et al.: Neural points: point cloud representation with neural fields for arbitrary upsampling. Proceedings of the IEEE/CVF Conference on Computer Vision and Pattern Recognition, pp. 18633–18642 (2022)
26. Dell'Eva, A., Orsingher, M., Bertozzi, M.: Arbitrary point cloud upsampling with spherical mixture of gaussians. In:2022 International Conference on 3D Vision (3DV), pp. 465–474 IEEE (2022)
27. He, Y., et al.: Grad-pu: arbitrary-scale point cloud upsampling via gradient descent with learned distance functions. Proceedings of the IEEE/CVF Conference on Computer Vision and Pattern Recognition, pp. 5354–5363 (2023)

Adaptive Non-local Means Filter Based on Multi-kernel for Complicated Noise

Qian long[1], Hongwei Qu[3(✉)], Yiping Wang[1], Gaihua Wang[1,2(✉)], and Bolun Zhu[1]

[1] College of Artificial Intelligence, Tianjin University of Science & Technology, Tianjin 300457, China
{longqian,wanggh}@tust.edu.cn
[2] Hubei Key Laboratory of Optical Information and Pattern Recognition, Wuhan Institute of Technology, Wuhan 430205, China
[3] Wuhan Electronic Information Institute, Wuhan 430019, China
394139525@qq.com

Abstract. In the paper, we propose a modified denoising filter based on multi-kernel for color images. To compare the similarity of patches, the patch standard deviation is taken to discriminate flat area and edges, which can capture local geometric structures. It gets rid of the effect of highly dissimilar image patches by setting the weights to zero. Then, we add multi-kernel weights to denoising filter. Different kernel parameters are used to remove complicated noise. The experimental results show that the proposed method has superior performance to existing approaches in terms of noise suppression and detail preservation, especially for the case of low signal-to-noise ratio (SNR). As our future research work, we intend to apply the method to speech and other intelligent recognition system.

Keywords: Non-local means · Multi-kernel · Gaussian noise · Adaptive filter

1 Introduction

Images are often corrupted by all kinds of noise. To remove noise and preserve the fine structures and textures, many approaches have been proposed, such as the total variation filter [1–3] and the wavelet filter [4]. However, these methods cannot be extended to color images. The vector median filter is a kind of traditional effective vector filter, which is used widely [5–7] to remove impulse noise. They have been developed with switching schemes [8–10] and detectors [11]. However, the effect is dropped dramatically with Gaussian noise.

Non-local means (NLM) [12], which operates on a non-local area, has attracted significant interest. Under the conditions of Gaussian noise contamination, the NLM filters outperform other classic filters. In [13, 14], it is an adaptive median filter based on NLM, which uses the piecewise function to compute weight. The paper [15] proposes modified NLM, which is based on unweighted Euclidean distance and integral image method, to denoise gravity datasets. The paper [16] makes full use of redundant texture and self-similarity of multidimensional data, which can obtain the estimated denoising result by the weighted average of pixels with similar neighborhood structures.

Above all these denoising methods can not consider texture feature effectively. When confronting with different level noise, the robust of these methods is worse. In this paper, we propose multi-kernel method to modify the NLM. First, we take a patch standard deviation to discriminate texture feature, and add weight strategic of similarity measure. Then we use the multi-kernel methods to remove the wide level noises. The proposed method is shown to have better performance than some popular methods through experiments.

2 Methodology

2.1 The Weight

For the NLM, weights of candidate patch are assigned solely based on similar measure between pixels, which may cause loss of fine structures and edge blurring. For example, suppose Fig. 1 (a) and (b) are neighbor patch window, and Fig. 1 (c) is central patch window. If only intensity similarity between corresponding pixels is considered, Fig. 1 (a) and (b) patch window have same weight for the NLM. But, in fact, Fig. 1 (a) has more similar property to Fig. 1 (c), and tends to edge area. To use local and non-local information, we add texture information to compare the similarity of patch image.

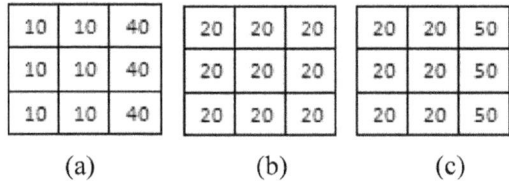

Fig. 1. The similarity properties of different patch windows

Given a patch standard deviation D. It is defined as.

$$D = \frac{1}{\sqrt{3}S} \sum_{s=0}^{S=1} \|f_p(x, y) - g_p\|_2 \tag{1}$$

Where g_p is the average of patch window, $f_p(x, y)$ is each pixel of patch window. It follows that the new weight of the NLM is.

$$w_0(x, y, x_0, y_0) = \exp\left(-\frac{(D_{x,y} - D_{x_0,y_0})^2}{h_3}\right) \tag{2}$$

where h_3 is a new parameter controlling the smooth degree.

Given thresholds T_1 and T_2, based on the idea of the paper [17], we are still setting the weights to zero when the Euclidean distances are quite large. It is expressed by.

$$w_0(x, y, x_0, y_0) = \begin{cases} 0, \text{IF } \sum_{s_1,s_2 \in S} \|f_p(x+s_1, y+s_2) - f_p(x_0+s_1, y_0+s_2)\|_2 \geq T_1 \text{ and } (D_{x,y} - D_{x_0,y_0})^2 \geq T_2 \\ w_0(x, y, x_0, y_0), \text{ otherwise} \end{cases} \quad (3)$$

It reflects the dissimilar properties from two parts, dissimilar properties between pixels and dissimilar properties on texture.

2.2 Multi-kernel NLM

To compensate the weakness of the NLM in removing the complicated noises, we use multi-kernel filter based on the GNLMKIM [20]. The similarity between two image patches $f_p(x+s_1, y+s_2)$ and $f_p(x_0+s_1, y_0+s_2)$ is expressed by.

$$K_i = \exp\left(\frac{\sum_{s_1,s_2 \in S} \|f_p(x+s_1, y+s_2) - f_p(x_0+s_1, y_0+s_2)\|_{2,\alpha}^2}{h_i^2}\right) \quad (4)$$

where h_i are the kernel parameter ($h_1, h_2 \in h_i$). We modify the weight of the NLM by.

$$w_0(x, y, x_0, y_0) = \sum_{t=1}^{2} \widehat{\lambda}_t K_t + w_0(x, y, x_0, y_0) \quad (5)$$

where $\widehat{\lambda}_t$ is the parameter of penalty, computed as.

$$\widehat{\lambda}_t = \frac{\exp\left(\frac{1}{P} \sum_{i \in S} \sum_{j \in N} \sum K_t(X_i, X_j)\right)}{\exp\left(\frac{1}{P}\right)\left(\sum_{i \in S} \sum_{j \in N} \sum K_t(X_i, X_j)\right)} \quad (6)$$

where P is a non-negative parameter controlling the degree of penalty for the $\widehat{\lambda}_t$. The new filtering output is expressed by.

$$g_p(x_0, y_0) = \frac{1}{\sum_{j \in N} w(x, y, x_0, y_0)} \sum_{j \in N} w(x, y, x_0, y_0) f_p(x, y) \quad (7)$$

We set $h_1 = 10$, $h_2 = 15$, $h_3 = 50$. . The proposed modified non-local means based on multi-kernel (MKNLM) algorithm is described as follows.

Input: The noisy image $f_p(x,y)$, with size of $H \times W \times 3$ Output: The restored image $g_p(x,y)$
1: Initialize (searching window) $N = 7 \times 7$, (patch window) $S = 3 \times 3$, $h_1 = 10$, $h_2 = 15$, $h_3 = 50$ 2: $D = \dfrac{1}{\sqrt{3}s} \sum_{s=0}^{S-1} \|f_p(x,y) - g_p\|_2 f_p(x,y) \in PatchWindow$ (Compute the standard deviation of each patch window).   3: for $x = 1$ to H; $y = 1$ to W 4:   for Searching window $n = 1$ to N 5:   for Patch Window $s = 1$ to S 6:   Use (4) to compute K_i 7:   Use (6) to compute $\hat{\lambda}_t$ 8:   end for   9:   Compute w_0, $w(x,y,x_0,y_0)$ according to (3) and (5)   10: end for   11: Use (7) to get the filtering value $g_p(x,y)$ of position (x_0, y_0) 12: end for   Output: The restored image $g_p(x,y)$

3 Experiments and Results

3.1 Quantitative Comparison

To compare the performance of the proposed algorithm, the experiments are tested. The execution time (in seconds) running on a desktop PC with 2.50GHz CPU and 4.0G RAM is measured.

We also give a quantitative comparison between the pro-posed algorithm and the recently methods through Peak Signal-to-Noise Ratio (PSNR), normalized mean square error (NMSE), mean squared error (MSE) and structural similarity (SSIM). The MSE and NMSE are represented in pixels, and PSNR is represented in decibels (dB). In this experiment, the public color images are from Matlab 7.0 and the database "google thing". We use the "image1" with 203 × 162 and "image2" with 150 × 150 in "google_things" (Fig. 2).

The results of performance are shown in Tables 1–2, the color images are degraded by Gaussian noise with zero means and different deviation. As is shown in Tables 1–2, the proposed method outperforms NLM, Bilateral Filter (BILF), FDNLM and GNLMKIM. The BILF is a non-linear filter. In Table 1, the variance of Gaussian noise ranges from 0.01 to 0.05. Our method did not experience a significant decline. For variance 0.05, the PSNR is 24.0002. The performance of BILF is worst. For the NLM and GNLMKIM,

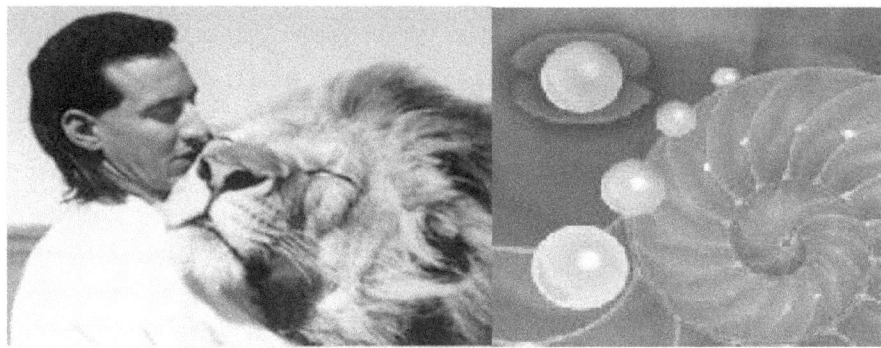

Fig.2. The original images: (a) "image1" (b) "image2"

they are effective at low noise level. When the variance is 0.05, the PSNR of NLM and GNLMKIM are 23.1770 and 23.1710. The FDNLM is mainly to denoise impulse noise and mixture noise. For Gaussian noise, the FDNLM is not better than the NLM.

3.2 Discussion

From experimental results, the NLM performs better than the BILF when the level of Gaussian noise increases. The FDNLM, GNLMKIM and the proposed method are modified methods based on the NLM. The GNLMKIM is a multi-kernel method that is more robust and effective in tackling complex problems than single-kernel ones. From Fig. 3, when the density of Gaussian noise increases from 0.01 to 0.03, the NLM has a better performance than BILF.

From Fig. 3, we can see that the similar neighbors in patch image are well identified and the weights are good enough to average the central pixel at low noise levels. The NLM and GNLMKIM can remove the low-level noise effectively. When noise is higher, the proposed method is best. Especially, the "image 1" in Fig. 3, when the noise level is higher, the performance of the proposed method doesn't drop dramatically. The robust of the proposed method is better.

Figure 4 shows the filtering outputs from "image1". Gaussian noise is added with mean of 0 and variance of 0.05. When the size of searching window is increasing, the blurring become more severe and the computational time is also increasing. For NLM, GNLMKIM and the proposed method, the size of the searching window is set to 7×7. And the size of the patch window is 3×3. For BILF, the filtering window is 3×3. For the FDNLM, the size of the searching window is 5×5 and the size of the patch window is 3×3. By comparing the result, it is obvious that the result of the BILF is bad, and the FDNLM is not effective to denoise Gaussian noise. The NLM, GNLMKIM and the proposed method have better results.

Table 1. Performance Comparison for the "image1" with different Gaussian noise

Noise Algorithms	Gaussian noise of mean 0 and variance 0.01					Gaussian noise of mean 0 and variance 0.02				
	PSNR	NMSE	MSE	SSIM	Time(s)	PSNR	NMSE	MSE	SSIM	Time(s)
NLM	25.4301	0.0066	186.2408	0.7379	11.45593	25.0926	0.0072	201.2910	0.7368	13.521567
BILF	22.0681	0.0144	403.8954	0.5841	**9.093267**	21.4976	0.0164	460.5993	0.5475	11.189882
FDNLM	24.3697	0.0085	237.7469	0.7228	12.86418	23.6930	0.0099	277.8306	0.6853	12.655751
GNLMKIM	25.4248	0.0066	186.4654	0.7437	9.956551	25.0819	0.0072	201.7876	0.7425	**10.474830**
MKNLM	**25.6321**	**0.0056**	**180.2258**	**0.7683**	11.73104	**25.3421**	**0.0062**	**190.1203**	**0.7522**	12.494737

Noise Algorithms	Gaussian noise of mean 0 and variance 0.03					Gaussian noise of mean 0 and variance 0.05				
	PSNR	NMSE	MSE	SSIM	Time(s)	PSNR	NMSE	MSE	SSIM	Time(s)
NLM	24.4861	0.0082	231.4592	0.7351	11.27403	23.1770	0.0111	312.8854	0.7306	11.523196
BILF	21.0864	0.0180 lePara>	506.3385	0.5135	22.03590	20.5120	0.0206	577.9309	0.4710	**8.9323334**
FDNLM	23.1144	0.0113	317.4252	0.6595	12.79744	22.0551	0.0144	404.1034	0.6019	13.178568
GNLMKIM	24.5859	0.0080	226.1989	0.7353	**9.709179**	23.1710	0.0111	313.3157	0.7341	10.110937
MKNLM	**25.0205**	**0.0070**	**217.8053**	**0.7517**	11.45487	**24.0020**	**0.0100**	**283.6257**	**0.7414**	11.873625

Table 2. Performance Comparison for the "image2" with different Gaussian noise

Noise Algorithms	Gaussian noise of mean 0 and variance 0.01					Gaussian noise of mean 0 and variance 0.02				
	PSNR	NMSE	MSE	SSIM	Time(s)	PSNR	NMSE	MSE	SSIM	Time(s)
NLM	27.1190	0.0078	126.2339	0.6890	7.65134	26.5247	0.0090	144.7470	0.6888	7.457209
BILF	24.8563	0.0132	212.5427	0.5849	**5.98015**	24.0521	0.0159	255.7824	0.5313	**6.011340**
FDNLM	26.8471	0.0083	134.3896	0.7060	8.72527	25.8025	0.0106	170.9352	0.6601	8.717982
GNLMKIM	27.1337	0.0078	125.8080	0.6863	6.56518	26.5494	0.0089	143.9279	0.6844	6.457455
MKNLM	**27.2863**	**0.0075**	**121.4639**	0.5970	7.69934	**26.6182**	**0.0088**	**141.6640**	**0.6897**	7.644170
Noise Algorithms	Gaussian noise of mean 0 and variance 0.03					Gaussian noise of mean 0 and variance 0.05				
	PSNR	NMSE	MSE	SSIM	Time(s)	PSNR	NMSE	MSE	SSIM	Time(s)
NLM	25.7482	0.0107	173.0848	0.6845	7.877205	23.7396	0.0171	274.8686	0.6839	7.608955
BILF	23.4217	0.0184	295.7384	0.4884	**6.149082**	22.5805	0.0223	358.9439	0.4308	**5.836560**
FDNLM	25.0970	0.0125	201.0842	0.6263	8.95965	23.3919	0.0185	297.7750	0.5386	8.592263
GNLMKIM	25.6979	0.0109	175.1037	0.6880	6.86835	23.7678	0.0169	273.0866	0.6786	6.588775
MKNLM	**25.8179**	**0.0106**	**170.3281**	**0.6935**	8.90800	**23.9617**	**0.0160**	**263.2485**	**0.6907**	7.589522

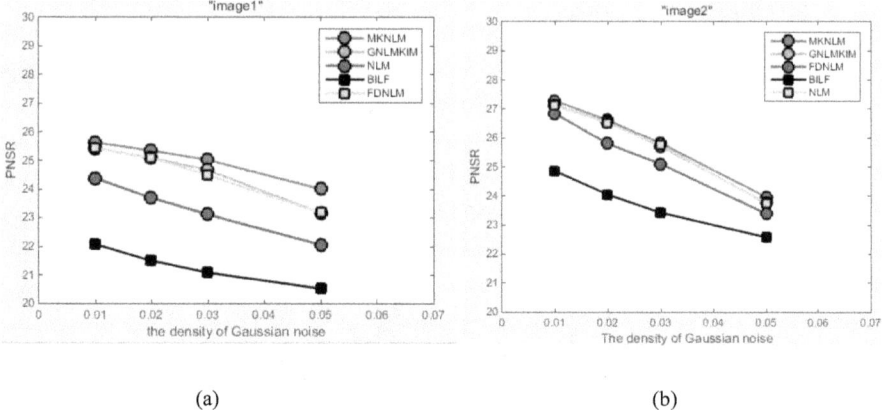

(a)   (b)

Fig.3. The results in PSNR (dB) from the different filters applied to the images: (a) PSNR for the "image1" (b) PSNR for the "image2"

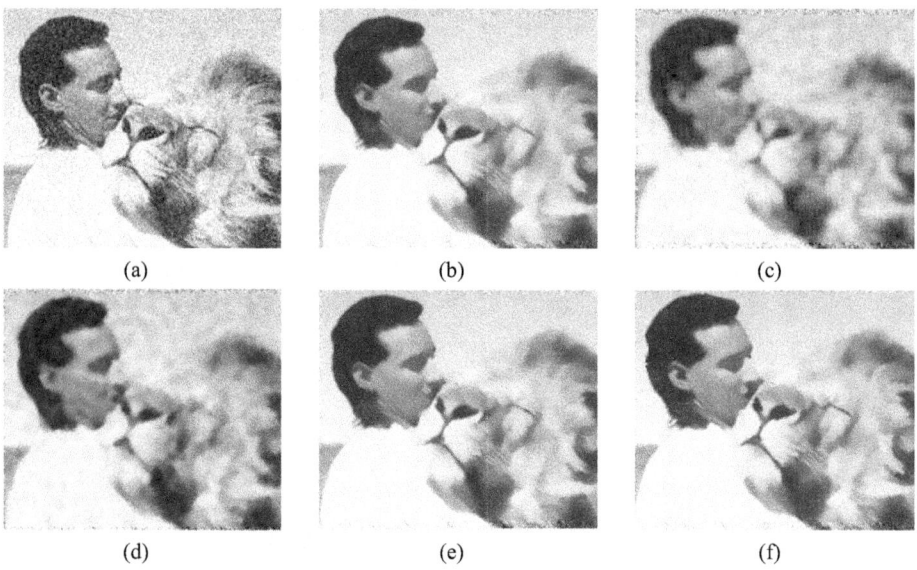

Fig.4. The output of "image1": (a) the "image1" with Gaussian noise of 0.05 variance (b) the output of NLM (c) the output of BILF (d) the output of FDNLM (e) the output of GNLMKIM (f) the output of the proposed algorithm

4 Conclusions

In this paper, we proposed a modified non-local means based on multi-kernel (MKNLM) filter for color image. Constructed by two individual kernel members, the multi-kernel methods can remove noises effectively. It calculates a weight by adding texture feature. And when the neighbor pixel is dissimilarity, the weight is set to zero. The proposed filter can remove Gaussian noise and preserve the image details effectively. Experimental results indicate that the proposed method has superior denoising performance to some classic filters. However, our method mainly aims to Gaussian noise. In the next work, we will further develop it to remove mixed noise and study its performance on real images.

Acknowledgments. This work is supported by the Open Foundation Project of Hubei Key Laboratory of Optical Information and Pattern Recognition, Wuhan Institute of Technology (grant No. 202306).

References

1. Srivastava, R., Gupta, J., Parthasarthy, H.: Comparison of PDE based and other techniques for speckle reduction from digitally reconstructed holographic images. Opt. Lasers Eng. **48**, 626–635 (2010)
2. Shih, Y., Rei, C., Wang, H.: A novel PDE based image restoration: convection diffusion equation for image denoising. J. Comput. Appl. Math. **231**, 771–779 (2009)
3. Liu, M., Vemuri, B.C., Deriche, R.: A robust variational approach for simultaneous smoothing and estimation of DTI. Neuro. Image **67**, 33–41 (2013)
4. Nowak, R.D.: Wavelet-based Rician noise removal for magnetic resonance imaging. IEEE Trans. Image Process. **10**(8), 1408–1419 (1999)
5. Astola, J., Haavisto, P., Neuvo, Y.: Vector median filters. Proc. IEEE **78**(4), 678–689 (1990)
6. Jin, L., Xiong, C., Li, D.: Adaptive center-weighted median filter. J. Huazhong Univ. Sci. Technol. **36**(8), 9–12 (2008)
7. Kang, C., Wang, W.: Fuzzy reasoning-based directional median filter design. Signal Process. **89**, 344–351 (2009)
8. Wang, G., et al.: Modified switching median filter for impulse noise removal. Signal Process. **90**(5), 3213–3218 (2010)
9. Chou, H., Hsu, L.: A noise-ranking switching filter for images with general fixed-value impulse noises. Signal Process. **106**, 198–208 (2015)
10. Wang, G., Liu, Y., Zhao, T.: Quaternion switching filter for suppression of impulse noise in color images. Signal Process. **102**(9), 216–225 (2014)
11. Luo, Z., Lu, P., Zhang, G.: Locally optimal detector design in impulsive noise with unknown distribution. EURASIP J. Adv. Signal Process. **2018**(1), 1–10 (2018). https://doi.org/10.1186/s13634-018-0560-x
12. Buades, A., Coll, B., Morel, J.M.: A review of image denoising algorithms with a new one. Multiscale Model. Simul. **2**(4), 490–530 (2005)
13. Sun, Z., Chen, S.: Modifying NLM to a universal filter. Opt. Commun. **285**, 4918–4926 (2012)
14. Zhang, X., Zhan, Y., et al.: Decision-based non-local means filter for removing impulse noise from digital images. Signal Process. **93**, 517–524 (2013)
15. Ai, H., Ahmad A., Ghanati, R.: Modified non-local means: a novel denoising approach to process gravity field data. Open Geosci. **15**(1), 20220551 (2022). https://doi.org/10.1515/geo-2022-0551
16. Li, J., Wang, Y., Xiao, L.: SNR enhancement with a non-local means image-denoising method for a Φ-OTDR system. Appl. Opt. **63**(9), 2283–2291 (2023)
17. Verma, R., Pandey, R.: Adaptive selection of search region for NLM based image denoising. Optik **147**, 151–162 (2017)

One-Stage Lightweight Network of Object Detection for Rectangular Panoramic Images

Yingying Lu[✉], Yun Tie, and Lin Qi

Zhengzhou University, Zhengzhou Henan 450000, China
luyingy2021@163.com

Abstract. Nowadays, object detection has developed rapidly and the application scenarios of panoramic image detection are increasing. Compared with ordinary images, panoramic images have a certain degree of distortion of the objects and the number of objects is greater. Therefore, the traditional target detection network designed for vanilla images will bring problems such as insufficient feature extraction and slow inference speed of object detection. In this paper, we proposed a one-stage detection network to solve the problems. First, we constructed the ELAN-P module with Partial Convolution (PConv) to reduce the computational complexity. Second, we introduced the bi-level attention mechanism Biformer into the network to improve the robustness of the detection network and better capture the distortion information. Finally, we made a panoramic dataset to train the detection model and evaluate the performance of the proposed model. The experiment results verified the effectiveness of our model compared to the popular networks.

Keywords: Object detection · Biformer · Partial Convolution · Panoramic images

1 Introduction

Currently, with the development of the high bandwidth and low latency with 5G, people have an increasing demand for wider image representation. The imperative of research based on panoramic videos has become increasingly pronounced. In daily life, panoramic video has made remarkable contributions in areas such as autonomous driving [1], VR [2], and video surveillance [3], leveraging its inherent advantages. As a fundamental task in computer vision, many researchers have begun to study object detection [4], semantic segmentation [5], and other basic tasks of image processing based on panoramic images. As shown in Fig. 1, the panoramic image contains more details and distorted parts compared to ordinary images, which greatly limits the application of target detection in panoramic images.

There are three difficulties that panoramic images face in object detection. First, the objects in panoramic images have various degrees of distortion to a certain extent, and the detection network's ability to recognize objects is weaker than that of conventional objects. Second, because the panoramic image includes all objects in the 360° angle of view, it makes the reasoning speed of the network correspondingly slow, the panoramic image needs a lighter network to improve the overall performance of the network. Third, the datasets of panoramic images with rectangular boxes are scarce, and it is necessary to build one.

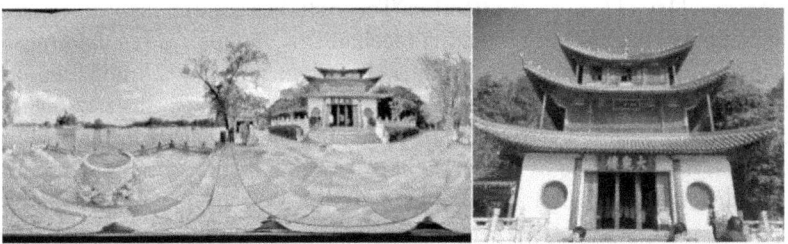

Fig. 1. Comparison between panoramic and vanilla images.

To crack the above nuts, we are dedicated to researching a fast and accurate panoramic image object detection network based on YOLOv7 architecture which is initially used for object detection of vanilla images and is not suitable for panoramic images. The main contributions are as follows:

1. **Effective fine-grained feature extraction.** An attention mechanism, Biformer is introduced to the basic network, which enables part of the vital features of the distorted graphics to be extracted effectively. Additionally, Biformer balances efficient feature extraction ability with computational complexity due to the designed bi-level routing attention architecture.
2. **Lower computational complexity.** The ELAN-P module with Partial Convolution (PConv) is introduced into our model to reduce the calculation complexity of the reasoning process and speed up the inference time. As a result, our model achieves a balance between computational efficiency and inference speed through the distinct design of both Biformer and ELAN-P with PConv.
3. **Self-build panoramic dataset**. To fill up the absence of a panoramic image dataset and train as well as evaluate the detection models, we established a panoramic dataset, namely Panowe. Finally, we conducted extensive experiments on both the public dataset and the self-built panoramic dataset. The experimental results show that the proposed model has better performance on the public dataset and self-build dataset.

2 Relate Work

According to the characteristics of panoramic images, researchers have devised several object detection frameworks, which can primarily be categorized into three categories. One is mapping panoramic images to the sphere to better extract object features, the second approach puts the focus on image pre-processing, and the last is based on the traditional detection algorithm [6–8]. In this paper, we design the network based on traditional algorithms, focusing on attention mechanisms and lightweight aspects.

The core idea of the attention mechanism is to mimic the human visual system, capable of automatically focusing on important parts of information. Its key structures include modules for computing attention weights and mechanisms for reallocating resources based on these weights. The design and implementation of these structures are crucial for the performance of the model. Currently, research on attention mechanisms encompasses various aspects such as channel attention [9], spatial attention, mixed channel-spatial attention [10, 11], and self-attention. These studies continuously advance the theory and practical applications of attention mechanisms, demonstrating their outstanding performance in different tasks and domains. The Transformer [12] model employs the Self-Attention mechanism as its core component to enable direct interactions between different positions within a sequence. To elaborate, traditional Recurrent Neural Networks (RNNs) face the issue of long-term dependency when processing sequential data. This means that the computational complexity of interactions between distant elements in a sequence increases with the distance between them. The Transformer addresses this by incorporating the Self-Attention mechanism, which allows for direct interaction between any two elements in the sequence, regardless of the distance separating them. This design facilitates information propagation in a single step, unlike the sequential transmission in RNNs, effectively resolving the problem of long-term dependencies. [13] is a transformer-based architecture designed for image recognition tasks. It represents a significant departure from the traditional convolutional neural network (CNN) approach that has dominated computer vision for many years.

Lightweight networks have always been a hot topic in the field of image processing. They maintain high accuracy while reducing the demand for computational resources. By employing knowledge distillation [14] to eliminate redundant information and preserve key insights, large complex models are compressed into smaller versions. Some studies have designed more efficient network structures, such as using depthwise separable convolution [15] to reduce the number of parameters and computations. Reference [16, 17] redesigns network layers to lower complexity. Several mature lightweight network models are already available, such as SqueezeNet, ShuffleNet, and MobileNet. Through innovations in these algorithms [18, 19], significant improvements in lightweight performance can also be achieved.

3 Proposed Method

The overall structure of the proposed model is shown in Fig. 2. In the feature extraction part, to reduce the parameters, the ELAN-P module with partial convolution is introduced. In the feature fusion part, the attention mechanism Biformer is introduced to realize more flexible calculation allocation and content awareness, and the distorted object features can be extracted more effectively.

3.1 Fine-Grained Feature Extraction

Due to the distortion of the object existing in the panoramic image, the vanilla object detection network has shown unsatisfactory detection effectiveness. Traditional convolution does not have enough representation ability to extract useful information from raw panoramic images. Currently, the multi-head self-attention (MHSA) mechanism is used in object detection to enhance representation capability. Compared to the normal convolution, MHSA has higher computational and storage requirements. However, an explosive amount of computation is inevitable in such a network.

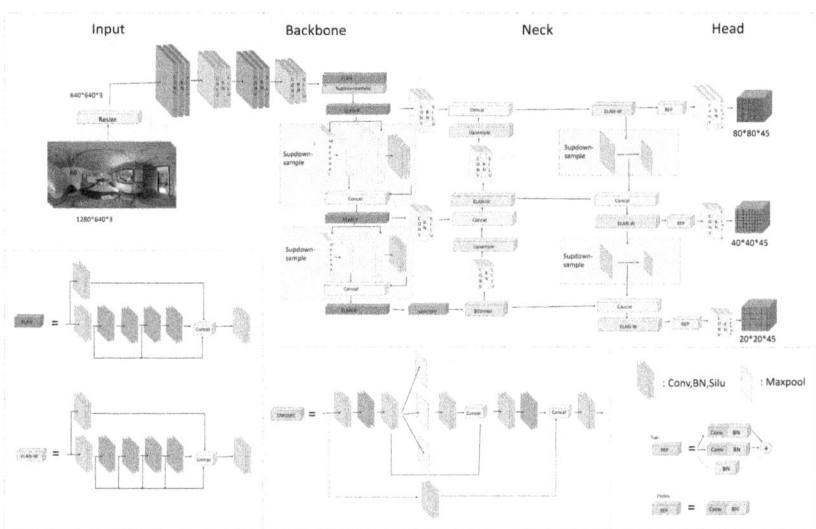

Fig. 2. The overall structure of the proposed model. The network includes three parts: backbone to extract the information, neck to fuse the information, and head to predict.

Therefore, inspired by MHSA, we introduce an effective module BiFormer to realize fine-grained feature extraction to maintain the feature extraction ability while accessing relatively little computation, which takes the feature representation capability and computation complexity into consideration. In particular, it adopts bi-level routing attention to speed up computation and employs a shortcut trick to maintain useful information.

To improve the feature extraction ability while accessing relatively little computation, a dynamic and query-aware sparse attention mechanism called BiFormer was introduced to our model. The fundamental concept of BiFormer is to filter out irrelevant key-value pairs at a coarse-grained region level, thereby retaining only a small subset that contains valuable information while eliminating redundancy. Additionally, BiFormer employs fine-grained token-to-token attention within these selected regions.

The structure of the BiFormer is shown in Fig. 3. It follows the common design of most vision transformer architectures, employing a four-level pyramid structure that achieves a downsampling factor of 32. In the first stage, BiFormer utilizes overlapping block embeddings, while in the second to fourth stages, block merging modules are employed to decrease the input spatial resolution while increasing the number of channels. Subsequently, a series of BiFormer blocks is used for feature transformation. Each Biformer block begins with a 3x3 depth-wise convolution to implicitly encode relative positional information. The BRA module and Multi-Layer Perceptron (MLP) module are then successively applied to the model positional relationships and embed information at each position. The most important construction of BiFormer is the BRA module. The BRA module includes the region-to-region routing step and token-to-token attention.

Equations (1), and (2) first calculate the semantic correlation between two regions and then filter out the most relevant regions. Among them, suppose that the feature map is divided into S*S non-overlapped regions. In the equation, $Q^r, K^r \in R^{S^2*C}, A^r \in R^{S^2*S^2}$. Equations (3), and (4) first gather the scattered key and value and then apply attention to the gathered key-value pairs. It collects key-value pairs from the top-k relevant windows and utilizes sparse operations to skip computations in the least relevant regions, thereby reducing parameter and computational costs. In the equation, $K^g, V^g \in R^{S^2*\frac{kHW}{S^2}*C}$, , LCE(V) [20] is used to enhance the local context.

$$A^r = Q^r(K^r)^T \tag{1}$$

$$I^r = topkIndex(A^r) \tag{2}$$

$$K^g = gather(K, I^r), V^g = gather(V, I^r) \tag{3}$$

$$O = Attention(Q, K^g, V^g) + LCE(V) \tag{4}$$

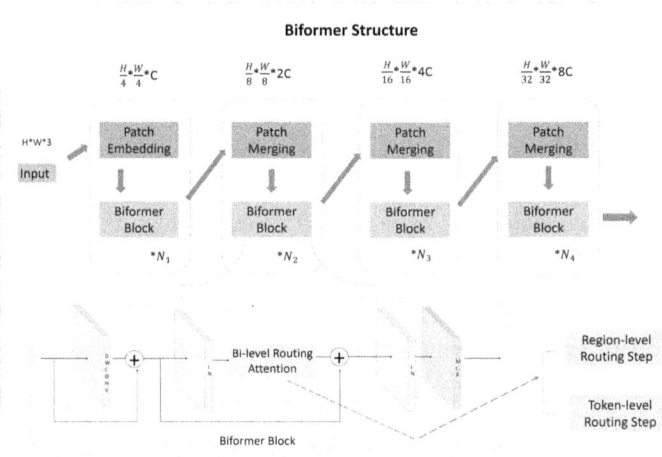

Fig. 3. The structure of the Biformer.

Due to the superior performance of the Biformer and the particularity of panoramic images, we introduced Bifomer into our module to improve the distortion characteristics feature extraction capability, and global dependency modeling capability.

3.2 Lightweight Operation

The task of object detection typically demands high real-time performance, particularly when applied to panoramic images, which encompass a 360-degree view of a scene.

Unlike standard images, panoramas inherently contain a greater number of objects, leading to an abundance of redundant information. Consequently, this results in excessive computations, leading to prolonged inference times and a reduction in the number of frames detected per second. Thus, the imperative arises to devise a lightweight network architecture to address this challenge.

Inspired by a novel technique called partial convolution in Faster Net, we reconstructed a module ELAN-P into our model. The introduction of the PConv addressed the issue of redundant computations and memory access while effectively extracting spatial features. PConv takes advantage of the high similarity among different channels in the feature map. It applies regular convolution selectively to a subset of input channels for spatial feature extraction while keeping the remaining channels unchanged. The structure of the PConv is shown on the right of Fig. 4. The researchers have found that the reduction in FLOPs does not always correspond to a proportional decrease in latency. This discrepancy primarily arises from the inefficiency of low-floating-point operations per second (FLOPS), which is caused by frequent memory access by operators. To facilitate contiguous or regular memory access, either the first or last contiguous channels are treated as representatives of the entire feature map during computation. Without loss of generality, it is assumed that the input and output feature maps have an equal number of channels. This approach greatly reduces the frequency of memory access by operators, resulting in faster and more efficient operation of neural networks. The FLOPs of a PConv are shown in Eq. (5), and the FLOPs of a Conv are shown in Eq. (6). The relationship between the c and c_p is shown in Eq. (7). We can see that the FLOPs of PConv are much less than Conv. Moreover, PConv demonstrates high efficacy in extracting spatial features.

$$FLOPs_{(Pconv)} = h * w * k^2 * c_p^2 \tag{5}$$

$$FLOPs_{(Conv)} = h * w * k^2 * c^2 \tag{6}$$

$$c_p = 1/4 * c \tag{7}$$

Considering the above characteristics of PConv, we constructed the module ELAN-P. In the ELAN-P, the convolution of the residual branch remains unchanged and in the other branch, we changed four ordinary convolutions into PConv. The structure of the ELAN-P is shown on the left of Fig. 4.

3.3 Loss Function

In the process of backpropagation of the neural network, the loss function plays an important part in network adaptive parameter updating. The loss function of the model includes confidence loss, localization loss, and classification loss. The contribution to the network of the three is different and the weight allocation is shown in Eq. (8). In the equation, $Loss_{con}$ stands for the confidence loss, $Loss_{cla}$ stands for the classification loss, $Loss_{loc}$ stands for the localization loss, Among them, the loss of confidence and classification is calculated by binary cross-entropy with Eq. (9), where N represents the

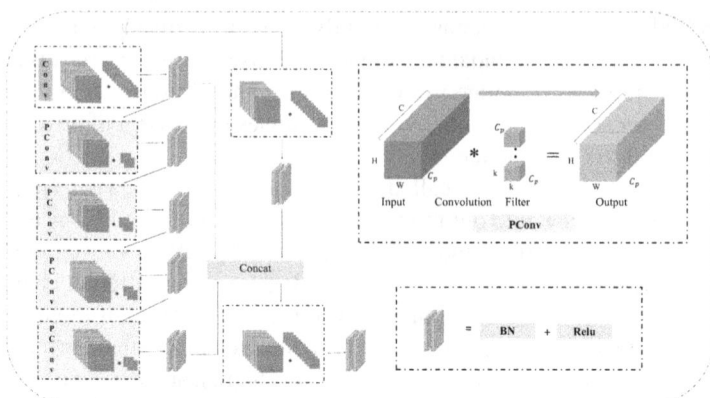

Fig. 4. The structure of the ELAN-P and PConv. The structure of ELAN-P is shown on the left, and the top right illustrates the convolution process of the PConv

categories, y_i is the binary label 0 or 1, and p_i is the probability that the output corresponds to the y label. The loss of localization is calculated by CIoU loss with Eq. (10), where IoU is used to measure the relevance between the prediction box and the real box, b and b^{gt} represents the center point of the prediction box and the real box respectively, and η represents the Euclidean distance between the two center points, c represents the diagonal length of the smallest external rectangle that can contain both the prediction box and the real box, α is the weight parameter, and υ is used to measure the consistency of the aspect ratio.

$$Loss_{total} = 0.1 * Loss_{con} + 0.125 * Loss_{cla} + 0.05 * Loss_{loc} \tag{8}$$

$$Loss = -\frac{1}{N}\sum_{i=1}^{N}[y_t log(p_t) + (1-y_i)log(1-p_i)] \tag{9}$$

$$L_{CIoU} = 1 - IoU + \frac{\eta^2(b, b^{gt})}{c^2} + \alpha\upsilon \tag{10}$$

4 Experiments

4.1 Implementation Details

The experimental setting is based on the Ubuntu20.04 platform, GTX1080Ti × 2 (12G) GPU, and Pytorch 1.10 library. In the training process, batch size and learning rate are set to 64 and 1e-3, respectively. Adam optimizer and weight decay are used for optimization. For experimental fairness and preciseness, the pre-trained strategy is employed in all models in this study.

To enhance the model's ability to swiftly learn the target features of objects within panoramic images, we adopted a transfer learning approach. Initially, we pre-trained the model on a publicly available dataset PASCAL VOC2007. Subsequently, since there is a large similarity in the information contained in the images. we employed this pre-trained model as the base for training on panoramic images.

4.2 Dataset

Due to the absence of a publicly available panoramic image object detection dataset, we created a self-built dataset named Panowe. This dataset is sourced from three primary origins: online searches, and images captured using KanDao four-eye and Teche six-eye cameras. The dataset includes images with three different resolutions: 9104x4552, 7680x3840, and 3840x1920.

To generate the panoramic images, the cameras were used to capture pictures from various angles. These images were then stitched together using KandaoStudio and TecheStudio software. Once the panoramic images were assembled, we used LabelImg to annotate them.

Panowe encompasses eight categories of objects found in both indoor and outdoor environments: person, chair, car, window, table, sofa, door, and bed, as illustrated in Fig. 5. The dataset consists of a total of 1,816 images, which were divided into training, validation, and test sets with a 7:2:1 ratio. This structured approach ensures a comprehensive and balanced dataset for developing and evaluating panoramic image object detection models.

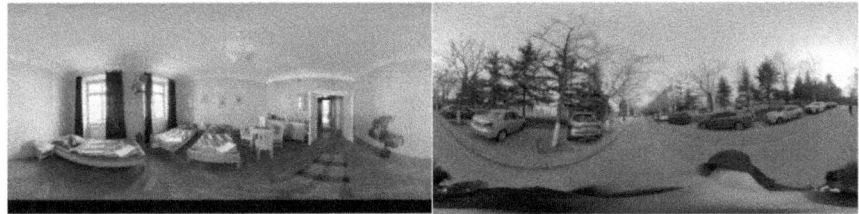

Fig. 5. Panoramic images in the Panowe dataset.

In addition, the public dataset VOC2007 is also employed in this study to ensure experimental fairness and evaluate the generalization of the models. The VOC2007 dataset contains 20 categories, and all of them are representative targets in object detection.

4.3 Baselines

To demonstrate the enhancement of our proposed method, we selected the YOLOv7 series as our baseline and conducted a comparative analysis. As shown in Table 1, our model exhibits significant improvements over YOLOv7 on the VOC2007 dataset. Specifically, our model has 3.5% fewer parameters, 4.46% less computation, and achieves a 0.92% higher mean Average Precision (mAP). Similarly, Table 2 presents a comparative evaluation of the Panowe dataset, where our model again outperforms the baselines, showing 3.5% fewer parameters, 3.8% less computation, and a 0.72% higher mAP than YOLOv7.

These experimental results clearly demonstrate the superiority and robustness of our proposed model, which integrates Biformer and ELAN-P with the Pconv module. The consistent performance improvements across different datasets underscore the efficacy of our enhancements in reducing computational complexity while boosting accuracy.

Table 1. Comparison with Baselines YOLOV7 on the VOC2007 dataset.

Model	Params(M)	FLOPs (G)	Size	mAP
YOLOv7	37.2	105.3	640*640	0.871
YOLOv7-X	71.5	189.9	640*640	0.887
YOLOv7-tiny	6.2	3.5	640*640	0.598
YOLOv7-E6	97.4	516.3	640*640	0.921
YOLOv7-E6E	152.3	846.2	640*640	0.936
Ours	35.89	100.6	640*640	0.879

Table 2. Comparison with Baselines YOLOV7 on the Panowe dataset.

Model	Params(M)	FLOPs (G)	Size	mAP
YOLOv7	37.2	106.7	640*640	0.839
YOLOv7-X	71.5	192.9	640*640	0.856
YOLOv7-tiny	6.2	3.8	640*640	0.573
YOLOv7-E6	97.4	526.3	640*640	0.908
YOLOv7-E6E	152.3	853.2	640*640	0.916
Ours	35.89	102.6	640*640	0.845

4.4 Comparison Study

To demonstrate the algorithm's effectiveness and applicability, we trained and tested the network model on the public dataset PASCAL VOC2007. We compared our model with other object detection algorithms, the results are shown in Table 3. From the results, we can see that although our model is designed for the detection of panoramic images, it also has a good performance on the ordinary object detection task. The detection accuracy and detection speed all have improved.

Table 3. Comparison of the popular object detection algorithms on the VOC2007 dataset.

Model	Image size	mAP	FPS
YOLOv5s	640*640	0.842	40
YOLOv7	640*640	0.871	51
YOLOv8s	640*640	0.867	47
Faster R-CNN	1000 * 600	0.732	7
SSD	512 * 512	0.767	18
Ours	640*640	0.879	53

Then the transfer learning method is adopted on the model we trained on the PASCAL VOC2007 dataset, we used it as our pre-trained model and then trained the model on the self-collected dataset Panowe. The comparison test results are shown in Table 4. From the table, we can see that the model we proposed performs best.

Table 4. Comparison of the popular object detection algorithms on the Panowe dataset.

Model	Image size	mAP	FPS	person	car	chair	window	table	sofa	door	bed
YOLOv5s	640*640	0.827	37	0.867	0.873	0.838	0.801	0.795	0.799	0.812	0.831
YOLOv7	640*640	0.839	48	0.919	0.927	0.833	0.77	0.799	0.809	0.819	0.836
YOLOv8s	640*640	0.823	45	0.911	0.917	0.77	0.782	0.778	0.805	0.803	0.818
Faster R-CNN	1000*600	0.722	6	0.829	0.843	0.63	0.668	0.671	0.698	0.711	0.726
SSD	512*512	0.745	15	0.814	0.826	0.706	0.722	0.699	0.709	0.725	0.759
Ours	640*640	0.845	50	0.928	0.941	0.801	0.792	0.813	0.811	0.823	0.851

4.5 Ablation Study

To explore the impact of different modules on network performance, we conducted ablation experiments, with results shown in Table 5. The introduction of Biformer significantly enhanced the feature extraction capability for distorted objects, thanks to its Bi-level routing attention, which effectively captures fine-grained information. However, this improvement also increased parameters and computational load.

ELAN-P addresses this issue by reducing computational complexity and improving detection speed through efficient convolution, significantly minimizing redundant operations. Panoramic images contain substantial extraneous information, and using standard convolution leads to redundancy. While PConv alone can reduce redundancy, it risks ignoring important features, particularly edges and text of distorted objects. Biformer effectively resolves this issue by maintaining critical feature extraction without excessive computation.

Table 5. Ablation study on Panowe dataset[1] with Biformer and ELAN-P.

Model	mAP	FPS	FLOPs(G)	Params(M)
Baseline	0.839	48	107.3	37.25
Baseline + B	0.847 (+0.008)	45 (−3)	133.6 (+26.3)	46.3 (+9.05)
Baseline + P	0.838 (−0.001)	54 (+6)	86.1 (−21.2)	32.9 (4.35)
Baseline + B + P (Ours)	0.845 (+0.006)	50 (+2)	102.6 (−4.7)	35.89 (−1.36)

---

[1] B represents Biformer and P represents ELAN-P.

To explore the best way to construct ELAN-P so that the detector performance is optimal, we combine the general convolution with the partial convolution. The model structure and experimental results are shown in Table 6. Since the ELAN-P network has a residual network connection at the input side, the convolution collocation with the proper structure makes the network play a better performance. It can effectively reduce the number of network parameters and make the model lighter with little loss in accuracy. From the experimental results, it can also be analyzed that keeping the original convolution at the initial end of the network tends to make the network more stable.

Table 6. Ablation study on ELAN-P modules[2] with different distributions of PConv.

Convolution permutation	mAP	FPS	FLOPs(G)	Params(M)
PPPPP	0.813	60	70.3	30.7
CPPPP (Ours)	0.828	54	86.1	32.9
CCPPP	0.826	48	97.3	35.9
PPPCC	0.824	49	96.6	34.8
PPPPC	0.821	53	87.4	33.1

5 Conclusion

In this study, we address two key challenges in panoramic image object detection: distortion and network lightweighting. To enhance effective information capture and better handle distorted objects in panoramic images, we incorporated Biformer into our model. To reduce computational complexity and improve detection speed, we introduced the ELAN-P module, which significantly reduces redundant computations while maintaining exceptional detection performance.

We created a panoramic image dataset named Panowe to train our model effectively. We evaluated our model's detection capabilities against popular algorithms, and the results demonstrated superior performance. Additionally, ablation studies were conducted to assess the impact of the different modules in our network. The results confirmed that both modules effectively address the identified challenges.

References

1. Kinzig, C., Cortés, I., Fernández, C., Lauer, M.: Real-time seamless image stitching in autonomous driving. In: 2022 25th International Conference on Information Fusion (FUSION), pp. 1–8. IEEE (2022)
2. Nieto-Escamez, F., Cortés-Pérez, I., Obrero-Gaitán, E., Fusco, A.: Virtual reality applications in neurorehabilitation: Current panorama and challenges (2023)

---

[2] In the table, P represents PConv and C represents Conv.

3. Gao, J., Hu, Z., Bian, K., Mao, X., Song, L.: Aq360: Uav-aided air quality monitoring by 360-degree aerial panoramic images in urban areas. IEEE Internet Things J. **8**(1), 428–442 (2020)
4. Kashika, P., Venkatapur, R.B.: Deep learning technique for object detection from panoramic video frames. Int. J. Comput. Theory Eng. **14**(1), 20–26 (2022)
5. Orhan, S., Bastanlar, Y.: Semantic segmentation of outdoor panoramic images. SIViP **16**(3), 643–650 (2022)
6. Lee, Y., Jeong, J., Yun, J., Cho, W., Yoon, K.J.: Spherephd: Applying cnns on a spherical polyhedron representation of 360deg images. In: Proceedings of the IEEE/CVF Conference on Computer Vision and Pattern Recognition, pp. 9181–9189 (2019)
7. Cao, M., Ikehata, S., Aizawa, K.: Field-of-view iou for object detection in 360° images. IEEE Trans. Image Process. (2023)
8. Tateno, K., Navab, N., Tombari, F.: Distortion-aware convolutional filters for dense prediction in panoramic images. In: Proceedings of the European Conference on Computer Vision (ECCV), pp. 707–722 (2018)
9. Hu, J., Shen, L., Sun, G.: Squeeze-and-excitation networks. In: Proceedings of the IEEE Conference on Computer Vision and Pattern Recognition, pp. 7132–7141 (2018)
10. Woo, S., Park, J., Lee, J.Y., Kweon, I.S.: Cbam: convolutional block attention module. In: Proceedings of the European Conference on Computer Vision (ECCV), pp. 3–19 (2018)
11. Zhang, Q.L., Yang, Y.B.: Sa-net: shuffle attention for deep convolutional neural networks. In: ICASSP 2021–2021 IEEE International Conference on Acoustics, Speech and Signal Processing (ICASSP), pp. 2235–2239. IEEE (2021)
12. Ł., Polosukhin, I.: Attention is all you need. Advances in neural information processing systems 30 (2017)
13. Dosovitskiy, A., et al.: An image is worth 16x16 words: Transformers for image recognition at scale. arXiv preprint arXiv:2010.11929 (2020)
14. Yang, Z., Zeng, A., Li, Z., Zhang, T., Yuan, C., Li, Y.: From knowledge distillation to self-knowledge distillation: a unified approach with normalized loss and customized soft labels. In: Proceedings of the IEEE/CVF International Conference on Computer Vision, pp. 17185–17194 (2023)
15. Chollet, F.: Xception: deep learning with depthwise separable convolutions. In: Proceedings of the IEEE Conference on Computer Vision and Pattern Recognition, pp. 1251–1258 (2017)
16. Gu, M., et al.: A lightweight convolutional neural network hardware implementation for wearable heart rate anomaly detection. Comput. Biol. Med. **155**, 106623 (2023)
17. Zhang, D., et al.: An efficient lightweight convolutional neural network for industrial surface defect detection. Artif. Intell. Rev. **56**(9), 10651–10677 (2023)
18. Ullah, N., Khan, J.A., El-Sappagh, S., El-Rashidy, N., Khan, M.S.: A holistic approach to identify and classify covid-19 from chest radiographs, ecg, and ct-scan images using shufflenet convolutional neural network. Diagnostics **13**(1), 162 (2023)
19. Kaya, Y., Gürsoy, E.: A mobilenet-based cnn model with a novel fine-tuning mechanism for covid-19 infection detection. Soft. Comput. **27**(9), 5521–5535 (2023)
20. Ren, S., Zhou, D., He, S., Feng, J., Wang, X.: Shunted self-attention via multi-scale token aggregation. In: Proceedings of the IEEE/CVF Conference on Computer Vision and Pattern Recognition, pp. 10853–10862 (2022)
21. Zhu, L., Wang, X., Ke, Z., Zhang, W., Lau, R.W.: Biformer: Vision transformer with bi-level routing attention. In: Proceedings of the IEEE/CVF Conference on Computer Vision and Pattern Recognition, pp. 10323–10333 (2023)

ISE-UFDS: A Dataset for Detecting the Degree of Danger to Vehicles in Urban Flooding and Performance Assessment

Jiwu Sun[1], Cheng Zhang[1], Cheng Xu[1], Pengfei Wang[1,2], and Hongzhe Liu[1(✉)]

[1] Beijing Key Laboratory of Information Service Engineering, Beijing Union University, Beijing, China
liuhongzhe@buu.edu.cn
[2] Big Data Center, Ministry of Emergency Management, Beijing, China

Abstract. As global warming and urbanisation continue to accelerate, resulting in the increasing likelihood and uncertainty of extreme rainstorms and floods, how to detect things in flooding scenarios and implement relevant rescue measures has become an urgent problem to be solved. Flooding scenarios are difficult and dangerous to obtain data, which leads to relatively few data sets dedicated to the detection of the degree of danger of vehicles in flooding scenarios. To this end, a dataset for vehicle hazard detection in urban flooding is proposed and the YOLOv8s algorithm is improved to increase the detection accuracy. The proposed dataset aims to provide realistic, diverse and challenging vehicle images in flooding scenarios, including different flood hazard scenarios and time periods. The dataset contains a total of 20,152 images, which are divided into training, validation and test sets in the ratio of 8: 1: 1 and evaluated and validated on the existing target detection algorithms. The authenticity and accuracy of the dataset is ensured by collecting data from real flooding sites.

Keywords: Vehicle Detection · Urban Waterlogging · Hazard Detection Dataset · YOLO · Performance Evaluation

1 Introduction

Several studies have shown that there is a complex interplay between urbanisation and flooding [1] With the acceleration of global warming and urbanisation, the likelihood and uncertainty of flooding triggered by extreme rainstorms is increasing [2]. Such disasters usually exhibit a chain development characteristic, where the initial heavy rainfall event may trigger a series of secondary disasters, such as ground subsidence, roadbed collapse, and house collapse, which further exacerbate the casualties and property losses, making the water safety situation in cities more complex and severe [3]. In flooded environments, roads and transport systems are often severely damaged, leading to disruption of traffic and rescue operations [4]. For example, in August 2023, Beijing, Tianjin, Hebei, Henan, and Shanxi were hit by frequent heavy rainstorms, which triggered frequent floods, posing a serious threat to the safety of people's lives and property and having a significant impact on the normal operation of cities [5]. In the process of coping with flooding, the rapid response of the rescue system and the effective execution of the rescue mission are crucial. Through in-depth research and development of advanced detection technologies, vehicle risks in flooding can be more accurately identified and assessed, thus providing timely and accurate information support for emergency decision-making, improving rescue efficiency, reducing casualties and property losses, and safeguarding the operational stability and safety of cities in the face of flooding [6].

However, current vehicle detection datasets generally suffer from insufficient coverage of flooding scenarios and lack of specialised design, which to a certain extent restricts the development and practical application of vehicle hazard detection algorithms in flooded environments. Existing datasets are usually based on conventional urban traffic environments, which cannot adequately simulate the environmental conditions and phenomena specific to flooding, such as water inundation, the refraction effect of light, and image blurring [7]. Therefore, in order to fill the gap of the vehicle hazard detection dataset in flooding scenarios and to promote the research and development of vehicle detection algorithms in this scenario, this paper proposes a dataset for the detection of vehicle hazards in urban flooding and applies a relevant target detection model to evaluate the performance of this dataset, aiming to provide a targeted data resource to support and optimise the development of vehicle detection technology in flooding environments, which in turn improves flood emergency response capability and public safety.

2 Related Works

Target detection is a key fundamental task in the field of deep learning computer vision and one of the hot topics in current academic research [8]. Its applications widely penetrate into many fields such as daily production and military, including important scenarios such as face recognition, aerospace, security and intelligent surveillance [9].

As a general tool for target detection, deep learning models show a wide range of application potential in vehicle detection tasks. For example, Zhang et al. [10] proposed an improved algorithm based on optimising the YOLO v5 network for the problem of misdetection or omission of vehicle targets due to occlusion, which is suitable for vehicle detection in various traffic scenarios.Dong et al. [11] were concerned about the problem of high computational load and low detection rate of YOLO v5, and their Neck network part of YOLO v5, introduced the C3Ghost and Ghost modules, aiming to reduce the floating-point operations in the feature channel fusion process, thus improving the feature representation performance and achieving more efficient vehicle detection. Pratama et al. [12] implemented real-time vehicle detection on the network by using the YOLOv8 algorithm, and their team constructed a large dataset of vehicle images for training the YOLOv8 model, to ensure that it is capable of recognising and track different types of vehicles.Chen et al. [13], on the other hand, proposed a modified SSD (single-shot multibox detector) algorithm, which is designed for fast vehicle detection in traffic scenarios, further improving detection speed and accuracy. These methods address specific problems in vehicle detection and provide more accurate and efficient solutions for vehicle detection in real traffic scenarios.

There are many datasets that can be used for vehicle detection. The COCO dataset is a large-scale dataset widely used for target detection, segmentation, and keypoint detection tasks, and it is one of the most influential and widely used datasets in the field of target detection [14]. Open Images contains more than 9 million images covering more than 60,000 different categories, and it provides an important resource for target detection algorithm research and evaluation [15]. The KITTI dataset is a widely used dataset for autonomous driving and computer vision research, containing data for tasks such as vehicle detection, target tracking, stereo vision, etc. [16]. The BDD100K dataset is a large-scale dataset for autonomous driving, containing high-definition images and videos from different cities [17]. These datasets provide specially designed images and annotation information for specific application scenarios and tasks, providing valuable benchmarks for related research work.

Numerous datasets and research works have emerged in the field of target detection, which provide rich content and standard references for algorithm training and performance evaluation. Due to the time-sensitive and potentially dangerous process of acquiring data in flooding scenarios, there is a lack of datasets in the field specifically designed for this scenario. Therefore, this paper proposes a dataset named Urban Flooding vehicle hazard Detection dataSet (ISE-UFDS), which is designed for vehicle hazard detection and risk assessment in flooding scenarios. In order to validate the effectiveness and practicality of the ISE-UFDS dataset, its performance will be evaluated by applying relevant detection algorithms in Chapter 4 of this paper.

3 Proposed Dataset

The proposed dataset implementation process is shown in Fig. 1.

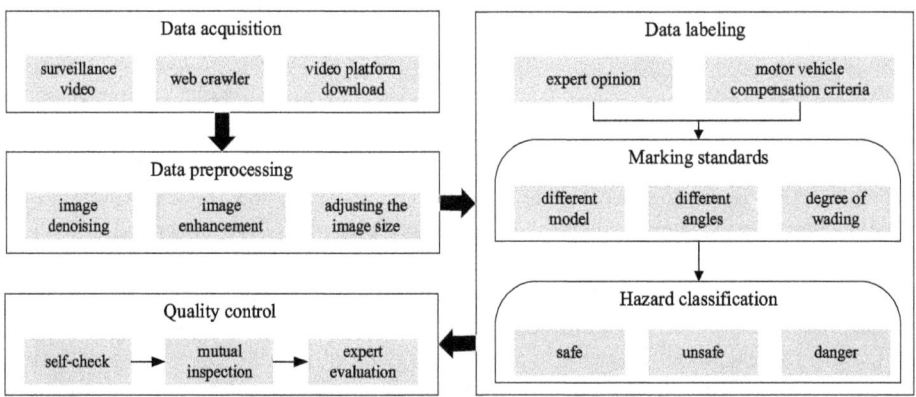

Fig. 1. Flow of dataset realization.

3.1 Data Acquisition

Given the difficulty in acquiring image data of flooded vehicles in flooding scenarios, the source data images in this study come from three main sources. Firstly, we use the road video monitoring privileges of the big data centre of the Ministry of Emergency Management and combine them with the national meteorological warning information to predict the areas where severe weather, such as heavy rainfall, is about to occur, so as to monitor and record the video in the areas where flooding or waterlogging of the roads is likely to occur. Secondly, we write Python crawler scripts to capture relevant video and image data on the web with the keywords of "urban flooding" and "flooded vehicles", and finally collect more than 10,000 images and 8G video clips. Finally, we also borrowed the videos of flooded vehicles taken by relevant bloggers on YouTube to supplement the data set moderately. Screenshots of some of the data clips are shown in Fig. 2, which were used as raw data for subsequent processing.

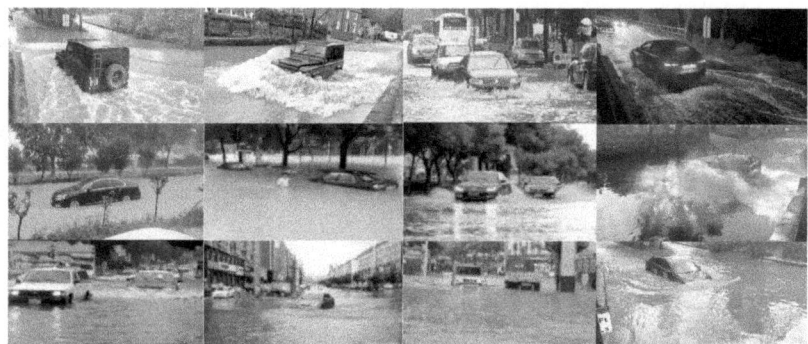

Fig. 2. Sample of some of the original images.

We decompose the acquired flood video data frame by frame, extracting one frame every 10 s, and then screen all the obtained image files to eliminate images that are too similar and irrelevant to the target to be detected. After the above operation screening, a total of 20, 152 images are retained for subsequent image annotation. At the same time, considering personal privacy issues, we blurred the positions involving faces and licence plate numbers before image annotation.

3.2 Hazard Classification and Data Labelling

Based on the compensation standards of some auto insurance companies for flooded vehicles, combined with professional knowledge of vehicle structures, and after consulting relevant experts and the Big Data Centre of the Ministry of Emergency Management, three labelling levels were developed for the vehicles targeted for detection in the dataset, using the side view perspective as an example:

(1) safe: A vehicle is considered to have no risk of flooding when the water level line is below the horizontal median line of the vehicle's wheel hub.
(2) unsafe: Vehicles are at risk of flooding when the water level line is above the median wheel level but still does not reach under the bonnet.
(3) danger: If the water line exceeds the bonnet of the vehicle, this indicates that flood water may have entered the engine of the vehicle and the vehicle is at serious risk of flooding and stalling.

Taking into account the differences in the water-wading capacity of different car models, the vehicles involved in this dataset were classified into three main categories: ordinary cars, sports cars (low chassis category) and SUVs (high chassis category). In addition, the labelling requirements were classified as side, front and rear of the vehicle according to the angle from which the vehicle enters the picture. The specific labelling requirements are described in detail in Table 1, including the labelling criteria and thresholds for each category of vehicle at different viewing angles.

Table 1. Dataset labelling requirements (based on water level line position)

	car side	car front	car rear
ordinary car	Lv. 1: wheel median Lv. 2: Above wheel median to below bonnet; Lv. 3: Above the bonnet	Lv. 1: below the lower edge of the body; Lv. 2: above the lower edge of the body to below the bonnet; Lv. 3: above the bonnet	Lv. 1: below the lower edge of the body; Lv. 2: above the lower edge of the body to below the upper edge of the for lights; Lv. 3: above the lower edge of the taillights
Sports car		Lv. 1: below the top edge of the licence plate frame; Lv. 2: above the top edge of the licence plate frame to below the bonnet; Lv. 3: above the bonnet	Lv. 1: below the lower edge of the licence plate frame Lv. 2: Above the lower edge of the licence plate frame to below the upper edge of the licence plate frame; Lv. 3: above the upper edge of the licence plate frame
SUV		Lv. 1: below the lower edge of the front end; Lv. 2: above the lower edge of the front end to below the bonnet; Lv. 3: above the bonnet	Lv. 1: below the lower edge of the vehicle body; Lv. 2: above the lower edge of the vehicle body to below the lower edge of the licence plate frame; Lv. 3: above the lower edge of the licence plate frame

Figure 3 provides a schematic representation of the labelling criteria for each type of vehicle at different angles, visually demonstrating how the type of labelling can be determined based on the position of the water level line relative to the critical parts of the vehicle.

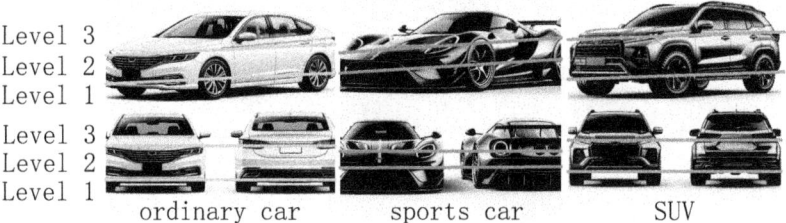

Fig. 3. Schematic diagram of the labelling standards for different angles of various types of vehicles.

In this study, we adjusted the labelling for special cases for the dataset of vehicle detection in flooding scenarios. For example, in the case of a transient water level line elevation caused by splashing water when the vehicle is travelling fast, we determine the actual water level line of the vehicle based on its position that is not obscured by splashing water. For passenger cars and lorries with large differences in size and structure, we adjusted the labelling criteria and simplified it to two water level classes: safe and unsafe, without creating a hazard class. In addition, in order to enhance the generalisation ability and adaptability of the dataset, we retained some images with lower image quality or partial occlusion and made fine annotations. Such treatment makes the model better adaptable to complex and changing real-world application scenarios.

The data labelling exercise was carried out after the pre-processing of the dataset was completed. The proposed dataset is labelled using LabelImg tool and the information is saved in YOLO format. Some of the data labelling results are shown in Fig. 4 and the sample distribution is shown in Fig. 5.

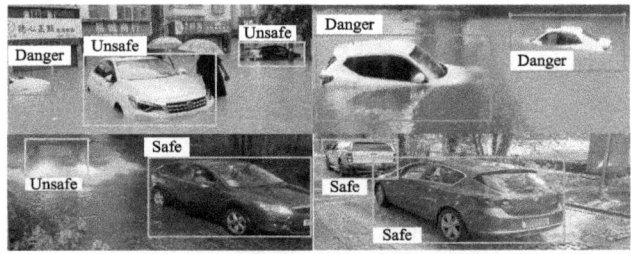

Fig. 4. Partial data labelling results.

3.3 Quality Control

When the data completed the labelling work for the relevant experimental tests, it was found that the detection effect deviated from the expected effect. In order to ensure

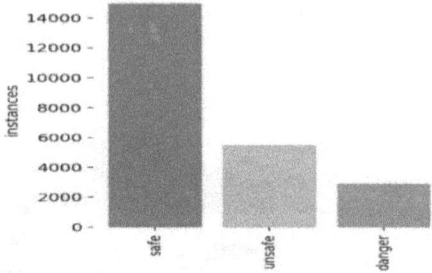

Fig. 5. Sample distribution.

the quality of the dataset annotation, the proposed dataset strictly adopts a three-step verification process for each annotation result:

Self-inspection by the annotator. The self-test can help the annotator to re-examine the results of his/her work, find deviations or errors, and correct the errors in advance to ensure the quality of the dataset.

Cross-checking between annotators. In the manual annotation work, the annotation results will often be affected by the subjective judgement of the annotator, in the cross-checking process, different annotators can check each other's errors, in order to reduce the impact of individual subjective judgement.

Validation by experts. By seeking experts in the relevant fields to evaluate the dataset, it helps to verify the validity of the dataset, and then the annotator modifies the annotation results based on the experts' opinions.

Through a careful review process, changes were made to some of the labelling results to ensure the quality of the labelling and consistency standards for this dataset, with an average improvement of 6.8 per cent in each metric compared to the initial experimental results.

4 Experiments

In order to verify the usability of the proposed dataset for the detection of vehicle hazard level in flooding scenarios, a more classical deep learning approach is used for evaluating the performance of the ISE-UFDS dataset [18]. All experiments were conducted utilizing an NVIDIA GeForce RTX 3090 GPU equipped with 24 GB of graphics memory for model training. The target detection models used were uniformly set to train for 200 epochs, with batch size set to 16, and were trained using the SGD optimiser with a learning rate of 0.001. The evaluation metrics used are precision (P), recall (R), F1-score, average accuracy (AP), and the mean of the AP of different categories of samples (mAP), which are calculated as shown in Eqs. (1)–(5), respectively.

$$Precision = \frac{TP}{TP+FP} \qquad (1)$$

$$Recall = \frac{TP}{TP+FN} \qquad (2)$$

$$F1 - score = 2 * \frac{P*R}{P+R} \qquad (3)$$

$$AP = S_{P-R} \quad (4)$$

$$mAP = \frac{\sum_{i=1}^{k} AP_i}{k} \quad (5)$$

where TP, FP and FN denote true cases, false positive cases and false negative cases, respectively, S_{P-R} denotes the area represented under the PR curve, and k is the number of all detection classes.

In order to verify the performance of the ISE-UFDS dataset, it is applied to the current mainstream target detection network models to verify the validity of the dataset, respectively. In this paper, the proposed dataset is respectively applied to the more classical target detection networks for performance testing to verify the quality of the dataset. The experimental results of multiple network models are shown in Table 2.

Table 2. Experimental results of multiple network models

Model	P	R	F1-score	mAP
YOLOv5s	0.663	0.668	0.665	0.676
YOLOv5s-BiFPN [19]	0.67	0.685	0.677	0.712
YOLOv5s-GIoU [20]	0.649	0.689	0.668	0.718
YOLOv8s	0.653	0.671	0.662	0.68
Faster R-CNN [21]	0.69	0.732	0.710	0.782
Cascade R-CNN [22]	0.70	0.75	0.724	0.789
Mask R-CNN [23]	0.725	0.763	0.744	0.796

The analysis of the experimental results shows that by comparing the performance of several other mainstream target detection algorithms on the ISE-UFDS dataset, the single-stage algorithm is able to achieve a mAP result of more than 0.6 and the two-stage algorithm is able to achieve a mAP result of more than 0.7, which further highlights the fact that the specialised dataset proposed in this study can be used for the detection of the hazardous level of flooded vehicles by the classical target detection network. Combined with the problems of vehicle detection in flooding scenarios, such as varying scales and water occlusion, in the case of the YOLOv5 network, a simple improvement is made by adding the BiFPN module, which alleviates the problem of multi-scale detection, and the GIoU loss function, which helps to solve the problem of occlusion, to the YOLOv5s network, respectively, and it is found that the mAPs are both improved to a certain extent.

Considering the need for high real-time performance in flood search and rescue scenarios, we will focus on the faster YOLOv8s algorithm with higher detection accuracy to improve it in order to balance the speed and accuracy of detection. The main problems encountered in the detection of vehicles in flooding scenarios from surveillance videos are due to the degree of occlusion of the vehicle by the water body i.e. the depth of the flooded vehicle and the presence of multi-scale target detection. In order to solve the above problems, we add the Efficient Multiscale Attention Module (EMA) [24],

Lightweight Generalised Upsampling Operator (CARAFE) [25], Bidirectional Feature Pyramid Network (BiFPN) [19], and Spatial Depth Converted Convolution (SPDConv) [26] one by one to the YOLOv8 base network, and the improved network diagram is shown in Fig. 6.

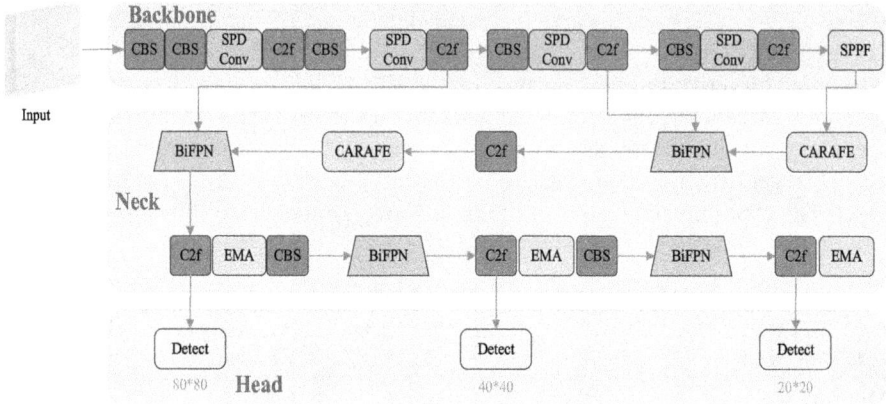

Fig. 6. Improved YOLOv8 network structure.

In this study, we adopt four key techniques to optimise vehicle detection in flooding scenarios: the EMA, CARAFE, BiFPN, and SPDConv. The EMA, as an attentional mechanism, is able to enhance the detection efficiency of small targets by optimising the information channel and reducing the computational overhead, especially when the target is partially occluded or of small size. The CARAFE, on the other hand, optimises feature continuity and detail through content aware up-sampling approach optimises the continuity and details of the features and improves the model's ability to distinguish between targets in complex environments. BiFPN, through its innovative feature fusion strategy, achieves an effective combination of features from different layers and enhances the model's ability to detect targets at different scales. Finally, SPDConv enhances the capture of spatial information by introducing spatial convolution, especially in the case where the target is partially occluded, to more accurately identify the edges and contours of the vehicle. Together, these techniques significantly improve the accuracy and efficiency of vehicle detection in flooding scenarios.

The results of the ablation experiments with the improved YOLOv8 model are shown in Table 3.

The baseline model YOLOv8s reached 0.68 in the mAP index. When we introduced EMA, the mAP was gradually increased to 0.689. Based on this, we introduced CARAFE, BiFPN and SPDConv one by one, and the mAP values were increased to 0.706, 0.694, and 0.724, respectively, which showed that each component had a positive effect. When we use the complete combination of EMA, CARAFE, BiFPN, and SPDConv, the mAP reaches up to 0.775, which is a 9.5% improvement compared to the baseline model.

Table 3. Ablation experiments with YOLOv8s as baseline

Method	EMA	CARAFE	BiFPN	SPDConv	mAP
Baseline	-	-	-	-	0.68
Ours	✓	-	-	-	0.689
	✓	✓	-	-	0.706
	✓	-	✓	-	0.694
	✓	-	-	✓	0.724
	✓	✓	✓	-	0.703
	✓	-	✓	✓	0.741
	✓	✓	✓	✓	0.775

Through the above ablation experiments, we validate the effectiveness of each component in improving the performance of the flooded vehicle detection model and demonstrate their potential in improving the accuracy of vehicle detection in complex scenarios. These findings provide a valuable reference for designing more efficient deep learning models in similar tasks in the future.

5 Future Challenges and Work

The proposed dataset has shown significant results in the application of vehicle hazard detection in flooded environments, however, the following challenges and improvement directions are worth further exploration:

(1) Balance of labelling classification: During the actual data labelling process, it is found that there is a significant gap between the number of samples in the first category of "safe" and the number of samples in the third category of "dangerous". Therefore, efforts should be made to reduce the difference between the number of samples in each category in the follow-up work.
(2) Response to complex environmental factors: Flooding is often accompanied by severe weather conditions such as cloudy skies or heavy rain, which brings challenges to the detection of water-related vehicles. Issues such as visual perception in low-light environments need to be addressed when assessing the hazard level of a vehicle, as well as improving the recognition ability in cases where the target is partially or completely obscured.
(3) Limitations of data collection: due to the difficulty of acquiring video surveillance data on urban roads, the number of video surveillance videos collected where flooding occurs is still relatively limited. In order to further improve the generalisation performance of the vehicle target detection model, it is necessary to collect more diverse video surveillance data.

6 Conclusion

In this paper, we investigate the key challenges of vehicle detection in flooding scenarios and propose a targeted dataset for flooded vehicle hazard level detection, aiming to fill the gaps of existing datasets in this specific context. By introducing a new dataset and improving the YOLOv8s algorithm, we conduct a series of ablation experiments on our home-built flooded vehicle detection dataset to evaluate the impact of different network components such as EMA, CARAFE, BiFPN and SPDConv. The experimental results show that the gradual addition of these components significantly improves the detection accuracy of the model, with the complete combination of configurations achieving the highest mAP value of 0.775, a 9.5% improvement over the baseline model. This result not only confirms the effectiveness of the components in improving vehicle detection performance in flooding scenarios, but also demonstrates their potential to improve vehicle detection accuracy in complex environments. Future work will focus on further optimising the model architecture and expanding the dataset to improve the generalisation ability and usefulness of the model in more complex scenarios.

Acknowledgments. This study was funded by the National Natural Science Foundation of China (Grant No. 62171042, 62102033), the R&D Program of Beijing Municipal Education Commission (Grant No. KZ202211417048), the Project of Construction and Support for high-level Innovative Teams of Beijing Municipal Institutions(Grant No. BPHR20220121), the National Key R&D Program of China (2022YFC3090603), the Beijing Natural Science Foundation(Grant No. 4232026, 4242020), the Academic Research Projects of Beijing Union University(No.ZKZD202302).

References

1. Tonne, C., Adair, L., Adlakha, D., et al.: Defining pathways to healthy sustainable urban development. Environ. Int. **146**, 106236 (2021)
2. Xiaotao, C., et al.: Evolutionary characteristics of flood risk and urban resilience enhancement strategies in changing environments. J. Water Resour. **53** (07), 757–768+778 (2022)
3. Zongxue, X.U., Chenlei, Y.E., Ruting, L.I.A.O.: Collaborative management of urban floods: research progress and application cases. Adv. Earth Sci. **38**(11), 1107–1120 (2023)
4. Kumar, V., Sharma, K.V., Caloiero, T., et al.: Comprehensive overview of flood modeling approaches: a review of recent advances. Hydrology **10**(7), 141 (2023)
5. Prakash, C., Barthwal, A., Acharya, D.: FLOODWALL: a real-time flash flood monitoring and forecasting system using IoT. IEEE Sens. J. **23**(1), 787–799 (2022)
6. Guofu, Z., et al.: Modelling and solution methods for dynamic scheduling problem of repair teams in disaster-affected road networks. Comput. Eng. **49**(06), 300–313 (2023)
7. Alam, F., Alam, T., Hasan, M.A., et al.: MEDIC: a multi-task learning dataset for disaster image classification. Neural Comput. Appl. **35**(3), 2609–2632 (2023)
8. Zhang, Y., Zhang, H., Huang, Q., et al.: DsP-YOLO: an anchor-free network with DsPAN for small object detection of multiscale defects. Expert Syst. Appl. **241**, 122669 (2024)
9. Li, C., Qu, Z., Wang, S., et al.: A method of cross-layer fusion multi-object detection and recognition based on improved faster R-CNN model in complex traffic environment. Pattern Recogn. Lett. **145**, 127–134 (2021)
10. Zhang, Y., Guo, Z., Wu, J., et al.: Real-time vehicle detection based on improved yolo v5. Sustainability **14**(19), 12274 (2022)

11. Dong, X., Yan, S., Duan, C.: A lightweight vehicles detection network model based on YOLOv5. Eng. Appl. Artif. Intell. **113**, 104914 (2022)
12. Pratama, V., et al.: Car detection over network using Yolov8 in forza horizon 4. In: 2023 17th International Conference on Telecommunication Systems, Services, and Applications (TSSA), 1–5. IEEE, 2023
13. Chen, Z., Guo, H., Yang, J., et al.: Fast vehicle detection algorithm in traffic scene based on improved SSD. Measurement **201**, 111655 (2022)
14. Lin, T Y., et al.: Microsoft coco: common objects in context. In: Computer Vision–ECCV 2014: 13th European Conference, Zurich, Switzerland, September 6-12, 2014, Proceedings, Part V 13. Springer International Publishing, 2014: 740-755. https://doi.org/10.1007/978-3-319-10602-1_48
15. Kuznetsova, A., Rom, H., Alldrin, N., et al.: The open images dataset v4: unified image classification, object detection, and visual relationship detection at scale. Int. J. Comput. Vision **128**(7), 1956–1981 (2020)
16. Geiger, A., Lenz, P., Stiller, C., et al.: Vision meets robotics: the kitti dataset. Int. J. Robot. Res. **32**(11), 1231–1237 (2013)
17. Yu, F., et al. Bdd100k: A diverse driving dataset for heterogeneous multitask learning. In: Proceedings of the IEEE/CVF Conference on Computer Vision and Pattern Recognition, 2636–2645 (2020)
18. Weikun, L., Linhui, W., Dian, Z., et al.: Mars surface image segmentation dataset and performance evaluation. Comput. Eng. **49**(05), 262–268 (2023)
19. Tan, M., Pang, R., Le, Q V.: Efficientdet: scalable and efficient object detection. In: Proceedings of the IEEE/CVF Conference on Computer Vision and Pattern Recognition, 10781–10790 (2020)
20. Rezatofighi, H., et al.: Generalized intersection over union: a metric and a loss for bounding box regression. In: Proceedings of the IEEE/CVF Conference on Computer Vision and Pattern Recognition, 658–666 (2019)
21. Ren, S., et al.: Faster r-cnn: towards real-time object detection with region proposal networks. Adv. Neural Inf. Process. Syst. 28 (2015)
22. Cai, Z., Vasconcelos, N.: Cascade R-CNN: high quality object detection and instance segmentation. IEEE Trans. Pattern Anal. Mach. Intell. **43**(5), 1483–1498 (2019)
23. He, K., et al.: Mask r-cnn. In: Proceedings of the IEEE International Conference on Computer Vision, 2961–2969 (2017)
24. Ouyang, D., et al.: Efficient multi-scale attention module with cross-spatial learning. In: ICASSP 2023–2023 IEEE International Conference on Acoustics, Speech and Signal Processing (ICASSP), 1–5. IEEE, 2023
25. Wang, J., et al.: Carafe: Content-aware reassembly of features. In: Proceedings of the IEEE/CVF International Conference on Computer Vision, 3007–3016 (2019)
26. Sunkara, R., Luo, T.: No more strided convolutions or pooling: a new CNN building block for low-resolution images and small objects. In: Joint European Conference on Machine Learning and Knowledge Discovery in Databases. Cham: Springer Nature Switzerland, 443–459, (2022). https://doi.org/10.1007/978-3-031-26409-2_27

Convergence and Divergence: A New Paradigm for Pedestrian Detection

Yueyan Zhu[1], Hai Huang[1,2(✉)], Shan Yue[1], Shu Zhang[1], and Aoran Chen[1]

[1] School of Information and Communication Engineering, Beijing University of Posts and Telecommunications, Beijing 100876, China
`huanghai@bupt.edu.cn`
[2] Key Laboratory of Interactive Technology and Experience System, Ministry of Culture and Tourism, Beijing 100876, China

Abstract. Complex backgrounds, scale and occlusion variance have long limited the accuracy of pedestrian detection. In this paper, we propose a pedestrian detector named Convergence and Divergence (CADNet). In "Convergence" network, we propose a cross-scale semantic alignment block (CSAB). CSAB effectively mitigates the background interference and resolves scale variance through multi-scale global contexts aggregation, without extensive computational overhead. In "Divergence" network, we propose a receptive field differentiation block (RFDB) to tackle the challenges of scale and occlusion variance. RFDB generates discriminative features with varying receptive fields, effectively capturing pedestrians across different scales and occlusion conditions. Due to the effectiveness of the proposed components, CADNet achieves an excellent performance of 8.47% and 2.16% MR^{-2} on a Reasonable subset of CityPersons and Caltech, respectively. Extensive experiments demonstrate the robustness and efficiency of CADNet, ensuring its superior performance in various scenarios.

Keywords: Object Detection · Pedestrian Detection · Cross-scale Semantic Alignment · Receptive Field Differentiation

1 Introduction

Computer vision has traditionally struggled with pedestrian detection. In intelligent transportation, pedestrian detection serves as an initial step. Traditional methods, relying on hand-crafted features, struggle to accurately detect pedestrians. The introduction of convolutional neural networks (CNNs) has yielded significant advancements. However, there still remains scope for enhancement in pedestrian detection.

Pedestrian detection has encountered limitations due to complex backgrounds, scale variance and occlusion variance, as shown in Fig. 1. Firstly, the complex background hinders detectors from learning discriminative features. The diverse attire worn by pedestrians, coupled with the inconsistency of low-level features, like color and texture, renders

---

Y. Zhu, H. Huang and S. Yue—Contribute equally to this work.

the reliance on these features for detection problematic. The semantic feature of pedestrians is appearance shape. However, objects such as trees and signage often exhibit shapes similar to human body and can interfere with detectors. It is crucial to weaken the background while strengthening the pedestrian's features. Some researchers leverage semantic labels or vision-language semantics to alleviate interference from surrounding context (e.g., [6, 11]). Whereas, this approach necessitates manual labeling efforts and computational overhead. Secondly, scale variance leads to inconsistent feature representations, with small-scale pedestrians often appearing as rectangular contours, lack of specific details. While large-scale pedestrians exhibit distinct body structures, such as heads and limbs. Previous approaches, such as [4], attempt to enhance feature details for small-scale pedestrians through feature fusion or super-resolution. These methods can not effectively address the issue of feature discrepancies caused by scale variance. Moreover, occlusion variance intensifies the problem of inconsistent features. The shape of pedestrians is relatively uniform when unobstructed. Its width is about 0.41 times of height. Whereas, occlusion results in the invisibility of certain body structures, altering their aspect ratios. Although several studies (e.g., [9, 21]) try to tackle occlusion problem, they still face challenges of intra-class discrepancies among pedestrians in heterogeneous occlusion scenarios. The diverse scales and shapes contribute to intra-class discrepancies, leading to degradation in detector performance.

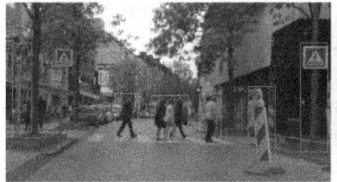 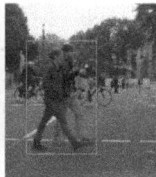 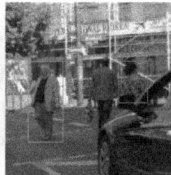

(a) Complex backgrounds   (b) Scale variance (c) Occlusion variance

Fig. 1. Examples of complex backgrounds, scale variance and occlusion variance. The area in the red box are objects that the detector tends to misrecognize.

In this paper, we propose a pedestrian detector, named convergence and divergence (CADNet). CADNet comprises 3 components, namely feature extract, feature convergence and feature divergence network. We use HRNet-W32 as the feature extraction network to enhance the feature details of small-scale pedestrians. For feature convergence network, we propose a cross-scale semantic alignment block (CSAB). Benefiting from recursive lightweight attention, CSAB effectively aggregates and reconfigures global contexts, thereby mitigating the interference of complex backgrounds without requiring semantic labeling or extensive computation. Natural images inherently exhibit cross-scale feature correlation. Leveraging this prior knowledge, CSAB expand the context from single scale to a multi-scale aspect through cross-scale feature-wise affinity. The established cross-scale convergence of features effectively addresses the scale variance issue. For feature divergence network, we propose a receptive field differentiation block (RFDB). Scale and occlusion discrepancy gives rise to diverse pedestrian patterns, necessitating the network to generate features that accurately capture these variations. RFDB generates a series of features with varying receptive fields by matching and combining multiple-branch convolutional layers, providing flexibility in receptive field shapes and diverse feature selection. Employing a two-layer and cross-branch design, RFDB enables feature reuse and multi-path fusion. Compared to traditional directly-connected multi-branch structure, RFDB achieves the same receptive field combinations with fewer model parameters and facilitates network learning.

Conclusively, this paper makes three contributions:

- We propose a cross-scale semantic alignment block (CSAB) to leverage dense contextual information across multiple scales and globally.
- We propose a receptive field differentiation block (RFDB) to generate a flexible and extensive feature selections to recognize pedestrians with intra-class disparities.
- Extensive experiments demonstrates that CADNet exhibits remarkable robustness and efficiency, ensuring its superior performance across various scenarios.

2 Related Work

2.1 Cross-Scale Visual Attention

Cross-scale visual attention has garnered significant attention across numerous study fields. CrossViT [1] comprises a dual-branch transformer that combines image patches of varying sizes to aid in the learning of multi-scale feature representations. CS-NL [15] is applied to image super resolution. It establishes a mapping between high and low resolution images through the inherent cross-scale feature correlation property in natural images. SMFE [20] introduces multi-scale deformable attention to pedestrian detection, aiming to explore its effectiveness in single-stage object detectors.

2.2 Adaptive Receptive Fields

There are two main approaches to form adaptive receptive fields, parallel multi-branch fusion and attention-based linear combination. RFBNet [12] uses multi-branch convolution to model the magnitude and eccentricity of RFs in human visual systems. SKNet [10], on the other hand, employs softmax attention to combine many branches with varied kernel size. This dynamic selection mechanism allows each neuron to modify its receptive field size based on various input information scales. ODConv [7] utilizes a multi-dimensional attention mechanism to learn a linear combination of convolutional kernels and weight them with input-dependent attention to expand the receptive field.

3 Method

3.1 Overview

The overall architecture of CADNet is illustrated in Fig. 2. CADNet comprises 3 components, feature extraction, feature convergence and feature divergence network. To effectively exploit the features of small-scale pedestrians, we employ HRNet-W32 [18] as the feature extract network. The 4 feature maps extracted from backbone are fed into the cross-scale semantic alignment block (CSAB). CSAB establishes feature correlations between multi-scale pedestrians and aggregates multi-scale contextual information through a cross-scale spatial attention mechanism. Processed by CSAB, the feature maps are concatenated for feature fusion. The fused feature map is then fed to the detection head. The detection head consists of three branches that predict the center, scale, and offset of pedestrians. The receptive field differentiation block (RFDB) is integrated in the center branch to facilitate locating pedestrians. During inference, the predictions of center, scale, and offset are combined to generate the detection results.

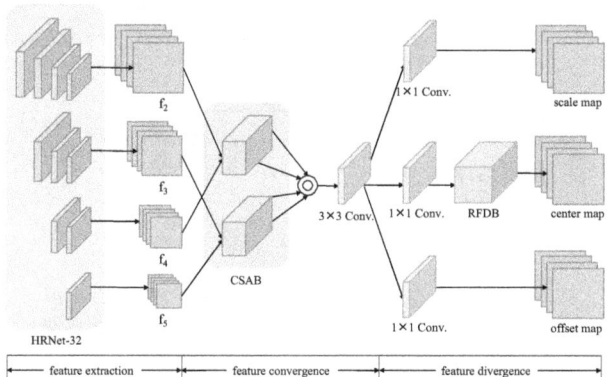

Fig. 2. The overall network architecture of CADNet.

3.2 Cross-Scale Semantic Alignment Block (CSAB)

The performance of pedestrian detectors is limited by the feature quality, both locally and globally. We propose a cross-scale semantic alignment block (CSAB) in the feature convergence network. The CSAB facilitates establishing feature correlations between cross-scale pedestrians and selectively integrates contexts based on a spatial attention map. Contexts and non-local features play a pivotal role in object detection, and CSAB extends their utilization to cross-scale, complementing non-local aggregation on the scale level. By effectively enhancing the feature self-similarity among multi-scale pedestrians, CSAB generates robust features to enhance the detector's performance.

Processing by the feature extraction network, 4 feature maps, denoted as f_2, f_3, f_4, and f_5 are output. The non-local computation [19], though effective, introduces space complexity due to dense feature sampling. To address this challenge, CADNet employs a two-by-two grouping strategy. Instead of performing simultaneous computations, it adopts a recursive sequential approach. This strategy forms two feature map pairs without concurrent computation, as illustrated in Fig. 3. Cross-scale attention is calculated between each pair of feature maps. During iter1, f_2 and f_3 form one pair, while f_4 and f_5 constitute another. This generates fused feature maps f_2' and f_3', f_4' and f_5'. In iter2, f_2' and f_5', with f_3' and f_4', are utilized as new pairs. This computation is conducted recursively, then outputs f_2'' and f_5'', f_3'' and f_4''. In iter3, f_2'' and f_4'' are paired together, while f_3'' and f_5'' form another pair, leading to the final output: $f_2''' \ f_3''' \ f_4'''$, and f_5'''.

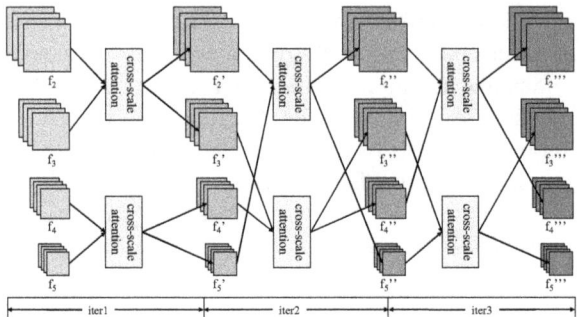

(a) The feature map grouping strategy during the 3 iters of CSAB.

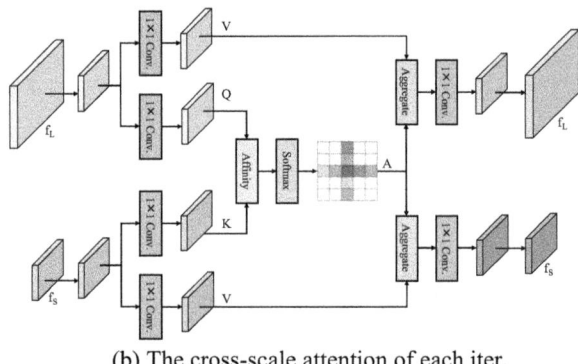

(b) The cross-scale attention of each iter.

Fig. 3. The network architecture of the cross-scale semantic alignment block (CSAB).

The cross-scale attention module is illustrated as Fig. 3. The large-scale feature map, denoted as f_L, serves as the query Q. The small-scale feature map, denoted as f_S, serves as the key K. Both feature maps are concurrently utilized as the value V. To enable affinity operations, the feature maps are resized by downsampling. Then, affinity is performed between Q and K to derive the attention map. A softmax layer is then applied to normalize the attention weights. This normalized attention map A is then used to guide feature aggregation with V. Then a 1×1 convolution is applied for feature reconfiguration. Afterward, f_L and f_S are reinstated to its original scales. Each attention computation focuses on aggregating contexts along criss-cross path, and through two recursive computations, contextual information is gathered for all pixels across the entire map [5]. This approach enables efficient aggregation of contextual information for each pixel across multiple scales while minimizing memory consumption.

After 3 iters, feature map $f_i \in \{f_2, f_3' f_4' f_5\}$ is semantically fused with other feature maps$\{f_j\}5\ j = 2, j \neq i$. This fusion ensures cross-scale information effectively integrated. For example, f_2 was fused with f_3 in iter1, and the output f_2' and f_3' both fused the contexts on the criss-cross paths of f_3. On this basis, f_3' was subjected to context aggregation with f_4' in iter2, and the output f_3'' and f_4'' still contain the contexts of f_3. Finally, f_2'' and f_4'' with f_3 features are computed in iter3, and a second recursive computation can aggregate the full context of f_3. The recursive pairwise computation allows the context of the initial feature map to pass along with the iterative computation, effectively generating a multi-scale attention pool. And it does not bring a large computational burden.

3.3 Receptive Field Differentiation Block (RFDB)

To mitigate the intra-class discrepancy caused by scale and occlusion variance, RFDB performs discriminative feature differentiation for pedestrians with various geometric structures. By matching and grouping, six convolutional branches with different receptive fields are formed. The advantage of RFDB is two-fold: 1) Constructing flexible receptive fields to extract pedestrian features of varying scales and occlusions. 2) Reusing shared features to jointly optimize parameters and save computational costs.

In RFDB, there are two stages of convolutional layers, as illustrated in Fig. 4. The multiplexing stage contains 2 branches, 3×1 and 5×3 general convolutions, respectively. A 1×1 convolutional layer is integrated to reduce the number of channels. The differentiation stage contains 3 branches of dilated convolutional layers. The convolutional kernels are 1×1, 3×3, and 3×3, and the dilation rates are set to 1×1, 2×1, and 3×1, respectively. The dilated convolution can be equivalent to a general convolution of size 1×1, 5×3, and 7×3, but with fewer parameters. The multiplexing stage generates two feature maps, which are fed to the differentiation stage to perform feature differentiation, ultimately generating 6 feature maps with heterogeneous receptive fields. The output 6 feature maps are concatenated and fed to 1×1 convolutional layer. A shortcut branch is added to facilitate gradient propagation. For computational simplicity, we replace large convolutions by stacking multiple small convolutions (e.g., 3×3).

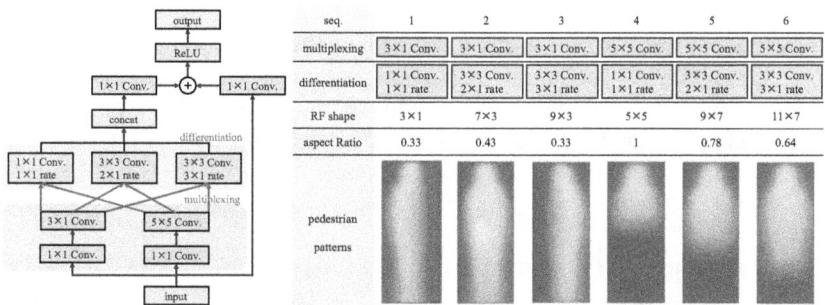

(a) The network architecture of RFDB. (b) The illustration of different receptive fields shapes.

Fig. 4. The network architecture of receptive field differentiation block (RFDB) and illustration of different receptive fields shapes. Pedestrian patterns are from the analysis of [22].

Based on statistics and analysis on pedestrian data [3, 22], it is known that about 80% of pedestrians have a maximum scale variance of 3 times. Having about 10 occlusion patterns, about 94% of pedestrians have aspects ratios from 0.3 to 1.0. By matching and combining the branches of the multiplexing and differentiation stages, we construct flexible convolutional combinations to generate receptive fields of various scales and aspects ratios, which are consistent with the scale and occlusion discrepancies of pedestrian data, as shown in the Fig. 4.

The multiplexing stage forms two shapes of receptive fields and generates reusable features for the differentiation stage. By effectively leveraging the output of the multiplexing stage, RFDB establishes a mechanism for information exchange and feature sharing, allowing for joint optimization of parameters. Typically, generating 6 parallel feature maps would necessitate 6 convolutional branches. While, RFDB's feature reuse mechanism enhances computational efficiency. By utilizing 3 × 3 general and dilated convolutions, RFDB only requires 6 convolutional layers to create 6 distinct receptive fields. In contrast, traditional multi-scale structure, for the same receptive fields, necessitates a six-way branching structure, totaling 18 layers of 3 × 3 convolution.

4 Experiments

4.1 Experiment Settings

Datasets. We evaluate CADNet on two datasets, Caltech [3] and CityPersons [22]. The Caltech dataset comprises approximately 10 h of video of urban scene. The frames of the video are partitioned into a training set, containing 42,500 images, and a validation set, including 4,024 images. The CityPersons dataset is a widely used benchmark. It includes 5,000 images captured from urban scenes, of which 2,975 images are allocated for training, 500 images for validation, and 1,525 images for testing.

Evaluation Metrics. We evaluate the performance using the evaluation criterion of Caltech evaluation measure [3], which is the log-average miss rate (MR-2) over false positive per image (FPPI) ranging from 10–2 to 100, denoted as MR-2. The lower MR-2 values indicate higher performance.

Implementation Details. For training, we employ the Adam optimizer, with $\beta 1$ and $\beta 2$ are set to 0.9 and 0.999. The initial learning rate is set to 1×10^{-4}. On Caltech, we use 8 NVIDIA A40 GPUs to train the network, with 16 images per GPU. Training is stopped after 10K iterations. On CityPersons, we use 2 NVIDIA A5000 GPUs, with 4 images per GPU. Training is stoped after 37.5K iterations.

4.2 Comparision with the State-Of-The-Art

CityPersons. We present the experimental results on CityPersons in Table 1. The results with best performance are highlighted in red. The results of the baseline method CSP are highlighted in green. CADNet achieves the outperformance in the Reasonable, Partial, and Small subsets. Compared to detectors designed for heavily occlusion, e.g., OAFNet, BGCNet, CADNet's performance in Heavy is impressive. Compared to VLPD and SOLIDER, CADNet does not leverage additional contextual and semantic labels. Compared to the baseline CSP, CADNet has performance improvement on all subsets, which demonstrates the effectiveness of CSAB and RFDB proposed. To visualize the performance of CADNet, we plot the detection results in Fig. 5 and compare them with CSP. It can be seen that CADNet has fewer false positives.

Caltech. We present the experimental results on Caltech, as shown in Table 2. The results with best performance are highlighted in red. The results of the baseline method CSP are highlighted in green. CADNet achieves MR-2 values of 2.16%, 51.47% and 38.31% on the Reasonable, All, and Occ subsets, respectively. CADNet outperforms existing methods in the Reasonable and All subsets. It performs slightly inferior to VLPD in the Occ subset, while VLPD leverages explicit semantic labels. Compared with baseline method CSP, CADNet achieves improvements in all subsets. The performance enhancement indicates that CADNet exhibits robust performance and the ability to facilitate detection in various scenarios.

Table 1. The performance comparison with other state-of-the-art methods on CityPersons dataset. Reason. is short for Reasonable. Med. is short for Medium.

Method	Backbone	Reason.	Heavy	Partial	Bare	Small	Med.	Large
FRCNN[22]	VGG-16	15.4	-	-	-	25.6	7.2	7.9
FRCNN+Seg[22]	VGG-16	14.8	-	-	-	22.6	6.7	8.0
OR-CNN[23]	VGG-16	12.8	-	-	-	-	-	-
TLL+MRF[16]	ResNet-50	14.4	52.0	15.9	9.2	-	-	-
ALFNet[13]	ResNet-50	12.0	51.9	11.4	8.4	19.0	5.7	6.6
CSP[14]	ResNet-50	11.0	49.3	10.4	7.3	16.0	3.7	6.5
BGCNet[8]	HRNet-W32	8.8	43.9	8.0	6.1	11.6	2.6	5.3
APD[21]	DLA-34	8.8	46.6	8.3	5.8	-	-	-
SMFE[20]	ResNet-50	10.9	38.6	-	-	-	-	-
OAFNet[9]	HRNet-W32	9.4	43.1	8.3	5.6	-	-	-
VLPD[11]	ResNet-50	9.4	43.1	8.8	6.1	-	-	-
SOLIDER[2]	Swin-B	9.7	39.4	-	-	-	-	-
CADNet(ours)	HRNet-W32	8.47	42.91	7.26	5.90	10.35	2.89	5.14

Table 2. The performance comparison with other state-of-the-art methods on Caltech dataset.

Method	Reasonable	All	Occ.
FRCNN[22]	8.7	62.6	53.1
OR-CNN[23]	4.1	58.8	45.0
ALFNet[13]	6.1	51.9	51.0
CSP[14]	4.5	56.9	45.8
BGCNet[8]	4.1	-	42.0
SMPD[6]	4.2	55.2	44.8
SMFE[20]	3.7	57.0	42.8
VLPD[11]	2.3	52.4	37.7
CADNet(ours)	2.16	51.47	38.31

4.3 Ablation Study

Component Evaluation. Ablation experiments are conducted on the CityPersons dataset to validate the component effectiveness. The experiments results are shown in Table 3. The optimal results are highlighted in red. The baseline uses ResNet-50 as the feature extraction network, and we replace with HRNet-W32. This improvement in performance is achieved on all 4 subsets. We integrate CSAB into the feature convergence network for cross-scale contextual semantic fusion. Experimental results show that CSAB reduces the MR^{-2} by 0.68%, 1.44%, 0.88%, and 0.32% in Reasonable, Heavy, Partial, and Bare subsets, respectively. It indicates the generality and effectiveness of CSAB. The introduction of RFDB enhances performance on all subsets. Especially on Heavy, RFDB brings significant improvement of 1.96% MR^{-2}. It demonstrates that RFDB effectively balances the intra-class variation caused by occlusion.

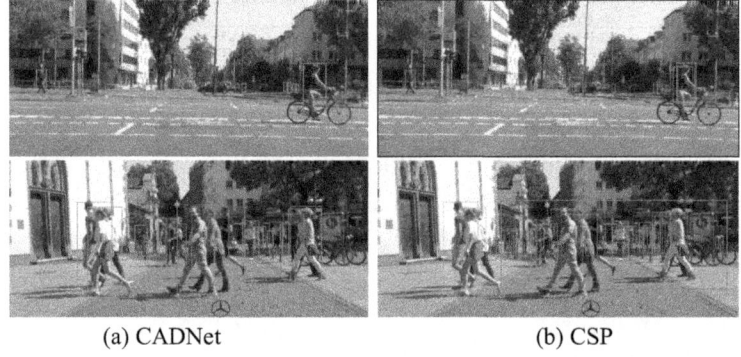

Fig. 5. The visualization of the detection results of CADNet and CSP.

Table 3. Ablation experiments on CityPersons dataset. Reason. is short for Reasonable.

Method	Backbone	CSAB	RFDB	Reason.	Heavy	Partial	Bare
Baseline	ResNet-50			10.90	48.73	10.15	7.22
CADNet	HRNet-W32			9.58	46.31	8.81	6.36
CADNet	HRNet-W32	✓		8.90	44.87	7.93	6.04
CADNet	HRNet-W32	✓	✓	8.47	42.91	7.26	5.90

Feature Map Grouping Strategy in CSAB. We explore the performance of different feature map grouping strategy in CSAB. Firstly, we evaluate the effectiveness of aggregating global contexts by performing criss-cross attention [5]. For this evaluation, we do not perform cross-scale operations, only single-scale self-attention. Experimental results are shown in the first row of Table 4, and "$f_i f_j$" indicates that f_i and f_j form a pair for contextual feature fusion, and (•) denotes one recursive iteration. Compared with baseline, the introduction of contexts brings performance improvement. Then, we evaluate the performance of cross-scale context fusion, as shown in Table 4. The experimental results show that in iter1, the optimal grouping is pairing f_2f_3 and f_4f_5. In iter2, the best configuration is grouping f_2f_5 and f_3f_4. In iter3, the best grouping is pairing f_2f_4 and f_3f_5. CADNet demonstrates performance enhancements on the Small and Reasonable, underscoring the significance of cross-scale contextual semantic fusion. Some of the grouping strategies fail to outperform, probably due to large gap of scale, which complicates feature similarity computation and hinders feature convergence.

Receptive Field Shapes in RFDB. To verify the effectiveness of RFDB, we conduct ablation experiments as shown in Table 5. Compared to RFB and P-RFB, which are also designed by the receptive fields concept, RFDB creates flexibility of receptive fields with less computation through the cross-combination of convolutional layers. The integration of RFDB achieves an MR^{-2} of 8.47% on Reasonable, also achieving excellent performance on other subsets. In contrast, RFB employs a square convolutional kernel and lacks a pedestrian-specific design, resulting in subpar performance. P-RFB falls short of RFDB in addressing heavily occluded pedestrians on Heavy subset. This may be because P-RFB's receptive fields adhere to a single aspect ratio, lack of diversity. These findings underscore the importance of flexible and comprehensive receptive field combinations in enhancing pedestrian detection performance.

Table 4. Ablation experiments of various grouping configurations in 3 iters.

Feature Map Pairs in 3 iters	Reasonable	Heavy	Small
$(f_2f_2, f_3f_3, f_4f_4, f_5f_5) \to (f_2f_2, f_3f_3, f_4f_4, f_5f_5)$	9.16	45.92	12.71
$(f_2f_5, f_3f_4) \to (f_2f_3, f_4f_5) \to (f_2f_4, f_3f_5)$	9.21	46.20	12.38
$(f_2f_5, f_3f_4) \to (f_2f_4, f_3f_5) \to (f_2f_3, f_4f_5)$	9.11	46.34	11.79
$(f_2f_4, f_3f_5) \to (f_2f_3, f_4f_5) \to (f_2f_5, f_3f_4)$	8.95	45.42	11.36
$(f_2f_4, f_3f_5) \to (f_2f_5, f_3f_4) \to (f_2f_3, f_4f_5)$	9.07	45.13	11.85
$(f_2f_3, f_4f_5) \to (f_2f_4, f_3f_5) \to (f_2f_5, f_3f_4)$	8.95	44.71	10.94
$(f_2f_3, f_4f_5) \to (f_2f_5, f_3f_4) \to (f_2f_4, f_3f_5)$	8.90	44.87	10.75

Table 5. Ablation experiments of receptive field shapes. Reason. is short for Reasonable.

Method	Receptive Field Shapes	Reason.	Heavy	Partial	Bare
RFB	(3×3),(9×9),(15×15)	8.65	43.85	7.62	5.95
P-RFB	(3×1),(7×3),(11×5)	8.53	44.36	7.43	6.01
RFDB(ours)	(3×1),(7×3),(9×3),(5×5),(9×7),(11×7)	8.47	42.91	7.26	5.90

5 Conclusion

In this paper, we introduce CADNet, a pedestrian detection method proposed to tackle the challenges posed by complex backgrounds, scale and occlusion variance. CADNet comprises 3 components: feature extraction, feature convergence, and feature divergence network. In the feature convergence network, we propose a cross-scale semantic alignment block, CSAB. This module aggregates contexts and non-local features across multi-scales, providing a comprehensive view for the detector. By establishing feature correlations, CSAB ensures feature consistency across scales. In the feature divergence network, we propose a receptive field differentiation block, RFDB. RFDB generates a series of feature maps with various receptive fields by combining multiple-branch convolutional layers. This module extracts diverse patterns to capture pedestrians of different scales and occlusion conditions. Extensive experiments conducted on the Caltech and CityPersons datasets demonstrate the robustness and effectiveness of CADNet.

Acknowledgments. This work was supported by the National Key R&D Program of China under Grant 2022YFF0904300.

References

1. Chen, C.F.R., Fan, Q., Panda, R.: Crossvit: cross-attention multi-scale vision transformer for image classification. In: ICCV, pp. 347–356 (2021)
2. Chen, W., et al.: Beyond appearance: a semantic controllable self-supervised learning frame work for human-centric visual tasks. In: CVPR, pp. 15050–15061 (2023)
3. Dollár, P., Wojek, C., Schiele, B., et al.: Pedestrian detection: an evaluation of the state of the art. IEEE Trans. Pattern Anal. Mach. Intell. **34**(4), 743–761 (2012)
4. Hsu, W.Y., Chen, P.C.: Pedestrian detection using stationary wavelet dilated residual super-resolution. IEEE Trans. Instrum. Meas. **71**, 1–11 (2022)
5. Huang, Z., et al.: Ccnet: criss-cross attention for semantic segmentation. In: ICCV, pp. 603–612 (2019)
6. Jiang, H., Liao, S., Li, J., et al.: Urban scene based semantical modulation for pedestrian detection. Neurocomputing **474**, 1–12 (2022)
7. Li, C., Zhou, A., Yao, A.: Omni-dimensional dynamic convolution. In: ICLR (2022)
8. Li, J., et al.: Box guided convolution for pedestrian detection. In: ACM MM, pp. 1615–1624 (2020)
9. Li, Q., Su, Y., Gao, Y., et al.: Oaf-net: an occlusion-aware anchor-free network for pedestrian detection in a crowd. IEEE Trans. Intell. Transp. Syst. **23**(11), 21291–21300 (2022)
10. Li, X., et al.: Selective kernel networks. In: CVPR, pp. 510–519 (2019)
11. Liu, M., et al.: Vlpd: context-aware pedestrian detection via vision-language semantic self-supervision. In: CVPR, pp. 6662–6671 (2023)
12. Liu, S., Huang, D., Wang, Y.: Receptive field block net for accurate and fast object detection. In: Ferrari, V., Hebert, M., Sminchisescu, C., Weiss, Y. (eds.) ECCV 2018. LNCS, vol. 11215, pp. 404–419. Springer, Cham (2018). https://doi.org/10.1007/978-3-030-01252-6_24
13. Liu, W., Liao, S., Weidong, H., Liang, X., Chen, X.: Learning efficient single-stage pedestrian detectors by asymptotic localization fitting. In: Ferrari, V., Hebert, M., Sminchisescu, C., Weiss, Y. (eds.) Computer Vision – ECCV 2018: 15th European Conference, Munich, Germany, September 8–14, 2018, Proceedings, Part XIV, pp. 643–659. Springer International Publishing, Cham (2018). https://doi.org/10.1007/978-3-030-01264-9_38

14. Liu, W., et al.: High-level semantic feature detection: a new perspective for pedestrian detection. In: CVPR, pp. 5182–5191 (2019)
15. Mei, Y., et al.: Image super-resolution with cross-scale non-local attention and exhaustive self-exemplars mining. In: CVPR, pp. 5689–5698 (2020)
16. Song, T., Sun, L., Xie, D., Sun, H., Shiliang, P.: Small-Scale Pedestrian Detection Based on Topological Line Localization and Temporal Feature Aggregation. In: Ferrari, V., Hebert, M., Sminchisescu, C., Weiss, Y. (eds.) Computer Vision – ECCV 2018: 15th European Conference, Munich, Germany, September 8–14, 2018, Proceedings, Part VII, pp. 554–569. Springer International Publishing, Cham (2018). https://doi.org/10.1007/978-3-030-01234-2_33
17. Tan, Y., et al.: Prf-ped: multi-scale pedestrian detector with prior-based receptive field. In: ICPR, pp. 6059–6064 (2020)
18. Wang, J., Sun, K., Cheng, T., et al.: Deep high-resolution representation learning for visual recognition. IEEE Trans. Pattern Anal. Mach. Intell. **43**, 3349–3364 (2021)
19. Wang, X., Girshick, R., Gupta, A., He, K.: Non-local neural networks. In: CVPR, pp. 7794–7803 (2018)
20. Yuan, J., Panagiotis, B., Stathaki, T.: Effectiveness of vision transformer for fast and accurate single-stage pedestrian detection. In: NIPS. (2022)
21. Zhang, J., Lin, L., Zhu, J., et al.: Attribute-aware pedestrian detection in a crowd. IEEE Trans. Multimedia **23**, 3085–3097 (2021)
22. Zhang, S., Benenson, R., Schiele, B.: Citypersons: a diverse dataset for pedestrian detection. In: CVPR, pp. 4457–4465 (2017)
23. Zhang, S., Wen, L., Bian, X., Lei, Z., Li, S.Z.: Occlusion-aware R-CNN: detecting pedestrians in a crowd. In: Ferrari, V., Hebert, M., Sminchisescu, C., Weiss, Y. (eds.) Computer Vision – ECCV 2018: 15th European Conference, Munich, Germany, September 8–14, 2018, Proceedings, Part III, pp. 657–674. Springer International Publishing, Cham (2018). https://doi.org/10.1007/978-3-030-01219-9_39

Improved YOLOv8-Based Lightweight Object Detection on Drone Images

Maoxiang Jiang, Zhanjun Si(✉), Ke Yang, and Yingxue Zhang

College of Artificial Intelligence, Tianjin University of Science and Technology, Tianjin 300457, China
szj@tust.edu.cn

Abstract. The target detection task of drones requires lightweight algorithms to fully utilize limited resources. Therefore, this paper proposes the YOLOv8-LD model. Firstly, propose the ASBiFPN neck network; Secondly, improve the detection head. Once again, introduce MPDIoU and improve the classification loss function to address the issue of imbalanced data samples. Finally, using pruning algorithms significantly reduces model volume. Improved YOLOv8-LD model in the VisDrone2019 dataset mAP@0.5 Improved by 21%. After pruning, compared with YOLOv8, the model parameters decreased by 81% and the volume decreased by 67%, mAP@0.5 increase by 3%.

Keywords: Object detection · Feature fusion · Pruning · YOLOv8

1 Introduction

In target detection tasks in drone scenarios, due to changes in viewpoint and height, the images in the scene contain the following features, there are many objects of different sizes, with small targets being the majority; The dense arrangement of objects; Lighting issues and complex background structures in images. The significance of the lightweight model is to enable UAVs to efficiently and effectively perform real-time multi-target detection, which is particularly important for missions such as aerial photography, surveillance and search and rescue [1]. A one-stage detector refers to predicting the position and category of the target directly from the input image, usually through dense anchor points or prior boxes for object detection. The advantage of one-stage detectors lies in real-time performance. Alam et al. [2] shift computational tasks from embedded processors to the cloud, alleviating computational pressure. Zhu et al. [3] proposed the TPH-YOLOv5 algorithm. Shao Y et al. [4] proposed target detection of UAV aerial images based on Aero-YOLO. Modern drones are equipped with high-performance processors with abundant computing resources, which deploy YOLO based object detection algorithms for real-time detection, recognition, and classification of task targets when the drone collects data. Even high-performance processors have inherent limitations, especially in terms of resource availability.

2 The Proposed Algorithm

2.1 YOLOv8-LD

This study chose YOLOv8 as the benchmark model. YOLOv8 is the latest version of the YOLO series algorithm. This paper proposes a lightweight object detection algorithm YOLOv8-LD (YOLOv8 Lightweight Target Detection Algorithm in UAV Scene) network for unmanned aerial vehicle scenarios, as shown in Fig. 1.

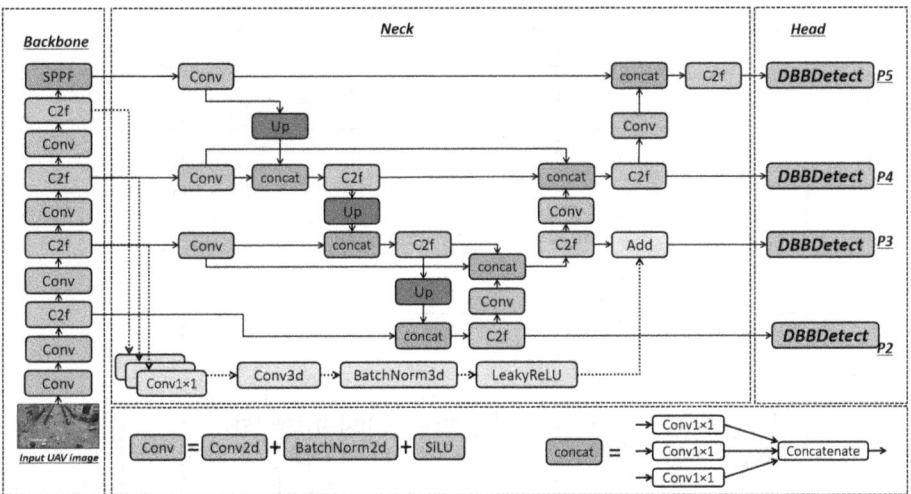

Fig. 1. Network chart of YOLOv8-LD

2.2 Improvement of the Neck Network

After passing through the backbone network, low-level features contain more positional and detailed information, while higher-level features have stronger linguistic information. How to further process and optimize features at different levels is crucial. In paper [5], different popular neck structures are described, as shown in Fig. 2. (a), (b), and (c).

Inspired by the neck network design of BiFPN and ASF-YOLO [6], We propose the ASBiFPN (A Specialized Shape Bidirectional Feature Pyramid Network for Small Target Detection) neck network structure, as shown in Fig. 2. (d) shown. We add detection heads for small targets in ASBiFPN. P4 and P5 are converted to channel number by 1 × 1 convolution, resized to the same size as P3 using interpolation operation, and spliced in the P3 dimension. The new feature maps are processed by passing them sequentially through 3D convolution, batch normalization layer and activation function, downscaled by 3D maximum pooling layer, compressed in the second dimension, and finally superimposed with the P3 detection layer. This approach exploits the application of 3D convolution in feature fusion in the target detection task, where the fused features can act directly on the P3 detection head by superimposing low-level features with semantic information and high-level features with more spatial information. The structure of the feature connection method used in this paper is shown as concat in Fig. 1. The feature mapping is added directly to the spatial and channel dimensions, which helps in the detection of small targets.

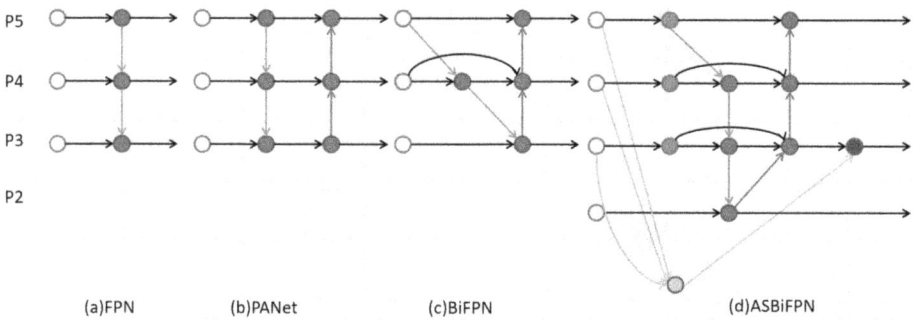

Fig. 2. Feature fusion method

2.3 Improved Detection Head

To improve the performance of convolutional neural networks, DBB convolution is introduced to form the DBBDetect module, as shown in Fig. 3. DBB(Diverse Branch Block) [7] module uses a structure-heavy parameterized design with a multi-branch topology, where each branch mainly consists of a 1×1 convolution, a 3×3 convolution, an average pooling (AVG), and a bulk normalization (BN) layer. The expressive power of a single convolution is enhanced by combining branches of different sizes and complexity (including tandem convolution, multi-scale convolution, and average pooling layers).

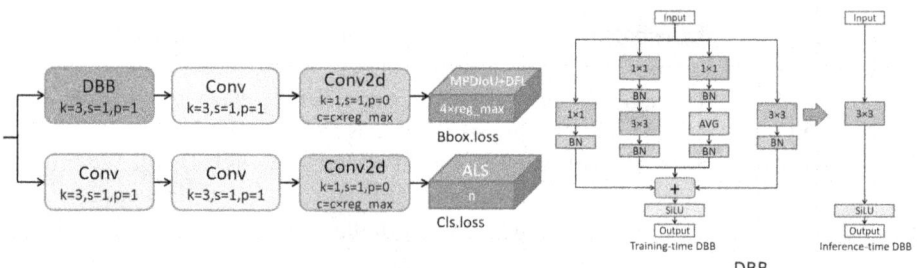

Fig. 3. DBBDetect

2.4 Improvement of the Loss Function

In target detection tasks in drone scenarios, difficult samples are relatively sparse, and samples near the boundaries often suffer significant losses. Reference [8] proposed Slide-Loss to solve this problem. Samples with values less than μ are assigned a negative label, while those with values greater than μ are assigned a positive label, as shown in Fig. 4.

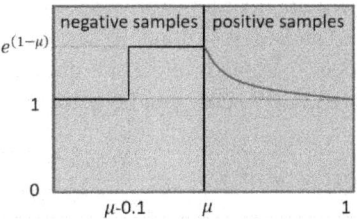

Fig. 4. Slide Loss

In order to enable the model to fully utilize the samples, EMA is introduced to solve the problem. EMA can adaptively adjust weights to better reflect trends. Calculate the exponential moving average of IOU values to smooth out changes in IOU, and then calculate adjustment weights to adjust losses based on different ranges of IOU values, forming the ASL (Average Sliding Loss) in this paper as follows:

$$new\alpha = init\alpha * \left(1 - e^{-\frac{updates}{2000}}\right) \quad (1)$$

$$\lambda = \alpha\lambda + (1 - \alpha)float(\mu.d) \quad (2)$$

$$\mu = \lambda \quad (3)$$

where (1) is the formula for the exponentially varying weighting α. μ.d denotes the detach operation on μ. The parameters as well as the current model parameters are weighted and summed by Eq. (2), and assigned to μ by Eq. (3).

In paper [9], MPDIoU includes all the factors that need to be considered in the loss function, namely overlapping or non overlapping regions, centroid distance, and width height deviation, while simplifying the calculation process. The formula is as follows:

$$d_1^2 = \left(x_1^B - x_1^A\right)^2 + \left(y_1^B - y_1^A\right)^2 \quad (4)$$

$$d_2^2 = \left(x_2^B - x_2^A\right)^2 + \left(y_2^B - y_2^A\right)^2 \quad (5)$$

$$MPDIoU = \frac{A \cap B}{A \cup B} - \frac{d_1^2 + d_2^2}{w^2 + h^2} \quad (6)$$

Where: where A is the real region, B is the predicted region, d_1 and d_2 are the distances corresponding to the upper left and lower right corners of regions A and B.

2.5 Pruning

In order to enable modern models to be deployed in environments with limited resources. We used multiple pruning methods to study the pruning experiment of YOLOv8-LD. The experimental results show that the LAMP (for amplitude based layer adaptive sparse pruning) [10] pruning method shows significant results in the proposed algorithm. To achieve a balance between performance and sparsity, LAMP proposes a pruning score based on layer adaptive amplitude. In order to provide a uniform definition of the LAMP score for both fully connected and convolutional layers, the LAMP method assumes that each weight tensor is expanded (or spread) into a one-dimensional vector. The u-th index of the weight tensor W of the LAMP score can be defined by the following Eq. 7:

$$score(u; W) := \frac{(W[u])^2}{\sum_{v \geq u}(W[v])^2}. \tag{7}$$

$$(W[u])^2 > (W[u])^2 \Rightarrow score(u; W) > score(v; W) \tag{8}$$

where: w[u] denotes the entry of w that indexes the u mapping. After calculating the LAMP score, the connection with the lowest global pruning score is selected until the desired global sparsity constraint is satisfied.

3 Experimental Results and Analysis

3.1 Hyperparameters and Evaluation Metrics

The network environment is Ubuntu, Python 3.9 and PyTorch 2.1.0, the GPU is RTX 4090 (24 GB), and the CUDA version is 12.1. In the hyperparameter setting, the batch is set to 8, and epoch is set to 200, In the hyperparameter settings, batch is set to 8, epoch is set to 200 and image size is 640 × 640. The main evaluation metrics set for the experiment are Param (number of parameters), GFLOPs (amount of computation), mAP@0.5, mAP@0.5-0.95.

3.2 Ablation Study

Table 1 shows the results of ablation experiments on the VisDrone2019 dataset [11]. It can be seen that the performance of each branch and component confirms the effectiveness and superiority of our proposed method.

Figure 5 shows the visualization comparison results of models in different scenarios. It can be seen that the improved YOLOv8-LD model in this paper has significantly improved performance under different environmental conditions (such as different lighting and weather conditions), especially in small object detection (such as pedestrians and vehicles of different categories), it has shown excellent performance. This further proves the effectiveness of the improved method in this paper.

Table 1. Ablation study

Methods	Param	GFLOPs	mAP@ 0.5	mAP@ 0.5-0.95
YOLOv8n	3.01	8.1	33.1	19.2
YOLOv8n+ASBiFPN	2.31	17.1	39.3	23.5
YOLOv8n+ASBiFPN+DBBDetect	2.31	17.1	39.6	23.6
YOLOv8n+ASBiFPN+DBBDetect+MPDIoU	2.31	17.1	39.7	23.6
YOLOv8n+ASBiFPN+DBBDetect+MPDIoU+Slide	2.31	17.1	39.7	23.5
YOLOv8n+ASBiFPN+DBBDetect+MPDIoU+ASL	2.31	17.1	39.9	23.8

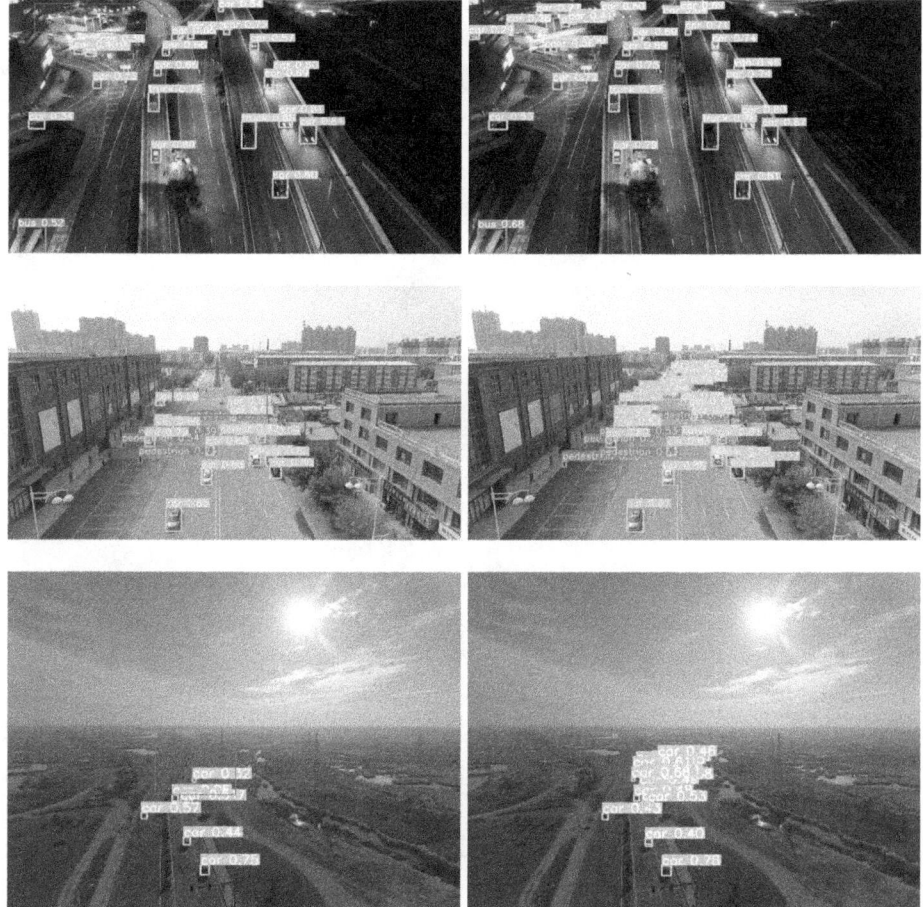

Fig. 5. On the left are the detection results of the YOLOv8 model; The detection results of the YOLOv8-LD model on the right

3.3 Comparative Experiments

To further evaluate the performance of the improved algorithm, comparisons were made in the VisDrone2019 dataset. As shown in Table 2, THP-YOLO is the SOTA algorithm of the YOLO series algorithm in the VisDrone challenge. In this experiment, the latest code released by the author of THP-YOLO is referenced to reproduce the THP-YOLOv5n version. YOLOv8-LD achieved the highest accuracy in different categories. This proves the effectiveness of the improved algorithm in this paper.

Table 2. Comparative experimental results with classical object detection algorithms

Methods	Pedestrian	People	Bicycle	Car	Van	Truck	Tricycle	Awning-tricycle	Bus	Motor	All
Faster R-CNN [12]	17.6	12.0	7.2	50.5	30.1	23.3	14.4	8.9	37.2	18.2	21.9
CenterNet [13]	22.6	20.6	14.6	59.7	24.0	21.3	20.1	17.4	37.9	23.7	26.2
YOLOv6n [14]	30.6	24.4	4.6	73.9	35.5	24.9	17.1	10.1	40.3	31.7	29.3
THP-YOLOv5n [3]	40.3	33.5	10.4	79.3	40.7	28.6	21.5	12.7	48.2	40.8	35.6
YOLOv8n	35.1	28.5	7.6	75.6	38.7	26.1	22.4	12.4	47.7	37.3	33.1
YOLOv8-LD	45.7	37.9	13.3	81.7	45.5	32.2	26.6	14.4	54.2	47.1	39.9

3.4 Pruning Experiments

As shown in Table 3, LAMP achieved the best experimental results compared to other pruning methods. As shown in Table 4, it can be seen that YOLOv8-LD in this paper has a better pruning effect than YOLOv8.

Table 3. Experimental results of different pruning algorithms

Methods	speed_up	Param	GFLOPs	ModelSize	mAP@0.5	mAP@0.5-0.95
LAMP [10]	2.0	0.60M	7.2	2.0 MB	34.1	20.1
group_hessian [15]	2.0	1.29M	7.2	3.4 MB	26.6	15.1
group_taylor [16]	2.0	1.15M	7.3	3.6 MB	26.7	15.0
random	2.0	0.75M	7.2	2.3 MB	31.3	17.9

Table 4. Experimental results of LAMP pruning algorithm

Methods	speed_up	Param	GFLOPs	mAP@0.5	mAP@0.5-0.95
YOLOv8	2.0	0.90M	4.0	32.3	18.7
YOLOv8-LD	2.5	0.43M	5.3	27.5	15.8
	2.0	0.60M	7.2	34.1	20.1

4 Conclusion

This paper proposes a lightweight object detection algorithm YOLOv8-LD suitable for drone scenarios. Proposed the ASBiFPN neck feature fusion network; Improve the detection head; Introducing MPDIoU loss; Propose ASL classification loss; Use pruning algorithms to reduce model volume. And verified the effectiveness of the proposed improvement plan in this paper.

References

1. Zhao, C., Liu, R.W., Qu, J., Gao, R.: Deep learning-based object detection in maritime unmanned aerial vehicle imagery: review and experimental comparisons. Eng. Appl. Artif. Intell. **128**, 107513 (2024)
2. Alam, M.S., Natesha, B.V., Ashwin, T.S., Guddeti, R.M.R.: UAV based cost-effective real-time abnormal event detection using edge computing. Multimed. Tools Appl. **78**(24), 35119–35134 (2019)
3. Zhu, X., Lyu, S., Wang, X., Zhao, Q.: TPH-YOLOv5: improved YOLOv5 based on transformer prediction head for object detection on drone-captured scenarios. In: Proceedings of the IEEE/CVF International Conference on Computer Vision 2021, Montreal, Canada, NJ, pp. 2778–2788. IEEE (2021)
4. Shao, Y., Yang, Z., Li, Z., Li, J.: Aero-YOLO: an efficient vehicle and pedestrian detection algorithm based on unmanned aerial imagery. Electronics **13**(7), 1190 (2024)
5. Tan, M., Pang, R., Le, Q.V.: EfficientDet: scalable and efficient object detection. In: Proceedings of the IEEE/CVF Conference on Computer Vision and Pattern Recognition 2020, Seattle, WA, USA, NJ, pp. 10781–10790. IEEE (2020)
6. Kang, M., Ting, C.M., Ting, F.F., Phan, R.C.W.: ASF-YOLO: a novel YOLO model with attentional scale sequence fusion for cell instance segmentation. Image Vis. Comput., 105057 (2024)
7. Ding, X., Zhang, X., Han, J., Ding, G.: Diverse branch block: building a convolution as an inception-like unit. In: Proceedings of the IEEE/CVF Conference on Computer Vision and Pattern Recognition 2021, Piscataway, Nashville, TN, USA, NJ, pp. 10886–10895. IEEE (2021)
8. Yu, Z., Huang, H., Chen, W., Su, Y., Liu, Y., Wang, X.: YOLO-FaceV2: a scale and occlusion aware face detector. arXiv preprint arXiv:2208.02019 (2022)
9. Siliang, M., Yong, X.: MPDIoU: a loss for efficient and accurate bounding box regression. arXiv preprint arXiv:2307.07662 (2023)
10. Lee, J., Park, S., Mo, S., Ahn, S., Shin, J.: Layer-adaptive sparsity for the magnitude-based pruning. arXiv preprint arXiv:2010.07611 (2020)

11. Cao, Y., et al.: VisDrone-DET2021: the vision meets drone object detection challenge results. In: Proceedings of the IEEE/CVF International Conference on Computer Vision 2021, Montreal, Canada, NJ, pp. 2847–2854. IEEE (2021)
12. Yu, W., Yang, T., Chen, C.: Towards resolving the challenge of long- tail distribution in UAV images for object detection. In: Winter Conference on Applications of Computer Vision 2021, Piscataway, pp. 3258–3267. Virtual. IEEE (2021)
13. Zhou, X., Wang, D., Krähenbühl, P.: Objects as points. arXiv preprint arXiv:1904.07850 (2019)
14. Li, C., et al.: YOLOv6: a single-stage object detection framework for industrial applications. arXiv preprint arXiv:2209. 02976 (2022)
15. LeCun, Y., Denker, J., Solla, S.: Optimal brain damage. In: Advances in Neural Information Processing Systems, vol. 2 (1989)
16. Molchanov, P., Mallya, A., Tyree, S., Frosio, I., Kautz, J.: Importance estimation for neural network pruning. In: Proceedings of the IEEE/CVF Conference on Computer Vision and Pattern Recognition 2019, Long Beach, CA, USA, NJ, pp. 11264–11272. IEEE (2019)

A Multi-dimensional Camera Image Stitching Method Under Large Parallax Conditions

Chuanlei Zhang[1], Yubo Li[1(✉)], Tianxiang Cheng[1], Jianrong Li[1], Haifeng Fan[1], Zhiqiang Zhao[2], Zhanjun Si[1], and Hui Ma[3]

[1] College of Artificial Intelligence, Tianjin University of Science and Technology, Tianjin 300457, China
`jaridli@163.com`
[2] Qinhuangdao Xinneng Energy & Equipment Co., Ltd., Qinhuangdao 066011, China
[3] Yunsheng Intelligent Technology Co., Ltd., Tianjin 300457, China

Abstract. Image stitching technology, as a critical link in digital image processing, can accurately combine numerous photos with overlapping sections into a panoramic image. Traditional image stitching typically demands that the input image have no parallax or very little parallax. However, in complex settings, spliced images produced by image splicing algorithms based on huge parallax are prone to issues such as ghosting and severe image distortion. This study provides an energy function optimization method for basic texture areas, as well as an enhanced seam quality evaluation algorithm to help with local seam alignment. Firstly, the entropy value based on the grey-scale covariance matrix is used to calculate the texture complexity, followed by region splitting, the penalty value of simple texture region is calculated based on the similarity of overlapping regions to obtain the energy function, secondly, the maximum flow minimum cut algorithm is used to locate the optimal seams, and finally, the simulated annealing algorithm is used to optimize the seam quality assessment algorithm for the algorithm suggested in this research performs well in picture fusion, as evidenced by experimental verification, which greatly enhances image fusion efficiency and final spliced image quality.

Keywords: Energy Function · Stitching Seam Quality Assessment · Local Seam Optimization · Optimal Splicing Seam

1 Introduction

In the real world, the field of vision of a single photo is limited by the physical restrictions of the viewing angles of various camera lenses. There are two approaches to improving it. One example is the employment of wide-angle lenses to directly record large-field images [1]. The second method is to capture numerous photographs using a general camera and then merge them using an image stitching technique to create a panoramic. The second option is more cost-effective.

Gao et al. [2] created an image calculation approach based on seams and found the optimal seams using the results of a seam evaluation algorithm. Li et al. [3] included sensory variables in the energy function, bringing the findings closer to the human sensory experience. Existing seam-cutting techniques [4] often bypass textured sections wherever possible. In this paper, a joint that can pass through simple texture areas is proposed, which can lead to higher overall quality joints.

Liao et al. [5] proposed in their study that traditional seam driving technology is not enough to find the most ideal seams in terms of feel. Therefore, they advocate calculating all points of the seam to obtain a better splicing effect. Liao et al. [6] proposed a local seam optimization strategy based on seam quality assessment, which can effectively reprocess local areas with poor seam processing. Since the seam quality assessment algorithm needs to calculate the quality of the entire seam, it takes a lot of time and affects the efficiency of local seam optimization. In this paper, a seam quality assessment algorithm optimized by a simulated annealing algorithm [7] is proposed, which significantly improves the efficiency of local seam optimization.

In this paper, we find a seam that can perfectly stitch together the left and right images under complex and variable large parallax conditions based on images taken by a multivariate camera, and optimize the efficiency of the algorithm to stitch as fast and well as possible. Our contributions can be summarized as follows:

(1) We propose an energy function optimization method for simple texture regions, which uses entropy value based on the grey-scale co-production matrix to calculate texture complexity, then performs region splitting, calculates the penalty value of simple texture regions based on the similarity of overlapping regions, obtains the energy function, and obtains the globally optimal seam through the graph cut algorithm.
(2) We use a simulated annealing algorithm to quickly find poorly spliced local regions for re-splicing, speeding up seam optimization.
(3) We conducted rich experiments to test the effectiveness of the optimized algorithm and compare it with mainstream algorithms.

2 Methods

The overall idea of our algorithm is to use a region separation algorithm [8] to find the texture simple region [9], followed by using entropy computation based on the grey-scale covariance matrix to improve the texture complexity term in the energy function, to determine the location with the smallest energy value as a seam, and then using simulated annealing algorithm to accelerate the seam quality assessment algorithm to locally optimize the seams, and finally smoothening to get the fused image.

We use a region-growing algorithm to find texture simple regions. Finally, several texture simple regions are obtained. The penalty term is then determined based on the region overlap similarity of the corresponding simple texture region [10]. At higher overlap similarity, it is considered that the seam passing through the simple texture region will be better and the penalty is smaller. At lower overlap similarity, the penalty term for this simple texture region is larger, reducing the seam line passing through the region. For the complex texture region, a smaller penalty term is set, mainly based on the color difference and gradient change can accurately guide the calculation of the seam.

Suppose I_0 and I_1 denote two images respectively, p and q represent a pair of pixel points with adjacent positions in the overlapping region Ω. The energy function is as follows:

$$E = \sum_{p \in \Omega} E_d(p, l_p) + \sum_{(p,q) \in \Omega} E_s(p, q, l_p, l_q) \tag{1}$$

where $E_d(p, l_p)$ represents the data term, $E_s(p, q, l_p, l_q)$ represents the smoothing term.

Then the texture complex term is integrated into the energy function, which is defined as follows:

$$E_s(p, q, l_p, l_q) = (E_c(p, q) + E_g(p, q))|ENT(p) + ENT(q)| \tag{2}$$

where $E_c(p, q)$ represents the grey-scale difference, $E_g(p, q)$ represents the gradient difference, and $|ENT(p) + ENT(q)|$ represents the image texture complexity term.

To solve the problem of low efficiency of the seam quality assessment algorithm, we use the simulated annealing algorithm to improve it and find the bad spots in the seams quickly. The simulated annealing process is shown in Algorithm 1.

Algorithm 1: Finding all bad pixels

Input: random init point set S, temperature set T, seam S_0, multiple B_0, Average of errors N_0
Output: all bad pixels
1: SPC = Sum(S_0), BP = ∅
2: for point in S do
3:   point_SSIM = calculate SSIM(point)
4:   for t in T
5:     if t > 0
6:       step = t * SPC
7:       point_left, point_right = step_instance(point)
8:       if point_left > point.left and point_right < point.right
9:         point_left_SSIM = calculate SSIM(point_left)
10:        point_right_SSIM = calculate SSIM(point_left)
11:        BP_candidate = max(point_SSIM, point_left_SSIM, point_right_SSIM)
12:        if BP_candidate > B_0 * N_0
13:          BP = BP ∪ BP_candidate
14:        End if
15:      End if
16:    End if
17: End for
18: End for
Return BP

After the simulated annealing algorithm, we get the location of several bad points, which are extended to the left and right sides to get several bad point segments. As shown in Fig. 1, splice recomputation is performed on these found bad segments using the splice cutting algorithm to get new seams. As shown in Fig. 2, finally image fusion is performed using a weighted average algorithm [11] which achieves smooth blending of pixels using the gradient for a natural transition.

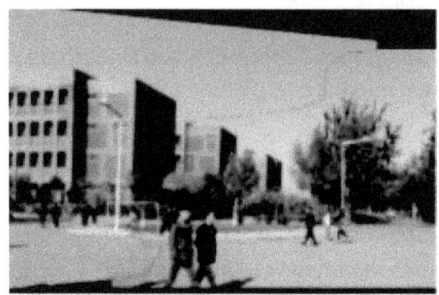 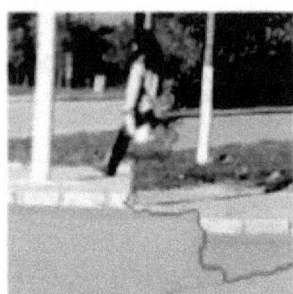

(a) Splice seams with bad pixel   (b) Local bad point segment

Fig. 1. Schematic diagram of a bad pixel segment.

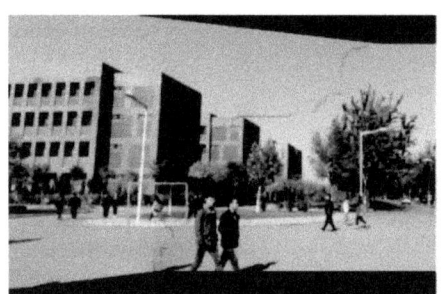 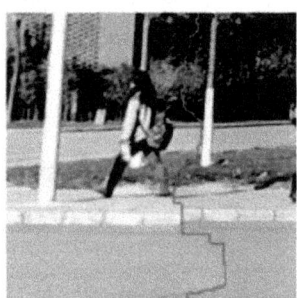

(a) Repaired spliced seam   (b) Localized seam

Fig. 2. Seam weight calculation.

3 Experiments

3.1 Experiments on Splicing Seams Based on Graph Cuts

To make the improved energy function in this paper to achieve the best effect, a series of data test experiments were done. First of all, we use the entropy value in the grey-scale covariance matrix can represent the texture complexity, the smaller the entropy value [12], the simpler the texture is, we need to get the simple texture region, we did some experiments for the definition of the simple texture and the complex texture, and got the following experimental results. As shown in Table 1.

From the experimental results, we can conclude that as the range of entropy values of simple texture regions increases, the number of simple texture regions increases and the total elapsed time is also increased. The result of seam quality assessment is maximum at maximum entropy value of 0.26 for simple texture region. The image is processed by the grey-scale covariance matrix and then the entropy value is used as a criterion for texture complexity. The texture with entropy value between 0 and 0.26, we consider this texture as simple texture region and the rest of the entropy value is considered as complex texture region.

Table 1. Defining the range of entropy values for simple texture regions.

Maximum entropy of a simple texture region	Number of simple texture areas	Total time consumption	Seam quality assessment
0.20	29	34.37	0.83
0.22	30	34.49	0.88
0.24	35	35.08	0.92
0.26	38	35.19	0.94
0.28	39	36.13	0.90
0.30	43	36.56	0.86

To determine the penalty term setting for simple texture areas, we conducted the following experiment. In the simple texture area, we use the contour matching algorithm [13] to measure the overlapping similarity. The higher the degree of contour matching in the simple texture area, the better the match between the two images. The higher the matching degree, the smaller the penalty term, and the greater the probability that the seam passes through this area. We assume that the overlapping similarity and the penalty term are linearly related, assuming that the linear ratio is k, and then we did some experiments to determine the value of this ratio. As shown in Table 2.

Table 2. Relationship between overlapping similarity and penalty terms.

Ratio k	Total time consumption	Seam quality assessment
0.75	36.13	0.90
0.85	36.46	0.93
0.95	36.27	0.91
1.05	35.96	0.90
1.15	35.78	0.85

From the experimental results, we can get the linear proportion k value between the penalty term and the overlapping similarity. It can be seen that the seam quality is the highest when k is near 0.85, and the relationship between the penalty term and the overlapping similarity is finally determined.

We also used the traditional energy function and the energy function improved based on the research in this article for splicing, and obtained the following experimental results. Figure 3 shows two images to be stitched. Figure 4 shows the splicing seam obtained based on the traditional energy function. The left image is the complete splicing seam, and the right image is the detailed display of the key areas of the splicing seam. Figure 5 shows the splicing seam obtained based on the improved energy function. The left image is the complete splicing seam, and the right image is the detailed display of the key areas of the splicing seam.

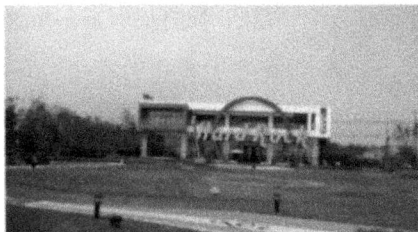 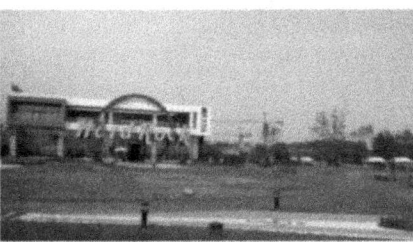

Fig. 3. Two images to be stitched.

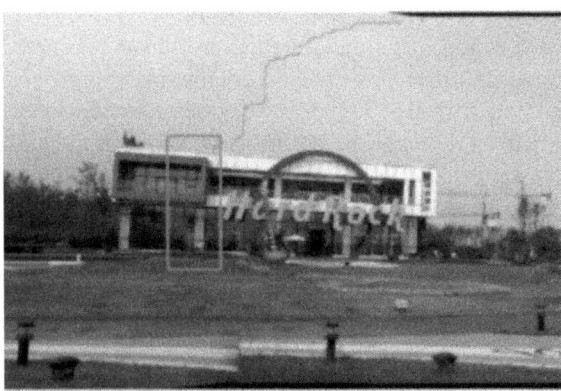 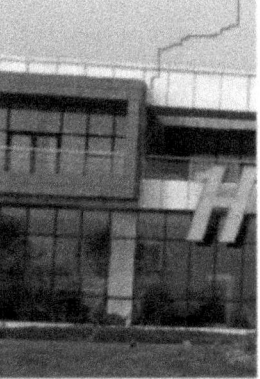

Fig. 4. Spliced seam based on the traditional energy function.

From Fig. 4, it can be seen that the seams obtained by the traditional energy function are more inclined to be along the edges of the object, which means that the search for the best splice seam is based on the structural gradient. From Fig. 5, it can be seen that the seams obtained by the improved energy function can be searched along the texture regularity and the region with uncomplicated texture, and there is no obvious error situation in the place where it enters and leaves the texture regularity region. In this paper, the improved splicing seam passes through areas with uncomplicated textures and can obtain seam splicing with lower energy values. Moreover, there is basically no difference in color and structural gradient after splicing in this part, the texture difference is smaller, and the splicing effect is better.

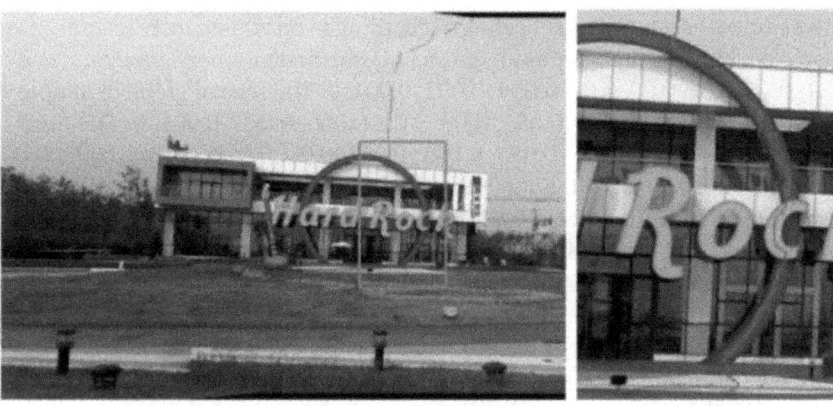

Fig. 5. Splice seams based on the improved energy function.

3.2 Improved Seam Quality Assessment Experiments

To improve the seam quality assessment algorithm to achieve the best results, a series of experiments were done to determine the values of some of these parameters. First of all, the number of random points we select will directly affect the efficiency of the algorithm, too few random points will lead to poor-quality seams, and the more random points we select, the more time will be consumed. We know that the longer the seam is, the more random points we need to select, so we need to determine a parameter d, indicating the number of d times the total length of the selected seam as the initial number of random points. To address these issues we did a series of experiments on the number of random points, and the results of the experiments are shown in Table 3.

Table 3. Proportion of random points d.

Ratio d	Total time	Seam quality assessment
0.005	3.963	0.885
0.008	4.204	0.906
0.011	4.437	0.922
0.014	4.869	0.930
0.017	5.671	0.931

From the experimental results, we can see that the higher the percentage of random points selected, the longer the algorithm takes and the higher the quality of the seams. We find that the time and seam quality performance is best when d is 0.011. So the final determination of the number of random points selected proportion is 0.011 times the total number of points of the seams.

The selection of temperature is the most important part of the simulated annealing, and whether the temperature is selected appropriately determines the efficiency and effectiveness of the simulated annealing. According to our experience, several groups of simulated annealing temperatures are given [14], the first group of temperatures are 0.3, 0.2, 0.1, 0.06, 0.03, 0.02, 0.01, 0.005, 0.002, 0.001, 0. The second group of temperatures are 0.25, 0.175, 0.125, 0.085, 0.055, 0.03, 0.01, 0.006, 0.003, 0.001, 0. The third set of temperatures were 0.2, 0.135, 0.085, 0.045, 0.025, 0.01, 0.008, 0.006, 0.003, 0.001, 0. Temperatures multiplied by the total length of the seam equaled the number of steps. We used 20 initial random points and did a series of experiments for each of these sets of temperatures, and the results are shown in Table 4.

The experimental findings show that the temperature in the first group has the maximum number of bad points and the best results. After analyzing the reason, it is found that because the temperature of the second and third groups is low, the random points across the local maximum worth of ability are weaker, resulting in fewer poor points. So, eventually, the temperature of the first group is determined.

Table 4. Effect of different temperature groups on the results.

Temperature	Total time	Number of bad points
group 1	4.147	5
group 2	4.104	3
group 3	4.203	2

3.3 Improved Seam Quality Assessment Experiments

The optimized algorithm in this paper is subjected to comparative experiments with algorithms involving seam-driven strategies [15]. We performed sufficient tests on this dataset, including 20 image pairs from [6], in which each image pair has overlapping parts and some parallax, and the dataset picture is shown in Fig. 6.

The method of this paper is compared with some commonly used panoramic image stitching methods, including APAP [16], and iterative seam estimation image stitching method based on quality assessment [17] (SEAGULL). A combination of subjective and objective evaluation is used to compare the different algorithms in the experimental results. The images to be spliced are shown in Fig. 7.

Figure 8 shows the comparison results, it can be seen that the APAP algorithm shows obvious ghosting, the staircase part of the SEAGULL algorithm is spliced unaligned, and the rest of the splicing is better. In addition, we use the information entropy (Entropy), root mean square error (RMSE), average gradient (AG), peak signal-to-noise ratio (PSNR) and program running time (Running Time) as evaluation indexes to objectively evaluate the effect of panorama splicing, and we get the results of Table 5.

From the experimental results, it can be seen that all the indexes of this paper's method perform well. The RMSE, AG and PSNR of this paper's method are the best among several methods. Entropy reacts to the richness of image information after fusion, and Entropy is only second to the SEAGULL method, and the gap between this value

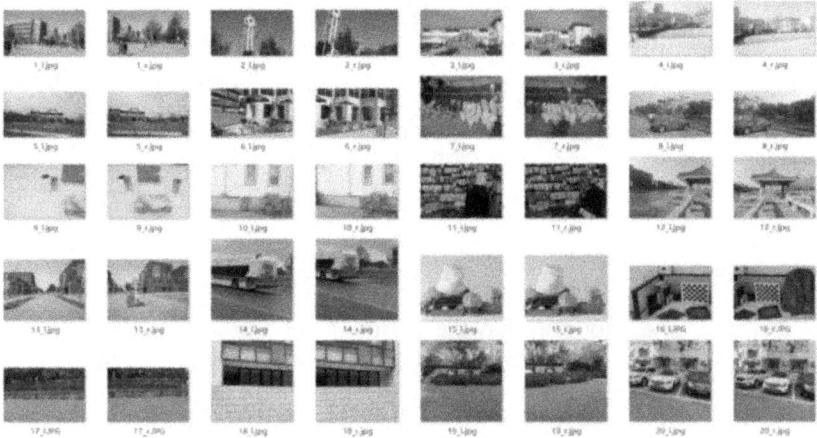

Fig. 6. Dataset Image.

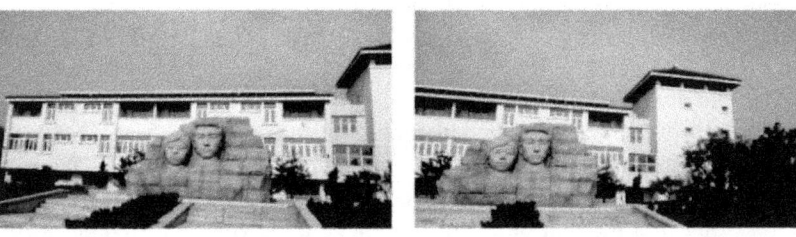

(a) The target images (b)The reference images

Fig. 7. Two images to be stitched.

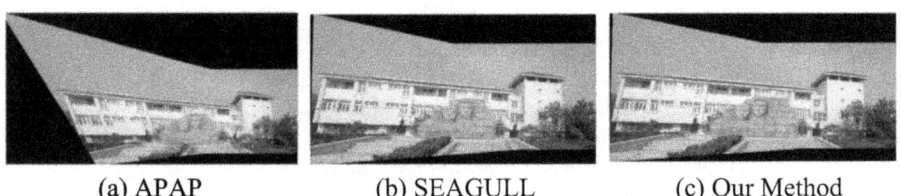

(a) APAP (b) SEAGULL (c) Our Method

Fig. 8. Experimental results of APAP, SEAGULL and our methods

and the best SEAGULL is very small, but this paper's algorithm takes a lot of time faster than that of SEAGULL. So the panoramic image obtained by the method of this paper is clearer and richer in image information.

The experimental data in this paper confirms that the proposed panoramic image stitching technique effectively handles the common phenomena of ghosting and ghosting, and at the same time can effectively smooth the transition region, thus generating high-quality panoramic images. Comprehensive subjective evaluation and objective

Table 5. Objective evaluation index of panorama stitching effect.

Method	Entropy	RMSE	AG	PSNR	Running Time (seconds)
APAP	8.57	3.31	7.96	18.69	50.56
SEAGULL	6.40	2.76	10.74	20.02	78.69
Our Method	6.46	2.73	11.13	20.39	39.67

analysis show that compared with other existing image stitching techniques, the method proposed in this study not only has the feasibility of practical application, but also demonstrates its unique advantages in terms of the overall stitching effect.

4 Conclusions

In this paper, we use a region separation algorithm to find simple texture regions, use entropy calculation based on gray-level co-occurrence matrices to improve the texture complexity term of the energy function, and find seams. Then the simulated annealing algorithm is used to quickly find the places with poor local seams and perform local re-stitching. Finally, the weighted average algorithm is used for image fusion, which significantly improves the efficiency and quality of image stitching.

Our method can handle the image stitching problem under large parallax well, but it still has limitations. Since there may be a certain amount of time between two captured images, resulting in a moving object in the image appearing at different locations in the overlapping region, this object may appear twice or zero times in the final stitching result, we hope that we can specify the number of times the moving object appears in the panorama by some methods. We leave this as our future work.

References

1. Gao, Z., et al.: Stereo camera calibration for large field of view digital image correlation using zoom lens. Measurement **185** (2021)
2. Gao, J., Li, Y., Chin, T.J., Brown, M. S.: Seam-driven image stitching. In: Eurographics (Short Papers), pp. 45–48 (2013)
3. Li, N., Liao, T., Wang, C.: Perception-based seam cutting for image stitching. SIViP **12**, 967–974 (2018)
4. Chen, J., Li, Z., Peng, C., Wang, Y., Gong, W.: UAV image stitching based on optimal seam and half-projective warp. Remote Sens. **14**(5), 1068 (2022). https://doi.org/10.3390/rs14051068
5. Liao, T., Chen, J., Xu, Y.: Quality evaluation-based iterative seam estimation for image stitching. SIViP **13**, 1199–1206 (2019)
6. Liao, T., Zhao, C., Li, L., Chao, H.: Seam-guided local alignment and stitching for large parallax images (2023). arxiv:2311.18564
7. Beneich, C., Douiri, S.M.: Solving the multi compartment vehicle routing problem using a hybridized simulated annealing algorithm. Int. J. Appl. Comput. Math. **9**(6), 127 (2023). https://doi.org/10.1007/s40819-023-01609-0

8. Zhang, Y., Yuan, Y.: ResNet-based surface normal estimator with multilevel fusion approach with adaptive median filter region growth algorithm for road scene segmentation. Int. J. Comput. Vis. Robot. **14**(1), 99–117 (2024)
9. Balling, J., Herold, M., Reiche, J.: How textural features can improve SAR-based tropical forest disturbance mapping. Int. J. Appl. Earth Obs. Geoinf. **124**, 103492 (2023)
10. Lhermitte, E., Hilal, M., Furlong, R., O'Brien, V., Humeau-Heurtier, A.: Deep learning and entropy-based texture features for color image classification. Entropy **24**(11), 1577 (2022). https://doi.org/10.3390/e24111577
11. Prabukumar, M., Shrutika, S.: Band clustering using expectation–maximization algorithm and weighted average fusion-based feature extraction for hyperspectral image classification. J. Appl. Remote. Sens. **12**(4), 046015 (2018)
12. Xie, C., Wang, J., Haase, D., Wellmann, T., Lausch, A.: Measuring spatio-temporal heterogeneity and interior characteristics of green spaces in urban neighborhoods: a new approach using gray level co-occurrence matrix. Sci. Total. Environ. **855**, 158608 (2023). https://doi.org/10.1016/j.scitotenv.2022.158608
13. Arulananth, T.S., Baskar, M., Sateesh, R.: Human face detection and recognition using contour generation and matching algorithm. Indonesian J. Electr. Eng. Comput. Sci. **16**(2), 709–714 (2019)
14. Shahrin, S.H., Hussin, M. S.: Comparisons of simulated annealing temperature schedule based on QAPLIB instances. In: AIP Conference Proceedings, vol. 1974. AIP Publishing (2018)
15. Chen, X., Mei, Y., Song, Y.: Optimized seam-driven image stitching method based on scene depth information. Electronics **11**(12), 1876 (2022). https://doi.org/10.3390/electronics11121876
16. Zaragoza J., Chin, T.J., Brown, M.S., Suter, D.: As-projective-as-possible image stitching with moving DLT. In: Proceedings of the IEEE Conference on Computer Vision and Pattern Recognition, pp. 2339–2346 (2013)
17. Lin, K., Jiang, N., Cheong, L F., Do, M., Lu, J.: SEAGULL: seam-Guided Local Alignment for Parallax-Tolerant Image Stitching. In: Leibe, B., Matas, J., Sebe, N., Welling, M. (eds.) Computer Vision – ECCV 2016. ECCV 2016. LNCS, vol. 9907. Springer, Cham (2016). https://doi.org/10.1007/978-3-319-46487-9_23

Harmonizing Stable Diffusion and GPT-4 for Mural Expansion with ArtExtend

Dufeng Chen[1], Yuqing Yang[2], Zehua Wang[2,3](✉), Zishan Xu[2], Jueting Liu[2], Tingting Xu[2], and Wei Chen[2]

[1] Beijing Geotechnical and Investigation Engineering Insititute, Beijing 100080, China
[2] School of Computer Science and Technology, China University of Mining and Technology, Xuzhou 221116, China
zehuaw@cumt.edu.cn
[3] Department of Electrical and Computer Engineering, The University of British Columbia, Vancouver, Canada

Abstract. The Dunhuang murals have a long history. Over the centuries, changes have made it hard to restore them. This study addresses the limitations of existing multimodal learning models in the lack of semantic information on the scene expansion of Dunhuang mural images. A total of 887 groups of Dunhuang mural patterns and their text descriptions were collected for this purpose. A method called ArtExtend was created based on the Stable Diffusion model. It uses BLIP-2 technology to encode keywords in mural images. It uses BLIP-2 technology to encode keywords from mural images and accurately represent mural image features in conjunction with image-text contrast loss. It then optimizes the GPT-4 large model expansion mural keywords through black-box prompt optimization (BPO) technology to generate scene descriptions. Finally, it fine-tunes the Stable Diffusion model and expands Dunhuang mural images with GPT-4 descriptions through LoRA technology. The experimental results show that the proposed method outperforms the benchmark model in terms of LPIPS metric reduction 28.5%, FID metric reduction 30.5%, and CLIPScore score improvement 16.6%. This makes the model better at understanding Dunhuang murals. This study combines deep language understanding and advanced image generation techniques in a new way. This approach reduces the time and cost of traditional restoration work and improves the use of large models in mural painting.

Keywords: Dunhuang Murals · Multimodal Learning · Text-to-Image · Stable Diffusion

1 Introduction

In the digital age, attention to the preservation of ancient murals has increased. These artworks are protected and revitalized through advanced technologies, which also foster the growth of cultural diversity. Digital mural technology applications: Ren et al.[1] applied neural networks for the digitalization of Dunhuang murals, and Xu et al.[2] used Generative Adversarial Networks (GANs) to enhance the precision and quality of the digitalization process. Wang et al.[3] integrated adaptive local convolution and arbitrary shape masks into GAN technology. Xu et al.[4] introduced a novel method based on a new diffusion model for digitizing Dunhuang murals. These studies showcase the application of various technologies in mural digitization.

In the field of image processing, outpainting presents a challenging task. Zhang et al.[5] introduced a new regularization method to encourage diversity sampling in conditional synthesis. Yang et al.[6] designed innovative modules to improve the realism and quality of the generated images. Zhang et al.[7] incorporated prior knowledge to enhance the inference ability of encoders for outpainting. Lu et al.[8] used contextual attention mechanisms and adversarial learning schemes for panorama outpainting. Gao et al.[9] the extrapolated visual context in all directions around the image. Van et al.[10] employed context encoders inspired by common image inpainting architectures and paradigms. Wang et al.[11] extended image borders with plausible structure and details. Zhuang et al.[12] introduced learnable task prompts and fine-tuning strategies, which can utilize different task prompts to accomplish various outpainting tasks.

The Stable Diffusion model[13] offers new ways to share ancient murals. But it still has problems. The expansion process might change the meaning of the generated content. This is because the model doesn't have enough information about the original murals. To make the model work better, we need to add more information. The pre-trained version of the model is not designed to reproduce the style of murals. This paper introduces an innovative approach called "ArtExtend." It employs the following strategies:

1. The multimodal image description function of BLIP-2 [14] and the language generation capability of GPT-4 are combined to provide detailed semantic guidance for Stable Diffusion, thereby ensuring that the generated images are technically advanced and faithful to the mural features. The specific process effects illustrated in Fig. 1.
2. The query is refined through the black-box prompt optimization (BPO) technique [15], thereby enhancing the text generated by GPT-4 and improving the performance and accuracy of Stable Diffusion. The performance and adaptability of Stable Diffusion will be evaluated.
3. The LoRA fine-tuning technique [16] will be employed to make specific adjustments to Stable Diffusion, to generate images that conform to the style of murals.

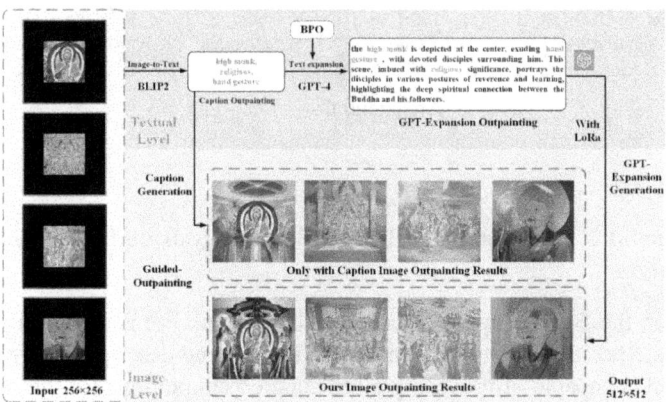

Fig. 1. ArtExtend flow effect diagram.

2 Method

This chapter introduces a comprehensive methodological framework named "ArtExtend" Fig. 2 illustrates that the framework consists of three core components: multimodal visual-language interaction analysis, query optimization, prompt engineering, and model fine-tuning tailored to specific requirements. Initially, large multimodal models are used for visual analysis and text description generation of murals. Then, BPO technology is utilized to optimize GPT-4, finding the optimal prompts that guide GPT-4 to generate the most accurate and relevant mural text descriptions. Subsequently, LoRA technology is applied for the specialized fine-tuning of the Stable Diffusion model to conform to the specific style of the murals. The goal of this comprehensive approach is to efficiently and accurately restore ancient murals, ensuring the preservation of their original artistic value. The specific network structure diagram is shown in Fig. 2.

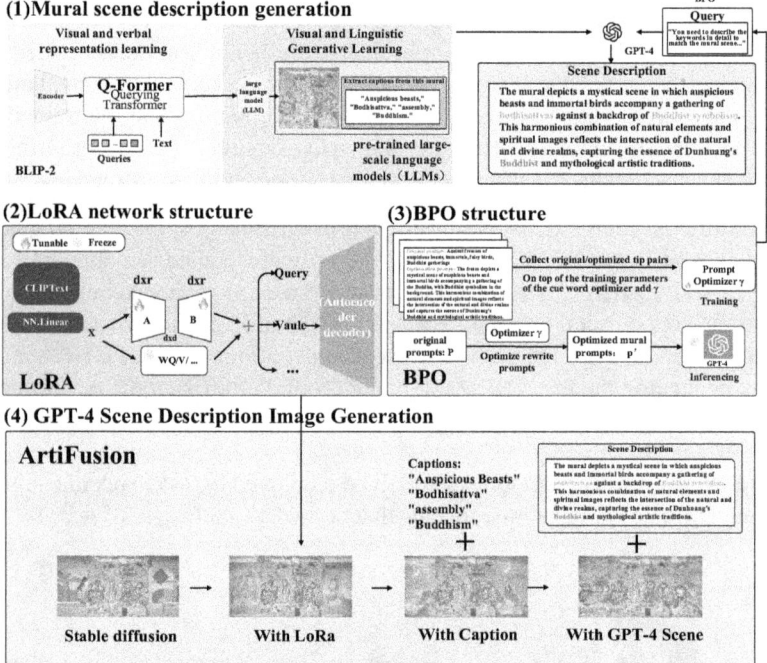

Fig. 2. ArtExtend flow effect diagram

2.1 Multimodal Visual Language Interaction Analysis and Description Generation

In this chapter, the BLIP-2 model is used to visually analyze ancient murals and identify keywords. Special datasets containing 887 images and descriptions are created. The BLIP-2 model is capable of providing more detailed annotations for the mural images, which assists in better understanding the images and generating more detailed descriptions. This is combined with a contrast loss function. The Image-Text Contrast Loss (ITM Loss) is aimed at making matched image-text pairs similar and mismatched pairs different, utilizing binary cross-entropy loss to achieve this objective.

$$L_{ITM} = -\frac{1}{N}\sum_{i=1}^{N}\left[y_i \log(\hat{y}_i) + (1 - y_i)\log(1 - \hat{y}_i)\right] \quad (1)$$

where N is the number of samples in the batch, y_i is the true label of the ith sample (1 for matching image-text pairs and 0 for mismatches), and $\hat{y}_i$ is the probability of matching predicted by the model. This process involves extracting the most important visual information from an image and turning it into a keyword description. Key elements in mural images can be identified by BLIP-2, and text descriptions are generated accordingly.

2.2 Query Optimization and Prompt Engineering

After obtaining captions, the next step is to make the queries better. At this stage, Blackbox Prompt Optimization technology is used to make simple queries more complex, specific, and information-rich. This process makes the queries better by evaluating the quality of the model's output. It aims to find the best prompts that can make GPT-4 generate the most accurate and relevant mural text descriptions. BPO technology makes queries more effective by adjusting external inputs. This leads to more precise and targeted prompts. This ensures that the prompts match the murals' visual and cultural characteristics and the research objectives. The target function CLIPLoss is used:

$$L = \frac{1}{N}\sum_{i=1}^{N} \log \frac{\exp(sim(i,i)/\tau)}{\sum_{j=1}^{N}\exp(sim(i,j)/\tau)} + \frac{1}{N}\sum_{i=1}^{N} \log \frac{\exp(sim(i,i)/\tau)}{\sum_{j=1}^{N}\exp(sim(j,i)/\tau)} \quad (2)$$

where $sim(i,j)$ represents the similarity between the ith image embedding and the jth text embedding and τ is the temperature parameter (a preset positive number used to control the smoothness of the distribution).

Using the Bayesian optimization algorithm, starting with basic prompts such as "Describe the theme of this mural" and "What story does this mural tell?", 35 iterations are set, with each iteration generating 5–10 prompts for evaluation and comparison. Based on the target function's score, the best prompt is selected for the next round of optimization. The prompts are refined to include information such as historical background and artistic style, with specific instructions like "Use professional terminology" or "Assume you are a Dunhuang mural historian" and diversity constraints to ensure the breadth and accuracy of the generated descriptions. The optimization process can be represented by the following formula:

$$Q_{opt} = BPO(Q_{init}, P, \gamma) \quad (3)$$

Here, Q_{init} is the initial keywords generated based on the formula, P is the auxiliary prompt, and γ represents the optimizer. The formula demonstrates how BPO technology optimizes queries. The key to this step is how effectively the original keywords are transformed into more specific and detailed descriptions of mural scenes, providing richer and more specific input for the textual expansion in the Stable Diffusion model.

2.3 Special Fine-Tuning for Mural Outpainting

To make the Stable Diffusion model match specific mural styles more precisely, we used LoRA technology to make fine adjustments. LoRA adds low-rank matrices to key parts of the model, allowing for efficient adjustments while keeping the majority of the pre-trained model's parameters unchanged. An auxiliary path is added alongside the original Stable Diffusion model, where only the dimensionality reduction matrix A and the dimensionality increasing matrix B are trained. The dimensions of the model stay the same, and the output of BA is combined with the parameters of Stable Diffusion. This fine-tuning strategy can be summarized by the following formula:

$$SD_{tuned} = LoRA(SD_{ori}, LRM, \beta) \tag{4}$$

where SD_{ori} represents the original Stable Diffusion model, LRM refers to the introduced low-rank matrices, β represents the adjustment parameters during the fine-tuning process, and SD_{tuned} is the model after fine-tuning. Through this method, we are able to effectively personalize the model without significantly changing its original structure, thereby generating images that conform more closely to specific artistic style requirements, such as Dunhuang mural style images.

We have created a way to turn text into images. This process involves converting detailed descriptions into images in the style of a mural. The process is as follows:

$$Image = Outpaint(SD_{tuned}, D, K) \tag{5}$$

D represents the detailed description, and K represents the keywords. These text inputs are used to make images. The Outpaint function makes images with specific features. Our Stable Diffusion model can generate images matching the style of Dunhuang murals and ensure the accuracy and richness of the images in terms of cultural and artistic content. This method opens new ways to represent and preserve cultural and artistic works like Dunhuang murals.

3 Experiment

This section explains the Dunhuang mural dataset that was collected to improve image generation technology. In this experiment, a dataset of Dunhuang murals and their descriptions was created. It was ensured that all the mural images had the same resolution to meet the experiment's quality requirements. A V100 GPU was used in the experiments. The experiments were conducted in stages to compare different technologies. The murals were restored through our approach, enhancing their visual and artistic value while preserving their artistic essence. These experiments demonstrated that our method works and can be used to preserve cultural heritage.

3.1 Unsupervised Image Expansion Comparative Experiment

This section presents a comparative experiment of our "ArtExtend" method under unsupervised conditions. We tested four image expansion techniques capable of extending images from a resolution of 512 × 512 to 1024 × 512. It was found that while the "SRN[11]," which optimizes based on image boundary structures, and "IOH-GAN[10]," based on inpainting architecture, performed well in standard tasks, they lacked semantic information during expansion. The "PowerPaint[12]" method, integrating task guidance and fine-tuning strategies, showed improvement but was limited in specific scenarios. In contrast, "ArtExtend" excelled in outpainting Dunhuang murals, generating precise images while retaining the original style, especially adept at handling complex themes. Further comparisons demonstrated the efficacy of "ArtExtend" combining Stable Diffusion technology, BLIP-2 for extracting key descriptions, BPO-optimized GPT-4, and LoRA style fine-tuning. As illustrated in Fig. 3, "ArtExtend" showcased its superior ability and potential value in the field of unsupervised image expansion of murals, offering more reasonable and precise scene generation.

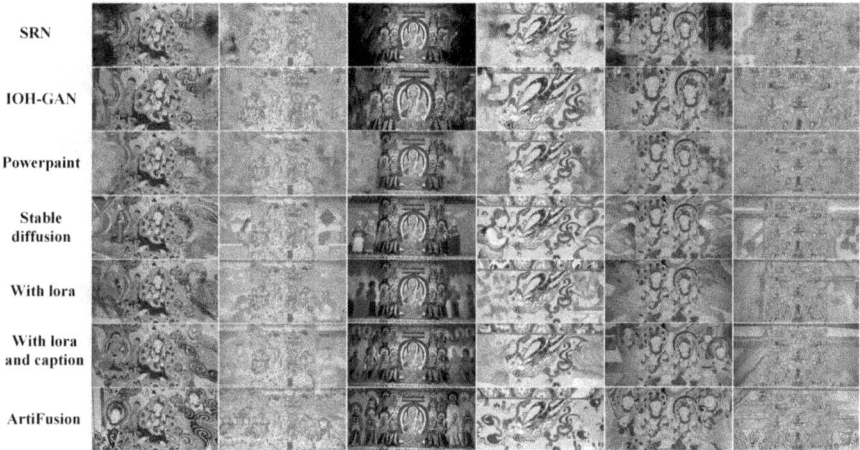

Fig. 3. Unsupervised image expansion comparative diagram

3.2 Comparative Analysis of Text-Guided Expansion Experiment

This section compares our "ArtExtend" mural image expansion technique with popular methods like "Wide-Context," "Image Outpainting," and "PowerPaint". The main goal was to outpaint 256 × 256 pixel images to 512 × 512 pixels and evaluate each model under the same training and testing conditions. A version of "PowerPaint" with prompt words was specifically tested, using LPIPS, FID, and CLIPscore as evaluation metrics. These metrics measure the quality of the generated images, their semantic consistency with the original images, and visual similarity, important criteria for assessing image generation model performance. Considering potential FID inflation due to sample limitations, "ArtExtend" ensures effective reflection of image quality and diversity even with limited samples by enhancing image details and overall consistency.

Detailed comparative analysis through Fig. 4 and Table 1 shows that, although some technologies perform well in general image expansion, they lack semantic information in

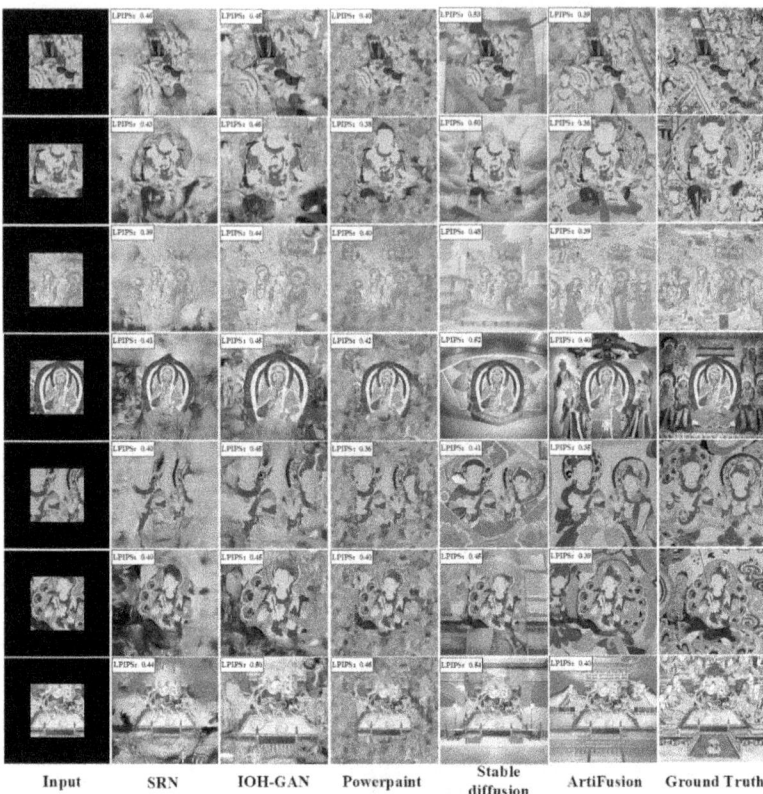

Fig. 4. Comparison diagram of results with other methods

Table 1. Comparative analysis table for evaluation of the effectiveness of outpainting

Methods	Lpips↓	Fid↓	Clipscore↑
Wide-Context	0.43	341	/
Image Outpainting	0.47	250	/
Powerpaint with Caption	0.40	259	26.32
Powerpaint with expantion	0.39	223	30.43
Stable Diffusion	0.49	285	/
ArtExtend	**0.35**	**198**	**31.50**

complex mural processing, compromising accuracy. "PowerPaint" attempts to enhance performance through mural keywords and descriptions but is limited in style and detail handling, demonstrating ArtExtend's superiority in specific scenarios and highlighting potential limitations of advanced technologies when facing challenges.

3.3 Comparative Ablation Study Experiment

This section evaluates the effects of Stable Diffusion, LoRA, BLIP-2, and GPT-4 optimized by BPO in mural image expansion tasks through ablation studies.

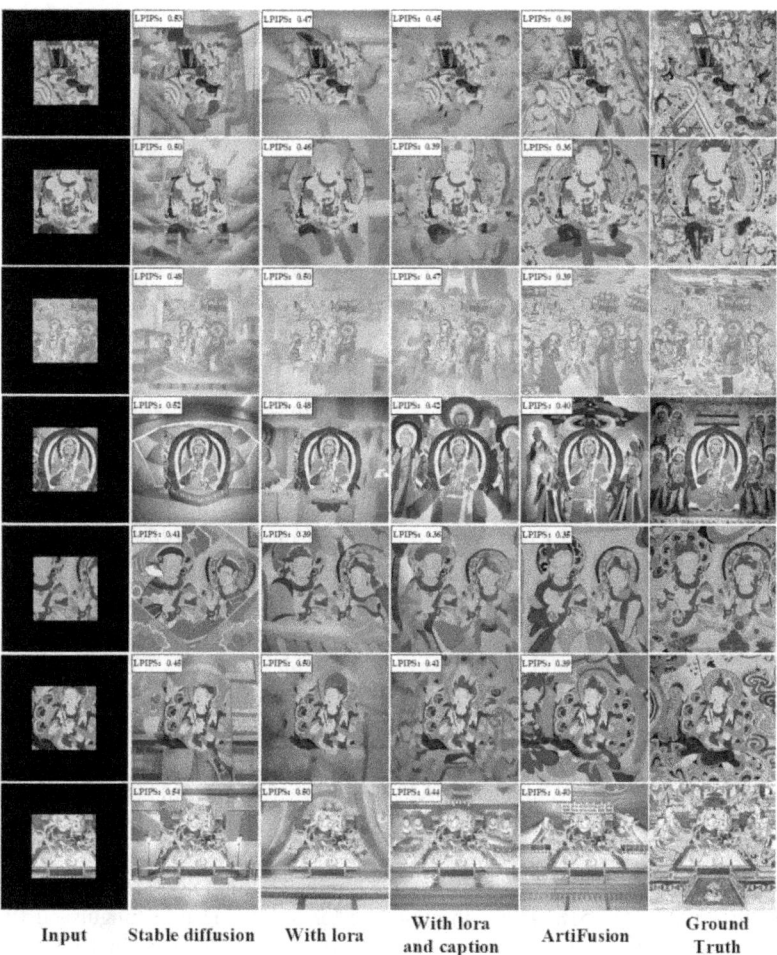

Fig. 5. Ablation experiment effect diagram

The results, displayed in Fig. 5, showcase the performance of each technology individually and in combination, confirming the outstanding effects of integrating GPT-4, BLIP-2, Stable Diffusion, and LoRA in mural expansion.The experiment demonstrates that GPT-4, optimized by BPO, can refine BLIP-2 text descriptions, effectively guiding Stable Diffusion and LoRA in image expansion to produce images that closely match the original mural style and are highly consistent visually and semantically. The results in Table 2 reflect the excellent performance of the "ArtExtend" method on FID, CLIP-Score, and LPIPS metrics, highlighting its strong capabilities in image quality, semantic relevance, and perceptual similarity, offering an efficient and creative solution for mural image expansion.

Table 2. Ablation comparison study effectiveness assessment table

	Lpips↓	Fid↓	Clipscore↑
Stable Diffusion	0.49	285	/
With LoRA	0.48	275	/
with Caption	0.42	231	27.02
ArtExtend	**0.35**	**198**	**31.50**

4 Conclusion

The main contribution of this study lies in combining deep language understanding with advanced image generation technology, offering a new perspective for the digital outpainting of ancient murals and paving a new technical path for the preservation and outpainting of cultural heritage. This research not only opens up new possibilities at a technical level but also provides fresh approaches and tools for the protection, education, and dissemination of global cultural heritage. However, ensuring cultural and historical accuracy remains a key challenge. Although artificial intelligence technology can restore and expand murals, it is crucial to ensure the authenticity and appropriateness of these works in cultural and historical aspects, which requires a deep understanding of the cultural background and historical context behind the murals. Additionally, the adaptability and universality of the technology pose another challenge, necessitating further development and optimization to ensure its applicability to ancient murals of various styles and periods. When using AI technology for cultural heritage preservation, it is imperative to respect and protect the integrity of the original art pieces.

Acknowledgments. This study was funded by the National Natural Science Foundation of China (grant number 52274160, 51874300), the Funding for the "Jiangsu Distinguished Professor" project in Jiangsu Province (grant number 140923070) and the Fundamental Research Funds for the Central Universities(2023QN1079).

Disclosure of Interests. The authors have no competing interests to declare that are relevant to the content of this paper.

References

1. Xiaokang, R., Peilin, C.: Murals inpainting based on generalized regression neural network. Comput. Eng. Sci. **39**, 1884–1889 (2017)

2. Xu, H., Kang, J., Zhang, J.: Digital mural inpainting method based on feature perception. Comput. Sci. **49**, 217–223 (2022)
3. Wang, N., Wang, W., Hu, W., Fenster, A., Li, S.: Thanka mural inpainting based on multi-scale adaptive partial convolution and stroke-like mask. IEEE Trans. Image Process. **30**, 3720–3733 (2021)
4. Xu, Z., et al.: Restoration of Dunhuang Murals on Large-scale pretraining. In: Proceedings of the 2023 6th International Conference on Signal Processing and Machine Learning, pp. 106–111 (2023)
5. Zhang, L., Wang, J., Shi, J.: Multimodal image outpainting with regularized normalized diversification. In: Proceedings of the IEEE/CVF Winter Conference on Applications of Computer Vision, pp. 3433–3442 (2020)
6. Yang, Z., Dong, J., Liu, P., Yang, Y., Yan, S.: Very long natural scenery image prediction by outpainting. In: Proceedings of the IEEE/CVF International Conference on Computer Vision, pp. 10561–10570 (2019)
7. Zhang, X., Chen, F., Wang, C., Tao, M., Jiang, G.-P.: Sienet: Siamese expansion network for image extrapolation. IEEE Signal Process. Lett. **27**, 1590–1594 (2020)
8. Lu, C.-N., Chang, Y.-C., Chiu, W.-C.: Bridging the visual gap: Wide-range image blending. In: Proceedings of the IEEE/CVF Conference on Computer Vision and Pattern Recognition, pp. 843–851 (2021)
9. Gao, P., et al.: Generalized image outpainting with U-transformer. Neural Netw. **162**, 1–10 (2023)
10. Van Hoorick, B.: Image outpainting and harmonization using generative adversarial networks. arXiv preprint arXiv:1912.10960 (2019)
11. Wang, Y., Tao, X., Shen, X., Jia, J.: Wide-context semantic image extrapolation. In: Proceedings of the IEEE/CVF Conference on Computer Vision and Pattern Recognition, pp. 1399–1408 (2019)
12. Zhuang, J., Zeng, Y., Liu, W., Yuan, C., Chen, K.: A task is worth one word: learning with task prompts for high-quality versatile image in painting. arXiv preprint arXiv:2312.03594 (2023)
13. Rombach, R., Blattmann, A., Lorenz, D., Esser, P., Ommer, B.: High-resolution image synthesis with latent diffusion models. In: Proceedings of the IEEE/CVF Conference on Computer Vision and Pattern Recognition, pp. 10684–10695 (2022)
14. Li, J., Li, D., Savarese, S., Hoi, S.: BLIP-2: bootstrapping language-image pre-training with frozen image encoders and large language models. In: International Conference on Machine Learning, pp. 19730–19742. PMLR (2023)
15. Cheng, J., et al.: Black-box prompt optimization: Aligning large language models without model training. arXiv preprint arXiv:2311.04155 (2023)
16. Hu, E.J., et al.: LoRA: Low-rank adaptation of large language models. arXiv preprint arXiv:2106.09685 (2021)

MuralRescue: Advancing Blind Mural Restoration via SAM-Adapter Enhanced Damage Segmentation and Integrated Restoration Techniques

Zishan Xu[1], Dufeng Chen[2], Qianzhen Fang[1], Wei Chen[1(✉)], Tingting Xu[1], Jueting Liu[1], and Zehua Wang[1]

[1] China University of Mining and Technology, Xuzhou 221116, China
chenwdavior@163.com

[2] Beijing Geotechnical and Investigation Engineering Insititute, Beijing 100080, China

Abstract. In this paper, we introduce an innovative method for blind mural restoration, named "MuralRescue," which demonstrates a systematic approach to progressively restore and enhance the quality of Dunhuang mural images by integrating damaged area segmentation, inpainting processing, and super-resolution techniques. In the process of mural damage segmentation, we employ the SAM-Adapter to optimize the "Segment Anything" model and to enhance the performance of mural damage segmentation. Specifically, we use an adapter module containing two layers of MLP to fine-tune the "Segment Anything" model, thereby increasing the accuracy of segmenting mural cracks. Through extensive experiments, we have proven the adapter's effectiveness in detecting small targets and fine-grained mural cracks. Additionally, by combining detected cracks with image restoration, we have significantly improved the superiority of blind image restoration tasks without reference.

Keywords: Segment Anything · Blind mural restoration · SAM-Adapter

1 Introduction

Mural images are a long-standing art form that records significant aspects of human history and reflects the uniqueness of different cultures. Despite their historical significance, many ancient murals have suffered severe damage due to natural and human factors. Traditionally, restoring these murals required extensive manual labor, and the results heavily depended on the skill of the restorers. With the rapid development of computer vision and deep learning technologies, new methods have emerged, offering possibilities to automate and improve the restoration process.

This paper introduces "MuralRescue," a comprehensive approach for automated blind mural segmentation and restoration. The method integrates area segmentation, advanced inpainting, and super-resolution techniques to systematically restore Dunhuang mural images. "MuralRescue" involves identifying and segmenting damaged areas, applying advanced inpainting technologies to fill these damages, and employing super-resolution techniques to enhance the clarity and detail of the images. The method leverages the Segment Anything Model (SAM) enhanced by a specially designed SAM-Adapter, which improves the accuracy of detecting fine cracks and segmentation of damaged areas.

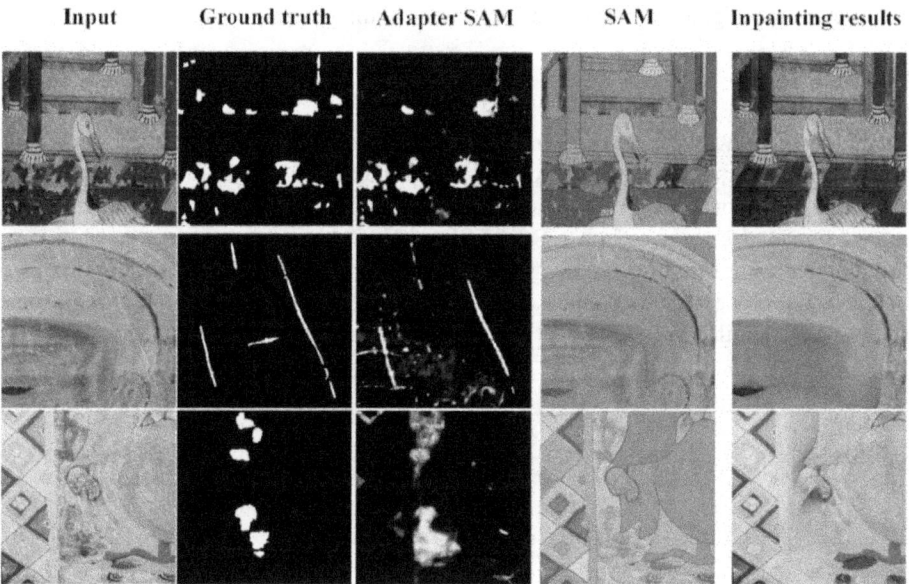

Fig. 1. The results of MuralRescue on Mural dataset, the ground truth is our marked damaged mask, and through Adapter SAM, the detected damage is more detailed, and the unmarked damage of the ground truth can also be detected so that the restored result is closer to reality.

Digital restoration of murals has gained attention globally. Initial digital restoration efforts by Pan et al. [1] have been refined by subsequent researchers such as Shen et al. [2], who utilized MCA decomposition for Tang Dynasty tomb murals. Further advancements were made using sequential similarity detection and cuckoo optimization by Chen et al. [3], and the disease extraction and in-painting algorithm for digital grotto murals by Zhang et al. [4]. Additional studies by Chen et al. [5] and Yang et al. [6] on improving algorithms for intricate disrepaired regions of murals have furthered the field. Moreover, Jiao et al. [7] have advanced mural inpainting based on an improved block matching algorithm.

The "Inpaint Anything" (IA) approach [9], which utilizes the Segment Anything Model (SAM) [10], combines state-of-the-art image painters and AI-generated content models for diverse restoration tasks. SAM's zero-shot performance has been demonstrated in a wide range of applications, including medical imaging [11–13], remote sensing [14], and camouflaged object detection [15]. SAM has also been adapted for non-Euclidean domains, which presents new research opportunities [16].

The results of MuralRescue are illustrated in Fig. 1. The main contributions of this paper are:

- Development and implementation of "MuralRescue," an automated mural restoration method that preserves the original texture and artistic style while improving the accuracy and efficiency of restoration.
- A novel blind image restoration method using the SAM-Adapter, which significantly enhances the segmentation and restoration of damaged mural areas.

2 Method

The main workflow of this study is implemented in three steps for the automatic restoration of murals: First, we use our designed SAM-adapter to segment the damaged areas in the murals; second, we employ the LAMA [20] inpainting algorithm to inpaint these damaged areas. Lastly, we choose Real-ESRGAN [21] to perform super-resolution on the inpainted mural images. The entire process is encapsulated within our "MuralRescue" method, presented in an end-to-end format. The implementation process of these three steps is detailed below. The structure of "MuralRescue" is illustrated in Fig. 2.

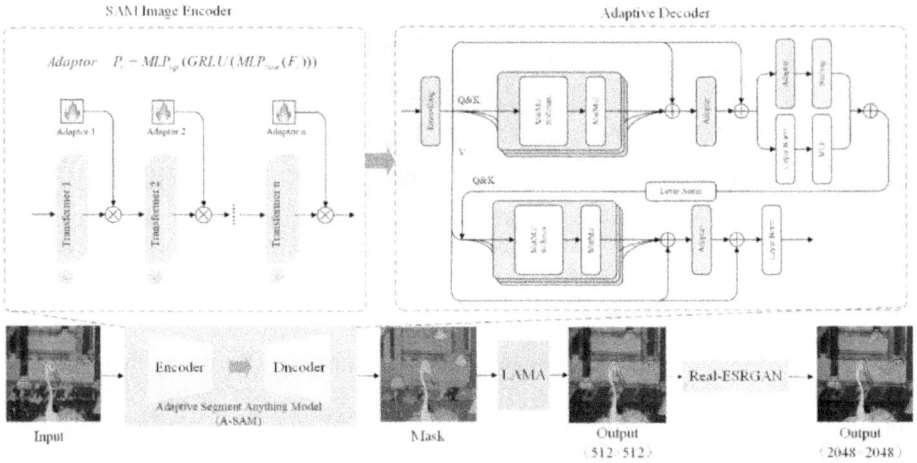

Fig. 2. The structure of MuralRescue

2.1 Segmentation of Damaged Areas

We input the mural image I into the model SAM and obtain the segmentation result S of the broken region:

$$S = SAM(I) \tag{1}$$

Segment Anything model (SAM) is used to accurately segment broken regions, We designed an Adapter to adapt to the specific needs of mural breakage detection. The adapter is a lightweight model that can be trained using relatively little data and inject task-specific bootstrap information into the SAM network. This information is communicated to the network through visual cues, demonstrating efficiency and effectiveness in adapting to many downstream tasks.

Specifically, SAM's image encoder used the ViT-H/16 model with a 14 × 14 window of attention and four uniformly distributed global attention blocks. We keep the weights of the original model frozen and add the adapter module between each transformer layer separately. Each adapter consists of two MLPs and an activation function. Specifically, the adapter receives task-related information F_i and then generates a cue P_i with the expression:

$$P_i = MLP_{up}(Gelu(MLP_{tune}(F_i))) \qquad (2)$$

In this formulation, MLP_{tune} denotes the linear layer used to generate task-specific cues for each Adapter, and MLP_{up} is an up-projection layer shared among all Adapters that adjusts the dimensionality of Transformer features. *Gelu* denotes the GELU activation function [8].

In SAM's mask decoder, we deploy three adapters for each ViT block. The first Adapter is deployed after cueing to the cross-attention of the image embedding, and it is fine-tuned to integrate the cueing information. The second Adapter is used to adapt the MLP-enhanced embedding. The third Adapter is deployed after the cross-attention of the image embedding to the cue, and then the final result is output by additional residual connections and layer normalization. The second decoder block and the mask prediction head are adapted to the given data.

For the training process, we used a dataset containing more than 5000 murals, of which 1000 murals containing broken regions were manually annotated with detailed semantics. In this way, our model can better learn and understand the features of the broken regions of the murals for more accurate segmentation.

2.2 Restoration of Damaged Areas

After completing the segmentation of the broken regions, we used the LAMA [20] algorithm to automate the repair of these regions. We input the original image I, and the segmentation results S into the LAMA algorithm to obtain the repaired image I':

$$I' = LAMA(I, S) \qquad (3)$$

LAMA is an algorithm with powerful restoration capability, which employs a multi-level texture synthesis and area expansion strategy to effectively restore the texture and colour of the mural while maintaining its original artistic style.

After obtaining the repaired image I' using the LAMA algorithm, we further enhance its resolution by employing the Real-ESRGAN [21] algorithm to upscale the image from 512 × 512 pixels to 2048 × 2048 pixels. This process is formulated as follows:

$$I'' = Real - ESRGAN(I') \qquad (4)$$

Image I'' is the final result of our blind restoration approach. The choice of the Real-ESRGAN method is motivated by its training on a real-world scene dataset, which, when combined with adversarial loss, improves the visual effects of super-resolution. This model is particularly suited for reconstructing lines, making it an ideal choice for enhancing mural lines which are critical to preserving the artistic integrity and details of the mural.

3 Experimental Results

In order to fully evaluate the performance of our proposed "MuralRescue" method on the mural restoration task, we designed and executed a series of detailed experiments. In this section, our experimental design, the obtained results, and the related data analysis are discussed in detail.

3.1 Experimental Setup and Dataset

The experiments were conducted on an A40 GPU. We collected and manually labelled a mural image dataset by ourselves, which was used as the data source for the experiments. The dataset includes more than 5000 images of frescoes, of which 1000 images have been manually annotated with detailed semantic annotations of the damaged areas. For model training and testing, we divided these data into a training set and a test set in the ratio of 80% : 20%.

3.2 Comparison Experiments

In our experiments (Fig. 3), we demonstrated the exceptional efficacy of our "MuralRescue" method in the automatic labeling and repair of defective mural areas, surpassing the performance of the popular inpaint anything approach. Our method, enhanced by integrating an adapter module into SAM for precise damage segmentation and employing the LAMA algorithm followed by Real-ESRGAN for super-resolution, produces high-resolution, high-quality mural restorations at 2048 × 2048 pixels. This approach ensures the restored murals exhibit significant improvements in texture, color fidelity, and line sharpness, closely mirroring their original state with superior detail and clarity. The final results set a new benchmark in digital heritage conservation, effectively preserving the intricate details and aesthetic values of ancient artworks.

3.3 Ablation Study

Ablation Study of Segment Model. We conducted ablation experiments to understand how our "MuralRescue" approach can improve mural restoration. We focused on segmenting defective areas using SAM with different adapter settings: (1) using SAM for mural segmentation only; (2) adding an adapter to the image encoder and training for 70 epochs; (3) adding an adapter to the image encoder and training for 100 epochs; (4) adding adapters to both the image encoder and mask decoder and training for 100 epochs. We examined and compared the defective areas of the murals under these four conditions (Table 1).

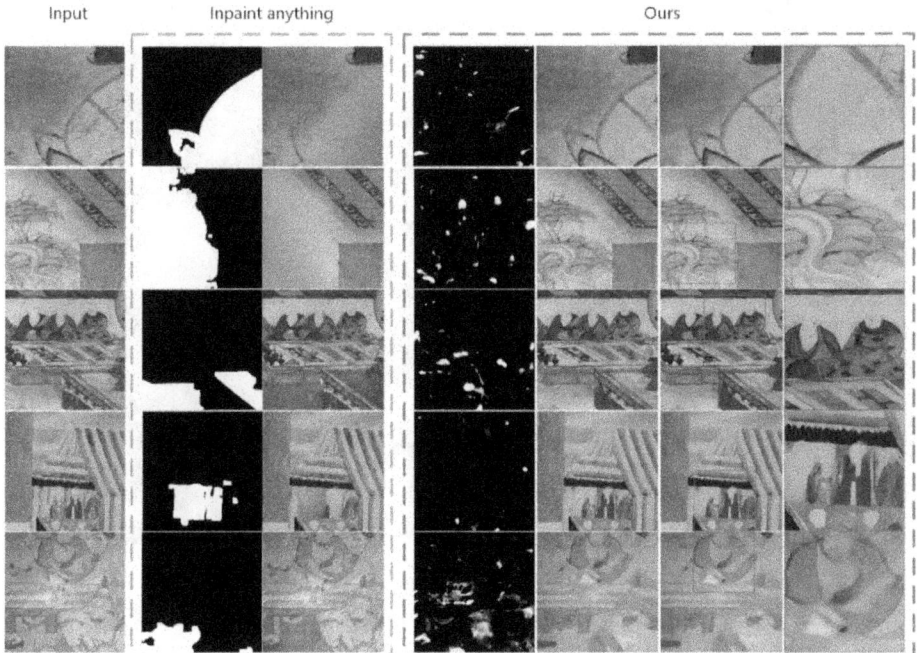

Fig. 3. The compare results with Inpainting-anything on Mural dataset

Table 1. Abaltion study of MuralRescue on Mural dataset (Frozen and Fintune)

Method	Epoch	Averge IoU score ↑	Average Dice Coeffcient ↑
Bring Old Life [19]		0.0790	0.5310
Encoder Adapter	70	0.1390	0.7610
Encoder Adapter	100	0.1366	0.7050
Encoder+Decoder Adapter	100	**0.1518**	**0.7459**

The results (Fig. 4) show that direct detection using the SAM method can segment many categories, but segmenting the damaged areas in the mural is challenging. The segmentation effect is greatly improved when we add the adapter to the image encoder in the SAM method. Not only can we bifurcate the damaged areas in the mural, but the damaged areas in the mural can also be segmented to a very detailed accuracy. The significant damages are peeling, scratching, fading, etc. When we add Adapter to SAM's mask decoder, our method achieves another significant improvement in segmenting the defective areas of the mural. Since many damaged areas of the mural are difficult to mark manually, but our "MuralRescue" can segment them, the semantic segmentation indexes IOU and DSI computed with ground truth are not of the reference value.

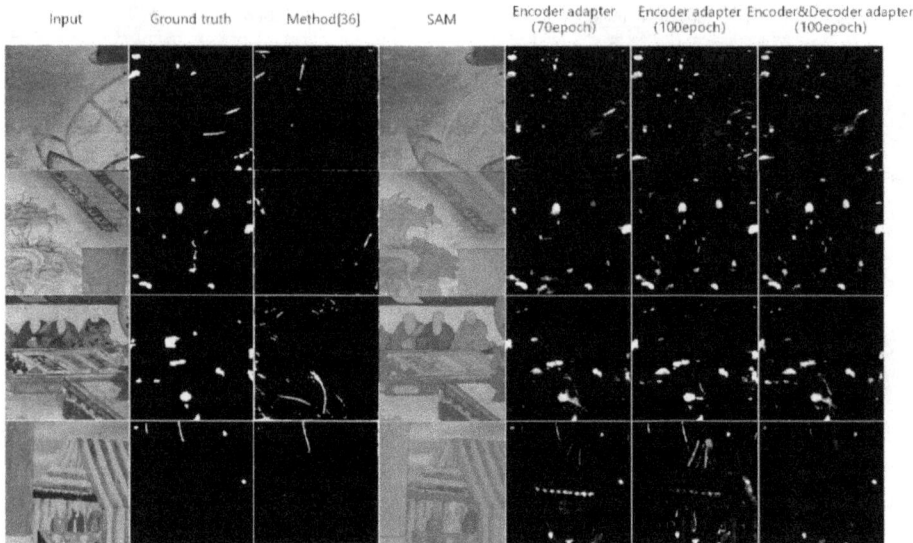

Fig. 4. The ablation study of Segment model on Mural dataset

4 Conclusion

In this paper, we introduce an innovative mural restoration method that combines the Segment Anything model and SAM-Adapter to improve the accuracy of mural restoration. Experimental results on a self-constructed mural dataset show that our method performs excellently on mural restoration tasks.

However, there is still room for improvement, including improving the accuracy of the segmentation stage and optimizing the restoration algorithm to enhance the visual effect. In the future, we plan to expand the application of this method to a broader range of restoration tasks, such as old building restoration, to achieve a greater impact in ancient art restoration work.

Acknowledgments. This study was funded by the National Natural Science Foundation of China (grant number 52274160, 51874300), the Funding for the "Jiangsu Distinguished Professor" project in Jiangsu Province (grant number 140923070).

Disclosure of Interests. The authors have no competing interests to declare that are relevant to the content of this paper.

References

1. Pan, Y.H., et al.: Digital Protection and Restoration of Dunhuang Mural. J. Syst. Simul. **15**(3), 310–314 (2003)

2. Jingni, S.H.E.N., et al.: Tang Dynasty Tomb Murals Inpainting Algorithm of MCA Decomposition. J. Front. Comput. Sci. Technol. **11**(11), 1826 (2017)
3. Chen, et al.: Dunhuang mural inpainting algorithm based on sequential similarity detection and cuckoo optimization. Laser Optoelectronics
4. Zhang, et al.: Research on disease extraction and inpainting algorithm of digital grotto murals. Appl. Res. Comput. **38**(08), 2495–2498+2504 (2021). https://doi.org/10.19734/j.issn.1001-3695.2020.09.0395
5. Yong, C., et al.: Inpainting Algorithm for Dunhuang Mural Based on Improved Curvature-Driven Diffusion Model. J. Comput.-Aided Des. Comput. Graph. **32**(5), 787–796 (2020)
6. Xiaoping, Y., Shuwen, W., et al.: Dunhuang mural inpainting in intricate disrepaired region based on improvement of priority algorithm. J. Comput.-Aided Des. Comput. Graph. **23**(2), 284–289 (2011)
7. Jiao, L.J., et al.: Wutai mountain mural inpainting based on improved block matching algorithm. J. Comput.-Aided Des. Comput. Graph. **31**(1), 118–125 (2019)
8. Hendrycks, D., Gimpel, K.: Gaussian error linear units (GELUs). arXiv preprint arXiv:1606.08415 (2016)
9. Yu, T., Feng, R., Feng, R., et al.: Inpaint anything: segment anything meets image inpainting. arXiv preprint arXiv:2304.06790 (2023)
10. Kirillov, A., Mintun, E., Ravi, N., et al.: Segment anything. arXiv preprint arXiv:2304.02643 (2023)
11. Ma, J., Wang, B.: Segment anything in medical images. arXiv preprint arXiv:2304.12306 (2023)
12. Zhang, K., Liu, D.: Customized segment anything model for medical image segmentation. arXiv preprint arXiv:2304.13785 (2023)
13. Roy, S., Wald, T., Koehler, G., et al.: SAM.MD: zero-shot medical image segmentation capabilities of the segment anything model. arXiv preprint arXiv:2304.05396 (2023)
14. Wang, D., Zhang, J., Du, B., et al.: Scaling-up remote sensing segmentation dataset with segment anything model. arXiv preprint arXiv:2305.02034 (2023)
15. Chen, T., Zhu, L., Ding, C., et al.: SAM fails to segment anything?–SAM-adapter: adapting SAM in underperformed scenes: camouflage, shadow, and more. arXiv preprint arXiv:2304.09148 (2023)
16. Jing, Y., Wang, X., Tao, D.: Segment anything in non-euclidean domains: challenges and opportunities. arXiv preprint arXiv:2304.11595 (2023)
17. Peng, J., Liu, D., Xu, S., Li, H.: Generating diverse structure for image inpainting with hierarchical VQ-VAE. In: Proceedings of the IEEE/CVF Conference on Computer Vision and Pattern Recognition, pp. 10775–10784 (2021)
18. Wan, Z., Zhang, J., Chen, D., Liao, J.: High-fidelity pluralistic image completion with transformers. arXiv preprint arXiv:2103.14031 (2021)
19. Wan, Z., Zhang, B., Chen, D., et al.: Bringing old photos back to life. In: Proceedings of the IEEE/CVF Conference on Computer Vision and Pattern Recognition, pp. 2747–2757 (2020)
20. Zhao, S., Cui, J., Sheng, Y., et al.: Large scale image completion via co-modulated generative adversarial networks. arXiv preprint arXiv:2103.10428 (2021)
21. Wang, X., Xie, L., Dong, C., et al.: Real-ESRGAN: training real-world blind super-resolution with pure synthetic data. In: Proceedings of the IEEE/CVF International Conference on Computer Vision, pp. 905–1914 (2021)

Full-Range Fusion Network with Local-Global Attention for Change Detection in Remote Sensing Images

Shuting Niu, Yingxue Zhang$^{(\boxtimes)}$, and Zhanjun Si

College of Artificial Intelligence,
Tianjin University of Science and Technology, Tianjin 300457, China
yxzhang@tust.edu.cn

Abstract. Remote sensing image change detection (CD) is an important technology used to monitor changes in surface features and objects over time, widely applied in fields such as land use planning, environmental monitoring, and disaster management. Although traditional change detection methods are effective in certain scenarios, they are often limited by high sensitivity to noise and computational complexity, making them unsuitable for the rapidly evolving demands of big data. In response, this paper proposes an efficient local-global context fusion network (LGCF-Net) based on a Siamese architecture, aimed at enhancing the accuracy and efficiency of change detection in remote sensing images. LGCF-Net incorporates efficient local-global context aggregator (ELGCA) module and cross fusion attention module (CFAM) to effectively improve the performance of change detection. The proposed method is evaluated on the SYSU-CD dataset, achieving accuracy and recall of 93.21% and 95.39%, respectively, which confirms the effectiveness of the proposed method.

Keywords: Remote sensing image · Change detection · Siamese architecture · Efficient Local-global context aggregator module · Cross fusion attention module

1 Introduction

Change detection(CD) in remote sensing images refers to the use of multitemporal remote sensing data to identify and analyze temporal and spatial changes in land surfaces or features, such as changes in land cover types, alterations in buildings, and impacts of natural disasters. This process aims to extract change information from remote sensing images, convert it into understandable data, and support applications across various fields [1].

Traditional methods of remote sensing image change detection primarily rely on pixel-level difference analysis or object-based change detection. However, inaccuracies often arise from factors such as seasonal variations in background colors, displacement changes caused by moving objects, and minor shooting errors between images. With the advancement of deep learning technologies, numerous deep learning-based methods have been proposed for change detection. SNUNet-CD [2] is a densely connected

Siamese network that reduces information loss during depth information loading by facilitating tight information transfer between the encoder and decoder. There are also networks that improve accuracy by incorporating an attention mechanism. STANet-CD [3] generates superior feature representations by capturing spatio-temporal dependencies at different scales through a spatio-temporal attention module. Similarly, DASNet [4] employs a dual attention mechanism to enhance the robustness of the model and addresses the sample imbalance problem by adjusting the loss function weights. And DSAMNet [5] combines the CBAM [6] attention mechanism with the metric module to improve the feature extraction capability and generate more useful features. In recent years, Transformer has garnered widespread attention in the field of remote sensing image change detection. ICIFNet [7] proposed an integrated CNN and Transformer network for intra-scale interaction and inter-scale feature fusion. WNet [8] combined CNNs and Transformers in a W-shaped dual-branch tiered network and developed a Differential Enhancement Module (DEM). BIT_CD [9] combined spatial attention and a Transformer encoder to convert images from different times into semantic labels, which were then remapped to the pixel space by the decoder, enhancing features to generate pixel-level change predictions.

The aforementioned methods demonstrate outstanding performance, yet some issues persist. Firstly, it remains challenging to suppress background interference in change detection while effectively capturing both global and local contextual information to detect subtle and significant structural changes between image pairs. Secondly, most current CD-based methods focus solely on the images themselves, overlooking temporal clues between images collected at different times. To overcome these challenges, we propose a change detection method based on the Siamese architecture named Efficient Local-Global Context Fusion Network (LGCF-Net). Specifically, we introduce a efficient local-global context aggregator (ELGCA) module [12] to capture contextual information, which uses various aggregation strategies for fine-grained optimization of features, enhancing the model's receptive field. To leverage temporal clues for addressing the change detection task, we further propose the cross fusion attention module (CFAM) that allows for the useful exchange and fusion of information between images taken at two different time points.

2 The Proposed Method

The proposed change detection framework mainly comprises a Siamese encoder, cross fusion attention module (CFAM), Dual Attention Module (DAM), and decoder, as illustrated in Fig. 1. The Siamese encoder takes a pair of satellite images as input, initially down-sampling them through a patch embedding layer, and then processing them through four pairs of encoding modules to output four pairs of multi-scale feature maps. Feature maps of the same size enter the CFAM, where fused feature maps are generated and subsequently sent to the DAM for further feature enhancement. The four feature maps enhanced by the DAM are fed into the fusion module, where simple linear projections, feature concatenation, and 1x1 convolution operations are performed to reduce the number of channels. Finally, these fused features are passed to the decoder module to produce more accurate change map predictions.

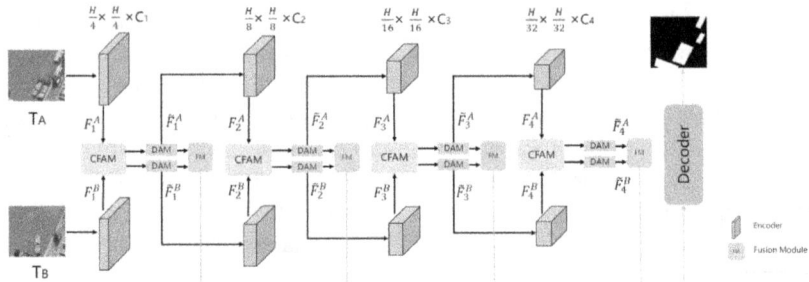

Fig. 1. Overall framework of the LGCF-Net

2.1 ELGCA Module

The encoding module consists of an efficient local-global context aggregator (ELGCA) module and an MLP module and utilizes a residual connection structure to mitigate the vanishing gradient problem. Our ELGCA module is designed to capture both local and global contextual information while reducing computational complexity, as illustrated in Fig. 2. The input features $f^i \in R^{H^i \times W^i \times C^i}$ are split into two halves channel-wise, resulting in f_{lo}^i and $f_{gl}^i \in R^{H^i \times W^i \times (C^i/2)}$. These are separately fed into individual context aggregators to obtain local and global contextual information, where H^i, W^i and C^i denote the width, height, and number of channels, respectively.

$$f_{lo}^i, f_{gl}^i = Split(f^i) \tag{1}$$

The X_{gl}^i feature of our ELGCA module initially undergoes a 1x1 convolution, dividing it into Z^i, Q^i, K^i and V^i features. Here, Z^i is used for multi-channel feature aggregation, while Q^i, K^i and V^i serve as the query, key, and value for the PT attention mechanism, aimed at capturing global contextual information. The PT attention mechanism first performs average pooling on the query Q^i and max pooling on K^i, capturing the average and maximum values of the input features. This process is designed to obtain feature representations $\overline{Q}^i$ and $\overline{K}^i$ that are robust to subtle changes, thereby more effectively capturing essential information from the input data. Subsequently, using the averaged features $\overline{Q}^i$, maximum features $\overline{K}^i$ and the value features V^i a transpose attention operation (G) is applied, resulting in the feature representation A_{att}^i.

$$A_{att}^i = V^i \times \left[\sigma \left(\overline{K}^{iT} \times \overline{Q}^i \right) \right] \tag{2}$$

The f_{lo}^i feature undergoes a 3x3 depthwise separable convolution, resulting in the locally aggregated contextual feature $\overline{f}_{lo}^i$. The purpose of this step is to capture local contextual information, and the use of depthwise separable convolution reduces both the number of model parameters and the computational complexity.

Finally, the feature A_{att}^i processed by the PT attention mechanism, the locally aggregated contextual feature $\overline{f}_{lo}^i$, and the multi-channel aggregated feature Z^i are concatenated. This results in a rich feature representation $\overline{f}^i$ that combines both local and global contextual information. This fusion of context information at different levels and through different methods provides a more comprehensive feature representation for subsequent full-range feature fusion.

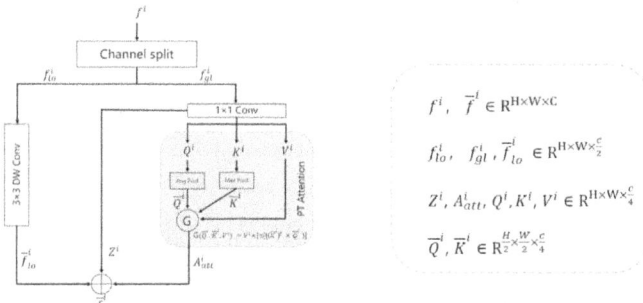

Fig. 2. Efficient local-global context aggregator (ELGCA) module

2.2 CFAM

Cross fusion attention module (CFAM) is shown in Fig. 3. Its primary function is to allow the useful exchange and fusion of information between bi-temporal remote sensing images. CFAM facilitates the mutual integration of information between two input data pairs, allowing the encoder processing Image A to concurrently consider information from Image B. This enables the encoder to comprehensively understand the relationship between images at different time points, thereby detecting change areas more accurately. For the input tensors $X, Y \in R^{H^i \times W^i \times C^i}$ they are fed into the CFAM for information interaction. In this module, we use a dot product operation to calculate the similarity matrix between the query Q from tensor X and the key K from tensor Y, and then normalize it using the softmax function. The purpose of this is to obtain normalized attention weights, allowing each pixel in tensor X to focus on important pixels in tensor Y. The process can be represented by the following formula:

$$Attention(X, Y) = softmax\left(\frac{Q_y K_x^T}{\sqrt{d_{kx}}}\right) V_x \qquad (3)$$

In the formula, d_k represents the dimension of the key K. For the fused features, we perform a linear transformation to map them to a higher-dimensional feature space. Then, the result of this linear transformation is added to the original query features of tensor X to retain the original feature information of image X, making the final feature representation richer. After the addition, we apply layer normalization to standardize the distribution of the features. Subsequently, a Multi-Layer Perceptron (MLP) is used to perform a nonlinear mapping of the features, enhancing their expressive power and distinctiveness. The same operations are performed for tensor Y. Ultimately, the CFAM outputs two cross-fused feature maps, each representing the remote sensing images at two different time points, and highlighting the common and differentiating features between them.

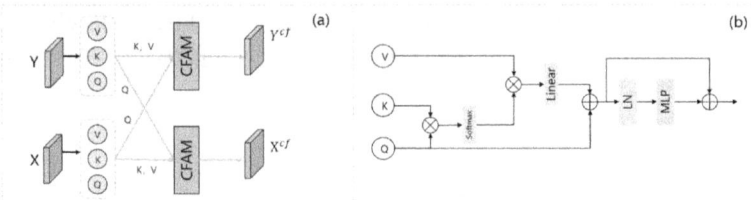

Fig. 3. Cross fusion attention module (CFAM)

2.3 Dam

For the two cross-fused feature maps, a Spatial and Channel Dual Attention Module is used to enhance the model's feature representation ability, effectively capturing and utilizing key features in the image to improve the model's ability to recognize and analyze changes in terrain. First, the channel attention module identifies which channels are more important by utilizing features from global average pooling and max pooling to generate a channel attention map. This map is used to adjust the response strengths of the individual channels. Next, the spatial attention module focuses on which areas within the feature map are more significant. It uses the previously channel-weighted feature map to perform max pooling and average pooling operations, creating a two-dimensional attention map that emphasizes important spatial regions in the feature map. Finally, the spatially attentive feature map is multiplied by the channel attentive feature map to produce a feature map with dual attention.

2.4 Decoder

The decoder is composed of convolutional and transposed convolutional layers, as shown in Fig. 4. Initially, four feature maps of different scales are merged along the channel dimension, and a 1x1 convolutional layer adjusts the number of channels and reorganizes the features. Subsequently, the transposed convolutional layer's upsampling operation increases the spatial resolution of the feature maps and restores image details, bringing the processed feature maps closer to the original image size. To further enhance feature expression, a residual block containing two 3x3 convolutional layers is introduced, where skip connections prevent information loss and ensure the accurate transfer of deep features. Moreover, the combination of transposed convolution and residual blocks is cascaded twice consecutively to progressively expand the spatial dimensions of the feature maps until they match the input size. This process not only improves spatial resolution but also enhances the feature hierarchy for change detection. The decoder ultimately outputs a binary change map through the convolutional layers.

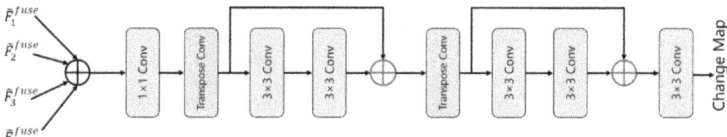

Fig. 4. Decoder

2.5 Loss Function

The cross-entropy loss function is used as shown in the following equation. The cross-entropy loss function is a method for measuring the difference between two probability distributions, primarily used to evaluate the proximity between model prediction results and true labels.

$$Loss = -\frac{1}{N}\Sigma_{i=1}^{N} q_n \log(P_n) + (1 - q_n)\log(1 - p_n) \tag{4}$$

where q_n represents the probability of the true label, P_n represents the model's predicted probability, N represents the total number of samples, and n represents the nth sample, with the value ranging from 1 to N.

3 Experimental Results

3.1 Dataset

The SYSU-CD [5] dataset consists of 20,000 pairs of image patches collected between 2007 and 2014, each with a size of 256 × 256, sourced from ortho-rectified aerial images in Hong Kong. The SYSU-CD dataset not only includes common change information in urban and suburban areas but also provides specific details regarding high-density building changes and marine construction changes, offering rich data support for spatial change research in the urbanization process. This dataset is randomly divided with 60% used for model training, and 20% each for model validation and testing.

3.2 Experimental Results

We employed four evaluation metrics: Precision (P), Recall (R), F1 score (F1), and Intersection over Union (IoU) to quantitatively assess the experimental results of our proposed network. To validate the effectiveness of our proposed network, we compare it with five mainstream deep learning-based change detection methods, including SNUNet [2], DSAMNet [5], LCDNet [10], GeSANet [11], and ELGC-Net [12]. From the results in Table 1, it is clear that our method has achieved improvements in all the metrics. For example, our LGCF-Net achieves 93.21% and 95.39% in precision and recall, respectively, successfully surpassing the existing methods being compared. It indicates that our model has a significant advantage in detecting changes in targets of different sizes in complex scenes.

Figure 5 presents a visual comparison of various methods on the SYSU-CD dataset, illustrating that our method visually outperforms others in detecting change areas. The

Table 1. Comparative experimental results of the SYSU-CD dataset

Method	P	R	F1	IoU
SNUNet [2]	82.86	74.87	78.50	64.16
DSAMNet [5]	83.86	73.32	78.24	64.25
LCDNet [10]	81.71	83.79	82.57	70.31
GeSaNet [11]	90.80	92.93	90.68	86.64
ELGCNet [12]	92.34	94.81	93.85	88.42
Ours	**93.21**	**95.39**	**93.97**	**88.63**

first row shows the changes in the road extension, and from the figure, it can be observed that some models incorrectly recognize the shadows as areas of change and there are missed detections. Our model, however, shows the most complete performance in detailed segmentation. The second displays the change comparison images for suburban expansion. It is evident that some models incorrectly identify the area in the middle of the houses as a changing area, while only our model provides the most accurate segmentation. The third row shows the change comparison for oceanic construction, revealing that for large and irregularly shaped change areas, most methods produce detection results that lack clarity in shape and contours, with significant missed areas. Our model, however, effectively maintains the integrity of large targets while somewhat restoring edge details. The fourth row displays the changes in newly constructed urban buildings, where the rooftop textures and contours of buildings are complex. The segmentation results from the other five methods are too coarse to accurately delineate the correct shapes. In contrast, our method identifies more detailed change information, generates change prediction maps with clear and continuous boundaries, and detects small targets missed by other methods. From the visual results, our model, by incorporating the ELGCA module, effectively captures both local and global information, thus expanding the model's receptive field. After introducing the CFAM, the model more effectively captures changes between two-time points, resulting in more precise segmentation of small objects. DAM effectively identifies hidden key information, further reducing the loss of edge details.

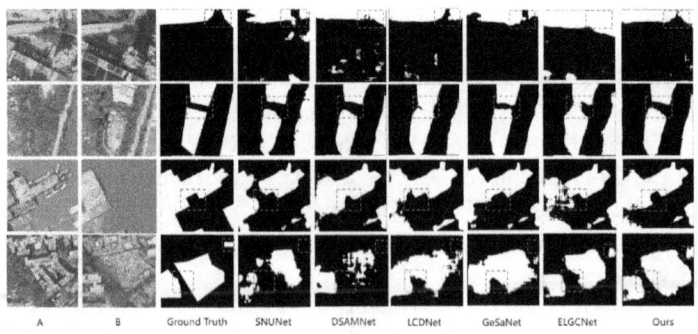

Fig. 5. Visualization results of the SYSU-CD dataset

4 Conclusions

In this paper, we introduce an Efficient Local-Global Context Fusion Network (LGCF-Net) based on the Siamese architecture. The ELGCA module leverages both local and global information to capture image changes more comprehensively. The CFAM enables dense fusion of bi-temporal features, while the DAM identifies hidden crucial information to improve feature extraction capabilities. Our method has been validated on the SYSU-CD dataset and demonstrates superior performance across multiple evaluation metrics compared to existing technologies. However, despite the excellent performance of our LGCF-Net in change detection, its high computational resource consumption is a significant drawback, leading to slower processing speeds. Future work will therefore explore lightweight models.

References

1. Bin, Y.A.N.G., et al.: Review of remote sensing change detection in deep learning: bibliometric and analysis. Nat. Remote Sens. Bull. **27**(9), 1988–2005 (2023)
2. Fang, S., et al.: SNUNet-CD: a densely connected Siamese network for change detection of VHR images. IEEE Geosci. Remote Sens. Lett. **19**, 1–5 (2021)
3. Chen, H., Shi, Z.: A spatial-temporal attention-based method and a new dataset for remote sensing image change detection. Remote Sens. **12**(10), 1662 (2020)
4. Chen, J., et al.: DASNet: dual attentive fully convolutional Siamese networks for change detection in high-resolution satellite images. IEEE J. Sel. Top. Appl. Earth Observations Remote Sens. **14**, 1194–1206 (2020)
5. Shi, Q., et al.: A deeply supervised attention metric-based network and an open aerial image dataset for remote sensing change detection. IEEE Trans. Geosci. Remote Sens. **60**, 1–16 (2021)
6. Woo, S., et al.: CBAM: convolutional block attention module. In: Proceedings of the European Conference on Computer Vision (ECCV) (2018)
7. Feng, Y., et al.: ICIF-Net: intra-scale cross-interaction and inter-scale feature fusion network for Bitemporal remote sensing images change detection. IEEE Trans. Geosci. Remote Sens. **60**, 1–13 (2022)
8. Tang, X., et al.: WNet: W-shaped hierarchical network for remote sensing image change detection. IEEE Trans. Geosci. Remote Sens. **61**, 1–14 (2023)
9. Chen, H., Qi, Z., Shi, Z.: Remote sensing image change detection with transformers. IEEE Trans. Geosci. Remote Sens. **60**, 1–14 (2021)
10. Li, J., Li, S., Wang, F.: LCDNet: lightweight change detection network with dual attention guidance and multiscale feature fusion for remote sensing images. IEEE Geosci. Remote Sens. Lett. **21**, 1–5 (2023)
11. Zhao, X., et al.: GeSANet: geospatial-awareness network for VHR remote sensing image change detection. IEEE Trans. Geosci. Remote Sens. **61**, 1–14 (2023)
12. Noman, M., et al.: ELGC-Net: efficient local-global context aggregation for remote sensing change detection. IEEE Trans. Geosci. Remote Sens. **62**, 1–11 (2024)

Author Index

C
Cao, Dehua 41
Cao, Fengping 77
Cao, Shitong 312
Chen, Aoran 414
Chen, Dufeng 124, 446, 456
Chen, Mengjie 345
Chen, Minglang 218
Chen, Siyi 279
Chen, Wei 446, 456
Chen, Zhanglu 15
Chen, Zhongyue 29
Cheng, Tianxiang 435

D
Deng, Ruting 15
Deng, Yifan 15
Dong, Chen 184
Dong, Feng 234
Dongye, Changlei 333
Du, Qiaoqiao 147
Duan, Wensi 41
Duan, Wen-Tao 134
Duan, Wentao 53

F
Fan, Bangkui 208
Fan, Haifeng 435
Fang, Qianzhen 456
Fu, Yaowen 300
Fu, Yutian 234

G
Gao, Lijun 89
Gao, Xueyan 300
Gong, Guoliang 172
Guo, Haozhe 345
Guo, Hui 218
Guo, Yitong 124

H
Hao, Weijie 147
He, Jie 218
Hu, Wei 53, 134
Huang, Hai 414
Huang, Lingfeng 266
Huang, Yangyang 65, 101
Huo, Wanli 29
Huo, Xiangzuo 197

J
Jiang, Maoxiang 426
Jiang, Peng 41
Jin, Xiao 89
Jin, Yu 41

K
Kang, Zhiqing 15
Kong, Xiangyu 369

L
Li, Aolun 197
Li, Cheng 41
Li, Jianrong 435
Li, Kaijiang 345
Li, Yachao 234
Li, Yubo 435
Li, Zhan 15
Li, Zhenhua 279
Lian, Zhe 53, 134
Liang, Dong 234, 266, 279
Liang, Qi 3
Lin, Yangde 323
Lin, Zhehao 184
Ling, Sai Ho 160
Liu, Hongzhe 402
Liu, Juan 41
Liu, Jueting 446, 456
Liu, Xiang 3
Long, Hang 15
Long, Qian 257

long, Qian   381
Lu, Huijuan   29
Lu, Yingying   390
Luo, Ronghua   65, 101
Lv, Pei   345
Lyu, Juan   160

M
Ma, Hui   435
Mei, Yijing   113, 124
Meng, Jinpeng   160
Meng, Xianghong   172
Mi, Zeng   134
Miao, Yi   77

N
Ni, Yuliang   357
Niu, Shuting   464

P
Pan, Gang   113, 124, 246
Pan, Xiangyu   246
Pang, Baochuan   41

Q
Qi, Lin   390
Qi, Tianyang   300
Qi, Xuan-Hao   134
Qi, Yaping   29
Qiu, Zhichao   15
Qu, Hongwei   257, 381

S
Shen, Sheng   323
Shi, Haoshan   300
Shi, Jinyu   291
Si, Zhanjun   291, 426, 435, 464
Su, Hao   345
Sun, Di   113, 124, 246, 323
Sun, Jiwu   402
Sun, Lin   160
Sun, Yue   266
Sun, Zeyang   89

T
Tang, Ying   29
Tian, Shengwei   197
Tie, Yun   390

W
Wan, Yuxuan   184
Wang, Daole   369
Wang, Gaihua   257, 381
Wang, Guibao   3
Wang, Jiahao   246
Wang, Jin   312
Wang, Lang   41
Wang, Lanmei   3
Wang, Lizhe   3
Wang, Pengfei   402
Wang, Qihang   323
Wang, Suran   89
Wang, Wenjun   369
Wang, Xiaoliang   172
Wang, Yiping   381
Wang, Yu   357
Wang, Yumei   333
Wang, Yunxiang   113
Wang, Zehua   446, 456
Wang, Zhihui   357
Wu, Pengnian   208
Wu, Weiye   65, 101

X
Xi, Xing   65, 101
Xie, Di   218
Xin, Qin   89
Xu, Caixu   218
Xu, Cheng   402
Xu, Qiaozhi   53
Xu, Tingting   446, 456
Xu, Yulong   208
Xu, Zishan   446, 456
Xue, Dong   208

Y
Yang, Ke   426
Yang, Na   53
Yang, Tingting   113, 246
Yang, Xinbin   291
Yang, Xinqi   172
Yang, Yuqing   446
Yao, Chaojie   124
Yao, Jingxuan   257
Ye, Minchao   29
Yin, Yan-Jun   134
Yin, Yanjun   53
Yu, Lei   53

Yu, Long 197
Yue, Shan 414

Z

Zeng, Zhiliang 323
Zhang, Cheng 402
Zhang, Chuanlei 435
Zhang, Ruiyu 208
Zhang, Shizhao 323
Zhang, Shu 414
Zhang, Wangyi 77
Zhang, Wenyin 147
Zhang, Xuejie 312
Zhang, Yingxue 291, 426, 464
Zhang, Youzhi 89
Zhang, Yu 160, 172
Zhang, Yue-Ning 134
Zhang, Zhaojuan 29
Zhang, Zhongwei 172
Zhao, Wenxiu 333
Zhao, Xiuyang 369
Zhao, Yanchen 147
Zhao, Zhiqiang 435
Zhi, Min 53, 134
Zhou, Bingming 197
Zhou, Xiaobing 312
Zhu, Bolun 257, 381
Zhu, Qi 266
Zhu, Yueyan 414
Zou, Yifei 300

Printed in the USA
CPSIA information can be obtained
at www.ICGtesting.com
CBHW051934180824
13382CB00003B/47